Procedural Dictations in Image-Guided Intervention

Bedros Taslakian · Aghiad Al-Kutoubi
Jamal J. Hoballah
Editors

Procedural Dictations in Image-Guided Intervention

Non-Vascular, Vascular and Neuro Interventions

Springer

Editors
Bedros Taslakian
Department of Radiology
New York University Langone Medical Center
New York
USA

Jamal J. Hoballah
Department of Surgery
American University of Beirut Medical Center
Beirut
Lebanon

Aghiad Al-Kutoubi
Department of Diagnostic Radiology
American University of Beirut Medical Center
Beirut
Lebanon

ISBN 978-3-319-40843-9 ISBN 978-3-319-40845-3 (eBook)
DOI 10.1007/978-3-319-40845-3

Library of Congress Control Number: 2016945110

Printed on acid-free paper

This Springer imprint is published by Springer Nature
The registered company is Springer International Publishing AG Switzerland

To my family, for their forbearance, love, support,
and guidance over the years;
To my patients, in gratitude for all they have taught me;
To my mentors, who encouraged my curiosity
and supported me;
To everyone who has taken the time to teach me
and from whom I have learned that, as physicians,
we are always students and teachers.

—Bedros Taslakian

To Nada, my wife and soul mate, who supported
me through thick and thin;
To my lovely children Dana, Masa, and Jude;
To my late father and my loving mother;
To everyone who contributed to my knowledge.
I hope this effort will perpetuate this knowledge
for posterity.

—Aghiad Al-Kutoubi

To Ali S. Hoballah with admiration and gratitude
for the love, support, and guidance throughout the years.

—Jamal J. Hoballah

To all interventionalists whose dedication throughout
the years has contributed to the advances made
in this specialty.

—Bedros Taslakian, Aghiad Al-Kutoubi and Jamal J. Hoballah

Preface

This book is designed to provide the practicing interventionalist with a comprehensive list of procedural reports that cover the vast majority of the currently performed interventional procedures outside the cardiac system, with up-to-date explanatory notes, synopsis of the indications, and potential complications in an organized and practical format that follows the various-body systems and progresses from the simple image-guided fine needle aspiration to the most complex procedures, incorporating at the same time the current societal guidelines. The book is divided for the ease of reference into three main parts: nonvascular, vascular, and neurovascular interventional procedures. This information is not currently available in any single publication.

The resident, the fellow, as well as the staff member will benefit from this unique, quickly accessible, detailed, and user-friendly resource for the documentation of image-guided interventional procedures that will facilitate their tasks, improve the standard of documentation, and reduce mistakes. The entries are vetted by recognized experts in the field of image-guided intervention.

There has been an exponential increase in the number and variety of image-guided interventions over the last decades, with increasing complexity in the vascular and nonvascular domains. Such wide variety and complexity comes with added obligations on the interventional team to ensure appropriate patient care. The interventional procedure report must be written in a timely manner and is a valuable and essential part of the patient's medical record. It should document the management decision process, including the indications and contraindications as well as the details of the procedure itself and post-procedural care. By doing so, communication with all members of the healthcare team is assured and clarity of the treatment pathway is detailed. Any subsequent management steps could then be decided in the light of the full record. In addition, the record of the procedure ensures appropriate reimbursement and reduces the possibility of any medico-legal issues resulting from the ambiguity in documentation.

This book is therefore a must-have for residents and fellows undergoing training and all specialists in image-guided intervention.

It is with a great deal of pride that we complete the first edition of this useful reference in the hope that it will encourage future generations of interventionalists to develop mutually productive relationships with other care providers.

We wish to acknowledge with sincere thanks the contribution of all authors and reviewers. Their efforts have greatly inspired us and strengthened our enthusiasm for bringing this edition to fruition.

New York, USA — Bedros Taslakian
Beirut, Lebanon — Aghiad Al-Kutoubi
Beirut, Lebanon — Jamal J. Hoballah

Note: The blank spaces and underlining that you will notice in each chapter indicate the items in the documentation that will vary depending upon the specific situation, for example: size of gauge, amount of radiation dose, amount of time, amount of fluid, etc. The chapters in the table of content are arranged alphabetically.

Contents

Contributors

Eric T. Aaltonen Department of Radiology, Division of Vascular and Interventional Radiology, New York University Langone Medical Center, New York, NY, USA

Maen Aboul Hosn Department of Vascular Surgery, University of Iowa Hospitals and Clinics, Iowa City, IA, USA

Murad M. Abusamra Department of Diagnostic Radiology, American University of Beirut Medical Center, Beirut, Lebanon

Mohammed Al-Garnawee Department of Surgery, Division of Neurosurgery, American University of Beirut Medical Center, Beirut, Lebanon

Faten El Ammar Department of Neurology, American University of Beirut Medical Center, Beirut, Lebanon

Sela Batouzian Coronary Care Unit (CCU), Clemenceau Medical Center (CMC), Beirut, Lebanon

Serine Baydoun Department of Radiology, University of Iowa Hospitals and Clinics, Iowa City, IA, USA

Abbas Chamsuddin Interventional Radiology, Balamand University Saint George University Medical Center, Beirut, Lebanon

Hearns W. Charles Department of Radiology, Division of Interventional Radiology, New York University Langone Medical Center, New York, NY, USA

Michele Fouad Chemali Department of Surgery, American University of Beirut Medical Center, Beirut, Lebanon

Jad Chokr Department of Diagnostic Radiology, Division of Neuroradiology, Banner University Medical Center, Tucson, AZ, USA

Anne M. Covey Department of Radiology, Division of Interventional Radiology, Memorial Sloan Kettering Cancer Center, Weill Cornell Medical College, New York, NY, USA

Houssein Darwish Department of Neurosurgery, University of Virginia Health System, Charlottesville, VA, USA

Keith G. DeSousa Department of Radiology, New York University Langone Medical Center, New York, NY, USA

Amy Deipolyi Department of Radiology, Division of Interventional Radiology, Memorial Sloan Kettering Cancer Center, New York, NY, USA

Mohamad Nasser Eddine Department of Surgery, Division of Orthopedic Surgery, American University of Beirut Medical Center, Beirut, Lebanon

Hiba Ezzeddine Department of General Surgery, American University in Beirut Medical Center, Beirut, Lebanon

Sandra Abi Fadel Department of Diagnostic Radiology, American University of Beirut Medical Center, Beirut, Lebanon

Sean Farquharson Department of Radiology, Division of Vascular and Interventional Radiology, New York University Langone Medical Center, New York, NY, USA

Jonathan S. Gross Department of Radiology, Division of Vascular and Interventional Radiology, New York University Langone Medical Center, New York, NY, USA

David H. Hoffman Department of Radiology, New York University Langone Medical Center, New York, NY, USA

Roula Hourani Department of Diagnostic Radiology, American University of Beirut Medical Center, Beirut, Lebanon

Nicole A. Lamparello Department of Radiology, New York University Langone Medical Center, New York, NY, USA

Naji S. Madi Department of Surgery, Division of Orthopedic Surgery, American University of Beirut Medical Center, Beirut, Lebanon

Karim Masrouha Department of Surgery, Division of Orthopedic Surgery, American University of Beirut Medical Center, Beirut, Lebanon

William Moore Department of Radiology, New York University Langone Medical Center, New York, NY, USA

Marc Mourad Department of Head and Neck and Endocrine Oncology, Moffitt Cancer Center, Tampa, FL, USA

Howayda Al Mrad Department of Diagnostic Radiology, American University of Beirut Medical Center, Beirut, Lebanon

Nadim Muallem Department of Radiology, Division of Interventional Radiology, Memorial Sloan Kettering Cancer Center, New York, NY, USA

Lara Nassar Department of Diagnostic Radiology, American University of Beirut Medical Center, Beirut, Lebanon

Roy A. Raad Department of Radiology, Division of Nuclear Medicine, New York University Langone Medical Center, New York, NY, USA

Eytan Raz Department of Radiology, Divisions of Neuroimaging and Neurointervention, New York University Langone Medical Center, New York, NY, USA

Karim Rebeiz Department of Radiology, Memorial Sloan Kettering Cancer Center, New York, NY, USA

Debkumar Sarkar Department of Radiology, Richard L. Roudebush VA Medical Center, Indianapolis, IN, USA

Peter Sawan Department of Radiology, Memorial Sloan Kettering Cancer Center, New York, NY, USA

Mikhael Georges Sebaaly Department of Diagnostic Radiology, American University of Beirut Medical Center, Beirut, Lebanon

Sahar Semaan Department of Radiology, Icahn School of Medicine at Mount Sinai, New York, NY, USA

Hiba H. Sharafeldeen Department of Neurosurgery, American University of Beirut Medical Center, Beirut, Lebanon

Divya Sridhar Department of Radiology, Division of Vascular and Interventional Radiology, New York University Langone Medical Center, New York, NY, USA

Tarek P. Sunna Department of Neurosurgery, University of Montreal, Montreal, QC, Canada

Bedros Taslakian Department of Radiology, New York University Langone Medical Center, New York, NY, USA

Joelle Wazen Department of Diagnostic Radiology, UMass Memorial Medical Center, Worcester, MA, USA

Arwa Zaghal Department of Diagnostic Radiology, American University of Beirut Medical Center, Beirut, Lebanon

Fahed Zairi Department of Neurosurgery, Lille University Hospital, Lille, France

Mehrzad Zarghouni Department of Radiology, Division of Vascular and Interventional Radiology, New York University Langone Medical Center, New York, NY, USA

Reviewers

Aghiad Al-Kutoubi Department of Diagnostic Radiology, American University of Beirut Medical Center, Beirut, Lebanon

Jamal J. Hoballah Department of Surgery, American University of Beirut Medical Center, Beirut, Lebanon

John A. Kaufman Oregon Health and Science University Hospital, Portland, OR, USA

Karen T. Brown Department of Radiology, Memorial Sloan Kettering Cancer Center, New York, NY, USA

Michel Elias Mawad The Neurological Institute, Cleveland Clininc Abu dhabi, Abu Dhabi, UAE

Part I

Non-vascular Interventional Procedures: Head and Neck

Introduction by Aghiad Al-Kutoubi, Section Reviewer

Percutaneous needle biopsy with imaging guidance is a well-established, safe, and effective technique for diagnosis of head and neck lesions. Percutaneous biopsies of head and neck lesions are usually performed with computed tomographic and/or ultrasonographic guidance because these modalities allow precise localization and documentation of the biopsy needle and target lesion. A thorough knowledge of the complex cross-sectional anatomy and good ultrasound scanning skills are essential for planning and performing the procedure.

This section provides a comprehensive list of procedural reports that covers the vast majority of the currently performed nonvascular interventional procedures in the head and neck region with up-to-date explanatory notes, synopsis of the indications and contraindications and potential complications in an organized and practical format.

Section Chapters

Core Biopsy of Cervical Lymph Node

1

Sahar Semaan and Marc Mourad

INTRODUCTION

Percutaneous needle biopsy of enlarged cervical lymph nodes using ultrasound or CT guidance is a relatively safe procedure for patients with a suspected pathologic cervical adenopathy and has low morbidity and mortality rates. It is important to monitor the patient following the procedure for a short period of time and to track the biopsy results to insure the safety and efficacy of the procedure.

COMMON INDICATIONS [1–3]

- Determination of the benign or malignant nature of the lymph node
- Microbiologic analysis in suspected infection
- Staging patients with known malignancy and suspected metastasis

COMMON CONTRAINDICATIONS [1, 3, 4]

There are no absolute contraindications. The relative contraindications to be considered include the following:

- Severe uncorrectable coagulopathy
- Hemodynamic instability
- Lack of a safe pathway to the lymph node
- Lack of patient cooperation

POSSIBLE COMPLICATIONS [1, 4]

- Vascular injury *(especially to the carotid arteries)*
- Tracheal injury
- Hemorrhage
- Superinfection
- Pneumothorax *(particularly in supraclavicular nodes)*
- Vasovagal reaction

PREPROCEDURAL ASSESSMENT AND PLANNING

- History, indications and physical examination *(Appendix 1* in Chap. 149*)*
- Evaluation of diagnostic imaging studies *(ultrasound, computed tomography, PET-CT, and/or magnetic resonance imaging)*: to

S. Semaan (✉)
Department of Radiology, Icahn School of Medicine at Mount Sinai, One Gustave L. Levy Place, New York, NY 10029-6574, USA
e-mail: saharsemaan@gmail.com

M. Mourad
Department of Head and Neck and Endocrine Oncology, Moffitt Cancer Center, 12902 USF Magnolia Drive, Tampa, FL 33612, USA
e-mail: marcmmourad@gmail.com

B. Taslakian et al. (eds.), *Procedural Dictations in Image-Guided Intervention*,
DOI 10.1007/978-3-319-40845-3_1

determine the location of the lymph node of interest and the relevant anatomy
- Periprocedural management of coagulation status *(Appendices 2* in Chap. 150 *and 3* in Chap. 151*)*
- Antibiotic prophylaxis: Not routinely recommended [5] *(Appendices 4* in Chap. 152 *and 5* in Chap. 153*)*
- Imaging modality for guidance: Ultrasound/CT guidance
- Positioning: Oblique/prone/supine *(depending on the location of the target lymph node)*

PROCEDURE NOTE

Procedure: CT/ultrasound-guided core biopsy of left/right cervical lymph node
Staff: [_]
Fellow: [_]
Resident: [_]
Clinical History and Indications: Describe history and list indications
Allergies: None known/Allergic to [specify/type of allergy]
Anesthesia: Local anesthesia/Conscious sedation
Medications: List any relevant medications used (sedation, antibiotics)
Field: Sterile
Procedure classification: Clean
Position: Supine/Oblique/Prone
Monitoring: Intravenous access line was secured and vital signs were continuously monitored by nursing staff/anesthesia team throughout the procedure
Cumulative radiation dose: (_) mGy

Description of Procedure:

The risks, benefits, and procedure itself were explained to the patient/patient's Power of Attorney/legal guardian, and informed written consent was obtained. The site of the procedure was identified and marked. Time out was performed to confirm the correct patient, procedure, and site.

The neck was evaluated using ultrasound/CT scan after placement of a radiopaque marker and showed enlarged lymph node(s) at level (s) [specify lymph node level(s)].

The skin was prepped and draped in the usual sterile fashion. Local anesthesia was administered. A small skin incision was made. Subsequently, a (_)-gauge core biopsy needle guide was advanced along the planned trajectory until the needle tip was within the target lymph node. Samples were obtained using the coaxial technique under direct ultrasound visualization/using planning CT information, placed in a formalin solution and sent for histopathological evaluation.

The patient was transferred to the floor/recovery room following the procedure in a stable condition. Staff was present for the entire procedure.

Intra-Procedure Findings: List all relevant findings.

Immediate Complications: None encountered during or directly after the procedure. List complications if any.

Post-Procedure Plan [1, 3, 4]**:**
- Follow-up histopathology results.
- Observe the patient in the recovery room following the procedure for 1 h.
- Discharge instructions:
  - Abstain from strenuous activities for 3 days.
  - Seek medical help if pain at the biopsy site lasts over one week, fever develops, erythema and edema develop at the biopsy site, or if there is purulent discharge.

Impression:
- Core biopsy of right/left cervical lymph node, as described above.
- The patient tolerated the procedure well and left the interventional unit in a stable condition.
- List any other relevant or important information/finding.

References

1. Pua B, Solomon S. Lymph node biopsy. In: Gervais D, Sabharwal T, editors. Interventional radiology procedures in biopsy and drainage. London: Springer; 2011. p. 73–9.
2. Gupta S, Madoff DC. Percutaneous needle biopsy in cancer diagnosis and staging. Tech Vasc Intervent Rad. 2007;10(2):88–101.

3. Screaton NJ, Berman LH, Grant JW. Head and neck lymphadenopathy: evaluation with US-guided cutting-needle biopsy. Radiology. 2002;224(1):75–81.
4. Smith EH. The hazards of fine-needle aspiration biopsy. Ultrasound Med Biol. 1984;10(5):629–34.
5. Venkatesan AM, Kundu S, Sacks D, Wallace MJ, Wojak JC, Rose SC, et al. Practice guidelines for adult antibiotic prophylaxis during vascular and interventional radiology procedures. J Vasc Interv Radiol. 2010;21(11):1611–30.

Core Biopsy of Neck Lesion

2

Sahar Semaan and Marc Mourad

INTRODUCTION

Imaging guided percutaneous needle biopsy of neck lesions is a minimally invasive and often safe procedure that can usually be done on outpatient basis. It is often used as a first line for characterization of neck masses reserving more invasive modes of biopsy for lesions that are not reachable or if samples are insufficient. Like any other minor procedure, percutaneous needle biopsy requires minimal post-procedure monitoring and is associated with few complications.

COMMON INDICATIONS

- Determination of the nature of the mass/lesion

COMMON CONTRAINDICATIONS [1, 2]

There are no absolute contraindications. The relative contraindications to be considered include the following:

- Severe uncorrectable coagulopathy
- Hemodynamic instability
- Lack of a safe pathway to the lesion
- Lack of patient cooperation

POSSIBLE COMPLICATIONS [1–3]

- Vascular injury
- Airway compromise
- Hemorrhage
- Superinfection
- Vasovagal reaction

PREPROCEDURAL ASSESSMENT AND PLANNING

- History, indications, and physical examination *(Appendix 1* in Chap. 149*)*
- Evaluation of diagnostic imaging studies *(ultrasound, computed tomography, PET/CT, and/or magnetic resonance imaging):* to determine the location of the cervical mass/lesion of interest and evaluate the relevant anatomy

S. Semaan (✉)
Department of Radiology, Icahn School of Medicine at Mount Sinai, One Gustave L. Levy Place, New York, NY 10029-6574, USA
e-mail: saharsemaan@gmail.com

M. Mourad
Department of Head and Neck and Endocrine Oncology, Moffitt Cancer Center, 12902 USF Magnolia Drive, Tampa, FL 33612, USA
e-mail: marcmmourad@gmail.com

B. Taslakian et al. (eds.), *Procedural Dictations in Image-Guided Intervention*,
DOI 10.1007/978-3-319-40845-3_2

- Periprocedural management of coagulation status *(Appendices 2* in Chap. 150 *and 3* in Chap. 151*)*
- Antibiotic prophylaxis: Not routinely recommended [4] *(Appendices 4* in Chap. 152 *and 5* in Chap. 153*)*
- Imaging modality for guidance: Ultrasound/CT guidance
- Positioning: Oblique/prone/supine

PROCEDURE NOTE

Procedure: CT/ultrasound-guided core biopsy of left/right/midline cervical mass/lesion
Staff: [_]
Fellow: [_]
Resident: [_]
Clinical History and Indications: Describe history and list indications
Allergies: None known/Allergic to [specify/type of allergy]
Anesthesia: Local anesthesia/Conscious sedation
Medications: List any relevant medications used (sedation)
Field: Sterile
Procedure classification: Clean
Position: Supine/Oblique/Prone
Monitoring: Intravenous access line was secured and vital signs were continuously monitored by nursing staff/anesthesia team throughout the procedure
Cumulative radiation dose: (_) mGy

Description of Procedure:

The risks, benefits, and procedure itself were explained to the patient/patient's Power of Attorney/legal guardian, and informed written/verbal consent was obtained. The site of the procedure was identified and marked. Time out was performed to confirm the correct patient, procedure, and site.
The neck was evaluated using ultrasound/CT scan after placement of a radiopaque marker and showed the target lesion at the left/right/midline aspect of the neck.
The skin was prepped and draped in the usual sterile fashion. Local anesthesia was administered. A small skin incision was made. Subsequently, a (_)-gauge core biopsy needle guide was advanced along the planned trajectory until the needle tip was within the target lesion. Samples were obtained using the coaxial technique, under direct ultrasound visualization/using planning CT information, placed in a formalin solution and sent for histopathological evaluation.
Post biopsy CT/ultrasound images were obtained.

The patient was transferred to the floor/recovery room following the procedure in a stable condition. Staff was present for the entire procedure.
Intra-Procedure Findings: List all relevant findings.
Immediate Complications: None encountered during or directly after the procedure. List complications if any.

Post-Procedure Plan [1–3, 5]**:**
- Follow-up histopathology results.
- Observe the patient in the recovery room following the procedure for 1 h.
- Discharge instructions:
  - Abstain from strenuous activities for 3 days.
  - Seek medical help if pain at the biopsy site lasts over one week, fever develops, erythema and edema develop at the biopsy site, or if there is purulent discharge.

Impression:

- Core biopsy of right/left/midline cervical mass/lesion, as described above.
- The patient tolerated the procedure well and left the interventional unit in a stable condition.
- List any other relevant or important information/finding.

References

1. Sherman PM, Yousem DM, Loevner LA. CT-guided aspirations in the head and neck: assessment of the first 216 cases. AJNR Am J Neuroradiol. 2004;25(9): 1603–7.
2. Sack MJ, Weber RS, Weinstein GS, Chalian AA, Nisenbaum HL, Yousem DM. Image-guided fine-needle aspiration of the head and neck: five years' experience. Arch Otolaryngol Head Neck Surg. 1998;124(10):1155–61.
3. Charboneau JW, Reading CC, Welch TJ. CT and sonographically guided needle biopsy: current techniques and new innovations. AJR Am J Roentgenol. 1990;154(1):1–10.
4. Venkatesan AM, Kundu S, Sacks D, Wallace MJ, Wojak JC, Rose SC, et al. Practice guidelines for adult antibiotic prophylaxis during vascular and interventional radiology procedures. J Vasc Interv Radiol. 2010;21(11):1611–30.
5. Gupta S, Madoff DC. Percutaneous needle biopsy in cancer diagnosis and staging. Tech Vasc Intervent Rad. 2007;10(2):88–101.

Core Biopsy of the Parotid Gland

3

Sahar Semaan and Marc Mourad

INTRODUCTION

Imaging guided biopsy of a parotid mass is a minimally invasive and safe procedure that allows for the pathologic characterization of parotid masses, with an accuracy rate reaching 97 %. Since the differentiation of benign and malignant parotid lesions is often difficult using imaging characteristics alone, percutaneous needle biopsy is useful in determining the nature of these lesions and hence to guide further management and avoid unnecessary surgery. The procedure is done on an outpatient basis and is associated with minimal morbidity and mortality.

COMMON INDICATIONS [1, 2]

- Determination of the benign or malignant nature of the parotid mass

COMMON CONTRAINDICATIONS [1–3]

There are no absolute contraindications. The relative contraindications to be considered include the following:

- Severe uncorrectable coagulopathy
- Lack of patient cooperation

POSSIBLE COMPLICATIONS [1–3]

- Vascular injury
- Facial nerve injury
- Hemorrhage
- Tumor seeding in the needle tract
- Infection
- Vasovagal reaction

PREPROCEDURAL ASSESSMENT AND PLANNING

- History, indications, and physical examination *(Appendix 1* in Chap. 149*)*
- Evaluation of diagnostic imaging studies to determine the location of the parotid mass and its relation with the surrounding anatomical structures
- Periprocedural management of coagulation status *(Appendices 2* in Chap. 150 *and 3* in Chap. 151*)*

S. Semaan (✉)
Department of Radiology, Icahn School of Medicine at Mount Sinai, One Gustave L. Levy Place, New York, NY 10029-6574, USA
e-mail: saharsemaan@gmail.com

M. Mourad
Department of Head and Neck and Endocrine Oncology, Moffitt Cancer Center, 12902 USF Magnolia Drive, Tampa, FL 33612, USA
e-mail: marcmmourad@gmail.com

B. Taslakian et al. (eds.), *Procedural Dictations in Image-Guided Intervention*,
DOI 10.1007/978-3-319-40845-3_3

- Antibiotic prophylaxis: Not routinely recommended [4, 5] *(Appendices 4* in Chap. 152 *and 5* in Chap. 153*)*
- Imaging modality for guidance: Ultrasound/CT guidance
- Positioning: Supine

PROCEDURE NOTE

Procedure: Core biopsy of left/right parotid lesion
Staff: [_]
Fellow: [_]
Resident: [_]
Clinical History and Indications: Describe history and list indications
Allergies: None known/Allergic to [specify/type of allergy]
Anesthesia: Local anesthesia/conscious sedation
Medications: List any relevant medications used (sedation)
Field: Sterile
Procedure classification: Clean
Position: Supine
Monitoring: Intravenous access line was secured and vital signs were continuously monitored by nursing staff/anesthesia team throughout the procedure
Cumulative radiation dose: (_) mGy

Description of Procedure:

The risks, benefits, and procedure itself were explained to the patient/patient's Power of Attorney/legal guardian, and informed written consent was obtained. The site of the procedure was identified and marked. Time out was performed to confirm the correct patient, procedure, and site.

The neck was evaluated using ultrasound/CT scan after placement of a radiopaque marker and showed the target lesion in the left/right parotid gland.

The skin was prepped and draped in the usual sterile fashion. Local anesthesia was administered. A small skin incision was made. Subsequently, a (_)-gauge core biopsy needle guide was advanced along the planned trajectory until the needle tip was within the target lesion. Samples were obtained using the coaxial technique, under direct ultrasound visualization/using planning CT information, placed in a formalin solution and sent for histopathological evaluation.

The patient was monitored for (_) minutes and subsequently discharged with the usual instructions. Staff was present for the entire procedure.
Intra-Procedure Findings: List all relevant findings.
Immediate Complications: None encountered during or directly after the procedure. List complications if any.

Post-Procedure Plan:

- Follow-up histopathology results.
- Discharge instructions: Seek medical help if pain at the biopsy site lasts over one week, erythema and edema develop at the biopsy site, if purulent discharge or fever occurs and in case of facial weakness or asymmetry is noted.

Impression:

- Percutaneous needle biopsy of right/left parotid mass, as described above.
- The patient tolerated the procedure well and left the interventional unit in a stable condition.
- List any other relevant or important information/finding.

References

1. Howlett DC. Diagnosing a parotid lump: fine needle aspiration cytology or core biopsy? Br J Radiol. 2006;79(940):295–7.
2. Layfield LJ, Glasgow BJ. Diagnosis of salivary gland tumors by fine-needle aspiration cytology: a review of clinical utility and pitfalls. Diagn Cytopathol. 1991;7(3):267–72.
3. Frable MA, Frable WJ. Fine-needle aspiration biopsy of salivary glands. Laryngoscope. 1991;101(3):245–9.
4. Taslakian B, Sebaaly MG, Al-Kutoubi A. Patient evaluation and preparation in vascular and interventional radiology: what every interventional radiologist should know (part 2: patient preparation and medications). Cardiovasc Intervent Radiol. 2016;39(4):489–99. doi:10.1007/s00270-015-1239-4. [Epub 2015 Nov 25].
5. Venkatesan AM, Kundu S, Sacks D, Wallace MJ, Wojak JC, Rose SC, et al. Practice guidelines for adult antibiotic prophylaxis during vascular and interventional radiology procedures. J Vasc Interv Radiol. 2010;21(11):1611–30.

Fine Needle Aspiration of Cervical Lymph Node

4

Sahar Semaan and Marc Mourad

INTRODUCTION

Fine needle aspiration of suspicious cervical lymph nodes using ultrasound guidance is a minimally invasive procedure for the classification of cervical lymph node disease. Although it is less sensitive than core biopsy, it is associated with less morbidity and mortality and requires only minimal post-procedure monitoring.

COMMON INDICATIONS [1, 2]

- Determination of the benign or malignant nature of the lymph node
- Microbiologic analysis in suspected infection
- Staging patients with known malignancy and suspected metastasis

COMMON CONTRAINDICATIONS [1, 3]

There are no absolute contraindications. The relative contraindications to be considered include the following:

- Uncorrectable coagulopathy
- Lack of a safe pathway to the lymph node
- Lack of patient cooperation

POSSIBLE COMPLICATIONS [1, 3]

- Hemorrhage
- Vascular injury
- Vasovagal reaction

PREPROCEDURAL ASSESSMENT AND PLANNING

- History, indications, and physical examination *(Appendix 1* in Chap. 149*)*
- Evaluation of diagnostic imaging studies *(ultrasound, computed tomography, PET-CT, and/or magnetic resonance imaging)*, to determine the location of the lymph node of interest and evaluate the relevant anatomy
- Periprocedural management of coagulation status *(Appendices 2* in Chap. 150 *and 3* in Chap. 151*)*

S. Semaan (✉)
Department of Radiology, Icahn School of Medicine at Mount Sinai, One Gustave L. Levy Place, New York, NY 10029-6574, USA
e-mail: saharsemaan@gmail.com

M. Mourad
Department of Head and Neck and Endocrine Oncology, Moffitt Cancer Center, 12902 USF Magnolia Drive, Tampa, FL 33612, USA
e-mail: marcmmourad@gmail.com

B. Taslakian et al. (eds.), *Procedural Dictations in Image-Guided Intervention*,
DOI 10.1007/978-3-319-40845-3_4

- Antibiotic prophylaxis: Not routinely recommended [4, 5] *(Appendices 4* in Chap. 152 *and 5* in Chap. 153*)*
- Imaging modality for guidance: Ultrasound/CT guidance
- Positioning: Oblique/prone/supine *(depending on the location of the target lymph node)*

PROCEDURE NOTE

Procedure: Fine needle aspirate of left/right cervical lymph node
Staff: [_]
Fellow: [_]
Resident: [_]
Clinical Information: Describe history and list indications
Allergies: None known/Allergic to [specify/type of allergy]
Anesthesia: Local anesthesia/conscious sedation
Medications: List any relevant medications used (sedation)
Field: Sterile
Procedure classification: Clean
Position: Supine/Prone/Oblique
Monitoring: IV access line was secured and vital signs were continuously monitored by nursing staff/anesthesia team throughout the procedure
Cumulative radiation dose: (_) mGy

Description of Procedure:

The risks, benefits, and procedure itself were explained to the patient/patient's Power of Attorney/legal guardian, and informed written consent was obtained. The site of the procedure was identified and marked. Time out was performed to confirm the correct patient, procedure, and site.
The neck was evaluated using ultrasound/CT scan after placement of a radiopaque marker and showed enlarged lymph node(s) at level (s) [specify lymph node level(s)].
The skin was prepped and draped in the usual sterile fashion. Local anesthesia was administered. Using a (_)-gauge needle attached to a (_) mL syringe, multipass aspiration of the lymph node at level [specify lymph node level] on the left/right was performed. The obtained material was placed on glass slides, smeared, and fixed using 95 % ethyl alcohol. The syringe was rinsed with normal saline to obtain any remaining aspirated material for cell block.
An adhesive plaster was applied to the needle entry site and the patient was advised to gently compress the area for 30 min. The patient was transferred to the floor/recovery room/discharged home following the procedure in a stable condition. Staff was present for the entire procedure.
Intra-Procedure Findings: List all relevant findings.
Immediate Complications: None encountered during or directly after the procedure. List complications if any.

Post-Procedure Plan [1, 3]**:**

- Follow-up cytopathology results.
- Discharge instructions:
  - Apply gentle manual compression to the site of entry for 30 min.
  - Seek medical help if neck swelling occurs following the procedure or significant shortness of breath or hemoptysis is noted.

Impression:

- Fine needle aspiration of the prominent right/left cervical lymph node at level [specify lymph node level], as described above.
- The patient tolerated the procedure well and left the interventional unit in stable condition.
- List any other relevant or important information/finding.

References

1. Pua B, Solomon S. Lymph node biopsy. In: Gervais D, Sabharwal T, editors. Interventional radiology procedures in biopsy and drainage. London: Springer; 2011. p. 73–9.
2. van den Brekel MWM, Castelijns JA, Stel HV, Golding RP, Meyer CJL, Snow GB. Modern imaging techniques and ultrasound-guided aspiration cytology for the assessment of neck node metastases: a prospective comparative study. Eur Arch Otorhinolaryngol. 1993;250(1):11–7.

3. Smith EH. The hazards of fine-needle aspiration biopsy. Ultrasound Med Biol. 1984;10(5):629–34.
4. Taslakian B, Sebaaly MG, Al-Kutoubi A. Patient evaluation and preparation in vascular and interventional radiology: what every interventional radiologist should know (part 2: patient preparation and medications). Cardiovasc Intervent Radiol. 2016;39(4):489–99. doi: 10.1007/s00270-015-1239-4. [Epub 2015 Nov 25].
5. Venkatesan AM, Kundu S, Sacks D, Wallace MJ, Wojak JC, Rose SC, et al. Practice guidelines for adult antibiotic prophylaxis during vascular and interventional radiology procedures. J Vasc Interv Radiol. 2010;21(11):1611–30.

Fine Needle Aspiration of Thyroid Nodule

5

Sahar Semaan and Marc Mourad

INTRODUCTION

Fine needle aspiration of thyroid nodules under real-time ultrasound guidance is a safe and minimally invasive procedure that generally provides sufficient samples for the characterization of suspicious nodules. As a minor outpatient procedure, it requires only minimal post-procedure monitoring and is associated with few complications.

COMMON INDICATIONS [1–4]

- Solid hypoechoic nodular lesion measuring ≥ 1 cm
- Nodular lesion of any size showing suspicious ultrasound features such as the following:
  - Microcalcifications
  - Irregular contour
  - Cross-sectional dimension < longitudinal dimension
  - Increased vascularity on color Doppler
  - Extension to adjacent soft tissues
  - Suspicion of lymph node metastasis
- Diffuse lesion showing nodular features or rapid gland enlargement in a background of Hashimoto thyroiditis
- Patients with high risk of thyroid cancer *(i.e., positive family history, MEN 2 syndrome, history of head and neck irradiation, isolated increased calcitonin levels)*

COMMON CONTRAINDICATIONS [4]

There are no absolute contraindications. The only relative contraindication to be considered is significant bleeding diathesis.

POSSIBLE COMPLICATIONS [2–4]

- Limited intrathyroidal bleeding
- Neck hematoma
- Local pain radiating to the ear
- Vasovagal reaction
- Tracheal injury
- Vascular injury

PREPROCEDURAL ASSESSMENT AND PLANNING

- History, indications, and physical examination *(Appendix 1* in Chap. 149*)*

S. Semaan (✉)
Department of Radiology, Icahn School of Medicine at Mount Sinai, One Gustave L. Levy Place, New York, NY 10029-6574, USA
e-mail: saharsemaan@gmail.com

M. Mourad
Department of Head and Neck and Endocrine Oncology, Moffitt Cancer Center, 12902 USF Magnolia Drive, Tampa, FL 33612, USA
e-mail: marcmmourad@gmail.com

B. Taslakian et al. (eds.), *Procedural Dictations in Image-Guided Intervention*,
DOI 10.1007/978-3-319-40845-3_5

- Evaluation of the thyroid gland using ultrasound to determine the location and features of the lesion of interest and its relation to the adjacent structures
- Periprocedural management of coagulation status *(Appendices 2* in Chap. 150 *and 3* in Chap. 151*)*
- Antibiotic prophylaxis: Not routinely recommended [5, 6] *(Appendices 4* in Chap. 152 *and 5* in Chap. 153*)*
- Imaging modality for guidance: Ultrasound guidance
- Positioning: Supine with the neck slightly extended

PROCEDURE NOTE

Procedure: Ultrasound-guided fine needle aspiration of thyroid nodule
Staff: [_]
Fellow: [_]
Resident: [_]
Clinical History and Indications: Describe history and list indications
Allergies: None known/Allergic to [specify/type of allergy]
Anesthesia: Local anesthesia/conscious sedation/none
Medications: List any relevant medications used (sedation, antibiotics)
Field: Sterile
Procedure classification: Clean
Position: Supine with the neck slightly extended
Monitoring: Vital signs were continuously monitored by nursing staff throughout the procedure

Description of Procedure:

The risks, benefits, and procedure itself were explained to the patient/patient's Power of Attorney/legal guardian, and informed written consent was obtained. The site of the procedure was identified and marked. Time out was performed to confirm the correct patient, procedure, and site.

The skin was prepped and draped in the usual sterile fashion. Local anesthesia was administered. Using a (_)-gauge needle attached to a (_) mL syringe, multipass aspiration of the target nodule(s) was performed. The obtained material was placed on glass slides, smeared, and fixed using 95 % ethyl alcohol. The syringe was rinsed with normal saline to obtain any remaining aspirated material for cell block.

An adhesive plaster was applied to the needle entry site and the patient was advised to gently compress the area for 30 min. The patient was transferred to the floor/discharged home following the procedure in a stable condition. Staff was present for the entire procedure.

Intra-Procedure Findings: List all relevant findings.
Immediate Complications: None encountered during or directly after the procedure. List complications if any.

Post-Procedure Plan:
- Follow-up cytopathology results.
- Discharge instructions:
  - Apply gentle manual compression to the site of entry for 30 min.
  - Seek medical help if neck swelling, significant shortness of breath, or hemoptysis occur following the procedure.

Impression:
- Fine needle aspiration of left/right/bilateral thyroid nodule(s).
- The patient tolerated the procedure well and left the interventional unit in a stable condition.
- List any other relevant or important information/finding.

References

1. Gharib H, Papini E, Paschke R, Duick DS, Valcavi R, Hegedüs L, et al. American Association of Clinical Endocrinologists, Associazione Medici Endocrinologi, and European Thyroid Association Medical guidelines for clinical practice for the diagnosis and management of thyroid nodules: executive summary of recommendations. Endocr Pract. 2010;16(3):468–75.
2. Frates MC, Benson CB, Charboneau JW, Cibas ES, Clark OH, Coleman BG, et al. Management of thyroid nodules detected at US: society of radiologists in ultrasound consensus conference statement. Radiology. 2005;237:794–800.

3. Kim MJ, Kim EK, Park SI, Kim BM, Kwak JY, Kim SJ, et al. US-guided fine-needle aspiration of thyroid nodules: indications, techniques, results. Radiographics. 2008;28(7):1869–86.
4. Hamburger JI. Diagnosis of thyroid nodules by fine needle biopsy: use and abuse. J Clin Endocrinol Metab. 1994;79:335–9.
5. Venkatesan AM, Kundu S, Sacks D, Wallace MJ, Wojak JC, Rose SC, et al. Practice guidelines for adult antibiotic prophylaxis during vascular and interventional radiology procedures. J Vasc Interv Radiol. 2010;21(11):1611–30.
6. Taslakian B, Sebaaly MG, Al-Kutoubi A. Patient evaluation and preparation in vascular and interventional radiology: what every interventional radiologist should know (part 2: patient preparation and medications). Cardiovasc Intervent Radiol. 2016;39(4):489–99. doi: 10.1007/s00270-015-1239-4. [Epub 2015 Nov 25].

Sialography

6

Roula Hourani

INTRODUCTION

Salivary duct stone and stenosis is a frequent phenomenon. Sialography is the radiologic investigation of choice for visualization of salivary gland ducts and establishing patency. It usually involves the injection of a small amount of contrast medium into the salivary duct of a single gland, followed by routine X-ray projections and/or CT scan [1, 2].

INDICATIONS [2]

- Sialolithiasis
- Obstruction/strictures
- Sialectasis
- Masses/tumors
- Infection
- Changes secondary to trauma

CONTRAINDICATIONS [2]

- Active inflammation/infection *(e.g., mumps)*
- Anticipated failure in cannulating duct orifice
- Anticipated thyroid investigations

R. Hourani (✉)
Department of Diagnostic Radiology, American University of Beirut Medical Center, Riad El Solh, Beirut 1107 2020, Lebanon
e-mail: rh64@aub.edu.lb

COMPLICATIONS [2]

- Infection, inflammation
- Swelling/bleeding of the salivary duct
- Extravasation of contrast media

PREPROCEDURAL ASSESSMENT AND PLANNING

- History, indications, and physical examination *(Appendix 1* in Chap. 149*)*
- Evaluation of diagnostic imaging studies
- Periprocedural management of coagulation status *(Appendices 2* in Chap. 150 *and 3* in Chap. 151*)*
- Preparation: 2–3 min before the procedure, give the patient sialogogue *(secretory stimulant)* or few drops of lemon [3]
- Imaging modality for guidance: Fluoroscopy
- Positioning: Supine

PROCEDURE NOTE

Procedure: Fluoroscopy-guided Sialography
Staff: [_]
Fellow: [_]
Resident: [_]
Clinical Information: <u>Describe history and list indications</u>
Allergies: <u>None known/Allergic to [specify/type of allergy]</u>

B. Taslakian et al. (eds.), *Procedural Dictations in Image-Guided Intervention*,
DOI 10.1007/978-3-319-40845-3_6

Anesthesia: Topical anesthesia
Medications: List any relevant medications used
Contrast Material: (_) mL of [type] contrast material was used for intra-ductal injection
Field: Sterile
Position: Supine
Total fluoroscopy time: (_) minutes
Cumulative radiation dose: (_) mGy

Description of the procedure:

The risks, benefits, alternatives, and the procedure itself were explained to the patient/patient's Power of Attorney/patient's legal guardian, and informed written consent was obtained. Time out was performed to confirm the correct patient, procedure, and site.

The orifice of the [name] duct was visualized and a small (_)-inch catheter/cannula was selected to cannulate the papilla and was introduced into the duct. The catheter/cannula was attached to a connecting tube.

A small piece of gauze was wrapped around the hub of the catheter/cannula which was placed in between the patient's teeth to hold the catheter/cannula in place during the injection of contrast with the guidance of fluoroscopy. Manual pressure was used to introduce the contrast into the glandular ducts and outline the ductal anatomy.

Radiograph/CT imaging was performed immediately after contrast injection. Post-procedure (delayed) radiographs were also obtained to confirm evacuation of contrast and demonstrate any residual contrast.

The patient was discharged home following the procedure in a stable condition. Staff was present for the entire procedure.

Intra-Procedure Findings: List all relevant findings.

Immediate Complications: None encountered during or directly after the procedure. List complications if any.

Post-Procedure Plan:

- Encourage patient to gently massage the salivary gland in order to express dye.

Impression:

- Sialography, as described above.
- The patient tolerated the procedure well and left the interventional unit in a stable condition.
- List any other relevant or important information/finding.

References

1. Brown JE. Interventional sialography and minimally invasive. Techniques in benign salivary gland obstruction. Semin Ultrasound CT MR. 2006;27(6):465–75.
2. Burke CJ, Thomas RH, Howlett D. Imaging the major salivary glands. Br J Oral Maxillofac Surg. 2011;49 (4):261–9.
3. Laudenbach P, Poncet JL, Carlier R, Doyon D. Imaging protocol in salivary pathology. J Radiol. 1994;75(11):585–96.

Part II

Non-vascular Interventional Procedures: Thorax

Introduction by Aghiad Al-Kutoubi, Section Reviewer

Percutaneous thoracic procedures were described before the advent of imaging. Leyden et al.[1] performed the first transthoracic needle lung biopsy in 1882 to confirm pulmonary infection. Percutaneous image-guided catheter drainage of intra-thoracic fluid collections was introduced in the late 70s using basic catheter-guidewire techniques. Recent developments in bronchoscopy and endobronchial ultrasound and advances in focal radiotherapy offer an expanded armamentarium in the diagnosis and treatment of intrathoracic diseases; however, image-guided procedures remain important tools in everyday practice. Imaging guidance, particularly with the development of digital fluoroscopy, CT fluoroscopy, and C-arm cone-beam CT that offers "CT-like" imaging and real-time fluoroscopy, offers a safe and minimally invasive alternative to surgical and endoscopic techniques in the appropriate clinical setting. Positron emission tomography (PET)-CT scanning also provides guidance on the targeting of the most likely component to provide a high diagnostic yield during percutaneous biopsy.

Pneumothorax and hemoptysis are the two most common complications but other more serious complications such as air embolus and cardiac tamponade, though very rare, should be kept in mind. Strategies for management of the complication should be formulated in every unit that performs intrathoracic interventions.

This section provides a comprehensive list of procedural reports that covers the vast majority of the currently performed nonvascular image-guided thoracic procedures with up-to-date explanatory notes, synopsis of the indications and contraindications, and potential complications in an organized and practical format.

Section Chapters

[1]Dtsch Med Wochenschr 1883;9:52–55.

Aspiration of Pleural Effusion

7

Bedros Taslakian, Roy A. Raad and William Moore

INTRODUCTION

A pleural effusion is classified as transudate or exudate according to its composition and underlying pathophysiology. Percutaneous image-guided aspiration of pleural effusion or thoracentesis is defined as the therapeutic evacuation or diagnostic sampling of pleural fluid during a single imaging session.

COMMON INDICATIONS [1–5]

- Diagnostic aspiration for fluid characterization
- Therapeutic aspiration for relief of symptoms

COMMON CONTRAINDICATIONS [2–4]

- Inability of the patient to tolerate the procedure
- Inability of the patient to be positioned for the procedure
- Lack of a safe route for needle insertion
- Significant coagulopathy that cannot be adequately corrected
- Hemodynamic instability
- Pregnancy in cases when imaging guidance involves ionizing radiation

POSSIBLE COMPLICATIONS [2–7]

- Hemorrhage due to intercostal vessel injury
- Superinfection of a sterile pleural effusion
- Pneumothorax
- Re-expansion pulmonary edema if more than 1500 mL of fluid is removed
- Organ laceration

PREPROCEDURAL ASSESSMENT AND PLANNING

- History, indications, and physical examination *(Appendix 1* in Chap. 149*)*
- Evaluation of diagnostic imaging studies to determine the location and amount of pleural effusion and relevant anatomy
- Periprocedural management of coagulation status *(Appendices 2* in Chap. 150 *and 3 in* Chap. 151*)*

B. Taslakian
Department of Radiology, New York University Langone Medical Center, 660 First Ave, New York, NY 10016, USA
e-mail: btaslakian@gmail.com

R.A. Raad
Department of Radiology, New York University Langone Medical Center, 660 First Ave, 3rd Floor, Rm 314, New York, NY 10016, USA
e-mail: roy.raad@nyumc.org

W. Moore (✉)
Department of Radiology, New York University Langone Medical Center, 660 First Ave, 3rd Floor, Rm 335, New York, NY 10016, USA
e-mail: William.moore@nyumc.org

B. Taslakian et al. (eds.), *Procedural Dictations in Image-Guided Intervention*,
DOI 10.1007/978-3-319-40845-3_7

- Antibiotic prophylaxis: Not routinely recommended, unless infection is suspected [8, 9] *(Appendices 4* in Chap. 152 *and 5* in Chap. 153*)*
- Imaging modality for guidance: Ultrasound, CT
- Positioning:
  - Sitting on the edge of the bed, leaning forward with the patient's arms resting on a bedside table *(facilitates US-guided thoracentesis)*
  - Oblique, lateral decubitus, or supine for CT-guided procedures and in critically ill patients

PROCEDURE NOTE

Procedure: CT/US-guided percutaneous aspiration of left/right pleural effusion
Staff: [_]
Fellow: [_]
Resident: [_]
Clinical Information: Describe history and list indications
Allergies: None known/Allergic to [specify/type of allergy]
Anesthesia: Local anesthesia/Conscious sedation
Medications: List any relevant medications used (sedation, antibiotics)
Field: Sterile
Procedure classification: Clean/dirty *(if empyema or infection is suspected)*
Position: Supine/Sitting/Left lateral decubitus/Right lateral decubitus/Oblique
Monitoring: Intravenous access line was secured and vital signs were continuously monitored by nursing staff/anesthesia team throughout the procedure
Cumulative radiation dose: (_) mGy

Description of Procedure:

The risks, benefits, alternatives, and the procedure itself were explained to the patient/patient's Power of Attorney/patient's legal guardian, and informed written consent was obtained. The site of the procedure was identified and marked. Time out was performed to confirm the correct patient, procedure, and site.

The right/left hemithorax was evaluated using CT imaging after placement of a radiopaque marker/grid/ultrasound and showed mild/moderate/large amount of free/loculated pleural effusion.

The skin was prepped and draped in the usual sterile fashion. Local anesthesia was administered. A small skin incision was made. Subsequently, a (_)-gauge [type] needle was advanced into the left/right pleural space under direct ultrasound visualization/using planning CT information. (_) mL of clear fluid/serosanguineous fluid/malodorous pus was aspirated, and sent to laboratory for culture/gram stain/cytology/chemistry.

(_) mL of fluid was drained for symptomatic relief after insertion of a (_)-French catheter over a (_)-inch [type] guidewire. The catheter/needle was removed and completion ultrasound/CT images were obtained.

The patient was transferred to the floor/recovery room/discharged home following the procedure in a stable condition. Staff was present for the entire procedure.

Intra-Procedure Findings: List all relevant findings.

Immediate Complications: None encountered during or directly after the procedure. List complications if any.

Post-Procedure Plan:

- Check vital signs every 15 min for 1 h, then every 30 min for 1 h during observation period.
- Inform interventional radiology team if systolic blood pressure <95 mm Hg, heart rate >100 beats per minute, or if any chest pain or shortness of breath develops.
- Follow-up laboratory results.
- Abstain from strenuous activities.

Impression:

- Percutaneous aspiration of right/left pleural effusion, as described above.
- The patient tolerated the procedure well and left the interventional unit in a stable condition.

- The patient was unstable and the procedure was canceled/terminated prematurely.
- List any other relevant or important information/finding.

References

1. Maslove DM, Chen BT, Wang H, Kuschner WG. The diagnosis and management of pleural effusions in the ICU. J Intensive Care Med. 2013;28(1):24–36.
2. Drainage of pleural effusions and empyemas. In: Burke CT, Dixon RG, Mauro MA, Murphy KPJ, Thomson KR, Venbrux AC, Zollikofer CL, editors. High yield imaging: interventional. Philadelphia: Saunders Elsevier; 2010. p. 495–7.
3. Lewandowski RJ, Desai SB, Nemcek AA. Treatment of effusions and abscesses. In: Mauro MA, Murphy KPJ, Thomson KR, Venbrux AC, Zollikofer CL, editors. Image-guided interventions. Philadelphi: Saunders Elsevier; 2008. p. 1615–27.
4. Patz EF, Erasmus JJ. Catheter drainage of intrathoracic collections. In: Kandarpa K, Machan L, editors. Handbook of interventional radiologic procedures. 4th ed. Philadelphia: Lippincott Williams & Wilkins; 2011. p. 486–94.
5. Yu H. Management of pleural effusion, empyema, and lung abscess. Semin Interv Radiol. 2011;28(1):75–86.
6. Klein JS, Schultz S, Heffner JE. Interventional radiology of the chest: image-guided percutaneous drainage of pleural effusions, lung abscess, and pneumothorax. AJR Am J Roentgenol. 1995;164(3):581–8.
7. Ault MJ, Rosen BT, Scher J, Feinglass J, Barsuk JH. Thoracentesis outcomes: a 12-year experience. Thorax. 2015;70(2):127–32.
8. Taslakian B, Sebaaly MG, Al-Kutoubi A. Patient evaluation and preparation in vascular and interventional radiology: what every interventional radiologist should know (part 2: patient preparation and medications). Cardiovasc Intervent Radiol. 2016;39(4):489–99. doi: 10.1007/s00270-015-1239-4. [Epub 2015 Nov 25].
9. Venkatesan AM, Kundu S, Sacks D, Wallace MJ, Wojak JC, Rose SC, et al. Practice guidelines for adult antibiotic prophylaxis during vascular and interventional radiology procedures. J Vasc Interv Radiol. 2010;21(11):1611–30.

Catheter Drainage of Lung Abscess

8

Bedros Taslakian, Roy A. Raad and William Moore

INTRODUCTION

Lung abscess is defined as parenchymal necrosis with confined cavitation in the lung. Percutaneous drainage of lung abscess is defined as the placement of a catheter using imaging guidance to provide continuous drainage.

COMMON INDICATIONS [1–5]

- Pyogenic lung abscess not responding to medical treatment with signs of persistent sepsis for 5–7 days
- Increase in the size of the abscess despite adequate antibiotic therapy
- Large lung abscess (>4–6 cm)
- Pyogenic lung abscess in pediatrics age group (younger than 7 years of age)
- Pyogenic lung abscess in immunocompromised or oncologic patients
- Temporizing measure before definitive surgery
- Complicated lung abscess with hemoptysis, bronchopleural fistula, or empyema
- Lung abscess in patients who lack adequate cough mechanism

COMMON CONTRAINDICATIONS [1, 6, 7]

- Significant coagulopathy that cannot be adequately corrected
- Hemodynamic instability
- Lack of a safe route to access the collection
- Inability of the patient to be adequately positioned for the procedure
- Presence of necrotic tissue requiring surgical debridement
- Necrotizing pneumonia in pediatrics age group *(risk of bronchopleural fistula and persistent pneumothorax).*
- Suspected hydatid (echinococcus) cyst *(increased risk of anaphylactic shock)*
- Pregnancy in cases when imaging guidance involves ionizing radiation

B. Taslakian
Department of Radiology, New York University Langone Medical Center, 660 First Ave, New York, NY 10016, USA
e-mail: btaslakian@gmail.com

R.A. Raad
Department of Radiology, New York University Langone Medical Center, 660 First Ave, 3rd Floor, Rm 314, New York, NY 10016, USA
e-mail: roy.raad@nyumc.org

W. Moore (✉)
Department of Radiology, New York University Langone Medical Center, 660 First Ave, 3rd Floor, Rm 335, New York, NY 10016, USA
e-mail: William.moore@nyumc.org

B. Taslakian et al. (eds.), *Procedural Dictations in Image-Guided Intervention*,
DOI 10.1007/978-3-319-40845-3_8

POSSIBLE COMPLICATIONS [1, 3, 6, 8]

- Pneumothorax, *2–10 %*
- Hemorrhage requiring transfusion, *1 %*
- Septic shock, 1–2 %
- Bronchopleural fistula
- Empyema
- Failure of drainage *(multiloculated abscess, abscess with thick wall and containing viscous material)*
- Tube malfunction requiring catheter exchange *(malposition, dislodgement, kinking, clotting)*
- Organ injury

PREPROCEDURAL ASSESSMENT AND PLANNING

- History, indications, and physical examination *(Appendix 1* in Chap. 149*)*
- Evaluation of diagnostic imaging studies to determine the location of the abscess, its size, and relevant anatomy. Contrast-enhanced CT is essential to differentiate a lung abscess from other similar pathologic conditions, such as empyema and necrotizing pneumonia
- Periprocedural management of coagulation status *(Appendices 2* in Chap. 150 *and 3* in Chap. 151*)*
- Antibiotic prophylaxis: Routinely recommended [9] *(Appendices 4* in Chap. 152 *and 5* in Chap. 153*)*
- Imaging modality for guidance: CT, ultrasound *(when the abscess is reaching the chest wall)*
- Positioning: Oblique, lateral decubitus, or supine. To avoid aspiration of pus, the patient should be positioned adequately with the abscess in a gravity-dependent location [1]

PROCEDURE NOTE

Procedure: CT-guided percutaneous catheter drainage of left/right/upper/middle/lower lobe abscess
Staff: [_]
Fellow: [_]
Resident: [_]
Clinical Information: Describe history and list indications
Allergies: None known/Allergic to [specify/type of allergy]
Anesthesia: Local anesthesia/Conscious sedation
Medications: List any relevant medications used (sedation, antibiotics)
Field: Sterile
Procedure classification: Dirty
Position: Supine/Left lateral decubitus/Right lateral decubitus/Oblique
Monitoring: Intravenous access line was secured and vital signs were continuously monitored by nursing staff/anesthesia team throughout the procedure
Cumulative radiation dose: (_) mGy

Description of Procedure:

The risks, benefits, alternatives, and the procedure itself were explained to the patient/patient's Power of Attorney/legal guardian, and informed written consent was obtained. The site of the procedure was identified and marked. Time out was performed to confirm the correct patient, procedure, and site.

The chest was evaluated using CT imaging after placement of a radiopaque marker/grid and showed a (_) cm cavity with air-fluid level in the left/right/upper/middle/lower lobe. The procedure was planned and the skin puncture site was marked using combined information from the preliminary CT images, the abscess location, and the radiopaque marker/grid. The angle of needle entry and the distance to the collection were calculated from the planning CT images.

The skin was prepped and draped in the usual sterile fashion. Local anesthesia was administered. A small skin incision was made. Subsequently, a (_)-gauge [type] needle was advanced into the abscess cavity using planning CT information. (_) mL of malodorous pus was aspirated, and sent for culture and gram stain. Then, a (_)-inch [type] guidewire was advanced through the needle into the abscess cavity and the tract was dilated up to the required size using (_)-French dilator(s). A (_)-French self-retaining [type/pigtail] catheter assembly with the metal stiffener was introduced over the guidewire to a satisfactory depth. The stiff trocar of the catheter was left within the shaft until the catheter was advanced just beyond the wall of the abscess. The guidewire and stiffener were removed after advancing the catheter into the abscess cavity. The catheter was locked, anchored to the skin, and attached to a drainage system. Following this, completion CT images were obtained through the drainage area to confirm correct position of the catheter. The catheter was then attached to a drainage system.

The patient was transferred to the floor/recovery room/intensive care unit following the procedure in a stable/critical condition. Staff was present for the entire procedure.

Intra-Procedure Findings: List all relevant findings.

Immediate Complications: None encountered during or directly after the procedure. List complications if any.

Post-Procedure Plan [1, 5, 10]:

- Follow-up laboratory results and adjust antibiotics treatment accordingly.
- Connect catheter to a self-contained suction system or under-water seal drainage system on low continuous suction *(20–30-cm water).*
- Abstain from strenuous activities.
- Start clear liquid diet for the first hour, then regular diet thereafter if tolerated and otherwise not contraindicated.
- Check vital signs every 15 min for 1 h, every 30 min for 1 h, and then every 60 min for 2 h.
- Inform interventional radiology team if systolic blood pressure <95 mm Hg, heart rate >100 beats per minute, or if any chest pain or shortness of breath develops.
- Daily catheter care:
  - Inspect catheter and make sure that the 3-way stopcock is open to the drainage system and the catheter has not been externally retracted.
  - Flush the catheter with 20 mL of bacteriostatic saline every 8 h; 10 mL toward the drainage system and 10 mL toward the collection.
  - Record the catheter outputs every 8 h.
  - Inform interventional radiology team if the draining amount decreases, or pericatheter leak or local skin complications occurs.
- Removal of catheter is safe after clinical improvement is documented and after resolution of the abscess on subsequent imaging studies.

Impression:

- Percutaneous drainage of right/left/upper/middle/lower lobe lung abscess, as described above
- The patient tolerated the procedure well and left the interventional unit in a stable condition.
- The patient was unstable and the procedure was canceled/terminated prematurely.
- List any other relevant or important information/finding.

References

1. Patz EF, Erasmus JJ. Catheter drainage of intrathoracic collections. In: Kandarpa K, Machan L, editors. Handbook of interventional radiologic procedures. 4th ed. Philadelphia: Lippincott Williams & Wilkins; 2011. p. 486–94.
2. Klein JS, Schultz S, Heffner JE. Interventional radiology of the chest: image-guided percutaneous drainage of pleural effusions, lung abscess, and pneumothorax. AJR Am J Roentgenol. 1995;164(3):581–8.
3. vanSonnenberg E, D'Agostino HB, Casola G, Wittich GR, Varney RR, Harker C. Lung abscess: CT-guided drainage. Radiology. 1991;178(2):347–51.
4. Wali SO, Shugaeri A, Samman YS, Abdelaziz M. Percutaneous drainage of pyogenic lung abscess. Scand J Infect Dis. 2002;34(9):673–9.
5. Yu H. Management of pleural effusion, empyema, and lung abscess. Semin Interv Radiol. 2011;28(1):75–86.
6. Wallace MJ, Chin KW, Fletcher TB, Bakal CW, Cardella JF, Grassi CJ, et al. Quality improvement

guidelines for percutaneous drainage/aspiration of abscess and fluid collections. J Vasc Interv Radiol. 2010;21(4):431–5.
7. Hoffer FA, Bloom DA, Colin AA, Fishman SJ. Lung abscess versus necrotizing pneumonia: implications for interventional therapy. Pediatr Radiol. 1999;29 (2):87–91.
8. Bakal CW, Sacks D, Burke DR, Cardella JF, Chopra PS, Dawson SL, et al. Quality improvement guidelines for adult percutaneous abscess and fluid drainage. J Vasc Interv Radiol. 2003;14(9 Pt 2): S223–5.
9. Venkatesan AM, Kundu S, Sacks D, Wallace MJ, Wojak JC, Rose SC, et al. Practice guidelines for adult antibiotic prophylaxis during vascular and interventional radiology procedures. J Vasc Interv Radiol. 2010;21(11):1611–30.
10. Drainage of pleural effusions and empyemas. In: Burke CT, Dixon RG, Mauro MA, Murphy KPJ, Thomson KR, Venbrux AC, Zollikofer CL, editors. High yield imaging: interventional. Philadelphia: Saunders Elsevier; 2010. p. 495–7.

Catheter Drainage of Pleural Effusion

9

Roy A. Raad, Bedros Taslakian and William Moore

INTRODUCTION

Percutaneous drainage is defined as the placement of a catheter using image guidance to provide continuous drainage of a fluid collection. Ultrasound is the preferred method for guidance providing a reliable tool for an easy, safe, radiation-free and real-time guidance along with the possibility to perform the procedure at bedside in critically ill patients.

COMMON INDICATIONS [1–6]

- Symptomatic pleural effusion
- Large malignant pleural effusion before starting chemotherapy
- Refractory or recurrent pleural effusion to facilitate subsequent pleurodesis
- Parapneumonic effusions or empyema *(pleural glucose <60 mg/dL or PH <7.2)*
- Hemothorax and hemopneumothorax
- Chylothorax
- Leakage into the pleural space from esophageal or gastric rupture

COMMON CONTRAINDICATIONS [2–5, 7]

The contraindications are relative and depend on the suitability of surgical or conservative alternatives.

- Airway obstruction with a central mass preventing lung re-expansion
- Complex loculated pleural fluid collections requiring insertion of several tubes
- Thick pleural fluid limiting the value of percutaneous drainage
- Significant coagulopathy that cannot be adequately corrected
- Hemodynamic instability
- Lack of a safe route for needle insertion
- Inability of the patient to tolerate the procedure
- Inability of the patient to be properly positioned for the procedure
- Pregnancy in cases when imaging guidance involves ionizing radiation

R.A. Raad
Department of Radiology, New York University Langone Medical Center, 660 First Ave, 3rd Floor, Rm 314, New York, NY 10016, USA
e-mail: roy.raad@nyumc.org

B. Taslakian
Department of Radiology, New York University Langone Medical Center, 660 First Ave, New York, NY 10016, USA
e-mail: btaslakian@gmail.com

W. Moore (✉)
Department of Radiology, New York University Langone Medical Center, 660 First Ave, 3rd Floor, Rm 335, New York, NY 10016, USA
e-mail: William.moore@nyumc.org

B. Taslakian et al. (eds.), *Procedural Dictations in Image-Guided Intervention*,
DOI 10.1007/978-3-319-40845-3_9

POSSIBLE COMPLICATIONS [2, 4–7]

- Bleeding from intercostal vessel injury
- Superinfection of a sterile pleural effusion
- Pneumothorax
- Subcutaneous emphysema
- Re-expansion pulmonary edema
- Bacteremia and septic shock *(empyema drainage)*
- Tube malfunction requiring catheter exchange *(malposition, dislodgement, kinking, clotting)*
- Failure of drainage *(multiloculated effusion, empyema containing viscous material)*
- Intercostal neuralgia due to injury to the neurovascular bundles
- Unintended organ injury

Preprocedural Assessment and Planning

- History, indications, and physical examination *(Appendix 1* in Chap. 149*)*
- Evaluation of diagnostic imaging studies to determine the location of the effusion, its severity and relevant anatomy
- Periprocedural management of coagulation status *(Appendices 2* in Chap. 150 *and 3* in Chap. 151*)*
- Antibiotic prophylaxis: Not routinely recommended for noninfected fluid; recommended for empyema [8, 9] *(Appendices 4* in Chap. 152 *and 5* in Chap. 153*)*
- Imaging modality for guidance: Ultrasound, CT
- Positioning:
  - Sitting on the edge of the bed, leaning forward with the patient's arms resting on a bedside table *(facilitates ultrasound-guided drainage).*
  - Oblique, lateral decubitus, or supine for CT-guided procedures and in critically ill patients.

PROCEDURE NOTE

Procedure: CT/ultrasound-guided percutaneous drainage of left/right pleural effusion
Staff: [_]
Fellow: [_]
Resident: [_]
Clinical Information: Describe history and list indications
Allergies: None known/Allergic to [specify/type of allergy]
Anesthesia: Local anesthesia/Conscious sedation
Medications: List any relevant medications used (sedation, antibiotics)
Field: Sterile
Procedure classification: Clean/Dirty (if empyema is suspected)
Position: Supine/sitting/left lateral decubitus/right lateral decubitus/oblique
Monitoring: Intravenous access line was secured and vital signs were continuously monitored by nursing staff/anesthesia team throughout the procedure.
Cumulative radiation dose: (_) mGy

Description of Procedure:

The risks, benefits, alternatives and procedure itself were explained to the patient/patient's Power of Attorney/patient's legal guardian, and informed written consent was obtained. The site of the procedure was identified and marked. Time out was performed to confirm the correct patient, procedure, and site.

The right/left hemithorax was evaluated using CT imaging after placement of a radiopaque marker/grid/ultrasound and showed mild/moderate/large amount of free/loculated pleural effusion.

The skin was prepped and draped in the usual sterile fashion. Local anesthesia was administered. A small skin incision was made. Subsequently, a (_)-gauge [type] needle was advanced into the left/right pleural space under direct ultrasound visualization/using planning CT information. (_) mL of clear fluid/serosanguineous fluid/blood/malodorous pus was aspirated, and sent for culture/gram stain/cytology/chemistry. A (_)-inch [type] guidewire was advanced through the needle into the pleural cavity and the tract was dilated up to the required size using (_)-French dilator(s). A (_)-French self-retaining [type/pigtail] catheter assembly with the metal stiffener was introduced over the guidewire to a satisfactory depth. The stiff trocar of the catheter was left within the shaft until the catheter was traversed the skin-chest wall. The guidewire and metal stiffener were removed, after advancing the catheter into the pleural cavity. The catheter was locked, anchored to the skin and attached to an under-water seal drainage system. Following this, ultrasound/CT images were obtained through the drainage area to confirm the position of the tube.

The patient was transferred to the floor/recovery room/discharged home following the procedure in a stable condition. Staff was present for the entire procedure.

Intra-Procedure Findings: List all relevant findings.

Immediate Complications: None encountered during or directly after the procedure. List complications if any.

Post-Procedure Plan [2, 4, 6]:

- Follow-up laboratory results if applicable.
- Connect catheter to an under-water seal drainage system and keep under dependent drainage or low continuous suction *(20–30 cm water)* as needed.
- Obtain postprocedure radiograph to confirm catheter position and allow subsequent comparison if needed.
- Abstain from strenuous activities.
- Start clear liquid diet for the first hour, then regular diet thereafter if tolerated and otherwise not contraindicated.
- Check vital signs every 15 min for 1 h, every 30 min for 1 h, and then every 60 min for 2 h.
- Inform interventional radiology team if systolic blood pressure <95 mm Hg, heart rate >100 beats per minute, or if any chest pain or shortness of breath develops.
- Daily catheter care:
  - Inspect catheter and make sure that the 3-way stopcock is open to the drainage system and the catheter has not been externally retracted.
  - Flush the catheter with 20 mL of bacteriostatic saline every 8 h; 10 mL toward the drainage system and 10 mL toward the pleural cavity.
  - Record the catheter outputs every 8 h.
  - Withhold drainage using a 3-way stopcock if draining amount is >500 mL per hour to avoid re-expansion pulmonary edema.
  - Obtain a chest radiograph if drainage decreases to 100–200 mL over 24 h.
- Inform interventional radiology team if the draining amount decreases, or pericatheter leak or local skin complications occurs.
- Removal of catheter:
  - Parapneumonic effusions and empyema: When drainage is minimal (<50 mL per 24 h), clinical improvement is noted and antibiotics are changed from intravenous to oral.
  - Malignant pleural effusions: When drainage decreases to 100–200 mL over 24 h and pleurodesis is performed.
  - Transudate effusions: When drainage decreases to 100–200 mL over 24 h, radiograph confirms resolution of the effusion and clinical improvement is noted.

Impression:

- Percutaneous drainage of right/left pleural effusion, as described above.
- The patient tolerated the procedure well and left the interventional unit in a stable condition.

- The patient was unstable and the procedure was canceled/terminated prematurely.
- List any other relevant or important information/finding.

References

1. Maslove DM, Chen BT, Wang H, Kuschner WG. The diagnosis and management of pleural effusions in the ICU. J Intensive Care Med. 2013;28(1):24–36.
2. Drainage of pleural effusions and empyemas. In: Burke CT, Dixon RG, Mauro MA, Murphy KPJ, Thomson KR, Venbrux AC, Zollikofer CL, editors. High yield imaging: interventional. Philadelphia: Saunders Elsevier; 2010. p. 495–7.
3. Lewandowski RJ, Desai SB, Nemcek AA. Treatment of effusions and abscesses. In: Mauro MA, Murphy KPJ, Thomson KR, Venbrux AC, Zollikofer CL, editors. Image-guided interventions. Philadelphia: Saunders Elsevier; 2008. p. 1615–27.
4. Patz EF, Erasmus JJ. Catheter drainage of intrathoracic collections. In: Kandarpa K, Machan L, editors. Handbook of interventional radiologic procedures. 4th ed. Philadelphia, PA: Lippincott Williams & Wilkins; 2011. p. 486–94.
5. Klein JS, Schultz S, Heffner JE. Interventional radiology of the chest: image-guided percutaneous drainage of pleural effusions, lung abscess, and pneumothorax. AJR Am J Roentgenol. 1995;164(3):581–8.
6. Yu H. Management of pleural effusion, empyema, and lung abscess. Semin Interv Radiol. 2011;28(1):75–86.
7. Wallace MJ, Chin KW, Fletcher TB, Bakal CW, Cardella JF, Grassi CJ, et al. Quality improvement guidelines for percutaneous drainage/aspiration of abscess and fluid collections. J Vasc Interv Radiol. 2010;21(4):431–5.
8. Taslakian B, Sebaaly MG, Al-Kutoubi A. Patient evaluation and preparation in vascular and interventional radiology: what every interventional radiologist should know (part 2: patient preparation and medications). Cardiovasc Intervent Radiol. 2016;39(4):489–99. doi: 10.1007/s00270-015-1239-4. [Epub 2015 Nov 25].
9. Venkatesan AM, Kundu S, Sacks D, Wallace MJ, Wojak JC, Rose SC, et al. Practice guidelines for adult antibiotic prophylaxis during vascular and interventional radiology procedures. J Vasc Interv Radiol. 2010;21(11):1611–30.

Core Biopsy of Chest Wall Lesion

10

William Moore and Bedros Taslakian

INTRODUCTION

Computed tomography is the primary imaging tool used for guidance for percutaneous needle biopsy of chest wall and pleural lesions. Ultrasound-guided biopsy is well suited for the sampling of superficial lesions where an adequate acoustic window is available.

COMMON INDICATIONS [1–3]

- Diagnosis of chest wall masses and rib lesions
- Diagnosis of focal or diffuse pleural thickening
- Evaluation of known or suspected infections refractory to antimicrobial therapy

COMMON CONTRAINDICATIONS [1–4]

- Uncooperative patients
- Hemodynamic instability
- Lack of a safe route to the lesion
- Significant coagulopathy that cannot be adequately corrected
- Pregnancy in cases when imaging guidance involves ionizing radiation
- Intractable cough *(increased risk of pneumothorax)*
- Patients on positive pressure ventilation *(increased risk of pneumothorax)*

POSSIBLE COMPLICATIONS [1–4]

- Bleeding due to intercostal vessel injury
- Chest wall hematoma
- Unintended organ injury
- Superinfection
- Pneumothorax
- Vasovagal reaction
- Malignant seeding along the needle tract *(rare)*

PREPROCEDURAL ASSESSMENT AND PLANNING

- History, indications, and physical examination *(Appendix 1* in Chap. 149*)*
- Evaluation of diagnostic imaging studies to determine the location of the lesion and relevant anatomy
- Periprocedural management of coagulation status *(Appendices 2* in Chap. 150 *and 3* in Chap. 151*)*

W. Moore (✉)
Department of Radiology, New York University Langone Medical Center, 660 1st Avenue, 3rd Floor, Room 335, New York 10016, USA
e-mail: William.moore@nyumc.org

B. Taslakian
Department of Radiology, New York University Langone Medical Center, 660 First Ave, New York, NY 10016, USA
e-mail: btaslakian@gmail.com

B. Taslakian et al. (eds.), *Procedural Dictations in Image-Guided Intervention*,
DOI 10.1007/978-3-319-40845-3_10

- Antibiotic prophylaxis: Not routinely recommended [5, 6] *(Appendices 4* in Chap. 152 *and 5* in Chap. 153*)*
- Imaging modality for guidance: Ultrasound, CT
- Positioning: Oblique, lateral decubitus, prone, or supine

PROCEDURE NOTE

Procedure: Percutaneous core biopsy of left/right/posterior/anterior chest wall/rib/pleural lesion
Staff: [_]
Fellow: [_]
Resident: [_]
Clinical Information: Describe history and list indications
Allergies: None known/Allergic to [specify/type of allergy]
Anesthesia: Local anesthesia/conscious sedation
Medications: List any relevant medications used (sedation, antibiotics)
Field: Sterile
Procedure classification: Clean
Position: Supine/Prone/Left lateral decubitus/Right lateral decubitus/Oblique
Monitoring: Intravenous access line was secured and vital signs were continuously monitored by nursing staff/anesthesia team throughout the procedure.
Cumulative radiation dose: (_) mGy

Description of Procedure:

The risks, benefits, alternatives and the procedure itself were explained to the patient/patient's Power of Attorney/patient's legal guardian, and informed written consent was obtained. The site of the procedure was identified and marked. Time out was performed to confirm the correct patient, procedure and site.

The right/left chest was evaluated using CT imaging after placement of a radiopaque marker/grid/ultrasound and showed a (_) cm round/oval/irregular soft tissue/rib/pleural lesion. The procedure was planned and the skin puncture site was marked using combined information from the location of the lesion and preliminary CT/ultrasound images. The angle of needle entry and the distance to the lesion were calculated from the planning images.

The skin was prepped and draped in the usual sterile fashion. Local anesthesia was administered. A small skin incision was made. Subsequently, using planning CT information/under direct ultrasound visualization, a (_)-gauge [type] needle guide was advanced along the planned trajectory until the needle tip reached the target lesion, confirmed by imaging. (_) samples were obtained using the coaxial technique, placed in a formalin solution and sent for histopathological evaluation. Following this, completion CT/ultrasound images were obtained.

The patient was transferred to the floor/recovery room/discharged home following the procedure in a stable condition. Staff was present for the entire procedure
Intra-Procedure Findings: List all relevant findings.
Immediate Complications: None encountered during or directly after the procedure. List complications if any.

Post-Procedure Plan [1–3]:

- Follow-up histopathology results.
- Observe the patient in the recovery room following the procedure for 2 h.
- Monitor vital signs every 30 min for 2 h.
- Keep patient recumbent with the puncture site down.
- Administer supplemental nasal oxygen *(if a small pneumothorax develops)*.
- If the patient's condition deteriorates, suspecting a large or expending pneumothorax during observation, obtain an immediate chest radiograph and inform interventional team.
- Discharge instructions:
  - Abstain from strenuous activities for 3 days and avoid vigorous cough.
  - Visit the nearest emergency room promptly if any chest pain or shortness of breath develops.
  - Start clear liquid diet for the first hour, then regular diet thereafter if tolerated and no complications occur.

Impression:

- Percutaneous core biopsy of right/left chest wall/rib/pleural lesion, as described above.
- The patient tolerated the procedure well and left the interventional unit in a stable condition.
- The patient was unstable and the procedure was canceled/terminated prematurely.
- List any other relevant or important information/finding.

References

1. Percutaneous biopsy of the thorax. In: Burke CT, Dixon RG, Mauro MA, Murphy KPJ, Thomson KR, Venbrux AC, Zollikofer CL, editors. High yield imaging: interventional. Philadelphia: Saunders Elsevier; 2010. p. 498–500.
2. Given MF, Thomson KR, Lyon SM. Percutaneous biopsy of the lung, mediastinum, and pleura. In: Mauro MA, Murphy KPJ, Thomson KR, Venbrux AC, Zollikofer CL, editors. Image-guided interventions. Philadelphia: Saunders Elsevier; 2008. p. 1628–32.
3. Cham MD, Henschke CI, Yankelevitz DF. Biopsy procedures of the lung, mediastinum, and chest wall. In: Kandarpa K, Machan L, editors. Handbook of interventional radiologic procedures. 4th ed. Philadelphia: Lippincott Williams & Wilkins; 2011. p. 478–85.
4. Müller NL, Bergin CJ, Miller RR, Ostrow DN. Seeding of malignant cells into the needle tract after lung and pleural biopsy. J Can Assoc Radiol. 1986;37:192–4.
5. Taslakian B, Sebaaly MG, Al-Kutoubi A. Patient evaluation and preparation in vascular and interventional radiology: what every interventional radiologist should know (part 2: patient preparation and medications). Cardiovasc Intervent Radiol. 2016;39(4):489–99. doi: 10.1007/s00270-015-1239-4. [Epub 2015 Nov 25].
6. Venkatesan AM, Kundu S, Sacks D, Wallace MJ, Wojak JC, Rose SC, et al. Practice guidelines for adult antibiotic prophylaxis during vascular and interventional radiology procedures. J Vasc Interv Radiol. 2010;21(11):1611–30.

Core Biopsy of Lung Lesion

11

Bedros Taslakian and William Moore

INTRODUCTION

Image-guided lung biopsy is an established, safe, and effective procedure for selected patients. It is used to obtain tissue for diagnosis and genetic and immunologic testing of cancer mutations, thus guiding the treatment of patients undergoing targeted chemotherapy.

COMMON INDICATIONS [1–5]

- Evaluation of a suspicious pulmonary nodule
- Evaluation of a solitary or multiple pulmonary nodules in a patient with known malignancy for staging
- Evaluation of focal pulmonary infections refractory to standard therapy
- Evaluation of suspicious centrally located pulmonary lesion after a failed or inconclusive bronchoscopy-guided biopsy or bronchial lavage

COMMON CONTRAINDICATIONS [1–3, 6–9]

- Uncooperative patients
- Hemodynamic instability
- Lack of a safe route to the lesion
- Significant coagulopathy that cannot be adequately corrected
- Pregnancy in cases when imaging guidance involves ionizing radiation
- Severe emphysema *(increased risk of pneumothorax)*
- Intractable cough *(increased risk of pneumothorax)*
- Patients on positive pressure ventilation *(increased risk of pneumothorax)*
- Suspected hydatid cysts *(risk of anaphylactic shock)*
- Suspected pulmonary arteriovenous malformation, vascular aneurysms, or pulmonary sequestration *(preprocedural contrast-enhanced CT scan is essential)*
- Pulmonary hypertension when a central biopsy is planned
- Severely limited pulmonary function *(relative contraindication, but feasible)*
- Contralateral pneumonectomy *(relative contraindication, but feasible)*

B. Taslakian
Department of Radiology, New York University Langone Medical Center, 660 First Ave, New York, NY 10016, USA
e-mail: btaslakian@gmail.com

W. Moore (✉)
Department of Radiology, New York University Langone Medical Center, 660 1st Avenue- 3rd Floor Room 335, New York, NY 10016, USA
e-mail: William.moore@nyumc.org

B. Taslakian et al. (eds.), *Procedural Dictations in Image-Guided Intervention*,
DOI 10.1007/978-3-319-40845-3_11

POSSIBLE COMPLICATIONS [1–3, 10, 11]

- Pneumothorax, *12–45 %* [11]
- Hemoptysis *(minor, 5–10 %)*, hemothorax, chest wall hematoma *(bleeding from intercostal, pulmonary, mediastinal vessel injury)*
- Superinfection
- Vasovagal reaction
- Unintended organ injury
- Air embolism, *0.06–0.07 %* [11]
- Cardiac tamponade, *rare*
- Malignant seeding along the needle tract, *rare*
- Fatal hemorrhage and massive hemoptysis, *rare*
- Lung torsion, *rare*

PREPROCEDURAL ASSESSMENT AND PLANNING [12–14]

- History, indications, and physical examination *(Appendix 1* in Chap. 149*)*
- Evaluation of diagnostic imaging studies to determine the location of the lesion and relevant anatomy
- Periprocedural management of coagulation status *(Appendices 2* in Chap. 150 and *3* in Chap. 151*)*
- Antibiotic prophylaxis: Not routinely recommended [12] *(Appendices 4* in Chap. 152 and *5* in Chap. 153*)*
- Imaging modality for guidance: CT, CT fluoroscopy, ultrasound *(for peripheral, pleural-based lesions)*, fluoroscopy *(rarely used)*
- Positioning: Oblique, lateral decubitus, prone, or supine

PROCEDURE NOTE

Procedure: Percutaneous core biopsy of left/right/upper/lower/middle lobe lung lesion
Staff: [_]
Fellow: [_]
Resident: [_]
Clinical Information: Describe history and list indications
Allergies: None known/Allergic to [specify/type of allergy]
Anesthesia: Local anesthesia/conscious sedation
Medications: List any relevant medications used (sedation, antibiotics)
Field: Sterile
Procedure classification: Clean
Position: Supine/Prone/Left lateral decubitus/Right lateral decubitus/Oblique
Monitoring: Intravenous access line was secured and vital signs were continuously monitored by nursing staff/anesthesia team throughout the procedure
Cumulative radiation dose: (_) mGy

Description of Procedure:
The risks, benefits, alternatives, and the procedure itself were explained to the patient/patient's Power of Attorney/patient's legal guardian, and informed written consent was obtained. The site of the procedure was identified and marked. Time out was performed to confirm the correct patient, procedure, and site.

The lungs were evaluated using CT imaging after placement of a radiopaque marker/grid/ultrasound showing a (_) cm round/oval/irregular lesion in the right/left/lower/upper/middle lobe. The procedure was planned and the skin puncture site was marked using combined information from the location of the lesion and preliminary CT/ultrasound images. The angle of needle entry and the distance to the lesion were calculated from the planning images.

The skin was prepped and draped in the usual sterile fashion. Local anesthesia was administered. A small skin incision was made. Subsequently, using planning CT information/using CT fluoroscopy/under direct ultrasound visualization, a (_)-gauge [type] needle guide was advanced along the planned trajectory until the needle tip reached the target lesion, confirmed by imaging. (_) samples were obtained using the coaxial technique, placed in a formalin solution and sent for histopathological evaluation. While obtaining samples, saline solution was placed in the hub of the reference (coaxial) needle to avoid air embolism. The biopsy track was plugged with autologous blood clot seal by injecting (_) mL of autologous blood/collagen plug while withdrawing the reference needle. Following this, immediate completion CT/ultrasound images were obtained at the level of the biopsy site.

The patient was transferred to the floor/recovery room/discharged home following the procedure in a stable condition. Staff was present for the entire procedure.

Intra-procedure Findings: List all relevant findings.

Immediate Complications: None encountered during or directly after the procedure. List complications if any.

Post-procedure Plan [1–3]**:**

- Follow-up histopathology results.
- Observe the patient in the recovery room following the procedure for 2 h.
- Monitor vital signs every 30 min for 2 h.
- Keep patient recumbent with the puncture site down.
- Obtain an upright chest radiograph immediately and 2 h after biopsy.
- Administer supplemental nasal oxygen *(if a small pneumothorax develops).*
- If the patient's condition deteriorates, suspecting a large or expending pneumothorax during observation, obtain an immediate chest radiograph and inform interventional team.
- Discharge instructions:
  - Abstain from strenuous activities for 3 days and avoid vigorous cough.
  - Visit the nearest emergency room promptly if any chest pain or shortness of breath develops.
  - Start clear liquid diet for the first hour, then regular diet thereafter if tolerated and no complications occur.

Impression:

- Percutaneous core biopsy of right/left/lower/upper/middle lobe lung lesion, as described above.
- The patient tolerated the procedure well and left the interventional unit in a stable condition.
- The patient was unstable and the procedure was canceled/terminated prematurely.
- List any other relevant or important information/finding.

References

1. Percutaneous biopsy of the thorax. In: Burke CT, Dixon RG, Mauro MA, Murphy KPJ, Thomson KR, Venbrux AC, Zollikofer CL, editors. High yield imaging: interventional. Philadelphia: Saunders Elsevier; 2010. p. 498–500.
2. Given MF, Thomson KR, Lyon SM. Percutaneous biopsy of the lung, mediastinum, and pleura. In: Mauro MA, Murphy KPJ, Thomson KR, Venbrux AC, Zollikofer CL, editors. Image-guided interventions. Philadelphia: Saunders Elsevier; 2008. p. 1628–32.
3. Cham MD, Henschke CI, Yankelevitz DF. Biopsy procedures of the lung, mediastinum, and chest wall. In: Kandarpa K, Machan L, editors. Handbook of interventional radiologic procedures. 4th ed. Philadelphia: Lippincott Williams & Wilkins; 2011. p. 478–85.
4. MacMahon H, Austin JH, Gamsu G, Herold CJ, Jett JR, Naidich DP, et al. Guidelines for management of small pulmonary nodules detected on CT scans: a statement from the Fleischner society. Radiology. 2005;237(2):395–400.
5. Naidich DP, Bankier AA, MacMahon H, Schaefer-Prokop CM, Pistolesi M, Goo JM, et al. Recommendations for the management of subsolid pulmonary nodules detected at CT: a statement from the Fleischner Society. Radiology. 2013;266(1):304–17.
6. Stampfel G. Anaphylactoid reaction, a rare complication after fine needle biopsy of the lung. Radiology. 1982;22(7):329–30.
7. Moore EH. Needle-aspiration lung biopsy: a comprehensive approach to complication reduction. J Thorac Imaging. 1997;12(4):259–71.
8. Khouri NF, Stitik FP, Erozan YS, Gupta PK, Kim WS, Scott WW Jr, et al. Transthoracic needle aspiration biopsy of benign and malignant lung lesions. AJR Am J Roentgenol. 1985;144(2):281–8.
9. Cronin CG, Sharma A, Digumarthy SR, Gilman MD, McLoud T, Muse VV, et al. Percutaneous lung biopsy after pneumonectomy: factors for improving success in the care of patients at high risk. AJR Am J Roentgenol. 2011;196(4):929–34.
10. Müller NL, Bergin CJ, Miller RR, Ostrow DN. Seeding of malignant cells into the needle tract after

lung and pleural biopsy. J Can Assoc Radiol. 1986;37:192–4.
11. Gupta S, Wallace MJ, Cardella JF, Kundu S, Miller DL, Rose SC. Quality improvement guidelines for percutaneous needle biopsy. J Vasc Interv Radiol. 2010;21(7):969–75.
12. Taslakian B, Sebaaly MG, Al-Kutoubi A. Patient evaluation and preparation in vascular and interventional radiology: what every interventional radiologist should know (part 1: patient assessment and laboratory tests). Cardiovasc Intervent Radiol. 2016; 39 (3):325–33.
13. Taslakian B, Sebaaly MG, Al-Kutoubi A. Patient evaluation and preparation in vascular and interventional radiology: what every interventional radiologist should know (part 2: patient preparation and medications). Cardiovasc Intervent Radiol. 2016;39(4):489–99. doi: 10.1007/s00270-015-1239-4. [Epub 2015 Nov 25].
14. Venkatesan AM, Kundu S, Sacks D, Wallace MJ, Wojak JC, Rose SC, et al. Practice guidelines for adult antibiotic prophylaxis during vascular and interventional radiology procedures. J Vasc Interv Radiol. 2010;21(11):1611–30.

Core Biopsy of Mediastinal Lesion

12

Bedros Taslakian and William Moore

Introduction

Image-guided percutaneous needle biopsy of mediastinal masses is a fairly safe and effective technique for obtaining tissue diagnoses. Although the presence of major vessels, bones, lung, and the airways may preclude an extrapleural needle placement, imaging guidance allows access to lesions in virtually all mediastinal locations. Different techniques allow extrapleural access including the parasternal, paravertebral, trans-sternal, and suprasternal approaches. When a direct extrapleural approach is not possible, advancing the needle through a pleural window created by an existing pleural effusion, an iatrogenic pneumothorax, hydro-dissection or pleural fluid, or using a transpulmonary approach, are feasible alternatives. Careful planning, post-procedure monitoring in addition to outcomes tracking is necessary to continue to improve the safety and efficacy of this procedure.

B. Taslakian
Department of Radiology, New York University Langone Medical Center, 660 First Ave, New York, NY 10016, USA
e-mail: btaslakian@gmail.com

W. Moore (✉)
Department of Radiology, New York University Langone Medical Center, 660 1st Avenue, 3rd Floor, Room 335, New York, NY 10016, USA
e-mail: William.moore@nyumc.org

COMMON INDICATIONS [1–3]

- Evaluation of suspicious mediastinal or hilar lesions
- To obtain material for microbiologic analysis in patients with suspected or known infections refractory to antimicrobial therapy

COMMON CONTRAINDICATIONS [1–3]

- Uncooperative patients
- Hemodynamic instability
- Lack of a safe pathway to the lesion
- Significant coagulopathy that cannot be adequately corrected
- Pregnancy in cases when imaging guidance involves ionizing radiation
- Severe emphysema *(increased risk of pneumothorax)*
- Intractable cough *(increased risk of pneumothorax)*
- Patients on positive pressure ventilation *(increased risk of pneumothorax)*

POSSIBLE COMPLICATIONS [1–5]

- Pneumothorax, *12–45 %* [5]
- Hemoptysis and alveolar hemorrhage, *5–10 %* [3]

B. Taslakian et al. (eds.), *Procedural Dictations in Image-Guided Intervention*,
DOI 10.1007/978-3-319-40845-3_12

- Hemothorax, chest wall hematoma, cardiac temponade
- Superinfection
- Vasovagal reaction
- Air embolism, *0.06–0.07* [5]
- Fatal hemorrhage and massive hemoptysis, *rare*
- Cardiac tamponade, *very rare*

PREPROCEDURAL ASSESSMENT AND PLANNING [6–8]

- History, indications, and physical examination *(Appendix 1* in Chap. 149*)*
- Evaluation of diagnostic imaging studies to determine the location of the lesion and relevant anatomy
- Periprocedural management of coagulation status *(Appendices* in Chap. 150 *and* in Chap. 151*)*
- Antibiotic prophylaxis: Not routinely recommended [6] *(Appendices* in Chap. 152 *and* in Chap. 153*)*
- Imaging modality for guidance: CT, CT fluoroscopy, ultrasound *(for anterior mediastinal lesions)* [3, 4]
- Positioning: Oblique, lateral decubitus, prone, or supine [4]

PROCEDURE NOTE

Procedure: Percutaneous core biopsy of anterior/middle/posterior mediastinal/subcarinal/right/left hilar lesion
Staff: [_]
Fellow: [_]
Resident: [_]
Clinical Information: Describe history and list indications
Allergies: None known/Allergic to [specify/type of allergy]
Anesthesia: Local anesthesia/conscious sedation
Medications: List any relevant medications used (sedation, antibiotics)
Field: Sterile
Procedure classification: Clean
Position: Supine/Prone/Left lateral decubitus/Right lateral decubitus/Oblique
Monitoring: Intravenous access line was secured and vital signs were continuously monitored by nursing staff/anesthesia team throughout the procedure.
Cumulative radiation dose: (_) mGy

Description of Procedure: *(extrapleural approach)* The risks, benefits, alternatives, and the procedure itself were explained to the patient/patient's Power of Attorney/patient's legal guardian, and informed written consent was obtained. The site of the procedure was identified and marked. Time out was performed to confirm the correct patient, procedure, and site.

The mediastinal lesion was evaluated using enhanced/plain CT imaging after placement of a radiopaque marker/grid/ultrasound showing a (_) cm mass in the anterior/middle/posterior mediastinum/subcarinal space/right/left hilar space. The procedure was planned and the skin puncture site was marked using combined information from the location of the mass and preliminary CT/ultrasound images. The angle of needle entry and the distance to the lesion were calculated from the planning images. An extrapleural parasternal, transsternal, paravertebral, suprasternal, subxiphoid approach was selected for access.

The skin was prepped and draped in the usual sterile fashion. Local anesthesia was administered. A small skin incision was made. Subsequently, using planning CT information/using CT fluoroscopy/under direct ultrasound visualization, a (_)-gauge [type] needle guide was advanced along the planned trajectory until the needle tip reached the target lesion, confirmed by imaging. (_) samples were obtained using the coaxial technique, placed in a formalin solution and sent for histopathological evaluation. Following this, immediate completion CT/ultrasound images were obtained at the level of the biopsy site.

The patient was transferred to the floor/recovery room following the procedure in a stable condition. Staff was present for the entire procedure.

Description of Procedure: *(Transpleural Approach, using a preexisting pleural effusion)*: The risks, benefits, alternatives, and the procedure itself were explained to the patient/patient's Power of Attorney/patient's legal guardian, and informed written consent was obtained. The site of the procedure was identified and marked. Time out was performed to confirm the correct patient, procedure, and site.

The mediastinal lesion was evaluated using enhanced/plain CT imaging after placement of a radiopaque marker/grid showing a (_) cm mass in the [specify location]. A transpleural approach was selected for access. The patient was positioned in the left/right lateral decubitus position to allow the preexisting free-flowing pleural fluid to flow into the medial pleural recess and create a "pleural window" for needle placement by displacing the intervening lung parenchyma. Repeat planning CT images were obtained. The procedure was planned and the skin puncture site was marked using combined information from the location of the mass and preliminary CT images. The angle of needle entry and the distance to the lesion were calculated from the planning images.

The skin was prepped and draped in the usual sterile fashion. Local anesthesia was administered. A small skin incision was made. Subsequently, using planning CT information/CT fluoroscopy, a (_)-gauge [type] needle guide was advanced along the planned trajectory until the needle tip reached the target lesion, confirmed by imaging. (_) samples were obtained using the coaxial technique, placed in a formalin solution and sent for histopathological evaluation. Following this, immediate completion CT images were obtained at the level of the biopsy site.

The patient was transferred to the floor/recovery room following the procedure in a stable condition. Staff was present for the entire procedure.

Description of Procedure: *(transpleural approach, using an intentionally injected intrapleural fluid)*: The risks, benefits, alternatives, and the procedure itself were explained to the patient/patient's Power of Attorney/patient's legal guardian, and informed written consent was obtained. The site of the procedure was identified and marked. Time out was performed to confirm the correct patient, procedure and site.

The mediastinal lesion was evaluated using enhanced/plain CT imaging after placement of a radiopaque marker/grid showing a (_) cm mass in the [specify location]. A transpleural approach was selected for access, through an intentionally injected intrapleural fluid.

The procedure was planned and the skin puncture site was marked using combined information from the location of the mass and preliminary CT images. The angle of needle entry and the distance to the lesion were calculated from the planning images.

The skin was prepped and draped in the usual sterile fashion. Local anesthesia was administered. A small skin incision was made. A (_)-gauge [trocar/type] needle with a blunt stylet was advanced through the parietal pleura slowly to displace the visceral pleura without puncturing it. (_) mL of sterile normal saline was then injected into the pleural space to collapse the lung. Subsequently, using planning CT information/CT fluoroscopy, a (_)-gauge [type] needle guide was advanced along the planned trajectory, through the created pleural window, until the needle tip reached the target lesion, confirmed by imaging. (_) samples were obtained using the coaxial technique, placed in a formalin solution and sent for histopathological evaluation. Following this, immediate completion CT images were obtained at the level of the biopsy site.

The patient was transferred to the floor/recovery room following the procedure in a stable condition. Staff was present for the entire procedure.

Description of Procedure: *(transpleural approach, using an iatrogenic pneumothorax)*: The risks, benefits, alternatives, and the procedure itself were explained to the patient/patient's Power of Attorney/patient's legal guardian, and informed written consent was obtained. The site of the procedure was identified and marked. Time out was performed to confirm the correct patient, procedure and site.

The mediastinal lesion was evaluated using enhanced/plain CT imaging after placement of a radiopaque marker/grid showing a (_) cm mass in the [specify location]. A transpleural approach was selected for access, through an intentionally injected intrapleural air.

The procedure was planned and the skin puncture site was marked using combined information from the location of the mass and preliminary CT images. The angle of needle entry and the distance to the lesion were calculated from the planning images.

The skin was prepped and draped in the usual sterile fashion. Local anesthesia was administered. A small skin incision was made. A (_)-gauge [trocar/type] needle with a blunt stylet was advanced through the parietal pleura slowly to displace the visceral pleura without puncturing it. (_) mL of air was then injected into the pleural space to collapse the lung. Subsequently, using planning CT information/CT fluoroscopy, a (_)-gauge [type] needle guide was advanced along the planned trajectory, through the created pleural window, until the needle tip reached the target lesion confirmed by imaging.

(_) samples were obtained using the coaxial technique, placed in a formalin solution and sent for histopathological evaluation. Following this, immediate completion CT images were obtained at the level of the biopsy site.

The patient was transferred to the floor/recovery room following the procedure in a stable condition. Staff was present for the entire procedure.

Description of Procedure: *(transpulmonary approach)* The risks, benefits, alternatives, and the procedure itself were explained to the patient/patient's Power of Attorney/patient's legal guardian, and informed written consent was obtained. The site of the procedure was identified and marked. Time out was performed to confirm the correct patient, procedure and site.

The mediastinal lesion was evaluated using enhanced/plain CT imaging after placement of a radiopaque marker/grid showing a (_) cm mass in the [specify location]. A transpulmonary approach was selected for access, due to inconvenience of any other alternative approach.

The procedure was planned and the skin puncture site was marked using combined information from the location of the mass and preliminary CT images. The angle of needle entry and the distance to the lesion were calculated from the planning images.

The skin was prepped and draped in the usual sterile fashion. Local anesthesia was administered. A small skin incision was made. Subsequently, using planning CT information/CT fluoroscopy, a (_)-gauge [type] needle guide was advanced along the planned trajectory, until the needle tip reached the target lesion confirmed by imaging. (_) samples were obtained using the coaxial technique, placed in a formalin solution and sent for histopathological evaluation. The biopsy track was plugged with autologous blood clot seal with the injection of ( ) mL of autologous blood/collagen plug while withdrawing the needle guide. Following this, immediate completion CT images were obtained at the level of the biopsy site.

The patient was transferred to the floor/recovery room following the procedure in a stable condition. Staff was present for the entire procedure.

Intra-Procedure Findings: List all relevant findings.

Immediate Complications: None encountered during or directly after the procedure. List complications if any.

Post-Procedure Plan [1–4]:

- Follow-up histopathology results.
- Observe the patient in the recovery room following the procedure for 2 h.
- Keep patient recumbent with the puncture site down.
- Obtain an upright chest radiograph immediately and 3 h after biopsy.
- Administer supplemental nasal oxygen *(if a small pneumothorax develops).*
- Monitor vital signs every 30 min for 2 h.
- If the patient's condition deteriorates, suspecting a large or expending pneumothorax during observation, obtain an immediate chest radiograph and inform interventional team.
- Discharge instructions:
  - Abstain from strenuous activities for 3 days and avoid vigorous cough.
  - Visit the nearest emergency room promptly if any chest pain or shortness of breath develops.
  - Start clear liquid diet for the first hour, then regular diet thereafter if tolerated and no complications occur.

Impression:

- Percutaneous core biopsy of anterior/middle/posterior mediastinal/subcarinal/right/left hilar lesion, as described above.
- The patient tolerated the procedure well and left the interventional unit in a stable condition.
- The patient was unstable and the procedure was canceled/terminated prematurely.
- List any other relevant or important information/finding.

References

1. Percutaneous biopsy of the thorax. In: Burke CT, Dixon RG, Mauro MA, Murphy KPJ, Thomson KR, Venbrux AC, Zollikofer CL, editors. High yield imaging: interventional. Philadelphia: Saunders Elsevier; 2010. p. 498–500.
2. Given MF, Thomson KR, Lyon SM. Percutaneous biopsy of the lung, mediastinum, and pleura. In: Mauro MA, Murphy KPJ, Thomson KR, Venbrux AC, Zollikofer CL, editors. Image-guided interventions. Philadelphia: Saunders Elsevier; 2008. p. 1628–32.
3. Cham MD, Henschke CI, Yankelevitz DF. Biopsy procedures of the lung, mediastinum, and chest wall. In: Kandarpa K, Machan L, editors. Handbook of interventional radiologic procedures. 4th ed. Philadelphia: Lippincott Williams & Wilkins; 2011. p. 478–85.
4. Gupta S, Seaberg K, Wallace MJ, Madoff DC, Morello FA Jr, Ahrar K, et al. Imaging-guided percutaneous biopsy of mediastinal lesions: different approaches and anatomic considerations. Radiographics. 2005 May-Jun;25(3):763–86.
5. Gupta S, Wallace MJ, Cardella JF, Kundu S, Miller DL, Rose SC. Quality improvement guidelines for percutaneous needle biopsy. J Vasc Interv Radiol. 2010;21(7):969–75.
6. Taslakian B, Sebaaly MG, Al-Kutoubi A. Patient evaluation and preparation in vascular and interventional radiology: what every interventional radiologist should know (part 1: patient assessment and laboratory tests). Cardiovasc Intervent Radiol. 2016;39(3):325–33.
7. Taslakian B, Sebaaly MG, Al-Kutoubi A. Patient evaluation and preparation in vascular and interventional radiology: what every interventional radiologist should know (part 2: patient preparation and medications). Cardiovasc Intervent Radiol. 2016;39(4):489–99. doi: 10.1007/s00270-015-1239-4. [Epub 2015 Nov 25].
8. Venkatesan AM, Kundu S, Sacks D, Wallace MJ, Wojak JC, Rose SC, et al. Practice guidelines for adult antibiotic prophylaxis during vascular and interventional radiology procedures. J Vasc Interv Radiol. 2010;21(11):1611–30.

Exchange of Chest Drain

13

Bedros Taslakian and William Moore

INTRODUCTION

Image-guided exchange of a drain, which is usually performed under fluoroscopy guidance, is a simple and safe procedure used in cases of blockage or malposition of or to upsize an existing catheter without the need for de novo puncture.

COMMON INDICATIONS [1]

- Tube malfunction *(malposition, dislodgement, kinking, clotting)*
- Exchange of a previously inserted catheter for a larger catheter

COMMON CONTRAINDICATIONS [2]

- Uncooperative patients
- Hemodynamic instability
- Pregnancy
- Complete dislodgment of the catheter

POSSIBLE COMPLICATIONS

- Superinfection of a sterile pleural effusion
- Catheter malfunction *(malposition, dislodgement, kinking, clotting)*

PREPROCEDURAL ASSESSMENT AND PLANNING

- History, indications, and physical examination *(Appendix 1* in Chap. 149*)*
- Evaluation of diagnostic imaging studies to determine the location of the effusion, its severity, the relevant anatomy and the position of the existing tube
- Periprocedural management of coagulation status *(Appendices 2* in Chap. 150 *and 3 in* Chap. 151*)*
- Antibiotic prophylaxis: Not routinely recommended unless the fluid is infected *(empyema, abscess)* [3] *(Appendices 4* in Chap. 152 *and 5* in Chap. 153*)*
- Imaging modality for guidance: Fluoroscopy [4]
- Positioning: Oblique, lateral decubitus, or supine

B. Taslakian
Department of Radiology, New York University Langone Medical Center, 660 First Ave, New York, NY 10016, USA
e-mail: btaslakian@gmail.com

W. Moore (✉)
Department of Radiology, New York University Langone Medical Center, 660 1st Avenue- 3rd Floor, Room 335, New York, NY 10016, USA
e-mail: William.moore@nyumc.org

B. Taslakian et al. (eds.), *Procedural Dictations in Image-Guided Intervention*,
DOI 10.1007/978-3-319-40845-3_13

PROCEDURE NOTE

Procedure: Fluoroscopy-guided left/right thoracic draining catheter exchange
Staff: [_]
Fellow: [_]
Resident: [_]
Clinical Information: Describe history and list indications
Allergies: None known/Allergic to [specify/type of allergy]
Anesthesia: Local anesthesia/conscious sedation
Medications: List any relevant medications used (sedation, antibiotics)
Contrast Material: ( ) mL of [type] contrast material was used for tubogram/Not required
Field: Sterile
Procedure classification: Clean/Dirty
Position: Supine/Left lateral decubitus/Right lateral decubitus/Oblique
Monitoring: Intravenous access line was secured and vital signs were continuously monitored by nursing staff/anesthesia team throughout the procedure.
Total fluoroscopy time: (_) minutes
Cumulative radiation dose: (_) mGy

Description of Procedure:

The risks, benefits, alternatives, and procedure itself were explained to the patient/patient's Power of Attorney/patient's legal guardian, and informed written consent was obtained. The site of the procedure was identified and marked. Time out was performed to confirm the correct patient, procedure, and site.

The skin and the existing catheter were prepared using standard sterile procedures. A plain radiograph was obtained to document the site of catheter entry through the patient's skin by placing a metal forceps over the site of the skin entry. A small amount of diluted contrast material was injected through the catheter to assess catheter patency, the size of the cavity, and the position of the catheter within the cavity. The catheter was then cut/unlocked by releasing the self-locking mechanism.

Then, a (_)-inch [type] guidewire was advanced through the existing catheter and coiled in the cavity. Once there was a sufficient length of guidewire within the cavity, the old catheter was withdrawn over the guidewire under fluoroscopic guidance. A new (_)-French self-retaining [type/pigtail] catheter assembly with the metal/plastic stiffener was advanced over the guidewire to a satisfactory depth. The guidewire and the stiffener were removed after advancing the catheter into the cavity. Following this, contrast material was injected through the catheter at the end of the procedure to confirm optimal catheter position and ensure that all side holes were placed within the cavity. The catheter was locked, anchored to the skin and attached to a drainage system.

The patient was transferred to the floor/recovery room/discharged home following the procedure in a stable condition. Staff was present for the entire procedure.

Intra-Procedure Findings: List all relevant findings.
Immediate Complications: None encountered during or directly after the procedure. List complications if any.

Post-Procedure Plan [4–6]:

- Connect the catheter to a self-contained suction system *(lung abscess)* or under-water seal drainage system on low continuous suction (20- to 30-cm water) *(lung abscess, pleural effusion, or empyema)*, as needed.
- Daily catheter care:
  - Inspect catheter and make sure that the 3-way stopcock is open to the drainage system and the catheter has not been externally retracted.
  - Flush the catheter with 20 mL of bacteriostatic saline every 8 h; 10 mL toward the drainage system and 10 mL toward the collection.
  - Record the catheter outputs every 8 h.
  - Inform interventional radiology team if the draining amount decreases, or pericatheter leak or local skin complications occurs.

- Removal of catheter:
  - Parapneumonic effusions and empyema: When drainage is minimal *(<50 mL per 24 h)*, clinical improvement is noted and antibiotics are changed from intravenous to oral.
  - Malignant pleural effusions: When drainage decreases to 100–200 mL over 24 h and pleurodesis is performed.
  - Transudate effusions: When drainage decreases to 100–200 mL over 24 h, radiograph confirms resolution of the effusion and clinical improvement is noted.
  - Lung abscess: When clinical improvement is documented and after resolution of the abscess on subsequent imaging studies.

Impression:

- Exchange of left/right chest drain, as described above.
- The patient tolerated the procedure well and left the interventional unit in a stable condition.
- The patient was unstable and the procedure was canceled/terminated prematurely.
- List any other relevant or important information/finding.

References

1. Nair AV, D'Agostino HR. Transcatheter fluid drainage. In: Valji K, editor. The practice of interventional radiology. Philadelphia: Saunders Elsevier; 2010. p. 106–25.
2. Wallace MJ, Chin KW, Fletcher TB, Bakal CW, Cardella JF, Grassi CJ, et al. Quality improvement guidelines for percutaneous drainage/aspiration of abscess and fluid collections. J Vasc Interv Radiol. 2010;21(4):431–5.
3. Venkatesan AM, Kundu S, Sacks D, Wallace MJ, Wojak JC, Rose SC, et al. Practice guidelines for adult antibiotic prophylaxis during vascular and interventional radiology procedures. J Vasc Interv Radiol. 2010;21(11):1611–30.
4. Patz EF, Erasmus JJ. Catheter drainage of intrathoracic collections. In: Kandarpa K, Machan L, editors. Handbook of interventional radiologic procedures. 4th ed. Philadelphia: Lippincott Williams & Wilkins; 2011. p. 486–94.
5. Drainage of pleural effusions and empyemas. In: Burke CT, Dixon RG, Mauro MA, Murphy KPJ, Thomson KR, Venbrux AC, Zollikofer CL, editors. High yield imaging: interventional. Philadelphia: Saunders Elsevier; 2010. p. 495–497.
6. Yu H. Management of pleural effusion, empyema, and lung abscess. Semin Intervent Radiol. 2011;28(1):75–86.

Fine Needle Aspiration of Lung Lesion

14

Bedros Taslakian and William Moore

INTRODUCTION

Percutaneous fine needle aspiration (FNA) is a minimally invasive percutaneous biopsy approach, causing minimal tissue disruption. The lesion is sampled via suction by passing the needle several times into the target. Smears are prepared and the specimen is often sent in a preservative. FNA biopsy has high cancer-specific diagnostic accuracy, but the accuracy of cancer-negative diagnoses is generally much lower.

COMMON INDICATIONS [1–4]

- Evaluation of a recently detected suspicious or growing solitary pulmonary nodule
- Evaluation of metabolically active suspicious pulmonary lesions on PET
- Evaluation of pulmonary lesions in a patient with known primary malignancy for staging
- Evaluation of focal pulmonary infections refractory to antimicrobial therapy *(cells/aspirate for microscopic examination, culture and gram stain)*

COMMON CONTRAINDICATIONS [1–3, 5]

- Uncooperative patients
- Hemodynamic instability
- Lack of a safe pathway to the lesion
- Significant coagulopathy that cannot be adequately corrected
- Pregnancy in cases when imaging guidance involves ionizing radiation
- Severe emphysema *(increased risk of pneumothorax)*
- Intractable cough *(increased risk of pneumothorax)*
- Patients on positive pressure ventilation *(increased risk of pneumothorax)*
- Suspected hydatid cysts *(risk of anaphylactic shock)*
- Suspected pulmonary arteriovenous malformation or vascular aneurysms *(preprocedural contrast-enhanced CT scan is essential)*
- Pulmonary hypertension
- Severely limited pulmonary function
- Contralateral pneumonectomy

B. Taslakian
Department of Radiology, New York University Langone Medical Center, 660 First Ave, New York, NY 10016, USA
e-mail: btaslakian@gmail.com

W. Moore (✉)
Department of Radiology, New York University Langone Medical Center, 660 First Ave, 3rd Floor, Rm 335, New York, NY 10016, USA
e-mail: william.moore@nyumc.org

B. Taslakian et al. (eds.), *Procedural Dictations in Image-Guided Intervention*,
DOI 10.1007/978-3-319-40845-3_14

POSSIBLE COMPLICATIONS [1–3, 6]

- Pneumothorax
- Hemoptysis, perilesional hemorrhage, hemothorax
- Superinfection
- Vasovagal reaction
- Air embolism, *rare*
- Cardiac tamponade, *rare*

PREPROCEDURAL ASSESSMENT AND PLANNING [7–9]

- History, indications and physical examination *(Appendix 1* in Chap. 149*)*
- Evaluation of diagnostic imaging studies to determine the location of the lesion and relevant anatomy
- Periprocedural management of coagulation status *(Appendices 2* in Chap. 150 *and 3* in Chap. 151*)*
- Antibiotic prophylaxis: Not routinely recommended [7] *(Appendices 4* in Chap. 152 *and 5* in Chap. 153*)*
- Imaging modality for guidance: CT, CT fluoroscopy, ultrasound *(for peripheral, pleural-based lesions)*
- Positioning: Oblique, lateral decubitus, prone or supine

PROCEDURE NOTE

Procedure: Percutaneous fine needle aspiration of left/right/lower/middle/upper lobe lung lesion
Staff: [_]
Fellow: [_]
Resident: [_]
Clinical Information: Describe history and list indications
Allergies: None known/Allergic to [specify/type of allergy]
Anesthesia: Local anesthesia/conscious sedation
Medications: List any relevant medications used (sedation, antibiotics)
Field: Sterile
Procedure classification: Clean
Position: Supine/Prone/Left lateral decubitus/Right lateral decubitus/Oblique
Monitoring: Intravenous access line was secured and vital signs were continuously monitored by nursing staff/anesthesia team throughout the procedure
Cumulative radiation dose: (_) mGy

Description of Procedure:
The risks, benefits, alternatives and the procedure itself were explained to the patient/patient's Power of Attorney/patient's legal guardian, and informed written consent was obtained. The site of the procedure was identified and marked. Time out was performed to confirm the correct patient, procedure and site.

The lungs were evaluated using CT imaging after placement of a radiopaque marker/grid/ultrasound showing a (_) cm round/oval/irregular lesion in the right/left/lower/upper/middle lobe. The procedure was planned and the skin puncture site was marked using combined information from the location of the lesion and preliminary CT/ultrasound images. The angle of needle entry and the distance to the lesion were calculated from the planning images.

The skin was prepped and draped in the usual sterile fashion. Local anesthesia was administered. A small skin incision was made. Subsequently, using planning CT information/under direct ultrasound visualization, a (_)-gauge reference [coaxial/type] needle was advanced along the planned trajectory until its tip reached the superficial edge of the lesion, confirmed by imaging. Samples were obtained using a (_)-gauge [type] longer needle placed coaxially through the reference needle (*coaxial technique*). Suction was generated using the syringe attached to the needle, which was passed through the target lesion using vigorous to-and-fro motion to obtain cells. The suction was then released and the needle was withdrawn. One drop of the aspirate was smeared on glass slides for on-site cytological assessment/and fixed in a preservative solution and the remainder were washed into a solution of formalin/saline. While obtaining samples, saline solution was placed in the hub of the needle guide to avoid air embolism. The biopsy track was plugged with autologous blood clot seal by injecting (_) mL of autologous blood/collagen plug while withdrawing the reference needle. Following this, immediate completion CT/ultrasound images were obtained at the level of the biopsy site.

The patient was transferred to the floor/recovery room following the procedure in a stable condition. Staff was present for the entire procedure.

Intra-Procedure Findings: List all relevant findings.

Immediate Complications: None encountered during or directly after the procedure. *List complications if any.*

Post-Procedure Plan [1–3]:

- Follow-up cytology results.
- Observe the patient in the recovery room following the procedure for 2 h.
- Keep patient recumbent with the puncture site down.
- Obtain an upright chest radiograph immediately and 2 h after biopsy.
- Administer supplemental nasal oxygen *(if a small pneumothorax develops).*
- Monitor vital signs every 30 min for 2 h.
- If the patient's condition deteriorates, suspecting a large or expending pneumothorax during observation, obtain an immediate chest radiograph and inform interventional team.
- Discharge instructions:
  - Abstain from strenuous activities for 3 days and avoid vigorous cough.
  - Visit the nearest emergency room promptly if any chest pain or shortness of breath develops.
  - Start clear liquid diet for the first hour, then regular diet thereafter if tolerated and no complications occur.

Impression:

- Percutaneous fine needle aspiration of right/left/lower/upper/middle lobe lung lesion, as described above.
- The patient tolerated the procedure well and left the interventional unit in a stable condition.
- The patient was unstable and the procedure was canceled/terminated prematurely.
- List any other relevant or important information/finding.

References

1. Gherardi G. Fine-needle biopsy of superficial and deep masses. Italy: Springer; 2009.
2. Cham MD, Henschke CI, Yankelevitz DF. Biopsy procedures of the lung, mediastinum, and chest wall. In: Kandarpa K, Machan L, editors. Handbook of interventional radiologic procedures. 4th ed. Philadelphia: Lippincott Williams & Wilkins; 2011. p. 478–85.
3. Percutaneous biopsy of the thorax. In: Burke CT, Dixon RG, Mauro MA, Murphy KPJ, Thomson KR, Venbrux AC, Zollikofer CL, editors. High yield imaging: interventional. Philadelphia: Saunders Elsevier; 2010. p. 498–500.
4. MacMahon H, Austin JH, Gamsu G, Herold CJ, Jett JR, Naidich DP, et al. Guidelines for management of small pulmonary nodules detected on CT scans: a statement from the Fleischner society. Radiology. 2005;237(2):395–400.
5. Stampfel G. Anaphylactoid reaction, a rare complication after fine needle biopsy of the lung. Radiology. 1982;22(7):329–30.
6. Wallace MJ, Krishnamurthy S, Broemeling LD, Gupta S, Ahrar K, Morello FA Jr, et al. CT-guided percutaneous fine-needle aspiration biopsy of small (< or = 1-cm) pulmonary lesions. Radiology. 2002;225(3):823–8.
7. Taslakian B, Sebaaly MG, Al-Kutoubi A. Patient evaluation and preparation in vascular and interventional radiology: what every interventional radiologist should know (part 1: patient assessment and laboratory tests). Cardiovasc Intervent Radiol. 2016;39(3):325–33.
8. Taslakian B, Sebaaly MG, Al-Kutoubi A. Patient evaluation and preparation in vascular and interventional radiology: what every interventional radiologist should know (part 2: patient preparation and medications). Cardiovasc Intervent Radiol. 2016;39(4):489–99. doi: 10.1007/s00270-015-1239-4. [Epub 2015 Nov 25].
9. Venkatesan AM, Kundu S, Sacks D, Wallace MJ, Wojak JC, Rose SC, et al. Practice guidelines for adult antibiotic prophylaxis during vascular and interventional radiology procedures. J Vasc Interv Radiol. 2010;21(11):1611–30.

Thermal Lung Ablation

15

Bedros Taslakian, Nadim Muallem and William Moore

Abbreviations

CT	Computed tomography
LITT	Laser induced thermotherapy
MWA	Microwave ablation
PCA	Patient-controlled analgesia
PET	Positron emission tomography
RF	Radiofrequency
RFA	Radiofrequency ablation
US	Ultrasound

INTRODUCTION

Image-guided percutaneous thermal lung ablation is a minimally invasive treatment consisting of the application of heat or cold in a precisely defined region for the purpose of cure and/or palliation of primary and metastatic lung cancer. There are various types of thermal ablation techniques which include Radiofrequency ablation (RFA), Microwave ablation (MWA) and laser induced thermotherapy (LITT) that generate heat and Cryoablation or Cryotherapy that generate cold. Regardless of technique, one or—if indicated—more than one probe with a built-in thermal applicator (RF electrode, Microwave antennae, Cryoprobe, optical fiber) is placed in the target lesion under imaging guidance. The applicator then generates heat or cold within a certain volume around the active applicator tip, the dimensions and geometry of which are determined by the probe type and manufacturer specifications. For effective heat-based ablation, the goal is to reach a target temperature between 60 and 100 °C through the target lesion and maintain the temperature for a few minutes.

B. Taslakian
Department of Radiology, New York University Langone Medical Center, 660 First Ave, New York, NY 10016, USA
e-mail: btaslakian@gmail.com

N. Muallem
Department of Radiology, Division of Interventional Radiology, Memorial Sloan Kettering Cancer Center, 1275 York Ave, New York 10065, NY, USA
e-mail: nadim.muallem@gmail.com

W. Moore (✉)
Department of Radiology, New York University Langone Medical Center, 660 First Ave, 3rd Floor, Rm 335, New York 10016, NY, USA
e-mail: William.moore@nyumc.org

B. Taslakian et al. (eds.), *Procedural Dictations in Image-Guided Intervention*,
DOI 10.1007/978-3-319-40845-3_15

Cryoablation causes irreversible cellular destruction through formation of intracellular ice crystal which is achieved at temperatures below −40 °C. Multiple alternating freeze and thaw cycles are required to obtain maximal cellular destruction.

In the specific setting of pulmonary ablation, the intrinsic characteristics of lung tissue may interfere with the electrical conductivity or thermal propagation more than in other tissues.

COMMON INDICATIONS [1–6]

Patient selection for ablation should be carefully performed by a multidisciplinary team. Ideally tumors should be smaller than 3.5 cm in diameter and completely surrounded by non-tumorous lung tissue/normal lung tissue. The following are some of the most commonly used indications for thermal ablation:

- Early stage biopsy-proven primary lung cancer in medically inoperable patients (FEV1 ≤ 50 %, DLCO ≤ 50 %) or in patients refusing surgical resection
- Early-stage biopsy-proven lung cancer with recurrence after surgery, chemotherapy or radiation therapy
- Limited metastatic lung disease (number of lesions ≤ 5) in medically inoperable patients or in patients refusing surgical resection
- Diffuse lung metastasis (number of lesions > 5) responding to systemic chemotherapy with a single nodule showing no response to systemic therapy
- Palliative therapy of painful malignant lung lesions

COMMON CONTRAINDICATIONS [1, 3, 6, 7]

Absolute contraindications:

- Significant coagulopathy that cannot be adequately corrected
- Bacteremia or active infections *(pneumonia)*
- Severe pulmonary arterial hypertension

Relative contraindications:

- Uncooperative patients
- Anatomic limitations with the target lesion adjacent to vital organs or vessels larger than 3 mm
- Severe emphysema
- Intractable cough
- Patients on positive pressure ventilation
- Severely limited pulmonary function
- Contralateral pneumonectomy *(ablation can be performed in the appropriate clinical setting, with the patient intubated and under general anesthesia. A chest tube kit should be ready on hand to be placed during the procedure if needed. The patient should also be closely monitored in recovery as well as admitted overnight for observation with a chest x-ray repeated the following morning)*
- Depending on the ablation technique used:
  - Patients with cardiac pacemakers and implantable defibrillators *(recommended to be deactivated during RFA; not applicable for cryoablation and LITT, slightly better safety profile for MWA but precaution should also be taken* [8]*)*
  - Metal implants *(small implants can potentially heat up due to the circuit created in RFA but are unlikely to be affected in MWA and certainly not affected in cryoablation and LITT)*

POSSIBLE COMPLICATIONS [1, 2, 6, 9, 10]

- Pneumothorax, *11–52 %*
- Chest tube placement, *6–29 %*
- Pleuritis manifested by:
  - Reactive pleural effusions *(usually small, resolve spontaneously), 6–19 %.* Usually due to pleuritis induced by thermal injury to pleura
  - Pleuritic chest pain secondary to thermal injury to pleura lasting up to 7 days and requiring oral analgesics, to prevent dyspnea

- Parenchymal hemorrhage, which tends to resolve spontaneously, *6–18 %*
- Hemoptysis, usually self-limiting, *3–9 %*
- Chest wall hematoma and hemothorax
- Delayed major hemorrhage, caused by the development of false pulmonary artery aneurysms
- Pericardial tamponade
- Neuropathy:
  - Due to thermal injury to adjacent nerves leading to phrenic nerve injury and diaphragmatic paralysis or dermatomal pain and/or paresthesia
  - Due to inappropriate positioning leading to brachial plexus nerve injury
- Postablation syndrome *(fever, cough, chills, pain, nausea, and malaise)*
- Superinfection or abscess formation, pneumonia
- Cavitation
- Chronic obstructive pulmonary disease exacerbation
- Tumor seeding along the needle tract, *rare*
- Bronchopleural fistula leading to intractable pneumothorax, *rare: 0.6 %*
- Vasovagal reaction
- Mortality, *rare*

PREPROCEDURAL ASSESSMENT AND PLANNING

- History, indications and physical examination *(Appendix 1* in Chap. 149*)*
- Evaluation of diagnostic imaging studies (CT, PET-CT) to assess indications and radiologically stage the tumor, and to determine the location of the lesion, the relevant anatomy, and develop trajectory route. It also serves as a baseline for follow-up [1, 6].
- Histopathologic diagnosis of the lesion should be generally obtained before the ablation, unless the patient is considered to be at very high risk, in which case biopsy and RFA could be performed in one setting [1, 6].
- Periprocedural management of coagulation status *(Appendices 2* in Chap. 150 *and 3* in Chap. 151*)*
- Antibiotic prophylaxis: No consensus; many practitioners continue to empirically use prophylaxis [1, 6, 11] *(Appendices 4* in Chap. 152 *and 5* in Chap. 153*)*
- Imaging modality for guidance: CT, CT fluoroscopy, ultrasound *(for chest wall and peripheral, pleural-based lesions)* [1, 6]
- Positioning: Lateral decubitus, prone or supine. Posterior approach with the patient prone provides a more consistent intercostal window *(preferred)*. Lateral approach should be avoided due to increased rib motion with breathing [6]. Place paddings in areas without important neurovascular bundles *(to avoid injury)* and dispersive grounding pads in a well-prepared *(shaved)* area to allow good contact with the skin [1, 6].

PROCEDURE NOTE

Procedure: Radiofrequency/Microwave/Cryo ablation of a left/right/lower/middle/upper lobe lung lesion and post-procedure radiographs
Staff: [_]
Fellow: [_]
Resident: [_]
Clinical Information: Specify existing diagnosis; Describe history and list indications
Allergies: None known/Allergic to [specify/type of allergy]
Anesthesia: Local anesthesia with conscious sedation/General anesthesia
Medications: List any relevant medications used (sedation, antibiotics)
Field: Sterile
Position: Supine/Prone/Left lateral decubitus/Right lateral decubitus/Oblique
Monitoring: Intravenous access line was secured and vital signs were continuously monitored by nursing staff/anesthesia team throughout the procedure
Cumulative radiation dose: (_) mGy

Description of Procedure:

The risks, benefits, alternatives and procedure itself were explained to the patient/patient's Power of Attorney/patient's legal guardian, and informed written consent was obtained. The site of the procedure was identified and marked. Time out was performed to confirm the correct patient, procedure and site.

Pre-procedure planning CT/ultrasound/MRI imaging was obtained and used to calculate the approach and distance to target lesion. One (or more) site of needle entry was determined and marked on the skin. The marked location(s) and surrounding skin area were prepped and draped in the usual sterile fashion.

Subcutaneous and pleural infiltration of local anesthetic was performed using a thin gauge needle. A small skin incision was made at the marked site(s). Under image guidance one (or more) applicator probe(s) was/were advanced along the planned trajectory and positioned into the target. No (one or more) repositioning was/were required. Ablation was performed by following the manufacturer's instructions until the target temperature was achieved/the perilesional ground-glass halo was visualized/the ice-ball was visualized to encase the targeted lesion within an acceptable margin.

Probe positioning, repositioning and ablation protocol are detailed below.

After completion, the tract of the lung parenchyma was cauterized using low-power application while withdrawing the radiofrequency/microwave electrode(s) from the lung.

After probe removal, immediate postprocedure CT images were obtained at the level of the lesion to evaluate the ablation zone, potential collateral damage and detect complications.

The patient was transferred to the inpatient unit/recovery room/discharged home following the procedure in a stable condition.

Preprocedural Planning and Approach

Target organ: Lung

Laterality: Right/Left

Reference scan/image for ablation target: CT dated [Month]/[Day]/[Year]. Series [series number] image [image number]

Target lesion size: Long axis: [_] cm, short axis: [_] cm

Specific target location: Right/Left lower/middle/upper lobe. Specify relationship to sensitive structures (pleura, vessels, nerves, etc.)

Target lesion appearance: Solid/Part-solid/Cavitary/Cystic

Patient position: Prone/Supine/Decubitus/Other

Approach: Posterior/Anterior/Lateral

Imaging guidance: Intra-procedural CT/CT-fluoroscopy/PET-CT/Ultrasound/MRI performed with/without multiplanar reconstruction confirming adequate positioning of the applicator within the target lesion

Ablation Technique

Ablation modality: Radiofrequency/Microwave/Cryoablation/Laser Ablation

Ablation device: Specify device brand/model, type, length, gauge, active length, single, multiple, tined etc.…

Number of applicators: If more than one applicator, specify locations; if single applicator with more that one repositioning, also specify different locations

Number of ablations: (number) overlapping/non-overlapping ablations *(list protocol details below)*

Protocol used: Device specific, but typically, power/wattage, duration, temperature achieved, and location if multiple probes or repositionings were needed

Eg. RFA *(single applicator—in this case the Valleylab/Covidien Cool-tip RFA probe—with multiple repositioning and overlapping ablation)*

Ablation #1: Cooled, 3 min, (_) degrees Celsius/Applicator #1 Posterior margin

Ablation #2: Cooled, 6 min, (_) degrees Celsius/Applicator #1 Superior margin proximal

Ablation #3: …

Eg. Cryoablation *(with multiple applicators)*

Ablation #1: 10 min freeze, 6 min active thaw, 10 min freeze, 8 min passive thaw, at 100 %, −(_) degrees Celsius/Applicator #1 superior margin

Ablation #2: 10 min freeze, 6 min active thaw, 10 min freeze, 8 min passive thaw, at 80 %, −(_) degrees Celsius/Applicator #2 inferior margin

Ablation #3: …

Post-Ablation Findings

Post ablation imaging: CT/MRI

Follow-up chest radiographs: (Immediate and) 2 h post procedure chest radiographs

Post-procedural imaging: (CT/MRI/PET-CT/ etc.…) was performed at the level of the target lesion. The ablation zone could not be clearly delineated/was clearly outlined consisting of ice-ball formation/ground-glass parenchymal attenuation encompassing the target tumor in its entirety with adequate margins extending (_) mm beyond the periphery of the lesion predictive of complete ablation/inadequate margins at the (_) border requiring additional targeted ablation [complement with additional details as needed].

Immediate post-procedure chest radiograph: No pneumothorax

Second chest radiograph findings: No pneumothorax

Immediate Complications: None encountered during or directly after the procedure. *List complications if any.*

Post-Procedure Plan [1, 6]:

- Assuming successful procedure with trace or no pneumothorax on post procedural imaging:
  - Transfer patient to recovery unit.
  - Observe in recovery unit for 2–4 h with continuous vital sign and pulse oximeter monitoring.
  - Complete bedrest and NPO for the duration of observation. Maintain patient recumbent with the puncture site down.
  - Post-procedure pain control as needed *(-consider PCA, and admission for pain control if needed).*
  - Administer supplemental nasal oxygen as needed *(O2 saturation less than baseline/ patient still sedated/presence of small pneumothorax…).*
  - Obtain chest x-ray at 2 h and prior to discharge to monitor for pneumothorax. Risk of delayed pneumothorax beyond 2 h decreases significantly [12].
- In the event of a small pneumothorax in an asymptomatic patient, consider obtaining follow up radiographs at 3–4 h to confirm stability prior to discharge.
- In the event of an expanding or symptomatic pneumothorax *(shortness of breath, pleuritic pain, …)*, a chest tube needs to be inserted (8–12 Fr pigtail sufficient) and depending on the hospital workflow, the patient can either be admitted for chest tube management or discharged home with a Heimlich valve [13] to follow up in clinic for chest tube removal.
- If the patient's condition deteriorates during observation, suspect pneumothorax primarily and obtain images of the chest immediately. Do not disregard other potential complications as well.
- *Discharge instructions*
  - Abstain from strenuous activities for 3 days.
  - Visit the nearest emergency room promptly if any chest pain or shortness of breath develops.
  - Start clear liquid diet for the first hour after discharge from observation, then regular diet thereafter if tolerated and no complications occur.
  - Take prescribed pain medications as needed.
  - Do not travel by air for at least 3 weeks or for 10 days with a repeat chest radiograph performed prior to travel date excluding the presence of a pneumothorax.
- *Follow-up imaging*
  - Obtain a new baseline contrast-enhanced CT scan within 1–3 months after the procedure.
  - Obtain repeat contrast-enhanced CT scan every 3 months to assess recurrence.
  - Note: To avoid the late diagnosis of incomplete ablation, PET-CT has been proposed in some centers, providing higher sensitivity and specificity than CT in depicting residual viable tumor. Fluorine-18 fluorodeoxyglucose uptake is highly increased 1–3 weeks after ablation, because of the post-treatment inflammatory reaction. Therefore, at least a 4 week interval is required to avoid false-positive results.

Impression:

- Percutaneous radiofrequency/microwave/cryo ablation of right/left/lower/upper/middle lobe lung lesion, as described above.

- The patient tolerated the procedure well and left the interventional unit in a stable condition.
- List any other relevant or important information/finding.
- The procedure was cancelled/abandoned.
- The primary operator (specify name) was present for the entire/key parts of the procedure.

References

1. Pua BB, Solomon SB. Radiofrequency ablation of pulmonary tumors. In: Kandarpa K, Machan L, editors. Handbook of interventional radiologic procedures. 4th ed. Philadelphia: Lippincott Williams & Wilkins; 2011. p. 494–502.
2. Guenette JP, Dupuy DE. Lung Ablation. In: Mauro M, Murphy K, Thomson K, Venbrux A, Morgan R, editors. Image-guided interventions. 2nd ed. Philadelphia: Saunders Elsevier; 2014. p. 1145–53.
3. Vogl TJ, Naguib NNN, Lehnert T, Nour-Eldin NE. Radiofrequency, microwave and laser ablation of pulmonary neoplasms: clinical studies and technical considerations—review article. Eur J Radiol. 2011;77(2):346–57.
4. Smith SL, Jennings PE. Lung radiofrequency and microwave ablation: a review of indications, techniques and post-procedural imaging appearances. Br J Radiol. 2015;88:20140598.
5. Quirk MT, Pomykala KL, Suh RD. Current readings: percutaneous ablation for pulmonary metastatic disease. Semin Thorac Cardiovasc Surg. 2014;26:239–48.
6. Gutierrez A, Abtin F, Suh R. Lung ablation. In: Hong K, Georgiades CS, editors. Percutaneous tumor ablation strategies and techniques. Stuttgart: Thieme Medical Publishers; 2010. p. 73–114.
7. Steinke K, Haghighi KS, Wulf S, Morris DL. Effect of vessel diameter on the creation of ovine lung radiofrequency lesions in vivo: preliminary results. J Surg Res. 2005;124:85–91.
8. Skonieczki BD, Wells C, Wasser EJ, Dupuy DE. Radiofrequency and microwave tumor ablation in patients with implanted cardiac devices: Is it safe? Eur J Radiol. 2011;79(3):343–6.
9. Borghol S, Alberti N, Frulio N, Crombe A, Marty M, Rolland A, et al. Pulmonary artery pseudoaneurysm after radiofrequency ablation: report of two cases. Int J Hyperth. 2015;31:1–4.
10. Hiraki T, Gobara H, Fujiwara H, Ishii H, Tomita K, Uka M, et al. Lung cancer ablation: complications. Semin Intervent Radiol. 2013;30:169–75.
11. Venkatesan AM, Kundu S, Sacks D, Wallace MJ, Wojak JC, Rose SC, et al. Practice guideline for adult antibiotic prophylaxis during vascular and interventional radiology procedures. J Vasc Interv Radiol. 2010;21(11):1611–30.
12. Brown KT, Brody LA, Getrajdman GI, Napp TE. Outpatient treatment of iatrogenic pneumothorax after needle biopsy. Radiology. 1997;205(1):249–52.
13. Gupta S, Hicks ME, Wallace MJ, Ahrar K, Madoff DC, Murthy R. Outpatient management of postbiopsy pneumothorax with small-caliber chest tubes: factors affecting the need for prolonged drainage and additional interventions. Cardiovasc Intervent Radiol. 2008;31(2):342–8.

Part III

Non-vascular Interventional Procedures: Breast

Introduction by Aghiad Al-Kutoubi, Section Reviewer

The development and widespread use of percutaneous image-guided breast biopsies has expanded the role of breast imaging and changed the management of breast disease. Minimally invasive core biopsies of breast lesions have replaced the surgical biopsy for most breast lesions requiring a tissue diagnosis after validation of the safety, accuracy, and cost-effectiveness of these biopsies combined with the smaller complication rate, lower cost, and faster recovery. Imaging of the specimen is a requirement in many centers to confirm and document the accuracy of the sampling procedure.

Tumor ablation by radiofrequency is an evolving treatment modality that might prove a useful adjunct in the treatment of breast cancer, the commonest malignant tumor in females.

This section provides a comprehensive list of procedural reports that covers the vast majority of the currently performed image-guided breast procedures with up-to-date explanatory notes, synopsis of the indications and contraindications, and potential complications in an organized and practical format.

Section Chapters

Fine Needle Aspiration of Axillary Lymph Node

16

Lara Nassar

INTRODUCTION

Axillary lymph node staging plays an important role in the planning of treatment to be delivered to a breast cancer patient. Fine needle aspiration allows preoperative assessment of thickened axillary lymph nodes, hence helping to plan the type of axillary surgery to be performed. Due to the sensitive neurovascular structures located in the axilla, core biopsy of axillary lymph nodes is rather infrequently performed.

COMMON INDICATIONS [1, 2]

- Assessment of suspicious axillary lymph nodes in the setting of known or highly suspected breast malignancy

CONTRAINDICATIONS [2]

- Inability to visualize the target or have a safe pathway for access
- Severe bleeding diathesis

L. Nassar (✉)
Department of Diagnostic Radiology, American University of Beirut Medical Center, Riad El-Solh, Beirut 1107 2020, Lebanon
e-mail: ln07@aub.edu.lb

POSSIBLE COMPLICATIONS [3]

These are very rare and include:

- Vasovagal reaction
- Bleeding
- Pain
- Infection
- Injury to neurovascular structures
- Pneumothorax
- Insufficient sampling

PREPROCEDURAL ASSESSMENT AND PLANNING [4–6]

- History, indications, and physical examination *(Appendix 1* in Chap. 149*)*
- Evaluation of diagnostic imaging studies: Previous mammogram, ultrasound, MRI, CT, or PET as available
- Periprocedural management of coagulation status *(Appendices 2* in Chap. 150 *and 3* in Chap. 151*)*
- Antibiotic prophylaxis: Not routinely recommended [4]
- Imaging modality for guidance: Ultrasound
- Positioning: Supine, supine oblique

PROCEDURE NOTE

Procedure: Ultrasound-guided fine needle aspiration of left/right axillary lymph node

B. Taslakian et al. (eds.), *Procedural Dictations in Image-Guided Intervention*,
DOI 10.1007/978-3-319-40845-3_16

Staff: [_]
Fellow: [_]
Resident: [_]
Clinical Information: Describe history and list indications
Allergies: None known/Allergic to [specify/type of allergy]
Anesthesia: Local anesthesia/conscious sedation
Medications: List any relevant medications used
Field: Sterile
Procedure classification: Clean
Position: Supine/Supine oblique
Monitoring: Vital signs were continuously monitored by nursing staff throughout the procedure

Description of Procedure:
The risks, benefits, alternatives, and the procedure itself were explained to the patient/patient's Power of Attorney/patient's legal guardian, and informed written consent was obtained. The site of the procedure was identified and marked. Time out was performed to confirm the correct patient, procedure, and site.

The left/right axilla was evaluated using ultrasound and a (_) cm round/oval/irregular lymph node was selected for biopsy. The procedure was planned and the skin puncture site was marked.

The skin was prepped and draped in the usual sterile fashion. Local anesthesia was administered. Under direct sonographic visualization, a (_)-gauge needle was advanced into the target left/right axillary lymph node. Suction was generated using the syringe attached to the needle, which was passed through the target lymph node using to-and-fro motion to obtain cells. Specimen was sent for cytological analysis.

The aspiration site was compressed; then a sterile dressing was applied. The patient was discharged home following the procedure in a stable condition.

Intra-Procedure Findings: List all relevant findings.
Immediate Complications: None encountered during or directly after the procedure. List complications if any.

Post-Procedure Plan:
- Abstain from strenuous activities.
- Check for redness, tenderness, hotness, fever, and induration and follow up with [specify team] in case any complication is noted.
- Follow up with [specify team] in (_) days for obtaining cytology results.

Impression:
- Ultrasound-guided fine needle aspiration of left/right axillary lymph node, as described above.
- The patient tolerated the procedure well and left the breast interventional unit in a stable condition.
- List any other relevant or important information/finding.

References

1. Koelliker SL, Chung MA, Mainiero MB, Steinhoff MM, Cady B. Axillary lymph nodes: US-guided fine needle aspiration for initial staging of breast cancer—correlation with primary tumor size. Radiology. 2008;246(1):81–9.
2. American College of Radiology. ACR practice parameter for the performance of ultrasound-guided percutaneous breast interventional procedures. Reston, VA: American College of Radiology; 2014.
3. Helvie MA, Ikeda DM, Adler DD. Localization and needle aspiration of breast lesions: complications in 370 cases. AJR Am J Roentgenol. 1991;157(4):711–4.
4. Taslakian B, Sebaaly MG, Al-Kutoubi A. Patient evaluation and preparation in vascular and interventional radiology: what every interventional radiologist should know (part 1: patient assessment and laboratory tests). Cardiovasc Intervent Radiol. 2016;39(3):325–33.
5. Taslakian B, Sebaaly MG, Al-Kutoubi A. Patient evaluation and preparation in vascular and interventional radiology: what every interventional radiologist should know (part 2: patient preparation and medications). Cardiovasc Intervent Radiol. 2016;39(4):489–99. doi: 10.1007/s00270-015-1239-4. [Epub 2015 Nov 25].
6. Venkatesan AM, Kundu S, Sacks D, Wallace MJ, Wojak JC, Rose SC, et al. Practice guidelines for adult antibiotic prophylaxis during vascular and interventional radiology procedures. J Vasc Interv Radiol. 2010;21(11):1611–30.

17 Fine Needle Aspiration of Breast Lesion

Lara Nassar

INTRODUCTION

Core needle biopsy has largely replaced fine needle aspiration (FNA) in the assessment of solid breast masses. This is due to limited ability of FNA in the characterization of hormonal receptor status of a tumor and in the differentiation of in situ versus invasive malignancy. In addition, core biopsy provides better sample size and has decreased the need for repeat biopsies due to insufficient samples. FNA remains however the modality of choice when evaluation of a cystic breast lesion is required.

COMMON INDICATIONS [1]

- Symptomatic simple or complicated cystic breast lesion
- Diagnosis and treatment of infected breast cysts or abscesses
- Important diagnostic information dictating patient management might be derived from documentation of evacuation

L. Nassar (✉)
Department of Diagnostic Radiology, American University of Beirut Medical Center, Riad El-Solh, Beirut 1107 2020, Lebanon
e-mail: ln07@aub.edu.lb

COMMON CONTRAINDICATIONS [1]

- Inability to visualize lesion on ultrasound
- Significant coagulopathy that cannot be corrected

POSSIBLE COMPLICATIONS [2]

- Vasovagal reaction
- Bleeding and pain
- Infection
- Pneumothorax

PREPROCEDURAL ASSESSMENT AND PLANNING [3–5]

- History, indications, and physical examination *(Appendix 1* in Chap. 149*)*
- Evaluation of diagnostic imaging studies to accurately localize the lesion, assess the need for aspiration, and determine that sonographic guidance is the most appropriate. Any previously eventual previously obtained biopsy at the site of interest should also be reviewed
- Periprocedural management of coagulation status *(Appendices 2* in Chap. 150 *and 3* in Chap. 151*)*
- Antibiotic prophylaxis: Not routinely recommended [3]
- Imaging modality for guidance: Ultrasound
- Positioning: Supine, supine oblique

B. Taslakian et al. (eds.), *Procedural Dictations in Image-Guided Intervention*,
DOI 10.1007/978-3-319-40845-3_17

PROCEDURE NOTE

Procedure: Ultrasound-guided FNA/drainage of left/right breast simple cyst/complicated cyst/abscess
Staff: [_]
Fellow: [_]
Resident: [_]
Clinical Information: Describe history and list indications
Allergies: None known/Allergic to [specify/type of allergy]
Anesthesia: Local anesthesia/conscious sedation
Medications: List any relevant medications used
Field: Sterile
Procedure classification: Clean
Position: Supine/Supine oblique
Monitoring: Vital signs were continuously monitored by nursing staff throughout the procedure

Description of Procedure:

The risks, benefits, alternatives, and the procedure itself were explained to the patient/patient's Power of Attorney/patient's legal guardian, and informed written consent was obtained. The site of the procedure was identified and marked. Time out was performed to confirm the correct patient, procedure, and site.

Ultrasound of the region of interest was performed, the target cyst/abscess was localized and marked.

The skin was prepped and draped in the usual sterile fashion. Local anesthesia was administered. Under direct sonographic visualization, a (_)-gauge needle was advanced into the left/right breast cyst/abscess. (_) mL of [specify color and consistency] fluid was retrieved. Specimen was sent for cytopathological/bacteriological analysis.

The puncture site was compressed; then a sterile dressing was applied. The patient was discharged home following the procedure in a stable condition.

Intra-Procedure Findings: List all relevant findings.

Immediate Complications: None encountered during or directly after the procedure. *List complications if any.*

Post-Procedure Plan:

- Abstain from strenuous activities.
- Check for redness, tenderness, hotness, fever, and induration and follow up with [specify team] in case any complication is noted.
- Follow up with [specify team] in (_) days for obtaining cytology results.

Impression:

- Ultrasound-guided FNA/drainage of left/right breast cyst/abscess as described above.
- The patient tolerated the procedure well and left the breast interventional unit in a stable condition.
- List any other relevant or important information/finding.

References

1. American College of Radiology. ACR practice parameter for the performance of ultrasound-guided percutaneous breast interventional procedures. Reston, VA: American College of Radiology; 2014.
2. Helvie MA, Ikeda DM, Adler DD. Localization and needle aspiration of breast lesions: complications in 370 cases. AJR Am J Roentgenol. 1991;157(4):711–4.
3. Taslakian B, Sebaaly MG, Al-Kutoubi A. Patient evaluation and preparation in vascular and interventional radiology: what every interventional radiologist should know (part 1: patient assessment and laboratory tests). Cardiovasc Intervent Radiol. 2016;39(3):325–33.
4. Taslakian B, Sebaaly MG, Al-Kutoubi A. Patient evaluation and preparation in vascular and interventional radiology: what every interventional radiologist should know (part 2: patient preparation and medications). Cardiovasc Intervent Radiol. 2016;39(4):489–99. doi: 10.1007/s00270-015-1239-4. [Epub 2015 Nov 25].
5. Venkatesan AM, Kundu S, Sacks D, Wallace MJ, Wojak JC, Rose SC, et al. Practice guidelines for adult antibiotic prophylaxis during vascular and interventional radiology procedures. J Vasc Interv Radiol. 2010;21(11):1611–30.

MRI-Guided Biopsy of Breast Lesion 18

Lara Nassar

INTRODUCTION

Magnetic resonance imaging (MRI) of the breasts is increasingly being used for several indications including but not limited to staging recently diagnosed cancers, following up cancers on neoadjuvant chemotherapy and screening high-risk patients. As a high sensitivity modality, MRI will detect mammographically and sonographically occult cancers and as such, facilities that offer breast MRI will also need to provide MRI-guided biopsy to target those MR-only visible cancers. Similar to other percutaneous biopsy techniques, it has an accuracy comparable to that of open surgical biopsy while resulting in less morbidity, less scarring, and improved cost effectiveness. MR-compatible metallic clip markers are almost always inserted following MRI-guided biopsy, they confirm proper sampling, allow post biopsy localization of a lesion that is mammographically and/or sonographically occult, and mark the location of the malignant lesion that will be treated by neoadjuvant chemotherapy.

L. Nassar (✉)
Department of Diagnostic Radiology, American University of Beirut Medical Center, Riad El-Solh, Beirut 1107 2020, Lebanon
e-mail: ln07@aub.edu.lb

COMMON INDICATIONS [1]

- Breast lesions classified as BI-RADS 4 or BI-RADS 5
- Lesions that are probably benign by imaging criteria classified as BI-RADS 3, for which it would be more appropriate to obtain tissue diagnosis for specific clinical indications or when a short-term follow up is difficult to obtain
- Repeat biopsy for nondiagnostic or discordant histologic result

COMMON CONTRAINDICATIONS [1]

- Inability to administer gadolinium *(e.g., end-stage renal disease, allergy, pregnancy)*
- Inability to perform MRI *(e.g., MR unsafe devices, severe claustrophobia, inability of the patient to remain still in prone position for the duration of the procedure)*
- Inability to identify the target lesion on planning MRI. This may happen in up to 13 % of cases. In this setting, the performing physician should make sure that the patient has received an adequate bolus of contrast and that contrast inflow is not impeded by excessive breast compression. A short-term follow-up MRI to ensure that the lesion is indeed absent is the proper course of action
- Bleeding diathesis or intake of medications such as antiplatelets or anticoagulants

B. Taslakian et al. (eds.), *Procedural Dictations in Image-Guided Intervention*,
DOI 10.1007/978-3-319-40845-3_18

POSSIBLE COMPLICATIONS [2]

- Inadequate/insufficient sampling
- Bleeding
- Infection

PREPROCEDURAL ASSESSMENT AND PLANNING [3–5]

- History, indications, and physical examination *(Appendix 1* in Chap. 149*)*
- Evaluation of diagnostic imaging studies to accurately localize the lesion, assess the need for biopsy, and determine that MRI guidance is the most appropriate. Any previously obtained biopsy at the site of interest should also be reviewed
- Periprocedural management of coagulation status *(Appendices 2* in Chap. 150 *and 3* in Chap. 151*)*
- Antibiotic prophylaxis: Not routinely recommended [3]
- Imaging modality for guidance: MRI
- Positioning: Prone/prone oblique

PROCEDURE NOTE

Procedure: MRI-guided biopsy of left/right breast suspicious focus/mass/non-mass enhancement.
Staff: [_]
Fellow: [_]
Resident: [_]
Clinical Information: Describe history and list indications
Allergies: None known/Allergic to [specify/type of allergy]
Anesthesia: Local anesthesia/conscious sedation
Medications: List any relevant medications used (sedation)
Field: Sterile
Procedure classification: Clean
Position: Prone/Prone oblique
Monitoring: Intravenous access line was secured and vital signs were continuously monitored by nursing staff/anesthesia team throughout the procedure.

Description of Procedure:
The risks, benefits, alternatives, and the procedure itself were explained to the patient/patient's Power of Attorney/patient's legal guardian, and informed written consent was obtained. Time out was performed to confirm the correct patient, procedure, and site.

The site of the procedure was identified and marked. The patient was positioned on the MRI biopsy table and a planning enhanced MRI acquisition was obtained to localize the target.

The left/right breast was prepped in the usual sterile fashion. Local anesthesia was administered. A small skin incision was made. A track was created using a trocar and a sheath was placed. Adequate position was documented by a confirmation scan. Subsequently, a (_)-gauge vacuum/automated needle was advanced. (_) cores were obtained. Specimen was sent for histopathological analysis. An MR-compatible metallic clip marker was inserted at the site of the biopsy and post-procedure mammograms were obtained. The clip was placed [describe location of the clip relative to the site of biopsy].

The biopsy site was compressed; then a sterile dressing was applied. The patient was discharged home following the procedure in a stable condition.

Intra-Procedure Findings: List all relevant findings.
Immediate Complications: None encountered during or directly after the procedure. List complications if any.

Post-Procedure Plan:

- Abstain from strenuous activities for 24 h.
- Keep incision site dry for 24 h.

- Check for redness, tenderness, hotness, fever, and induration and follow up with [specify team] in case any complication is noted.
- Follow up with [specify team] in (_) days for obtaining pathology results.

Impression:

- MRI-guided biopsy of left/right breast focus/mass/non-mass enhancement as described above.
- The patient tolerated the procedure well and left the MRI unit in a stable condition.
- List any other relevant or important information/finding.

References

1. American College of Radiology. ACR practice parameter for the performance of magnetic resonance imaging-guided breast interventional procedures. Reston, VA: American College of Radiology; 2014.
2. Imschweiler T, Haueisen H, Kampmann G, Rageth L, Seifert B, Rageth C, et al. MRI-guided vacuum-assisted breast biopsy: comparison with stereotactically guided and ultrasound-guided techniques. Eur Radiol. 2014;24(1):128–35.
3. Taslakian B, Sebaaly MG, Al-Kutoubi A. Patient evaluation and preparation in vascular and interventional radiology: what every interventional radiologist should know (part 1: patient assessment and laboratory tests). Cardiovasc Intervent Radiol. 2016;39(3):325–33.
4. Taslakian B, Sebaaly MG, Al-Kutoubi A. Patient evaluation and preparation in vascular and interventional radiology: what every interventional radiologist should know (part 2: patient preparation and medications). Cardiovasc Intervent Radiol. 2016;39(4):489–99. doi: 10.1007/s00270-015-1239-4. [Epub 2015 Nov 25].
5. Venkatesan AM, Kundu S, Sacks D, Wallace MJ, Wojak JC, Rose SC, et al. Practice guidelines for adult antibiotic prophylaxis during vascular and interventional radiology procedures. J Vasc Interv Radiol. 2010;21(11):1611–30.

Needle Localization of Breast Lesion 19

Lara Nassar

INTRODUCTION

The different imaging modalities of the breast have an important role not only in diagnosis of breast pathologies and guidance of biopsy, but also in preoperative localization of breast lesions, namely those that are not palpable. By allowing real-time visualization of the needle and being more comfortable for the patient, ultrasound guidance is the preferred modality whenever a breast lesion can be identified sonographically. Otherwise, the lesion needs to be localized using the imaging modality that best depicts it, such as mammography, or MRI. Two or more wires may sometimes need to be inserted when bracketing of a rather extended breast pathology is needed.

COMMON INDICATIONS [1]

- Non palpable breast lesions requiring surgical excision

COMMON CONTRAINDICATIONS

- No need for wire localization in palpable lesions or when the patient is scheduled for mastectomy

POSSIBLE COMPLICATIONS [2–4]

- Vasovagal reactions
- Suboptimal positioning of the wire
- Migration or inadvertent dislodgment of the wire
- Bleeding and pain
- Pneumothorax

PREPROCEDURAL ASSESSMENT AND PLANNING [5–7]

- History, indications, and physical examination *(Appendix 1* in Chap. 149*)*
- Evaluation of diagnostic imaging studies to accurately localize the lesion and determine the most appropriate imaging modality for guidance and best pathway for access
- Periprocedural management of coagulation status *(Appendices 2* in Chap. 150 *and 3* in Chap. 151*)*
- Antibiotic prophylaxis: Not routinely recommended [5]
- Imaging modality for guidance: Mammography, ultrasound, or MRI

L. Nassar (✉)
Diagnostic Radiology, American University of Beirut Medical Center, Riad El-Solh, Beirut 1107 2020, Lebanon
e-mail: ln07@aub.edu.lb

B. Taslakian et al. (eds.), *Procedural Dictations in Image-Guided Intervention*,
DOI 10.1007/978-3-319-40845-3_19

- Positioning: Prone, sitting, supine, oblique, or decubitus

PROCEDURE NOTE

Procedure: Mammography/ultrasound/MRI-guided localization of left/right breast lesion
Staff: [_]
Fellow: [_]
Resident: [_]
Clinical Information: Describe history and list indications
Allergies: None known/Allergic to [specify/type of allergy]
Anesthesia: Local anesthesia/conscious sedation
Medications: List any relevant medications used
Field: Sterile
Procedure classification: Clean
Position: Prone/Sitting/Supine/Oblique/Left lateral decubitus/Right lateral decubitus
Monitoring: Vital signs were continuously monitored by nursing staff team throughout the procedure
Cumulative radiation dose: (_) mGy/cm

Description of Procedure:

The risks, benefits, alternatives, and the procedure itself were explained to the patient/patient's Power of Attorney/patient's legal guardian, and informed written consent was obtained. Time out was performed to confirm the correct patient, procedure, and site.

The site of the procedure was identified and marked. The patient was positioned and a medio-lateral mammographic view/latero-medial mammographic view/craniocaudal mammographic view/ultrasound/planning enhanced MRI acquisition was obtained for localization of the lesion.

The skin was prepped in the usual sterile fashion. Local anesthesia was administered. A small skin incision was made. Subsequently, a [type] wire was advanced into the left/right breast target lesion. Craniocaudal and lateral mammographic views/confirmation ultrasound images/confirmation MRI acquisitions were obtained to document adequate positioning of the wire. A sterile dressing was applied and a post-procedure mammogram was obtained and submitted to the surgical team.

The patient was then transferred to the recovery/operating room in a stable condition.
Immediate Complications: None encountered during or directly after the procedure. List the complication if any.

Post-Procedure Plan:

- Abstain from movements that may dislodge the wire.

Impression:

- Mammography/ultrasound/MRI-guided localization of left/right breast mass/distortion/calcification, as described above.
- The patient tolerated the procedure well and left the breast interventional unit in a stable condition.
- List any other relevant or important information/finding.

References

1. Philpotts LE. Needle localisation for surgical procedures. In: Dershaw D, editor. Imaging guided interventional breast techniques. New York: Springer-Verlag; 2003. p. 31–52.
2. Helvie MA, Ikeda DM, Adler DD. Localization and needle aspiration of breast lesions: complications in 370 cases. AJR Am J Roentgenol. 1991;157(4):711–4.
3. Bristol JB, Jones PA. Transgression of localizing wire into the pleural cavity prior to mammography. Br J Radiol. 1981;54(638):139–40.
4. Owen AW, Kumar EN. Migration of localizing wires used in guided biopsy of the breast. Clin Radiol. 1991;43(4):251.
5. Taslakian B, Sebaaly MG, Al-Kutoubi A. Patient evaluation and preparation in vascular and interventional radiology: what every interventional radiologist should know (part 1: patient assessment and laboratory tests). Cardiovasc Intervent Radiol. 2016;39(3):325–33.
6. Taslakian B, Sebaaly MG, Al-Kutoubi A. Patient evaluation and preparation in vascular and interventional radiology: what every interventional radiologist should know (part 2: patient preparation and medications). Cardiovasc Intervent Radiol. 2016;39(4):489–99. doi: 10.1007/s00270-015-1239-4. [Epub 2015 Nov 25].
7. Venkatesan AM, Kundu S, Sacks D, Wallace MJ, Wojak JC, Rose SC, et al. Practice guidelines for adult antibiotic prophylaxis during vascular and interventional radiology procedures. J Vasc Interv Radiol. 2010;21(11):1611–30.

20 Stereotactic Core Biopsy of Breast Lesion

Lara Nassar

INTRODUCTION

Stereotactically guided breast biopsy is the procedure of choice when tissue diagnosis of a mammographic abnormality is deemed necessary. It has an accuracy comparable to that of open surgical biopsy while resulting in less morbidity, less scarring, and improved cost effectiveness. According to the available equipment, this can be performed in either prone or sitting position, noting that prone tables have a maximum weight capacity and this has to be considered in patients with high body mass index. The biopsy procedure can be performed with either automated gun or vacuum biopsy needles, the former being the most favored. When the targeted lesion contains calcifications, specimen radiograph is very helpful in confirming adequate sampling by demonstrating the targeted calcifications within the retrieved cores. Metallic clip markers are very frequently inserted after a stereotactic biopsy; they confirm proper sampling, allow localization of a lesion that has been largely removed by the biopsy or a lesion that might be difficult to visualize, and mark malignant lesions that will be treated by neoadjuvant chemotherapy.

L. Nassar (✉)
Department of Diagnostic Radiology, American University of Beirut Medical Center, Riad El-Solh, Beirut 1107 2020, Lebanon
e-mail: ln07@aub.edu.lb

COMMON INDICATIONS [1]

- Breast lesions classified as BI-RADS 4 or BI-RADS 5
- Lesions that are probably benign by imaging criteria classified as BI-RADS 3, for which it would be more appropriate to obtain tissue diagnosis in specific clinical situations or when a short term follow up is difficult to obtain
- Suspected multifocal or multicentric breast cancer for planning of treatment
- Mammographic lesion correlating with an area of suspicious contrast enhancement on MRI
- Repeat biopsy of a mammographic lesion for non-diagnostic or discordant histologic result

COMMON CONTRAINDICATIONS [1]

- Inability to adequately localize lesion on mammography
- Significant bleeding disorder
- Inability to remain still in a prone position for the duration of the procedure
- Benefits versus risks need to be assessed on a case by case basis in the setting of pregnancy

POSSIBLE COMPLICATIONS [2]

- Minor discomfort and bruising
- Bleeding
- Infection

B. Taslakian et al. (eds.), *Procedural Dictations in Image-Guided Intervention*,
DOI 10.1007/978-3-319-40845-3_20

- Need for repeat biopsy in cases of insufficient sample, discordance of imaging and pathology findings and in some specific histological diagnoses

PREPROCEDURAL ASSESSMENT AND PLANNING [3–5]

- History, indications and physical examination *(Appendix 1* in Chap. 149*)*
- Evaluation of diagnostic imaging studies to accurately localize the lesion, assess the need for biopsy and determine that stereotactic guidance is the most appropriate. Any previously obtained biopsy at the site of interest should also be reviewed.
- Periprocedural management of coagulation status *(Appendices 2* in Chap. 150 *and 3* in Chap. 151*)*
- Antibiotic prophylaxis: Not routinely recommended [3]
- Imaging modality for guidance: Mammography
- Positioning: Prone, sitting or decubitus

PROCEDURE NOTE

Procedure: Stereotactic-guided biopsy of left/right breast mass/distortion/calcification
Staff: [_]
Fellow: [_]
Resident: [_]
Clinical Information: Describe history and list indications
Allergies: None known/Allergic to [specify/type of allergy]
Anesthesia: Local anesthesia/conscious sedation
Medications: List any relevant medications used
Field: Sterile
Procedure classification: Clean
Position: Sitting position/Left lateral decubitus/Right lateral decubitus/Prone
Monitoring: Vital signs were continuously monitored by nursing staff team throughout the procedure
Cumulative radiation dose: (_) mGy

Description of Procedure:
The risks, benefits, alternatives and the procedure itself were explained to the patient/patient's Power of Attorney/patient's legal guardian, and informed written consent was obtained. Time out was performed to confirm the correct patient, procedure and site.

The site of the procedure was identified and marked. The patient was positioned on the biopsy table, a scout view and $+15^{\circ}/-15^{\circ}$ stereotactic pair images were obtained for localization of the lesion in question.

The skin was prepped in the usual sterile fashion. Local anesthesia was administered. A small skin incision was made. Subsequently, a (_)-gauge vacuum/automated needle was advanced into the left/right breast. A pre-fire stereo pair was obtained confirming adequate direction. The needle was fired and post-fire stereo pair was obtained for confirmation of adequate targeting. (_) cores were obtained. Specimen radiograph showed calcifications in the cores. Specimen was sent for histopathological analysis. A metallic clip marker was inserted at the site of the biopsy and post-procedure mammograms were obtained showing the clip to be [describe location of the clip relative to the site of biopsy].

The biopsy site was compressed then a sterile dressing was applied. The patient was discharged home following the procedure in a stable condition.
Immediate Complications: None encountered during or directly after the procedure. List complications if any.
Post-Procedure Plan:

- Abstain from strenuous activities.
- Keep incision site dry for 24 h.
- Check for redness, tenderness, hotness, fever and induration and follow up with [specify team] in case any complication is noted.
- Follow up with [specify team] in (_) days for obtaining pathology results.

Impression:

- Stereotactic biopsy of left/right breast mass/distortion/calcification, as described above.
- The patient tolerated the procedure well and left the breast interventional unit in a stable condition.

- List any other relevant or important information/finding.

References

1. American College of Radiology. ACR practice parameter for the performance of stereotactic-guided breast interventional procedures. Reston, VA: American College of Radiology; 2014.
2. Liberman L. Stereotactic core biopsy. In: Dershaw D, editor. Imaging guided interventional breast techniques. New York: Springer; 2003. p. 87–118.
3. Taslakian B, Sebaaly MG, Al-Kutoubi A. Patient evaluation and preparation in vascular and interventional radiology: what every interventional radiologist should know (part 1: patient assessment and laboratory tests). Cardiovasc Intervent Radiol. 2016;39(3):325–33.
4. Taslakian B, Sebaaly MG, Al-Kutoubi A. Patient evaluation and preparation in vascular and interventional radiology: what every interventional radiologist should know (part 2: patient preparation and medications). Cardiovasc Intervent Radiol. 2016;39(4):489–99. doi: 10.1007/s00270-015-1239-4. [Epub 2015 Nov 25].
5. Venkatesan AM, Kundu S, Sacks D, Wallace MJ, Wojak JC, Rose SC, et al. Practice guidelines for adult antibiotic prophylaxis during vascular and interventional radiology procedures. J Vasc Interv Radiol. 2010;21(11):1611–30.

Ultrasound-Guided Core Biopsy of Breast Lesion

21

Lara Nassar

INTRODUCTION

Ultrasound-guided breast biopsy is the procedure of choice when tissue diagnosis of a sonographic abnormality *(e.g., solid mass, calcification)* is deemed necessary. It has an accuracy comparable to that of open surgical biopsy, while resulting in less morbidity, less scarring, and improved cost effectiveness. When compared to stereotactic guidance, ultrasound guidance offers the advantage of patient comfort, efficiency, economy, absence of ionizing radiation, and real-time visualization of the needle during the procedure. Metallic clip markers may be inserted after an ultrasound-guided biopsy to confirm proper sampling, allow localization of a lesion that has been largely removed by the biopsy or a lesion that might be difficult to visualize. Clips are also used to mark malignant lesions that will be treated by neoadjuvant chemotherapy.

L. Nassar (✉)
Department of Diagnostic Radiology, American University of Beirut Medical Center, Riad El-Solh, Beirut 1107 2020, Lebanon
e-mail: ln07@aub.edu.lb

COMMON INDICATIONS [1]

- Breast lesions classified as BI-RADS 4 or BI-RADS 5
- Lesions that are probably benign by imaging criteria classified as BI-RADS 3, for which it would be more appropriate to obtain tissue diagnosis in specific clinical indications or when a short-term follow up is difficult to obtain
- Suspected multifocal or multicentric breast cancer for planning of treatment
- Targeted second-look ultrasound shows a lesion correlating with an area of suspicious contrast enhancement on MRI
- Repeat biopsy of a lesion for nondiagnostic or discordant histologic result

COMMON CONTRAINDICATIONS [1]

- Inability to visualize lesion on ultrasound
- Inability of the patient to cooperate
- Significant bleeding disorder

POSSIBLE COMPLICATIONS [2, 3]

- Inadequate/insufficient sampling
- Bleeding
- Infection
- Pneumothorax

B. Taslakian et al. (eds.), *Procedural Dictations in Image-Guided Intervention*,
DOI 10.1007/978-3-319-40845-3_21

PREPROCEDURAL ASSESSMENT AND PLANNING [4–6]

- History, indications and physical examination *(Appendix 1* in Chap. 149*)*
- Evaluation of diagnostic imaging studies to accurately localize the lesion, assess the need for biopsy, and determine that ultrasound guidance is the most appropriate. Any previously obtained biopsy at the site of interest should also be reviewed.
- Periprocedural management of coagulation status *(Appendices 2* in Chap. 150 *and 3* in Chap. 151*)*
- Antibiotic prophylaxis: Not routinely recommended [4]
- Imaging modality for guidance: Ultrasound
- Positioning: Supine, oblique, decubitus

PROCEDURE NOTE

Procedure: Ultrasound-guided biopsy of left/right breast mass/calcification
Staff: [_]
Fellow: [_]
Resident: [_]
Clinical History and Indications: Describe history and list indications
Allergies: None known/Allergic to [specify/type of allergy]
Anesthesia: Local anesthesia/conscious sedation
Medications: List any relevant medications used
Field: Sterile
Procedure classification: Clean
Position: Supine/Oblique/Right lateral decubitus, Left lateral decubitus
Monitoring: Vital signs were continuously monitored by nursing staff throughout the procedure

Description of Procedure:

The risks, benefits, alternatives, and procedure itself were explained to the patient/patient's Power of Attorney/patient's legal guardian, and informed written consent was obtained. The site of the procedure was identified and marked. Time out was performed to confirm the correct patient, procedure, and site.

Ultrasound of the region of interest was performed, and the mass/calcification was localized. The skin was prepped and draped in the usual sterile fashion. Local anesthesia was administered. A small skin incision was made. Under direct sonographic visualization a (_)-gauge vacuum/automated needle was advanced into the left/right breast lesion. (_) cores were obtained. Specimen radiograph was performed showing calcifications in the obtained cores. Specimen was sent for histopathological analysis. A metallic clip marker was inserted at the site of the biopsy and post-procedure ultrasound and mammogram were obtained showing the clip to be [describe location of the clip relative to the site of biopsy].

The biopsy site was compressed and a sterile dressing was applied. The patient was discharged home following the procedure in a stable condition.

Immediate Complications: None encountered during or directly after the procedure. List the complication if any.

Post-Procedure Plan:

1. Abstain from strenuous activities for 24 h.
2. Keep incision site dry for 24 h.
3. Check for redness, tenderness, hotness, fever, and induration and follow up with [specify team] in case any complication is noted.
4. Follow up with [specify team] in (_) days for obtaining pathology results.

Impression:

- Ultrasound-guided biopsy of left/right breast mass/calcification, as described above.
- The patient tolerated the procedure well and left the breast interventional unit in stable condition.
- List any other relevant or important information/finding.

References

1. American College of Radiology. ACR practice parameter for the performance of ultrasound-guided percutaneous breast interventional procedures. Reston, VA: American College of Radiology; 2014.
2. Parker SH, Burbank F, Jackman RJ, Aucreman CJ, Cardenosa G, Cink TM, et al. Percutaneous large-core breast biopsy: a multi-institutional study. Radiology. 1994;193(2):359–64.
3. Meyer JE, Smith DN, Lester SC, Kaelin C, DiPiro PJ, Denison CM, et al. Large-core needle biopsy of nonpalpable breast lesions. JAMA. 1999;281(17):1638–41.
4. Taslakian B, Sebaaly MG, Al-Kutoubi A. Patient evaluation and preparation in vascular and interventional radiology: what every interventional radiologist should know (part 1: patient assessment and laboratory tests). Cardiovasc Intervent Radiol. 2016;39(3):325–33.
5. Taslakian B, Sebaaly MG, Al-Kutoubi A. Patient evaluation and preparation in vascular and interventional radiology: what every interventional radiologist should know (part 2: patient preparation and medications). Cardiovasc Intervent Radiol. 2016;39(4):489–99. doi: 10.1007/s00270-015-1239-4. [Epub 2015 Nov 25].
6. Venkatesan AM, Kundu S, Sacks D, Wallace MJ, Wojak JC, Rose SC, et al. Practice guidelines for adult antibiotic prophylaxis during vascular and interventional radiology procedures. J Vasc Interv Radiol. 2010;21(11):1611–30.

Part IV

Non-vascular Interventional Procedures: Gastrointestinal

Introduction by Aghiad Al-Kutoubi, Section Reviewer

Gastrointestinal intervention has seen many changes over the last couple of decades with a shift towards endoscopic applications by gastroenterologists.

Whereas stenting of the esophagus, duodenum, or colon was initially performed by interventionalists under fluoroscopy guidance, it is now mostly performed under endoscopy guidance. However, the role of the interventionalists remains well established particularly when it comes to the placement of the various tubes for feeding purposes.

Gastrostomy and gastrojejunostomy catheters are as amended well-accepted means of providing access for enteric feeding in patients with inadequate oral intake. Different placement techniques have been described including surgical, percutaneous endoscopic, and percutaneous radiologic techniques. Fluoroscopically guided gastrostomy was first reported in 1981 and the use of gastropexy devices (T-fasteners) was first reported in 1986.

This section provides a comprehensive list of procedural reports that covers the vast majority of the currently performed image-guided, non-vascular gastrointestinal procedures with up-to-date explanatory notes, synopsis of the indications and contraindications, and potential complications in an organized and practical format.

Section Chapters

Colorectal Stent Placement

22

Murad M. Abusamra

INTRODUCTION

Colorectal cancer is the third most common cancer in the United States and is the most common cause of colonic obstruction. Colorectal stenting is a minimally invasive procedure for gaining colon decompression to allow bridging to elective surgery or for palliation. Colorectal stent placement can be performed through the transanal route under fluoroscopic guidance, colonoscopy, or combination of both.

COMMON INDICATIONS [1–4]

- Decompression of acute colorectal obstructive tumor before curative surgery
- Benign colonic strictures due to Crohn's disease, radiation therapy, and diverticular disease
- Inoperable malignant colorectal obstruction to achieve colonic decompression
- Closure of ileocolic, colovesical, or colocutaneous fistulae

M.M. Abusamra (✉)
Department of Diagnostic Radiology, American University of Beirut Medical Center, Riad Elsolh, Beirut 1107 2020, Lebanon
e-mail: muradabusamra@gmail.com

COMMON CONTRAINDICATIONS [2, 3]

- Perforation or peritonitis
- Uncorrectable coagulopathy
- Small bowel obstruction
- Rectal cancer extending to the anal sphincter
- Long segment colonic stricture *(relative contraindication)*

POSSIBLE COMPLICATIONS [2–4]

- Bowel perforation
- Stent obstruction and restenosis
- Stent migration
- Luminal bleeding and abdominal/anorectal pain

PREPROCEDURAL ASSESSMENT AND PLANNING [5–6]

- History, indications, and physical examination *(Appendix 1* in Chap. 149*)*
- Evaluation of diagnostic imaging studies *(barium studies and computed tomography)*: to determine the location of the stenosis, as well as its severity and extent
- Antibiotics prophylaxis: Not routinely recommended
- Preparation: The patient should be fasting for 8 h; perform cleansing enema to clear the distal colon
- Imaging modality for guidance: Fluoroscopy
- Positioning of the patient: Left lateral decubitus

B. Taslakian et al. (eds.), *Procedural Dictations in Image-Guided Intervention*,
DOI 10.1007/978-3-319-40845-3_22

PROCEDURE NOTE

Procedure: Fluoroscopy-guided colorectal stent placement
Staff: [_]
Fellow: [_]
Resident: [_]
Clinical Information: Describe history and list indications
Allergies: None known/Allergic to [specify/type of allergy]
Anesthesia: Topical anesthesia/conscious sedation
Medications: List any relevant medications used (sedation, antibiotics)
Contrast Material: (_) mL of [type] contrast material was used for colonography
Field: Sterile
Procedure classification: Dirty
Position: Left lateral decubitus
Monitoring: Intravenous access line was secured and vital signs were continuously monitored by nursing staff/anesthesia team throughout the procedure
Total fluoroscopy time: (_) minutes
Cumulative radiation dose: (_) mGy

Description of Procedure:

The risks, benefits, alternatives, and the procedure itself were explained to the patient/patient's Power of Attorney/legal guardian, and informed written consent was obtained. Time out was performed to confirm the correct patient, procedure, and site.

The patient was placed in a left lateral decubitus position. Then a (_)-inch [type] guidewire and a (_)-French [type] catheter were inserted through the anus, across the obstruction, into the proximal part of the obstruction. Water-soluble [type] contrast was injected to outline the anatomy, locate the stricture, and measure its length and skin markers were placed. Following that a (_)-inch [type/stiff] guidewire was inserted through the catheter and looped in a stable location beyond the stricture. A stent delivery system [type/size] was introduced over the guidewire, and after confirming the position of the stent, it was deployed under direct fluoroscopic visualization. Completion colonography was performed to rule out perforation and to assess stent position and patency.

The patient was transferred to the floor/recovery room/discharged home following the procedure in a stable condition. Staff was present and scrubbed for the entire procedure.

Intra-Procedure Findings: List all relevant findings.
Immediate Complications: None encountered during or directly after the procedure. List complications if any.

Post-Procedure Plan [1–4]:

- Assess for resolution of symptoms periodically.
- Perform water-soluble enema 1 day following the procedure.
- Advise the patient to consume a low-residue diet and mineral oil.

Impression:

- Colorectal stent placement, as described above.
- The patient tolerated the procedure well and left the interventional unit in stable condition.
- The procedure was canceled/terminated prematurely.
- List any other relevant or important information/finding.

References

1. Bonin EA, Baron TH. Update on the indications and use of colonic stents. Curr Gastroenterol Rep. 2010;12(5):374–82.
2. Kim JH, Song HY, Shin JH. Colorectal Stent placement. In: Kandarpa K, Machan L, editors. Handbook of interventional radiologic procedures. 4th ed. Philadelphia: Lippincott Williams & Wilkins; 2011. p. 572–6.
3. De Gregorio MA, Mainar A, Rodriguez J, Alfonso ER, Tejero E, Herrera M, et al. Colon stenting: a review. Semin Interv Radiol. 2004;21(3):205–16.
4. Hong SP, Kim TI. Colorectal stenting: an advanced approach to malignant colorectal obstruction. World J Gastroenterol. 2014;20(43):16020–8.
5. Taslakian B, Sebaaly MG, Al-Kutoubi A. Patient evaluation and preparation in vascular and interventional radiology: what every interventional radiologist should know (part 1: patient assessment and laboratory tests). Cardiovasc Intervent Radiol. 2016;39(3):325–33.
6. Taslakian B, Sebaaly MG, Al-Kutoubi A. Patient evaluation and preparation in vascular and interventional radiology: what every interventional radiologist should know (part 2: patient preparation and medications). Cardiovasc Intervent Radiol. 2016;39(4):489–99. doi: 10.1007/s00270-015-1239-4. [Epub 2015 Nov 25].

Conversion Gastrojejunostomy

23

Bedros Taslakian

INTRODUCTION

Percutaneous transgastric jejunostomy *(gastrojejunostomy)* provides access for enteral nutrition in patients for whom oral intake is either impossible or unsafe, by the placement of a feeding tube in the jejunum through the stomach. Using double lumen tubes will allow gastric decompression with simultaneous jejunal feeding in patients with high risk of gastroesophageal reflux or aspiration. It also allows the administration of specific medication only absorbed by the stomach through the gastric lumen of the tube. The procedure can be performed as an initial feeding tube placement *(primary gastrojejunostomy)* or by converting a previously inserted mature gastrostomy to gastrojejunostomy *(conversion gastrojejunostomy).*

COMMON INDICATIONS [1–5]

Decompression of gastroenteric contents with simultaneous jejunal tube feeding in patients who could not tolerate gastric feeding through the gastrostomy tube as a result of:

- Worsening gastroparesis resulting in large gastric residual
- Proximal small bowel obstruction
- Severe gastroesophageal reflux
- Recurrent aspiration pneumonia
- Gastrostomy-related complications *(i.e. peristomal leakage and skin irritation)*

COMMON CONTRAINDICATIONS [1, 2]

- Hemodynamic instability
- Uncorrectable coagulopathy
- Surgical or endoscopy-guided gastrostomy tube *(conversion can be challenging)*
- Anatomic distortion due to prior gastric surgery
- Immature tract in the absence of gastropexy

POSSIBLE COMPLICATIONS [1–3]

- Failure of the procedure due to anatomic distortion or unfavorable angle of entry
- Wound infection *(peristomal infection)*
- Gastrointestinal perforation
- Tube malfunction *(retrograde tube migration into duodenum or stomach, malposition, kinking, clogging)*
- Ileus
- Buried bumper syndrome

B. Taslakian (✉)
Department of Radiology, New York University Langone Medical Center, 660 First Ave, New York, NY 10016, USA
e-mail: btaslakian@gmail.com

B. Taslakian et al. (eds.), *Procedural Dictations in Image-Guided Intervention*,
DOI 10.1007/978-3-319-40845-3_23

PREPROCEDURAL ASSESSMENT AND PLANNING [6–8]

- History, indications, and physical examination *(Appendix 1* in Chap. 149*)*
- Evaluation of diagnostic imaging studies to determine the location of gastrostomy tube and the relevant anatomy
- Periprocedural management of coagulation status *(Appendices 2* in Chap. 150 *and 3* in Chap. 151*)*
- Antibiotic prophylaxis: No consensus [6] *(Appendices 4* in Chap. 152 *and 5* in Chap. 153*)*
- Imaging modality for guidance: Fluoroscopy
- Positioning: Supine

PROCEDURE NOTE

Procedure: Conversion of percutaneous gastrostomy to gastrojejunostomy
Staff: [_]
Fellow: [_]
Resident: [_]
Clinical Information: Describe history and list indications
Allergies: None known/Allergic to [specify/type of allergy]
Anesthesia: Local anesthesia/conscious sedation
Medications: List any relevant medications used (sedation, antibiotics)
Contrast Material: (_) mL of [type] contrast material/Not required
Field: Sterile
Procedure classification: Clean-contaminated
Position: Supine
Monitoring: Intravenous access line was secured and vital signs were continuously monitored by nursing staff/anesthesia team throughout the procedure
Total fluoroscopy time: (_) minutes
Cumulative radiation dose: (_) mGy

Description of Procedure:

The risks, benefits, alternatives, and procedure itself were explained to the patient/patient's Power of Attorney/patient's legal guardian, and informed written consent was obtained. The site of the procedure was identified and marked. Time out was performed to confirm the correct patient, procedure, and site.

The skin and previously inserted gastrostomy tube were prepped and draped in the usual sterile fashion. A (0.035)-in. [type] guidewire was advanced through the gastrostomy tube and looped in the stomach. Once there was a sufficient length of guidewire within the stomach, a (_) French peel-away sheath was advanced over the guidewire into the stomach. Through the sheath, a (_) French [Torqueable/type] catheter was used for manipulation and a (0.035)-in. [type] guidewire was advanced into the small intestine beyond the ligament of Treitz followed by the catheter. Subsequently, the initial guidewire was replaced for a (_)-inch [stiff/type] exchange guidewire, and its tip was looped within the jejunum. Through the sheath, a (_)-French [pigtail-retained/type] dual-lumen gastrojejunostomy feeding tube was advanced over the guidewire and positioned under fluoroscopy guidance. Completion spot fluoroscopy image was obtained after contrast administration to document the tube position for future reference. The sheath was removed and the tube was anchored to the skin and sterile dressing was applied. The tube was flushed with normal saline.

The patient was transferred to the floor/recovery room/discharged home following the procedure in a stable condition. Staff was present for the entire procedure.

Intra-Procedure Findings: List all relevant findings.

Immediate Complications: None encountered during or directly after the procedure. List complications if any.

Post-Procedure Plan [1, 4]**:**

- Perform serial abdominal examination if peritonitis is suspected in the setting of an immature tract.
- Start feeding from the jejunal lumen post-insertion if the abdominal exam is

benign, with an initial infusion rate of 5 mL per hour, increased as tolerated by 5 mL per shift to reach the goal rate determined by the nutritional support team.

- Gastric lumen should be clamped or connected to a gravity drainage bag for the first 24 h *(immature tract).*
- To prevent tube clogging, medications should be administered through the gastrostomy port when possible.
- Keep the catheter always fixed in place and apply sterile dressing after disinfecting the skin with chlorhexidine-based preparation.
- When not in use, flush the feeding tube with 30–50 mL of distilled water every 8 h to keep patency.
- Flush the feeding tube with 30–50 mL of distilled water before and after each use to keep patency.
- If the catheter is clogged, flush the catheter with warm or carbonated water.
- If the patient complains of skin irritation or breakdown at the insertion site, evaluate for infection, and treat with antibiotics as appropriate.
- Inform interventional team if tube malfunction or dislodgment is suspected, peristomal leak or skin irritation occurs, or when abdominal pain or feeding intolerance *(vomiting, diarrhea)* is observed.

Impression:

- Conversion of percutaneous gastrostomy to gastrojejunostomy, as described above.
- The patient tolerated the procedure well and left the interventional unit in a stable condition.
- The patient was unstable and the procedure was canceled/terminated prematurely.
- List any other relevant or important information/finding.

References

1. Shin J, Lieberman J, Song H, Brown DB. Percutaneous gastrostomy, percutaneous gastrojejunostomy, jejunostomy, and cecostomy. In: Kandarpa K, Machan L, editors. Handbook of interventional radiologic procedures. 4th ed. Philadelphia: Lippincott Williams & Wilkins; 2011. p. 555–66.
2. Power S, Lee MJ. Gastrostomy and gastrojejunostomy. In: Murphy KPJ, Thomson KR, Venbrux AC, Morgan RA, editors. Image-guided interventions. 2nd ed. Philadelphia: Saunders Elsevier; 2014. p. 969–75.
3. Itkin M, DeLegge MH, Fang JC, McClave SA, Kundu S, Janne d'Othee B, et al. Multidisciplinary practical guidelines for gastrointestinal access for enteral nutrition and decompression from the Society of Interventional Radiology and American Gastroenterological Association (AGA) Institute, with endorsement by Canadian Interventional Radiological Association (CIRA) and Cardiovascular and Interventional Radiological Society of Europe (CIRSE). J Vasc Interv Radiol. 2011;22(8):1089–106.
4. Lyon SM, Pascoe DM. Percutaneous gastrostomy and gastrojejunostomy. Semin Interv Radiol. 2004;21 (3):181–9.
5. Shin KH, Shin JH, Song HY, Yang ZQ, Kim JH, Kim KR. Primary and conversion percutaneous gastrojejunostomy under fluoroscopic guidance: 10 years of experience. Clin Imaging. 2008;32(4):274–9.
6. Taslakian B, Sebaaly MG, Al-Kutoubi A. Patient evaluation and preparation in vascular and interventional radiology: what every interventional radiologist should know (part 1: patient assessment and laboratory tests). Cardiovasc Intervent Radiol. 2016;39(3):325–33.
7. Taslakian B, Sebaaly MG, Al-Kutoubi A. Patient evaluation and preparation in vascular and interventional radiology: what every interventional radiologist should know (part 2: patient preparation and medications). Cardiovasc Intervent Radiol. 2016;39(4):489–99. doi: 10.1007/s00270-015-1239-4. [Epub 2015 Nov 25].
8. Venkatesan AM, Kundu S, Sacks D, Wallace MJ, Wojak JC, Rose SC, et al. Practice guidelines for adult antibiotic prophylaxis during vascular and interventional radiology procedures. J Vasc Interv Radiol. 2010;21(11):1611–30.

24 Esophageal Balloon Dilation and Stent Placement

Murad M. Abusamra

INTRODUCTION

Balloon dilation and esophageal stenting are safe options for the nonsurgical management of dysphagia due to esophageal or esophagogastric malignancy. Fluoroscopically guided balloon dilation and esophageal stenting may be used for temporary benign esophageal conditions such as postsurgical, post-sclerotherapeutic, and corrosive strictures and fistulae and are associated with lower morbidity and mortality rates when comparted to surgical correction.

COMMON INDICATIONS [1–5]

Balloon dilatation:

- Benign esophageal stenosis
  Esophageal stenting with or without balloon dilatation:
- Non-resectable esophagogastric tumor
- Iatrogenic esophageal perforation
- Enteral feeding prior to surgery or chemoradiation
- Esophagorespiratory fistula
- Esophagogastric and esophagojejunal anastomotic leak
- Benign esophageal strictures not responding to balloon dilation

COMMON CONTRAINDICATIONS [1, 5]

- Tumor of the upper esophageal sphincter
- Severe vocal cord paralysis
- Severe uncorrectable coagulopathy
- Active esophageal perforation *(absolute contraindication to balloon dilatation)*
- Severe cardiorespiratory disease

POSSIBLE COMPLICATIONS [1–5]

- Chest pain after stent placement, *12–14 %**
- Stent obstruction due to tumor ingrowth, overgrowth, or food impaction, *17–33 %**
- Esophageal perforation, *0–5 %**
- Bleeding, *3–8 %**
- Stent migration, *4–9 % (bare stents), 25–32 % (covered stents)**
- Compression of the trachea
- Gastroesophageal reflux, *4 %**
- Fistula formation, *3 %**
- Mortality, *0.5–2.0 %**
  *Complication rates for esophageal stenting

M.M. Abusamra (✉)
Department of Diagnostic Radiology, American University of Beirut Medical Center, Riad El solh, Beirut 1107 2020, Lebanon
e-mail: muradabusamra@gmail.com

B. Taslakian et al. (eds.), *Procedural Dictations in Image-Guided Intervention*,
DOI 10.1007/978-3-319-40845-3_24

PREPROCEDURAL ASSESSMENT AND PLANNING [6, 7]

- History, indications, and physical examination *(Appendix 1* in Chap. 149*)*
- Evaluation of diagnostic imaging studies *(barium studies and computed tomography)*: to determine the location of the stenosis, its severity and the relevant anatomy
- Periprocedural management of coagulation status *(Appendices 2* in Chap. 150 *and 3* in Chap. 151*)*
- Antibiotic prophylaxis: Not routinely recommended
- Imaging modality for guidance: Fluoroscopy
- Positioning: Supine, left anterior oblique position

PROCEDURE NOTE

Procedure: Fluoroscopy-guided esophageal balloon dilatation and stent placement
Staff: [_]
Fellow: [_]
Resident: [_]
Clinical Information: Describe history and list indications
Allergies: None known/Allergic to [specify/type of allergy]
Anesthesia: Topical anesthesia/conscious sedation
Medications: List any relevant medications used
Contrast Used: (_) mL of [type] contrast material was used for esophagogram
Field: Sterile
Procedure classification: Clean contaminated
Position: Supine/Left anterior oblique
Monitoring: Intravenous access line was secured and vital signs were continuously monitored by nursing staff/anesthesia team throughout the procedure.
Total fluoroscopy time: (_) minutes
Cumulative radiation dose: (_) mGy

Description of Procedure:

The risks, benefits, alternatives, and procedure itself were explained to the patient/patient's Power of Attorney/patient's legal guardian, and informed written consent was obtained. Time out was performed to confirm the correct patient, procedure, and site.

With the patient in the supine/left anterior oblique position, the pharynx was topically anesthetized. A mouth guard was placed and a (_)-French [type] catheter was inserted over a (_)-inch [type] guidewire through the mouth guard into the esophagus and the catheter was positioned proximal to the site of the stricture/fistula/leak. Then water-soluble [type] contrast medium was injected through the catheter to delineate the esophageal anatomy and measure the length of stricture. The location of the stricture/fistula/leak was marked on the patient's skin under fluoroscopic control. The catheter and guidewire were used to bypass the stricture and positioned in a stable location in the stomach. The guidewire was then exchanged for a (_)-inch [type/stiff] guidewire which was looped in the stomach. The catheter was removed, leaving the guidewire in place. Then a (_) mm/(_)-cm-long [type] balloon was advanced over the guidewire and positioned at the site of the stricture and balloon dilatation of the stricture was performed. Following adequate dilatation, a preloaded stent delivery system [type/size] was passed over the guidewire into the esophagus and advanced until the markers on the stent corresponded to the skin markers and the distal end of the stent reached a satisfactory location distal to the stricture/fistula/leak. The introducing sheath was slowly removed over the pusher, allowing the stent to expand. The delivery system and guidewire were then retracted. Completion water-soluble esophagogram was performed to confirm the location and patency of the stent, and absence of complications. The catheter was then removed.

The patient was transferred to the floor/recovery room/discharged home following the procedure in a stable condition. Staff was present for the entire procedure.
Intra-Procedure Findings: List all relevant findings.
Immediate Complications: None encountered during or directly after the procedure. List complications if any.

Post-Procedure Plan [1, 2]:

- Bed rest for 3 h, in a semi-erect position.
- Pain control.
- Obtain chest radiograph during observation period.
- Discharge the patient after 4–5 h of observation.
- Keep patient fasting after stent placement.
- Perform esophagography 24 h after stent placement to verify the position and patency of the stent, then gradually resume soft food intake according to tolerance, progressing to normal food *(proper chewing should be advised).*

Impression:

- Esophageal balloon dilatation and stent placement, as described.
- The patient tolerated the procedure well and left the interventional unit in stable condition.
- The patient was unstable and the procedure had to be canceled/terminated prematurely.
- List any other relevant or important information/finding.

References

1. Song HY, Shin JH, Yoon CJ. Esophageal stents. In: Kandarpa K, Machan L, editors. Handbook of interventional radiologic procedures. 4th ed. Philadelphia: Lippincott Williams & Wilkins; 2011. p. 510–6.
2. Therasse E, Oliva VL, Lafontaine E, Perreault P, Giroux MF, Soulez G. Balloon dilation and stent placement for esophageal lesions: indications, methods, and results. Radiographics. 2003;23(1):89–105.
3. Catalano O, De Bellis M, Sandomenico F, de Lutio di Castelguidone E, Delrio P, Petrillo A. Complications of biliary and gastrointestinal stents: MDCT of the cancer patient. AJR Am J Roentgenol. 2012;199 (2):W187–96.
4. Kochar R, Shah N. Enteral stents: from esophagus to colon. Gastrointest Endosc. 2013;78(6):913–8.
5. Riley S, Attwood S. Guidelines on the use of oesophageal dilatation in clinical practice. Gut. 2004;53(Suppl 1):i1–6.
6. Taslakian B, Sebaaly MG, Al-Kutoubi A. Patient evaluation and preparation in vascular and interventional radiology: what every interventional radiologist should know (part 1: patient assessment and laboratory tests). Cardiovasc Intervent Radiol. 2016;39(3):325–33.
7. Taslakian B, Sebaaly MG, Al-Kutoubi A. Patient evaluation and preparation in vascular and interventional radiology: what every interventional radiologist should know (part 2: patient preparation and medications). Cardiovasc Intervent Radiol. 2016;39 (4):489–99. doi: 10.1007/s00270-015-1239-4. [Epub 2015 Nov 25].

25 Gastroduodenal Stent Placement

Murad M. Abusamra

INTRODUCTION

Gastroduodenal obstruction is the most common complication of advanced distal gastric, periampullary, pancreatic, hepatobiliary, or duodenal malignancy. Palliative bypass surgery is the traditional treatment to provide enteral feeding. Fluoroscopic or endoscopic placement of a gastroduodenal metal stent is an effective and minimally invasive alternative palliative treatment of malignant gatroduodenal obstruction. In addition, it has a lower mortality and morbidity rates, in comparison to surgical gastroenterostomy.

COMMON INDICATIONS [1–3]

- Non-resectable cancer causing gastroduodenal obstruction
- Enteral feeding prior to surgery or chemoradiation therapy
- Malignant or postsurgical fistula

COMMON CONTRAINDICATIONS [2, 3]

- Gastrointestinal perforation
- Distal gastrointestinal obstruction *(relative contraindication)*

M.M. Abusamra (✉)
Department of Diagnostic Radiology, American University of Beirut Medical Center, Riad El solh, Beirut 1107 2020, Lebanon
e-mail: muradabusamra@gmail.com

POSSIBLE COMPLICATIONS [1–3]

- Perforation
- Bleeding
- Ulceration
- Stent migration
- Food impaction
- Biliary obstruction
- Stent obstruction due to tumor ingrowth, overgrowth, or food impaction

PREPROCEDURAL ASSESSMENT AND PLANNING [4, 5]

- History, indications, and physical examination *(Appendix 1* in Chap. 149*)*
- Evaluation of diagnostic imaging studies *(barium studies and computed tomography)* to determine the location of the stenosis, its severity, and the relevant anatomy
- Periprocedural management of coagulation status *(Appendices 2* in Chap. 150 *and 3* in Chap. 151*)*
- Antibiotic prophylaxis: Not routinely recommended
- The patient should be fasting for 8 h
- Imaging modality for guidance: Fluoroscopy
- Positioning: Right lateral decubitus

B. Taslakian et al. (eds.), *Procedural Dictations in Image-Guided Intervention*, DOI 10.1007/978-3-319-40845-3_25

PROCEDURE NOTE

Procedure: Fluoroscopy-guided gastroduodenal stent placement
Staff: [_]
Fellow: [_]
Resident: [_]
Clinical Information: Describe history and list indications
Allergies: None known/Allergic to [specify/type of allergy]
Anesthesia: Topical anesthesia/conscious sedation
Medications: List any relevant medications used
Contrast Material: (_) mL of [type] contrast material
Field: Sterile
Procedure classification: Clean-contaminated
Position: Right lateral decubitus
Monitoring: Intravenous access line was secured and vital signs were continuously monitored by nursing staff/anesthesia team throughout the procedure
Total fluoroscopy time: (_) minutes
Cumulative radiation dose: (_) mGy

Description of Procedure:

The risks, benefits, alternatives, and the procedure itself were explained to the patient/patient's Power of Attorney/legal guardian, and informed written consent was obtained. Time out was performed to confirm the correct patient, procedure and site.

The patient's neck was extended and an oral guard was used to facilitate the procedure. With the patient in the right lateral decubitus position, the pharynx was topically anesthetized. A (_)-inch [type] guidewire was inserted, with the help of a (_)-French [angiographic/type] catheter, through the mouth into the antrum. A small amount of diluted [type] contrast material was injected to identify the location and length of the stricture and the location was marked on the patient's skin. The stricture was then traversed using a (_)-French curved [type/angiographic] catheter and a (_)-inch [type] guidewire. The catheter was advanced distal to the stricture into the first portion of the jejunum. A (_)-inch exchange [type/stiff] guidewire was then advanced through the catheter and looped in a stable position distal to the stricture. The catheter was removed, leaving the guidewire in place. A preloaded stent delivery system [type/size] was passed over the guidewire and advanced until the distal end of the stent reached an adequate position distal to the stricture. The position of the stent relative to the stricture was confirmed with contrast injection. The introducing sheath was slowly withdrawn over the pusher in a continuous motion, deploying the stent in place. The delivery system and guidewire were then removed. Completion contrast injection confirmed good positioning and patency of the stent as well as absence of complications.

The patient was transferred to the floor/recovery room/discharged home following the procedure in a stable condition. Staff was present for the entire procedure.

Intra-Procedure Findings: List all relevant findings.
Immediate Complications: None encountered during or directly after the procedure. List complications if any.

Post-Procedure Plan [2, 3]:

- Allow liquid diet 1 h after the procedure.
- Perform a follow-up upper gastrointestinal study the next day after stent placement to verify the position and patency of the stent.
- Advance diet after confirming stent expansion and position, and absence of complications.
- Dietary counseling; advice proper chewing of food, and use of carbonated drinks to reduce risk of food impaction.

Impression:

- Gastroduodenal stent insertion, as described above.
- The patient tolerated the procedure well and left the interventional unit in stable condition.
- The patient was unstable and the procedure was canceled/terminated prematurely.
- List any relevant findings.

References

1. Shi D, Qiu XM, Feng TY. Current status of metal stents for malignant gastro-duodenal obstruction. J Gastroint Dig Syst. 2013;3:3.
2. Lopera JE, Brazzini A, Gonzales A, Castaneda-Zuniga WR. Gastroduodenal stent placement: current status. Radiographics. 2004;24(6):1561–73.
3. Patz EF, Erasmus JJ. Gastroduodenal stent placement. In: Kandarpa K, Machan L, editors. Handbook of interventional radiologic procedures. 4th ed. Philadelphia: Lippincott Williams & Wilkins; 2011. p. 567–72.
4. Taslakian B, Sebaaly MG, Al-Kutoubi A. Patient evaluation and preparation in vascular and interventional radiology: what every interventional radiologist should know (part 1: patient assessment and laboratory tests). Cardiovasc Intervent Radiol. 2016;39(3):325–33.
5. Taslakian B, Sebaaly MG, Al-Kutoubi A. Patient evaluation and preparation in vascular and interventional radiology: what every interventional radiologist should know (part 2: patient preparation and medications). Cardiovasc Intervent Radiol. 2016;39(4):489–99. doi: 10.1007/s00270-015-1239-4. [Epub 2015 Nov 25].

Nasal/Oral Feeding Tube Insertion

26

Bedros Taslakian

INSTRUCTIONS

Feeding tubes can be temporarily placed through natural orifices (i.e., nose, mouth). Their use is recommended for short-term use (i.e., few days to 6 weeks). Image-guided temporary feeding tube insertion has been increasingly used for accurate placement of the tube in the required location within the gastrointestinal tract and to decrease complications associated with malpositioning. The gastric route is the most common artificial nutrition route used for feeding; however, patients who are unable to tolerate gastric feeding should receive distal post-pyloric feeding.

COMMON INDICATIONS [1–3]

Indications for temporary gastric feeding tube insertion:

- Inadequate oral intake with malnutrition
- Neurologic disorders with severe dysphagia and recurrent aspiration
- Extensive burns, comatose, and trauma patients
- Administration of radiographic contrast
- Venting gastric tube for decompression

Indications for temporary distal (duodenal or jejunal) tube insertion:

- Delayed gastric emptying
- Hyperemesis gravidarum
- Acute pancreatitis
- Partial gastric outlet or duodenal obstruction
- Gastric or duodenal fistula *(consider jejunostomy feeding)*
- Patients at high risk of aspiration
- Chemotherapy induced nausea
- Severe gastric mucositis
- Gastrectomy and gastro-enteric anastomosis

COMMON CONTRAINDICATIONS [3, 4]

- Maxillofacial disorders or surgery *(consider oroenteric tube feeding)*
- Abnormal nasal anatomy or nasal injury *(consider oroenteric tube feeding)*
- Skull fractures *(consider oroenteric tube feeding)*
- Laryngectomy
- Oral/pharyngeal tumors or after oropharyngeal surgery
- Patients receiving nasal Continuous Positive Airway Pressure
- Esophageal varices
- Preexisting sinusitis *(consider oroenteric tube feeding)*
- High output small bowel fistula
- Expending descending thoracic aortic aneurysm

B. Taslakian (✉)
Department of Radiology, New York University Langone Medical Center, 660 First Ave, New York, NY 10016, USA
e-mail: btaslakian@gmail.com

B. Taslakian et al. (eds.), *Procedural Dictations in Image-Guided Intervention*,
DOI 10.1007/978-3-319-40845-3_26

POSSIBLE COMPLICATIONS [2–5]

- Malposition: tracheal intubation, pneumothorax, intracranial placement *(rare when using fluoroscopy)*
- Inadvertent dislodgment
- Pulmonary aspiration
- Nosocomial rhinitis, sinusitis, and otitis media
- Hoarseness
- Epistaxis
- Perforation of the esophagus, stomach, or small bowel
- Esophageal mucosal injury with submucosal false tunnel creation
- Esophageal stricture
- Tracheoesophageal fistula
- Aortoesophageal fistula
- Variceal rupture

PREPROCEDURAL ASSESSMENT AND PLANNING [6, 7]

- History, indications, and physical examination *(Appendix 1* in Chap. 149*)*
- Evaluation of available diagnostic imaging studies to determine the relevant anatomy
- Imaging modality for guidance: Fluoroscopy
- Positioning: Supine, right lateral decubitus position to facilitate the passage of the tube through the pylorus

PROCEDURE NOTE

Procedure: Fluoroscopic-guided nasal- / oral-gastric/duodenal/jejunal feeding tube insertion
Staff: [_]
Fellow: [_]
Resident: [_]
Clinical Information: Describe history and list indications
Allergies: None known/Allergic to [specify/type of allergy]
Anesthesia: Topical anesthesia/conscious sedation
Medications: List any relevant medications used
Contrast Material: (_) mL of [type] contrast material was used
Field: Sterile
Position: Supine/Right lateral decubitus
Monitoring: Vital signs were continuously monitored by nursing staff/anesthesia team throughout the procedure
Total fluoroscopy time: (_) minutes
Cumulative radiation dose: (_) mGy

Description of Procedure: *(straightforward procedure)*

The risks, benefits, alternatives, and procedure itself were explained to the patient/patient's Power of Attorney/patient's legal guardian, and informed written consent was obtained *(might not be needed, depending on the institutional guidelines)*. The entry site was identified. Time out was performed to confirm the correct patient, procedure, and site.

The patient was positioned supine/in the right lateral decubitus position to facilitate the passage of the tube. Under direct fluoroscopy visualization, a (_) French, (_) cm-long radiopaque [type] feeding tube was advanced through the nose/mouth/over a (_)-inch [type] guidewire, and the tip was positioned within the [specify location]. The guidewire was withdrawn under fluoroscopy visualization, keeping the tube in position. Completion spot fluoroscopy image was obtained after contrast injection to document the tube position for future reference. The tube was secured to the side of the face by a hypoallergenic adherent dressing and looped over the ear.

The patient was transferred to the floor/recovery room following the procedure in a stable condition. Staff was present for the entire procedure.

Description of Procedure: *(Difficult procedure, with gastric/enteral obstruction, surgery, stricture, or leak)*

The risks, benefits, alternatives, and procedure itself were explained to the patient/patient's Power of Attorney/patient's legal guardian, and informed written/verbal consent was obtained. The entry site was identified. Time out was performed to confirm the correct patient, procedure and site.

The patient was positioned supine/in the right lateral decubitus position to facilitate the passage of the tube. Under direct fluoroscopy visualization, a (_) French, [type] manipulation catheter was advanced through the nose/mouth over a (_)-inch [hydrophilic/type] guidewire, and the site of leak/anastomosis/obstruction/stricture at the [specify location] was crossed with careful manipulation of the catheter and guidewire. Following this, the catheter was advanced to [specify location] and the [hydrophilic/type] guidewire was exchanged for a (_)-inch [stiff/type] guidewire. Once there was a sufficient length of guidewire within the system, the catheter was exchanged for a (_) French, (_) cm-long radiopaque [type] feeding tube and the tip was positioned within the [specify location]. The guidewire was withdrawn under fluoroscopy visualization, keeping the tube in position. Completion spot fluoroscopy image was obtained after contrast injection to document the tube position for future reference. The tube was secured to the side of the face by a hypoallergenic adherent dressing and looped over the ear.

The patient was transferred to the floor/recovery room following the procedure in a stable condition. Staff was present for the entire procedure.

Intra-Procedure Findings: List all relevant findings.

Immediate Complications: None encountered during or directly after the procedure. List complications if any.

Post-Procedure Plan:

- Start feeding with an initial infusion rate of 5–10 mL per hour, increased as tolerated by 10 mL per shift to reach the goal rate determined by the nutritional support team.
- Feeding via a nasojejunal tube should not routinely be administered as a bolus, as the jejunum does not have the capacity for bolus feeding. Bolus feeding carries a risk of pain, diarrhea, and a dumping-like syndrome.
- Nurse the patient at a 30° angle or higher, if not contraindicated, to decrease the risk of aspiration.
- Keep the catheter always fixed in place. Secure the tube to the patient's nostril and make sure that it is well adhered but not causing pressure on the nostril; localized cyanosis and necrosis can occur if blood flow is impaired.
- When not in use, flush the feeding tube with 30–50 mL of distilled water every 8 h to keep patency.
- Flush the feeding tube with 30–50 mL of distilled water before and after each use to keep patency.
- If the catheter is clogged, flush the catheter with warm or carbonated water.
- Note (jejunal feeding): No aspirate is normally obtainable from the jejunum. The absence of aspirate is not a contraindication to feeding and routine aspiration is not required. If the patient is nauseated or vomiting, the jejunal tube should be aspirated and if an aspirate is obtained, this may indicate that the tip of the tube has migrated to the stomach. Any feed or medication being administered through the tube at this time should be stopped until imaging is performed to document position.

Impression:

- Temporary feeding tube insertion, as described above.
- The patient tolerated the procedure well and left the interventional unit in a stable condition.
- The patient was unstable and the procedure was canceled/terminated prematurely.
- List any other relevant or important information/finding.

References

1. Ciocon JO. Indications for tube feedings in elderly patients. Dysphagia. 1990;5(1):1–5.

2. Ciocon JO, Silverstone FA, Graver LM, Foley CJ. Tube feedings in elderly patients. Indications, benefits, and complications. Arch Intern Med. 1988;148(2):429–33.
3. Pearce CB, Duncan HD. Enteral feeding. Nasogastric, nasojejunal, percutaneous endoscopic gastrostomy, or jejunostomy: its indications and limitations. Postgrad Med J. 2002;78(918):198–204.
4. Spurrier EJ, Johnston AM. Use of nasogastric tubes in trauma patients–a review. J R Army Med Corps. 2008;154(1):10–3.
5. Prabhakaran S, Doraiswamy VA, Nagaraja V, Cipolla J, Ofurum U, Evans DC, et al. Nasoenteric tube complications. Scand J Surg. 2012;101(3):147–55.
6. Taslakian B, Sebaaly MG, Al-Kutoubi A. Patient evaluation and preparation in vascular and interventional radiology: what every interventional radiologist should know (part 1: patient assessment and laboratory tests). Cardiovasc Intervent Radiol. 2016;39(3):325–33.
7. Taslakian B, Sebaaly MG, Al-Kutoubi A. Patient evaluation and preparation in vascular and interventional radiology: what every interventional radiologist should know (part 2: patient preparation and medications). Cardiovasc Intervent Radiol. 2016;39(4):489–99. doi: 10.1007/s00270-015-1239-4. [Epub 2015 Nov 25].

Percutaneous Cecostomy

27

Bedros Taslakian

INTRODUCTION

Described recently, cecostomy is the creation of an opening in the cecum to provide decompression *(decompressive cecostomy)* or to use for antegrade cleansing enema *(lavage cecostomy).* Cecostomy tubes can be placed surgically or percutaneously with either imaging or endoscopic guidance. Anterior intraperitoneal approach is used.

COMMON INDICATIONS [1–6]

- Massive ascites
- Fecal incontinence due to neurologic disease
- Colonic pseudo-obstruction *(Ogilvie syndrome)*
- Cecal volvulus
- Overflow incontinence secondary to colonic obstruction and chronic refractory constipation
- Preanastomotic decompression *(to relieve acute distention of the colon in patients with malignant colonic obstruction before surgical resection)*
- Impending perforation of the colon
- Antegrade placement of colonic stents through a percutaneous route

COMMON CONTRAINDICATIONS [3]

- Respiratory compromise
- Bowel necrosis
- Bowel perforation
- Uncorrectable coagulopathy
- Hemodynamic instability

POSSIBLE COMPLICATIONS [1, 4–6]

- Hemorrhage
- Peritonitis and sepsis
- Wound infection *(peristomal infection), 25–40 %*
- Peristomal leakage
- Intestinal perforation
- Tube malfunction *(displacement, malposition, kinking, clogging)*
- Excessive granulation tissue formation surrounding the tube
- Inadvertent placement into the terminal ileum

PREPROCEDURAL ASSESSMENT AND PLANNING [7, 8]

- History, indications, and physical examination *(Appendix 1* in Chap. 149*)*

B. Taslakian (✉)
Department of Radiology, New York University Langone Medical Center, 660 First Ave, New York, NY 10016, USA
e-mail: btaslakian@gmail.com

B. Taslakian et al. (eds.), *Procedural Dictations in Image-Guided Intervention*,
DOI 10.1007/978-3-319-40845-3_27

- Evaluation of diagnostic imaging studies to determine the relevant anatomy
- Periprocedural management of coagulation status *(Appendices 2* in Chap. 150 *and 3 in* Chap. 151*)*
- Antibiotic prophylaxis: Recommended before and after the procedure [4]
- Imaging modality for guidance: Fluoroscopy, combined CT, or ultrasound/fluoroscopy-based technique for puncture in difficult cases
- Positioning: Supine
- Enteral preparation:
  - Keep patient fasting for 8 h
  - Perform enema with water soluble contrast, if not contraindicated, before the procedure to identify the location of the cecum

PROCEDURE NOTE

Procedure: Percutaneous cecostomy tube insertion
Staff: [_]
Fellow: [_]
Resident: [_]
Clinical Information: Describe history and list indications
Allergies: None known/Allergic to [specify/type of allergy]
Anesthesia: Local anesthesia/conscious sedation
Medications: List any relevant medications used (sedation, antibiotics)
Contrast Material: (_) mL of [type] contrast material
Field: Sterile
Procedure classification: Contaminated
Position: Supine
Monitoring: Intravenous access line was secured and vital signs were continuously monitored by nursing staff/anesthesia team throughout the procedure
Total fluoroscopy time: (_) minutes
Cumulative radiation dose: (_) mGy

Description of Procedure:
The risks, benefits, alternatives, and procedure itself were explained to the patient/patient's Power of Attorney/patient's legal guardian, and informed written consent was obtained. The site of the procedure was identified and marked. Time out was performed to confirm the correct patient, procedure, and site.

The skin of the right lower quadrant was prepped and draped in the usual sterile fashion. Air was insufflated into the cecum under fluoroscopy guidance via a Foley catheter placed through the rectum until adequate cecal distention was achieved. After air insufflation, frontal and lateral views of the lower abdomen were obtained to determine the depth of the anterior cecal wall. The puncture site was determined, local anesthesia was administered and a small skin incision was made. The anterior wall of the cecum was punctured under direct fluoroscopy visualization using a (_)-gauge [type] needle preloaded with an anchor system; the needle position was confirmed by aspiration of air into a syringe and injection of contrast outlining the cecum. The T-fastener was loaded using a (_)-inch [Amplatz stiff/type] guidewire. The needle was removed leaving the guidewire in place. Another puncture was performed to load the second, 3rd and 4th T-fastener (s). The retention sutures were pulled and used to fix the anterior cecal wall to the lower abdominal wall, the tract was dilated to the required size using a (_)-French [type] dilator introduced over the guidewire and then a (_)-French [type] cecostomy tube was inserted. Spot fluoroscopy image was obtained after contrast administration to document the tube position for future reference. The tube was anchored to the skin and attached to an external drainage system and sterile dressing was applied.

The patient was transferred to the floor/recovery room following the procedure in a stable condition. Staff was present for the entire procedure.

Intra-Procedure Findings: List all relevant findings.

Immediate Complications: None encountered during or directly after the procedure. List complications if any.

Post-Procedure Plan:

- Monitor vital sign every 30 min for 2 h, then every 60 min for 2 h.
- Perform serial abdominal examination if peritonitis is suspected.
- Keep tube connected to a gravity drainage bag for decompression.
- Keep the catheter always fixed in place and apply sterile dressing after disinfecting the skin with chlorhexidine-based preparation.
- Flush the catheter twice daily with 30–50 mL of distilled water.
- If the patient complains of skin irritation/breakdown at the insertion site, evaluate for infection and treat with antibiotics as appropriate.
- Inform interventional team if tube malfunction or dislodgment is suspected; peristomal leak or skin irritation occurs, or when abdominal pain is observed.

Impression:

- Fluoroscopy-guided percutaneous cecostomy tube insertion, as described above.
- The patient tolerated the procedure well and left the interventional unit in a stable condition.
- The patient was unstable and the procedure was canceled/terminated prematurely.
- List any other relevant or important information/finding.

References

1. Shin J, Lieberman J, Song H, Brown DB. Percutaneous gastrostomy, percutaneous gastrojejunostomy, jejunostomy, and cecostomy. In: Kandarpa K, Machan L, editors. Handbook of interventional radiologic procedures. 4th ed. Philadelphia: Lippincott Williams & Wilkins; 2011. p. 555–66.
2. Zollikofer CL. Preoperative and palliative colonic stenting. In: Murphy KPJ, Thomson KR, Venbrux AC, Morgan RA, editors. Image-guided interventions. 2nd ed. Philadelphia: Saunders Elsevier; 2014. p. 958–68.
3. Varghese JC, Lee MJ. Percutaneous cecostomy. Semin Interv Radiol. 1996;13(4):351–4.
4. Chait PG, Shlomovitz E, Connolly BL, Temple MJ, Restrepo R, Amaral JG, et al. Percutaneous cecostomy: updates in technique and patient care. Radiology. 2003;227(1):246–50.
5. Itkin M, DeLegge MH, Fang JC, McClave SA, Kundu S, Janne d'Othee B, et al. Multidisciplinary practical guidelines for gastrointestinal access for enteral nutrition and decompression from the Society of Interventional Radiology and American Gastroenterological Association (AGA) Institute, with endorsement by Canadian Interventional Radiological Association (CIRA) and Cardiovascular and Interventional Radiological Society of Europe (CIRSE). J Vasc Interv Radiol. 2011;22 (8):1089–106.
6. Tewari SO, Getrajdman GI, Petre EN, Sofocleous CT, Siegelbaum RH, Erinjeri JP, et al. Safety and efficacy of percutaneous cecostomy/colostomy for treatment of large bowel obstruction in adults with cancer. J Vasc Interv Radiol. 2015;26(2):182–8.
7. Taslakian B, Sebaaly MG, Al-Kutoubi A. Patient evaluation and preparation in vascular and interventional radiology: what every interventional radiologist should know (part 1: patient assessment and laboratory tests). Cardiovasc Intervent Radiol. 2016;39(3):325–33.
8. Taslakian B, Sebaaly MG, Al-Kutoubi A. Patient evaluation and preparation in vascular and interventional radiology: what every interventional radiologist should know (part 2: patient preparation and medications). Cardiovasc Intervent Radiol. 2016;39(4):489–99. doi: 10.1007/s00270-015-1239-4. [Epub 2015 Nov 25].

28 Percutaneous Direct Jejunostomy

Bedros Taslakian

INTRODUCTION

Permanent enteral access can be established surgically or percutaneously with imaging or endoscopic guidance. Direct percutaneous jejunostomy is considered in patients where percutaneous gastrostomy or gastrojejunostomy is not feasible. Primary percutaneous jejunostomy is technically more challenging because of the mobility and collapsibility of the jejunum. Secondary jejunostomy is performed to reestablish a previously created jejunostomy and is performed under fluoroscopy guidance.

COMMON INDICATIONS [1–7]

- Prolonged enteral feeding in patients with gastrectomy and complete gastric outlet or duodenal obstruction
- Prolonged enteral feeding in patients whose stomach is inaccessible for gastrostomy or gastrojejunostomy tube insertion
- Small bowel decompression in cases of bowel obstruction
- To establish access for biliary interventions in patients with biliary-enteric anastomosis

B. Taslakian (✉)
Department of Radiology, New York University Langone Medical Center, 660 First Ave, New York, NY 10016, USA
e-mail: btaslakian@gmail.com

COMMON CONTRAINDICATIONS [4, 7]

- Massive ascites
- Respiratory compromise
- Uncorrectable coagulopathy
- Hemodynamic instability
- Absence of safe access to the jejunum

POSSIBLE COMPLICATIONS [2, 4, 6–8]

- Hemorrhage
- Peristomal leak and skin irritation
- Intraperitoneal leak and peritonitis
- Jejunal volvulus
- Small bowel/colonic perforation
- Wound infection *(peristomal infection)*
- Abdominal wall abscess
- Tube malfunction *(displacement, malposition, kinking, clogging)*
- Laceration of abdominal viscera *(rare)*
- Persistent enterocutaneous fistula after tube removal
- Pressure-induced jejunal mucosal ulcerations

PREPROCEDURAL ASSESSMENT AND PLANNING [4, 7, 9–11]

- History, indications, and physical examination *(Appendix 1* in Chap. 149*)*

B. Taslakian et al. (eds.), *Procedural Dictations in Image-Guided Intervention*,
DOI 10.1007/978-3-319-40845-3_28

- Evaluation of diagnostic imaging studies to determine the relevant anatomy
- Periprocedural management of coagulation status *(Appendices 2* in Chap. 150 *and 3 in* Chap. 151*)*
- Antibiotic prophylaxis: No consensus [4, 9]
- Imaging modality for guidance: Fluoroscopy, combined CT or ultrasound/fluoroscopy-based technique for puncture in difficult cases [4, 7]
- Positioning: Supine

PROCEDURE NOTE

Procedure: Percutaneous direct jejunostomy tube insertion
Staff: [_]
Fellow: [_]
Resident: [_]
Clinical Information: Describe history and list indications
Allergies: None known/Allergic to [specify/type of allergy]
Anesthesia: Local anesthesia/conscious sedation
Medications: List any relevant medications used (sedation, antibiotics)
Contrast Material: (_) mL of [type] contrast material was used for injection
Field: Sterile
Procedure classification: Clean-contaminated
Position: Supine
Monitoring: Intravenous access line was secured and vital signs were continuously monitored by nursing staff/anesthesia team throughout the procedure
Total fluoroscopy time: (_) minutes
Cumulative radiation dose: (_) mGy

Description of Procedure: *(Fluoroscopy-guided Jejunostomy)*
The risks, benefits, alternatives, and procedure itself were explained to the patient/patient's Power of Attorney/patient's legal guardian, and informed written consent was obtained. The site of the procedure was identified and marked. Time out was performed to confirm the correct patient, procedure, and site.

The skin of the abdomen was prepped and draped in the usual sterile fashion. A (_)-French angled [angiographic/type] catheter was introduced through the nostril over a (0.035)-inch [type] guidewire, and directed into the jejunum under direct fluoroscopic guidance. The jejunal loops were dilated by slow saline/contrast injection and the catheter tip was located in a proximal jejunal loop close to the anterior abdominal wall using frontal and lateral fluoroscopic guidance/ultrasound. The distended jejunal loop was punctured using a (_)-gauge [Chiba/type] needle preloaded with a suture anchor. After confirming the intraluminal position of the needle by injecting a small amount of contrast, the T-fastener was delivered to secure the loop against the anterior abdominal wall. A (_)-inch [type] guidewire was then advanced through the needle as far as possible into the jejunum, the tract was serially dilated, and a (_)-French [type] jejunostomy tube was placed over the guidewire under fluoroscopy. Spot fluoroscopy image was obtained after contrast administration to document the tube position for future reference. The tube was anchored to the skin and sterile dressing was applied.

The patient was transferred to the floor/recovery room following the procedure in a stable condition. Staff was present for the entire procedure.

Description of Procedure: *(CT assisted puncture)*
The risks, benefits, alternatives, and procedure itself were explained to the patient/patient's Power of Attorney/patient's legal guardian, and informed written consent was obtained. The site of the procedure was identified and marked. Time out was performed to confirm the correct patient, procedure, and site.

The abdomen was evaluated using CT imaging after placement of a radiopaque marker. The procedure was planned and the skin puncture site was marked using combined information from the location of the target jejunal loop and preliminary CT images. The angle of needle entry and the distance to the jejunal loop were calculated from the planning images.

The skin was prepped and draped in the usual sterile fashion. Local anesthesia was administered. A small skin incision was made. Subsequently, using planning CT information/CT fluoroscopy, a (_)-gauge [Chiba/type] needle preloaded with a suture anchor was advanced along the planned trajectory until the needle tip reached the target jejunal loop. After confirming the intraluminal position of the needle by injecting a small amount of contrast and repeat CT imaging, the T-fastener was delivered to secure the loop against the anterior abdominal wall. Another puncture was performed to load the second T-fastener. A (_)-inch [type] guidewire was then advanced through the needle as far as possible into the jejunum using fluoroscopy guidance, the tract was serially dilated, and a (_)-French [type] jejunostomy tube was placed over the guidewire under fluoroscopy. Spot fluoroscopy image was obtained after contrast administration to document the tube position for future reference. The tube was anchored to the skin and sterile dressing was applied.

The patient was transferred to the floor/recovery room following the procedure in a stable condition. Staff was present for the entire procedure.

Intra-Procedure Findings: List all relevant findings.

Immediate Complications: None encountered during or directly after the procedure. List complications if any.

Post-Procedure Plan [4]:

- Monitor vital sign every 30 min for 2 h, then every 60 min for 2 h.
- Perform serial abdominal examination looking for signs of peritonitis.
- Keep tube clamped or connected to a gravity drainage bag for the first 24 h.
- Start feeding after 24 h post-insertion if the abdominal exam is benign, with an initial infusion rate of 5 mL per hour, increased as tolerated by 5 mL per shift to reach the goal rate determined by the nutritional support team.
- Keep the catheter always fixed in place and apply sterile dressing after disinfecting the skin with chlorhexidine-based preparation.
- When not in use, flush the feeding tube with 30–50 mL of distilled water every 8 h to keep patency.
- Flush the feeding tube with 30–50 mL of distilled water before and after each use to keep patency.
- If the catheter is clogged, flush the catheter with warm or carbonated water.
- If the patient complains of skin irritation or breakdown at the insertion site, evaluate for infection and treat with antibiotics as appropriate.
- Inform interventional team if tube malfunction or malposition/dislodgment is suspected; peristomal leak or skin irritation occurs, or when abdominal pain, feeding intolerance *(vomiting, diarrhea)* is observed.

Impression:

- Percutaneous direct jejunostomy tube insertion, as described above.
- The patient tolerated the procedure well and left the interventional unit in a stable condition.
- The patient was unstable and the procedure was canceled/terminated prematurely.
- List any other relevant or important information/finding.

References

1. Shin J, Lieberman J, Song H, Brown DB. Percutaneous gastrostomy, percutaneous gastrojejunostomy, jejunostomy, and cecostomy. In: Kandarpa K, Machan L, editors. Handbook of interventional radiologic procedures. 4th ed. Philadelphia: Lippincott Williams & Wilkins; 2011. p. 555–66.
2. Power S, Lee MJ. Gastrostomy and gastrojejunostomy. In: Murphy KPJ, Thomson KR, Venbrux AC, Morgan RA, editors. Image-guided interventions. 2nd ed. Philadelphia: Saunders Elsevier; 2014. p. 969–75.
3. van Overhagen H, Ludviksson MA, Laméris JS, Zwamborn AW, Tilanus HW, Dees J, et al. US and fluoroscopic-guided percutaneous jejunostomy: experience in 49 patients. J Vasc Interv Radiol. 2000;11 (1):101–6.
4. Overhagen Hv, Schipper J. Percutaneous jejunostomy. Semin Interv Radiol. 2004;21(3):199–204.
5. Hallisey MJ, Pollard JC. Direct percutaneous jejunostomy. J Vasc Interv Radiol. 1994;5(4):625–32.

6. Cope C, Davis AG, Baum RA, Haskal ZJ, Soulen MC, Shlansky-Goldberg RD. Direct percutaneous jejunostomy: techniques and applications—ten years experience. Radiology. 1998;209(3):747–54.
7. Sparrow P, David E, Pugash R. Direct percutaneous jejunostomy—an underutilized interventional technique? Cardiovasc Interv Radiol. 2008;31(2):336–41.
8. Itkin M, DeLegge MH, Fang JC, McClave SA, Kundu S, Janne d'Othee B, et al. Multidisciplinary practical guidelines for gastrointestinal access for enteral nutrition and decompression from the Society of Interventional Radiology and American Gastroenterological Association (AGA) Institute, with endorsement by Canadian Interventional Radiological Association (CIRA) and Cardiovascular and Interventional Radiological Society of Europe (CIRSE). J Vasc Interv Radiol. 2011;22(8):1089–106.
9. Venkatesan AM, Kundu S, Sacks D, Wallace MJ, Wojak JC, Rose SC, et al. Practice guidelines for adult antibiotic prophylaxis during vascular and interventional radiology procedures. J Vasc Interv Radiol. 2010;21(11):1611–30.
10. Taslakian B, Sebaaly MG, Al-Kutoubi A. Patient evaluation and preparation in vascular and interventional radiology: what every interventional radiologist should know (part 1: patient assessment and laboratory tests). Cardiovasc Intervent Radiol. 2016;39 (3):325–33.
11. Taslakian B, Sebaaly MG, Al-Kutoubi A. Patient evaluation and preparation in vascular and interventional radiology: what every interventional radiologist should know (part 2: patient preparation and medications). Cardiovasc Intervent Radiol. 2016;39(4):489–99. doi: 10.1007/s00270-015-1239-4. [Epub 2015 Nov 25].

29 Percutaneous Feeding Tube Replacement

Bedros Taslakian

INSTRUCTIONS

Percutaneous feeding tubes may require replacement as a result of breakage, occlusion, or dislodgment. Preventive maintenance includes elective change at a fixed period of time (usually 3–6 months). Gastrojejunostomy tubes may require more frequent maintenance and replacement because of their smaller diameter and complicated configurations. Image-guided exchange of a feeding tube is a simple and safe procedure, performed under fluoroscopy guidance without the need for de novo puncture.

COMMON INDICATIONS [1–4]

- Breakage, occlusion, or dislodgment of previously inserted feeding tube
- Inadvertent tube removal if a mature tract is present
- Preventive maintenance
- Infected and colonized feeding tubes
- Exchange for a longer tube in case of significant post-procedural weight gain

B. Taslakian (✉)
Department of Radiology, New York University Langone Medical Center, 660 First Ave, New York, NY 10016, USA
e-mail: btaslakian@gmail.com

COMMON CONTRAINDICATIONS

- Uncorrectable coagulopathy *(bleeding risk is low after tract maturation)*
- Hemodynamic instability

POSSIBLE COMPLICATIONS [1–3]

- Peristomal infection
- Peristomal leakage *(rare when a mature tract is present)*
- Tube malfunction *(displacement, breakage, and occlusion)*

PREPROCEDURAL ASSESSMENT AND PLANNING [5, 6]

- History, indications, and physical examination *(Appendix 1* in Chap. 149*)*
- Evaluation of diagnostic imaging studies to determine the tube location and relevant anatomy
- Periprocedural management of coagulation status *(Appendices 2* in Chap. 150 *and 3 in* Chap. 151*)*
- Antibiotic prophylaxis: Not routinely recommended unless infection is present
- Imaging modality for guidance: Fluoroscopy
- Positioning: Supine

B. Taslakian et al. (eds.), *Procedural Dictations in Image-Guided Intervention*,
DOI 10.1007/978-3-319-40845-3_29

PROCEDURE NOTE

Procedure: Percutaneous gastrostomy/gastrojejunostomy/jejunostomy tube replacement
Staff: [_]
Fellow: [_]
Resident: [_]
Clinical Information: Describe history and list indications
Allergies: None known/Allergic to [specify/type of allergy]
Anesthesia: Local anesthesia/conscious sedation
Medications: List any relevant medications used (sedation, antibiotics)
Contrast Material: (_) mL of [type] contrast material was used for injection
Field: Sterile
Procedure classification: Clean-contaminated
Position: Supine
Monitoring: Intravenous access line was secured and vital signs were continuously monitored by nursing staff/anesthesia team throughout the procedure.
Total fluoroscopy time: (_) minutes
Cumulative radiation dose: (_) mGy

Description of Procedure *(old tube is in place and a guidewire can be advanced):*
The risks, benefits, alternatives, and procedure itself were explained to the patient/patient's Power of Attorney/patient's legal guardian, and informed written consent was obtained. The site of the procedure was identified and marked. Time out was performed to confirm the correct patient, procedure, and site.

The skin and the previously inserted tube were prepped and draped in the usual sterile fashion. Under fluoroscopy visualization, a (0.035)-inch [type] guidewire was inserted through the old tube and its tip was looped in the stomach/jejunum. Once there was a sufficient length of guidewire within the system, a new (_)-French self-retaining [type/pigtail] feeding tube [assembly with a plastic stiffener] was introduced over the guidewire to a satisfactory depth. The guidewire/and stiffener was/were removed after sliding the tube over the guidewire into the stomach/jejunum. Following this, contrast material was injected through the tube at the end of the procedure to confirm optimal position and ensure that all side holes were placed correctly. The feeding tube was locked, anchored to the skin, and capped. Sterile dressing was applied.

The patient was transferred to the floor/recovery room/discharged home following the procedure in a stable condition. Staff was present for the entire procedure.

Description of Procedure *(old gastrostomy tube is dislodged or totally occluded preventing guidewire insertion):*
The risks, benefits, alternatives, and procedure itself were explained to the patient/patient's Power of Attorney/patient's legal guardian, and informed written consent was obtained. The site of the procedure was identified and marked. Time out was performed to confirm the correct patient, procedure, and site.

The old tube was removed. The skin of the left subcostal area and epigastrium were prepped and draped in the usual sterile fashion. Under fluoroscopy visualization, a (0.035)-inch [hydrophilic/type] guidewire, and a (_)-French [type] catheter were advanced gently through the mature tract into the stomach. Once there was a sufficient length of guidewire within the stomach, a new (_)-French self-retaining [type/pigtail] gastrostomy tube [assembly with a plastic stiffener] was introduced over the guidewire to a satisfactory depth. The guidewire/and stiffener was/were removed after sliding the tube over the guidewire into the stomach. Following this, contrast material was injected through the tube at the end of the procedure to confirm optimal position and ensure that all side holes were placed correctly. The gastrostomy tube was locked, anchored to the skin, and capped. Sterile dressing was applied.

The patient was transferred to the floor/recovery room/discharged home following the procedure in a stable condition. Staff was present for the entire procedure.

Description of Procedure *(old gastrojejunostomy tube is dislodged or totally occluded preventing guidewire insertion):*

The risks, benefits, alternatives, and procedure itself were explained to the patient/patient's Power of Attorney/patient's legal guardian, and informed written consent was obtained. The site of the procedure was identified and marked. Time out was performed to confirm the correct patient, procedure, and site.

The old tube was removed. The skin of the left subcostal area and epigastrium were prepped and draped in the usual sterile fashion. Under fluoroscopy visualization, a (0.035)-inch [hydrophilic/type] guidewire, and a (_)-French [type] catheter were advanced gently through the mature tract into the stomach. Once there was a sufficient length of guidewire within the stomach, a (_)-French peel-away vascular sheath was advanced over the guidewire into the stomach. Through the sheath, a (_) French [angled/type] catheter was used for manipulation and a (0.035)-inch [type] guidewire was advanced into the small intestine beyond the ligament of Treitz followed by the catheter. Subsequently, the initial guidewire was replaced for a (_)-inch [stiff/type] exchange guidewire, and its tip was looped within the jejunum. A (_)-French tapered dilator was introduced over the guidewire to dilate the tract to the required size, after which a (_)-French [pigtail-retained/type] dual-lumen gastrojejunostomy feeding tube was advanced and positioned under fluoroscopy guidance. Completion spot fluoroscopy image was obtained after contrast administration to document the tube position for future reference. The tube was anchored to the skin and sterile dressing was applied.

The patient was transferred to the floor/recovery room/discharged home following the procedure in a stable condition. Staff was present for the entire procedure.

Intra-Procedure Findings: List all relevant findings.

Immediate Complications: None encountered during or directly after the procedure. List complications if any.

Post-Procedure Plan [1, 2]:

- Monitor vital sign every 30 min for 2 h.
- Perform serial abdominal examination if peritonitis is suspected.
- Start feeding post-insertion if the abdominal exam is benign and the tract was mature with no detected complications during the procedure.
- Keep the catheter always fixed in place and apply sterile dressing after disinfecting the skin with chlorhexidine-based preparation.
- When not in use, flush the feeding tube with 30–50 mL of distilled water every 8 h to keep patency.
- Flush the feeding tube with 30–50 mL of distilled water before and after each use to keep patency.
- If the catheter is clogged, flush the catheter with warm or carbonated water.
- If the patient complains of skin irritation or breakdown at the insertion site, evaluate for infection and treat with antibiotics as appropriate.
- Inform interventional team if tube malfunction or malposition/dislodgment is suspected; peristomal leak or skin irritation occurs, or when abdominal pain, feeding intolerance *(vomiting, diarrhea)* is observed.

Impression:

- Percutaneous gastrostomy/jejunostomy/gastrojejunostomy tube replacement, as described above.
- The patient tolerated the procedure well and left the interventional unit in stable condition.
- The patient was unstable and the procedure was canceled/terminated prematurely.
- List any other relevant or important information/finding.

References

1. Shin J, Lieberman J, Song H, Brown DB. Percutaneous gastrostomy, percutaneous gastrojejunostomy, jejunos-

tomy, and cecostomy. In: Kandarpa K, Machan L, editors. Handbook of interventional radiologic procedures. 4th ed. Philadelphia: Lippincott Williams & Wilkins; 2011. p. 555–66.
2. Power S, Lee MJ. Gastrostomy and gastrojejunostomy. In: Murphy KPJ, Thomson KR, Venbrux AC, Morgan RA, editors. Image-guided interventions. 2nd ed. Philadelphia: Saunders Elsevier; 2014. p. 969–75.
3. Itkin M, DeLegge MH, Fang JC, McClave SA, Kundu S, Janne d'Othee B, et al. Multidisciplinary practical guidelines for gastrointestinal access for enteral nutrition and decompression from the Society of Interventional Radiology and American Gastroenterological Association (AGA) Institute, with endorsement by Canadian Interventional Radiological Association (CIRA) and Cardiovascular and Interventional Radiological Society of Europe (CIRSE). J Vasc Interv Radiol. 2011;22(8):1089–106.
4. Lyon SM, Pascoe DM. Percutaneous gastrostomy and gastrojejunostomy. Semin Interv Radiol. 2004;21 (3):181–9.
5. Taslakian B, Sebaaly MG, Al-Kutoubi A. Patient evaluation and preparation in vascular and interventional radiology: what every interventional radiologist should know (part 1: patient assessment and laboratory tests). Cardiovasc Intervent Radiol. 2016;39(3):325–33.
6. Taslakian B, Sebaaly MG, Al-Kutoubi A. Patient evaluation and preparation in vascular and interventional radiology: what every interventional radiologist should know (part 2: patient preparation and medications). Cardiovasc Intervent Radiol. 2016;39(4):489–99. doi: 10.1007/s00270-015-1239-4. [Epub 2015 Nov 25].

30 Percutaneous Gastrojejunostomy

Bedros Taslakian

INTRODUCTION

Percutaneous gastrojejunostomy *(transgastric jejunostomy)* is the creation of an artificial access to the jejunum through a puncture of the stomach wall under fluoroscopic guidance. Using double lumen tubes will allow gastric decompression and the administration of specific medication only absorbed by the stomach through the gastric lumen with simultaneous jejunal feeding in patients with high risk of gastroesophageal reflux or aspiration. The procedure can be performed as an initial feeding tube placement *(primary gastrojejunostomy)* or by converting a previously inserted mature gastrostomy to gastrojejunostomy *(conversion gastrojejunostomy)*. To facilitate placement of the gastrojejunostomy, puncture of the stomach is performed in the direction of the pylorus.

COMMON INDICATIONS [1–5]

- Decompression of gastroenteric contents with concurrent jejunal tube feeding in patients who cannot tolerate gastric feeding as a result of:
  - Gastroparesis
  - Gastric outlet or duodenal obstruction
  - Gastric or duodenal fistula
  - Proximal small bowel obstruction
  - Severe gastroesophageal reflux
  - Recurrent aspiration pneumonia
- Prevention of gastroesophageal reflux in cases of disrupted gastrointestinal tract

COMMON CONTRAINDICATIONS [1–3]

- Absence of a safe access to the stomach *(hepatosplenomegaly, interposed colon)*
- Hemodynamic instability and respiratory compromise
- Uncorrectable coagulopathy
- Anatomic distortion due to prior gastric surgery
- Recent gastrointestinal bleed from peptic ulcer disease with visible vessel or from esophageal varices
- Gastric varices
- Massive ascites *(higher risk for bacterial peritonitis, uncontrolled bleeding, impaired tract maturation)*
- Ventriculoperitoneal shunts *(higher risk of ascending meningitis)*
- Morbidly obese patients with a panniculus *(higher risk of tube dislodgment)*
- Inflammatory, neoplastic, or infectious involvement of the abdominal or gastric wall
- Active peritonitis
- Intestinal ischemia

B. Taslakian (✉)
Department of Radiology, New York University Langone Medical Center, 660 First Ave, New York, NY 10016, USA
e-mail: btaslakian@gmail.com

B. Taslakian et al. (eds.), *Procedural Dictations in Image-Guided Intervention*,
DOI 10.1007/978-3-319-40845-3_30

POSSIBLE COMPLICATIONS [1–3]

- Hemorrhage
- Peritonitis
- Peristomal infection, leakage, and skin irritation
- Fungal colonization or infection of tube leading to malfunction/degradation
- Prolonged ileus and feeding intolerance
- Tube malfunction, *53–84 %*; due to retrograde tube migration into the stomach *(27–42 %)*, kinking, clogging, and/or occlusion *(3.5–35 %)*
- Aspiration pneumonia
- Laceration of the spleen, liver, or pancreas
- Gastroenteric fistula
- Gastrointestinal perforation
- Gastric ulcer
- Necrotizing fasciitis
- Mortality

PREPROCEDURAL ASSESSMENT AND PLANNING [6–8]

- History, indications, and physical examination *(Appendix 1* in Chap. 149*)*
- Evaluation of diagnostic imaging studies to determine the relevant anatomy
- Periprocedural management of coagulation status *(Appendices 2* in Chap. 150 *and 3 in* Chap. 151*)*
- Antibiotic prophylaxis: No consensus for "push" technique [6] *(Appendices 4* in Chap. 152 *and 5* in Chap. 153*)*
- Imaging modality for guidance: Fluoroscopy, combined CT, or ultrasound/fluoroscopy-based technique for puncture in difficult cases [1, 2]
- Positioning: Supine
- Enteral preparation [1, 2]:
  – Keep patient fasting for 8 h *(required)*
  – Unless contraindicated, insert a nasogastric tube the evening before the procedure to decompress the stomach and help insufflation of air during the procedure
  – Unless contraindicated, administer 200 mL of dilute barium suspension via the nasogastric tube 12 h before the procedure to outline the colon

PROCEDURE NOTE

Procedure: Percutaneous gastrojejunostomy tube insertion
Staff: [_]
Fellow: [_]
Resident: [_]
Clinical Information: Describe history and list indications
Allergies: None known/Allergic to [specify/type of allergy]
Anesthesia: Local anesthesia/Conscious sedation
Medications: List any relevant medications used (sedation, antibiotics)
Contrast Material: (_) mL of [type] contrast material was used for injection
Field: Sterile
Procedure classification: Clean-contaminated
Position: Supine
Monitoring: Intravenous access line was secured and vital signs were continuously monitored by nursing staff/anesthesia team throughout the procedure
Total fluoroscopy time: (_) minutes
Cumulative radiation dose: (_) mGy

Description of Procedure:

The risks, benefits, alternatives, and procedure itself were explained to the patient/patient's Power of Attorney/patient's legal guardian, and informed written consent was obtained. The site of the procedure was identified and marked. Time out was performed to confirm the correct patient, procedure, and site.

Preliminary CT/ultrasound examination was performed to mark the edge of the left hepatic lobe and identify the spleen and transverse colon.

The skin of the left subcostal area and epigastrium was prepped and draped in the usual sterile fashion. Air was insufflated into the stomach via the previously inserted nasogastric tube until adequate gastric distention was achieved. After air insufflation, frontal and lateral views of the upper abdomen were obtained to determine the depth of the anterior gastric wall and location of the transverse colon. The puncture site was determined, local anesthesia was administered and a small skin incision was made. The anterior wall of the distal gastric body was punctured under direct fluoroscopy visualization using a (_) gauge [type] needle preloaded with an anchor system; the needle position was confirmed by aspiration of air into a syringe and injection of contrast outlining gastric rugal folds. The T-fastener was loaded and used to fix the anterior gastric wall to the abdominal wall. Another puncture was performed to load the second, third and fourth T-fastener(s). After gastropexy was achieved, the anterior fixed gastric wall was punctured using the needle and position was confirmed by injecting contrast. A (0.035)-inch [J-tipped/stiff/type] guidewire was inserted and looped in the stomach. Once there was a sufficient length of guidewire within the stomach, the tract was dilated up to the required size using (_)-French dilator(s) and a (_) French peel-away sheath was advanced. Through the sheath, a (_) French [Torqueable/type] catheter was used for manipulation and a (0.035)-inch [type] guidewire was advanced into the small intestine beyond the ligament of Treitz followed by the catheter. Subsequently, the initial guidewire was replaced for a (_)-inch [stiff/type] exchange guidewire, and its tip was looped within the jejunum. A (_)-French [pigtail-retained/type] dual-lumen gastrojejunostomy feeding tube was advanced over the guidewire into the jejunum. Completion fluoroscopy image was obtained after contrast administration to document the tube position for future reference. The sheath was removed and the tube was locked and anchored to the skin. The gastrostomy port was attached to a gravity drainage bag. Sterile dressing was applied.

The patient was transferred to the floor/recovery room/discharged home following the procedure in a stable condition. Staff was present for the entire procedure.

Intra-Procedure Findings: List all relevant findings.

Immediate Complications: None encountered during or directly after the procedure. List complications if any.

Post-Procedure Plan [1, 2]:

- Monitor vital sign every 30 min for 2 h then every 60 min for 2 h.
- Perform serial abdominal examination if peritonitis is suspected.
- Start feeding in the **jejunal lumen** post-insertion if the abdominal exam is benign, with an initial infusion rate of 5 mL per hour, increased as tolerated by 5 mL per shift to reach the goal rate determined by the nutritional support team.
- Gastric lumen should be clamped or connected to a gravity drainage bag *(cannot be used)* for the first 24 h.
- The gastric lumen can be used 24 h post-insertion if the abdominal exam is benign.
- Keep the catheter always fixed in place and apply sterile dressing after disinfecting the skin with chlorhexidine-based preparation.
- When not in use, flush the feeding tube with 30–50 mL of distilled water every 8 h to keep patency.
- Flush the feeding tube with 30–50 mL of distilled water before and after each use to keep patency.
- If the catheter is clogged, flush the catheter with warm or carbonated water.
- If the patient complains of skin irritation or breakdown at the insertion site, evaluate for infection and treat with antibiotics as appropriate.
- Inform interventional team if tube malfunction or malposition/dislodgment is suspected; peristomal leak or skin irritation occurs, or when abdominal pain or feeding intolerance *(vomiting, diarrhea)* is observed.

Impression:

- Percutaneous gastrojejunostomy tube insertion, as described above.
- The patient tolerated the procedure well and left the interventional unit in a stable condition.

- The patient was unstable and the procedure was canceled/terminated prematurely.
- List any other relevant or important information/finding.

References

1. Shin J, Lieberman J, Song H, Brown DB. Percutaneous gastrostomy, percutaneous gastrojejunostomy, jejunostomy, and cecostomy. In: Kandarpa K, Machan L, editors. Handbook of interventional radiologic procedures. 4th ed. Philadelphia: Lippincott Williams & Wilkins; 2011. p. 555–66.
2. Power S, Lee MJ. Gastrostomy and gastrojejunostomy. In: Murphy KPJ, Thomson KR, Venbrux AC, Morgan RA, editors. Image-guided interventions. 2nd ed. Philadelphia: Saunders Elsevier; 2014. p. 969–75.
3. Itkin M, DeLegge MH, Fang JC, McClave SA, Kundu S, Janne d'Othee B, et al. Multidisciplinary practical guidelines for gastrointestinal access for enteral nutrition and decompression from the Society of Interventional Radiology and American Gastroenterological Association (AGA) Institute, with endorsement by Canadian Interventional Radiological Association (CIRA) and Cardiovascular and Interventional Radiological Society of Europe (CIRSE). J Vasc Interv Radiol. 2011;22(8):1089–106.
4. Lyon SM, Pascoe DM. Percutaneous gastrostomy and gastrojejunostomy. Semin Interv Radiol. 2004;21 (3):181–9.
5. Shin KH, Shin JH, Song HY, Yang ZQ, Kim JH, Kim KR. Primary and conversion percutaneous gastrojejunostomy under fluoroscopic guidance: 10 years of experience. Clin Imaging. 2008;32(4):274–9.
6. Venkatesan AM, Kundu S, Sacks D, Wallace MJ, Wojak JC, Rose SC, et al. Practice guidelines for adult antibiotic prophylaxis during vascular and interventional radiology procedures. J Vasc Interv Radiol. 2010;21(11):1611–30.
7. Taslakian B, Sebaaly MG, Al-Kutoubi A. Patient evaluation and preparation in vascular and interventional radiology: what every interventional radiologist should know (part 1: patient assessment and laboratory tests). Cardiovasc Intervent Radiol. 2016;39(3):325–33.
8. Taslakian B, Sebaaly MG, Al-Kutoubi A. Patient evaluation and preparation in vascular and interventional radiology: what every interventional radiologist should know (part 2: patient preparation and medications). Cardiovasc Intervent Radiol. 2016;39(4):489–99. doi: 10.1007/s00270-015-1239-4. [Epub 2015 Nov 25].

31 Percutaneous Gastrostomy

Bedros Taslakian

INTRODUCTION

Percutaneous gastrostomy is the creation of an artificial access into the stomach through a small incision in the abdominal wall. The transabdominal "push" technique has a lower rate of peristomal infection when compared to transoral "pull" technique.

COMMON INDICATIONS [1–4]

- Inadequate oral intake due to dysphagia with high risk of aspiration *(stroke or neurologic disorders)*
- Inadequate oral intake due to dysphagia resulting from esophageal, head, neck, and mediastinal malignancies
- Traumatic or iatrogenic esophageal leaks for diversion
- Small bowel pathology leading to intestinal malabsorption *(e.g., inflammatory bowel disease, radiation enteritis, scleroderma)*
- Long-term supplementary enteral nutrition *(e.g., cystic fibrosis, significant burns, eating disorders, profound depression)*

COMMON CONTRAINDICATIONS [1–4]

- Absence of a safe access to the stomach *(hepatosplenomegaly, interposed colon)*
- Hemodynamic instability and respiratory compromise
- Uncorrectable coagulopathy
- Anatomic distortion due to prior gastric surgery
- Recent gastrointestinal bleed from peptic ulcer disease with visible vessel or from esophageal varices
- Gastric varices
- Massive ascites *(has higher risk for bacterial peritonitis, uncontrolled bleeding, and impaired tract maturation)*
- Severe gastroesophageal reflux *(consider gastrojejunostomy or jejunostomy)*
- Ventriculoperitoneal shunts *(higher risk of ascending meningitis)*
- Morbidly obese patients with a panniculus *(higher risk of tube dislodgment)*
- Inflammatory, neoplastic, or infectious involvement of the abdominal or gastric wall
- Active peritonitis
- Intestinal ischemia

POSSIBLE COMPLICATIONS [1–4]

- Hemorrhage. *0–2.5 %*
- Peritonitis, *0.5–1.3 %*

B. Taslakian (✉)
Department of Radiology, New York University
Langone Medical Center, 660 First Ave, New York,
NY 10016, USA
e-mail: btaslakian@gmail.com

B. Taslakian et al. (eds.), *Procedural Dictations in Image-Guided Intervention*,
DOI 10.1007/978-3-319-40845-3_31

- Peristomal infection, *5.4–30 %*
- Stomal leakage and skin irritation, *1–2 %*
- Fungal colonization or infection of tube leading to malfunction/degradation
- Prolonged ileus, *1–2 %*
- Tube malfunction *(displacement, malposition, kinking, clogging)*
- Buried bumper syndrome, *0.3–2.4 %*
- Aspiration pneumonia, *0.3–1 %*
- Laceration of the spleen, liver or pancreas
- Gastroenteric fistula, *0.3–6.7 %*
- Gastrointestinal perforation
- Gastric ulcer, *0.3–1.2 %*
- Necrotizing fasciitis, *rare*
- Implantation of head and neck cancer at the stoma site when "pull" technique is used, *rare*
- Mortality, *0–2.1 %*

PREPROCEDURAL ASSESSMENT AND PLANNING [5–7]

- History, indications, and physical examination *(Appendix 1* in Chap. 149*)*
- Evaluation of diagnostic imaging studies to determine the relevant anatomy
- Periprocedural management of coagulation status *(Appendices 2* in Chap. 150 *and 3* in Chap. 151*)*
- Antibiotic prophylaxis: Recommended for "pull" technique, no consensus for "push" technique [5] *(Appendices 4* in Chap. 152 *and 5* in Chap. 153*)*
- Imaging modality for guidance: Fluoroscopy, combined CT or ultrasound/fluoroscopy-based technique for puncture in difficult cases [1, 2]
- Positioning: Supine
- Enteral preparation [1, 2]:
  - Keep patient fasting for 8 h *(required)*
  - Unless contraindicated, insert a nasogastric tube the evening before the procedure to decompress the stomach and help insufflation of air during the procedure
  - Unless contraindicated, administer 200 mL of dilute barium suspension via the nasogastric tube 12 h before the procedure to outline the colon

PROCEDURE NOTE

Procedure: Percutaneous gastrostomy tube insertion
Staff: [_]
Fellow: [_]
Resident: [_]
Clinical Information: Describe history and list indications
Allergies: None known/Allergic to [specify/type of allergy]
Anesthesia: Local anesthesia/conscious sedation
Medications: List any relevant medications used (sedation, antibiotics)
Contrast Material: (_) mL of [type] contrast material was used for injection
Field: Sterile
Procedure classification: Clean-contaminated
Position: Supine
Monitoring: Intravenous access line was secured and vital signs were continuously monitored by nursing staff/anesthesia team throughout the procedure
Total fluoroscopy time: (_) minutes
Cumulative radiation dose: (_) mGy

Description of Procedure *(Push-type gastrostomy):*

The risks, benefits, alternatives, and procedure itself were explained to the patient/patient's Power of Attorney/patient's legal guardian, and informed written consent was obtained. The site of the procedure was identified and marked. Time out was performed to confirm the correct patient, procedure, and site.

Preliminary CT/ultrasound examination was performed to mark the edge of the left hepatic lobe and identify the spleen and transverse colon.

The skin of the left subcostal area and epigastrium was prepped and draped in the usual sterile fashion. Air was insufflated into the stomach via the previously inserted nasogastric tube until adequate gastric distention was achieved. After air insufflation, frontal and lateral views of the upper abdomen were obtained to determine the depth of the anterior gastric wall and location of the transverse colon. The puncture site was determined, local anesthesia was administered and a small skin incision was made. The anterior wall of the distal body of the stomach was punctured under direct fluoroscopy visualization using a (_) gauge [type] needle preloaded with an anchor system; the needle position was confirmed by aspiration of air into a syringe and injection of contrast outlining gastric rugal folds. The T-fastener was loaded and used to fix the anterior gastric wall to the abdominal wall. Another puncture was performed to load the second, third, and fourth T-fastener(s). After gastropexy was achieved, the anterior fixed gastric wall was punctured using the needle and position was confirmed by injection of contrast. A (0.035)-in. [J-tipped/stiff/type] guidewire was inserted and looped in the stomach. The tract was dilated up to the required size using (_)-French dilator(s). A (_)-French [pigtail-retained/type] gastrostomy feeding tube assembly with the metal stiffener was introduced over the guidewire to a satisfactory depth. The stiff trocar of the tube was left within the shaft until the catheter was advanced just beyond the abdominal and anterior gastric wall. The guidewire and stiffener were removed after advancing the tube into the stomach. Completion fluoroscopy image was obtained after contrast administration to document the tube position for future reference. The tube was locked, anchored to the skin, and attached to a gravity drainage bag. Sterile dressing was applied.

The patient was transferred to the floor/recovery room following the procedure in a stable condition. Staff was present for the entire procedure.

Description of Procedure *(Pull-type gastrostomy/per-oral image guided gastrostomy):*

The risks, benefits, alternatives, and procedure itself were explained to the patient/patient's Power of Attorney/patient's legal guardian, and informed written consent was obtained. The site of the procedure was identified and marked. Time out was performed to confirm the correct patient, procedure and site.

Preliminary CT/ultrasound examination was performed to mark the edge of the left hepatic lobe and identify the spleen and transverse colon.

The skin of the left subcostal area and epigastrium was prepped and draped in the usual sterile fashion. Air was insufflated into the stomach via the previously inserted nasogastric tube until adequate gastric distention was achieved. After air insufflation, frontal and lateral views of the upper abdomen were obtained to determine the depth of the anterior gastric wall and location of the transverse colon. The puncture site was determined, local anesthesia was administered and a small skin incision was made. The anterior wall of the distal body of the stomach was punctured under direct fluoroscopy visualization using a (_) gauge [type] needle; the needle position was confirmed by aspiration of air into a syringe and injection of contrast outlining gastric rugal folds.

Following this, a (_)-in. [type] guidewire was advanced into the stomach, the needle was removed and a (_)-French [type/angiographic] catheter was inserted over the guidewire and used to cross the gastroesophageal junction from the stomach to the esophagus. The catheter and guidewire were advanced in a retrograde direction and pulled out of the patient's mouth. The guidewire was exchanged for a (_)-in. [exchange-length/type] guidewire, and a (_)-French mushroom-retained gastrostomy tube was introduced coaxially, passing in an antegrade direction down the mouth into the esophagus and out the anterior abdominal wall. The tapered tip of the gastrostomy tube was then cut to the desired length. The tube was affixed externally at the skin and sterile dressing was applied. Completion fluoroscopy image was obtained after contrast administration to document the tube position for future reference. The tube was attached to a gravity drainage bag.

The patient was transferred to the floor/recovery room following the procedure in a stable condition. Staff was present for the entire procedure.

Description of Procedure *(Button gastrostomy device insertion):*

The risks, benefits, alternatives, and procedure itself were explained to the patient/patient's Power of Attorney/patient's legal guardian, and informed written consent was obtained. The site of the procedure was identified and marked. Time out was performed to confirm the correct patient, procedure, and site.

Preliminary CT/ultrasound examination was performed to mark the edge of the left hepatic lobe and identify the spleen and transverse colon.

The skin of the left subcostal area and epigastrium was prepped and draped in the usual sterile fashion. Air was insufflated into the stomach via the previously inserted nasogastric tube until adequate gastric distention was achieved. After air insufflation, frontal and lateral views of the upper abdomen were obtained to determine the depth of the anterior gastric wall and location of the transverse colon. The puncture site was determined, local anesthesia was administered and a small skin incision was made. The anterior wall of the distal body of the stomach was punctured under direct fluoroscopy visualization using a (_) gauge [type] needle preloaded with an anchor system; the needle position was confirmed by aspiration of air into a syringe and injection of contrast outlining gastric rugal folds. The T-fastener was loaded and used to fix the anterior gastric wall to the abdominal wall. Another puncture was performed to load the second, third, and fourth T-fasteners. After gastropexy was achieved, the anterior fixed gastric wall was punctured at the center point of the square-configured gastropexy, using a (_)-gauge needle and position was confirmed by injection of contrast. A (_)-in. [Amplatz super-stiff/type] guidewire was inserted through the needle and coiled in the stomach. Accurate measurement of gastrostomy tract length was performed using an angioplasty balloon catheter. The angioplasty balloon catheter was passed over the super-stiff guide wire into the stomach. The balloon was inflated manually in the gastric lumen and pulled back until it abutted the anterior gastric wall. The balloon catheter was held between the operator's thumb and forefinger at the skin insertion site. The angioplasty balloon was deflated and the catheter was withdrawn over the guide wire until the balloon was fully visible. The balloon was then reinflated and the tract length was measured.

The angioplasty balloon catheter was then reinserted into the gastrostomy tract and inflated to dilate it/A (_)-French dilator was inserted over the guidewire for complete dilation of the gastrostomy tract.

Following adequate dilatation of the tract, a (_)-French dilator was passed through the center of a (_)-French, (_)-cm long button gastrostomy catheter which was inserted over the super-stiff guidewire with use of abundant lubrication. After placing the button gastrostomy, the guide wire was removed and the dilator was pulled back so that its tip resided in the proximal lumen of the gastrostomy button. Contrast material was injected to confirm intra-gastric position and the button balloon was inflated with (_) mL of normal saline solution. Sterile dressing was applied.

The patient was transferred to the floor/recovery room following the procedure in a stable condition. Staff was present for the entire procedure.

Intra-Procedure Findings: List all relevant findings.

Immediate Complications None encountered during or directly after the procedure. List complications if any.

Post-Procedure Plan [1, 2]:

- Monitor vital sign every 30 min for 2 h then every 60 min for 2 h.
- Perform serial abdominal examination looking for signs of peritonitis.
- Keep the tube clamped or connected to a gravity drainage bag for the first 24 h.
- Start feeding 24 h post-insertion if the abdominal exam is benign, with an initial infusion rate of 10 mL per hour, increased as

tolerated by 10 mL per shift to reach the goal rate determined by the nutritional support team.

- Remove T-fasteners 7 days after the procedure.
- Keep the catheter always fixed in place and apply sterile dressing after disinfecting the skin with chlorhexidine-based preparation.
- When not in use, flush the feeding tube with 30–50 mL of distilled water every 8 h to keep patency.
- Flush the feeding tube with 30–50 mL of distilled water before and after each use to keep patency.
- If the catheter is clogged, flush the catheter with warm or carbonated water.
- If the patient complains of skin irritation or breakdown at the insertion site, evaluate for infection and treat with antibiotics as appropriate.
- Inform interventional team if tube malfunction or malposition/dislodgment is suspected; peristomal leak or skin irritation occurs, or when abdominal pain or feeding intolerance *(vomiting, diarrhea)* is observed.

Impression:

- Fluoroscopy-guided percutaneous gastrostomy tube insertion, as described above.
- The patient tolerated the procedure well and left the interventional unit in a stable condition.
- The patient was unstable and the procedure was canceled/terminated prematurely.
- List any other relevant or important information/finding.

References

1. Shin J, Lieberman J, Song H, Brown DB. Percutaneous gastrostomy, percutaneous gastrojejunostomy, jejunostomy, and cecostomy. In: Kandarpa K, Machan L, editors. Handbook of interventional radiologic procedures. 4th ed. Philadelphia: Lippincott Williams & Wilkins; 2011. p. 555–66.
2. Power S, Lee MJ. Gastrostomy and gastrojejunostomy. In: Murphy KPJ, Thomson KR, Venbrux AC, Morgan RA, editors. Image-guided interventions. 2nd ed. Philadelphia: Saunders Elsevier; 2014. p. 969–75.
3. Itkin M, DeLegge MH, Fang JC, McClave SA, Kundu S, Janne d'Othee B, et al. Multidisciplinary practical guidelines for gastrointestinal access for enteral nutrition and decompression from the Society of Interventional Radiology and American Gastroenterological Association (AGA) Institute, with endorsement by Canadian Interventional Radiological Association (CIRA) and Cardiovascular and Interventional Radiological Society of Europe (CIRSE). J Vasc Interv Radiol. 2011;22(8):1089–106.
4. Lyon SM, Pascoe DM. Percutaneous gastrostomy and gastrojejunostomy. Semin Intervent Radiol. 2004;21 (3):181–9.
5. Venkatesan AM, Kundu S, Sacks D, Wallace MJ, Wojak JC, Rose SC, et al. Practice guidelines for adult antibiotic prophylaxis during vascular and interventional radiology procedures. J Vasc Interv Radiol. 2010;21(11):1611–30.
6. Taslakian B, Sebaaly MG, Al-Kutoubi A. Patient evaluation and preparation in vascular and interventional radiology: what every interventional radiologist should know (part 1: patient assessment and laboratory tests). Cardiovasc Intervent Radiol. 2016;39(3): 325–33.
7. Taslakian B, Sebaaly MG, Al-Kutoubi A. Patient evaluation and preparation in vascular and interventional radiology: what every interventional radiologist should know (part 2: patient preparation and medications). Cardiovasc Intervent Radiol. 2016;39(4):489–99. doi: 10.1007/s00270-015-1239-4. [Epub 2015 Nov 25].

Part V

Non-vascular Interventional Procedures: Hepatobiliary-Liver

Introduction by Karen T. Brown, Section Reviewer

Three types of procedure are commonly performed that involve insertion of needles, applicators, or catheters into the liver parenchyma either for diagnosis; needle biopsy or treatment; ablation of a tumor or drainage of an abscess. In fact, core needle biopsy of the liver is one of the most common biopsy procedures performed, either nontargeted, to diagnose underlying generalized liver disease or stage cirrhosis, or targeted to diagnose a liver mass. Primary liver cancer [hepatocellular carcinoma, HCC] rarely requires biopsy when appropriate imaging features are present in a patient with typical clinical history (hepatitis B or C, for example) but may be indicated in cases without classic clinical/ imaging presentation, or for investigational studies. Many transplant centers prefer to avoid biopsy in cases with appropriate clinical and imaging findings so as to avoid the possibility of tumor seeding. The main complication after liver biopsy is bleeding and, fortunately, significant bleeding though uncommon can be easily treated by embolization of the offending vessel.

Alcohol ablation of HCC [percutaneous ethanol injection therapy, PEIT] is the most "low-tech" way of treating HCC. It is used in the well-circumscribed HCC because the tumor is "soft" compared to the background cirrhotic liver, and small tumors are often encapsulated. This is not the case for most metastatic tumors, and as a result PEIT has limited applicability for metastatic disease. PEIT is limited to treatment of small HCC, and often requires repeat treatment, making it less cost-effective. For this reason, PEIT has largely been supplanted by other ablative methods. Thermal ablation of liver tumors can be performed with a variety of devices causing either extreme cooling (cryoablation) or heating (radio-frequency or microwave ablation) resulting in tumor cell death. Irreversible electroporation uses high-voltage direct current to create multiple holes in the tumor cell membrane that irreversibly damages the cell's homeostatic mechanism, leading to instant cell death. These percutaneous methods all require percutaneous placement of one or more applicators and are subject to individual limitations. These techniques are appropriately used in tumors <3 cm in size; beyond that the risk of recurrence can be 30 % or higher. It is best if the individual practitioner becomes familiar with the performance of one or two devices, understanding the mechanism of action, stated size of the "kill zone," factors that may limit this "kill zone," risk for collateral damage with the device, and general limitations. Using a devise repeatedly and becoming familiar with its use will likely result in the most successful outcome for the patient.

Liver abscesses often result from ascending infection via the portal venous system from a bowel source and can occur in patients with appendicitis, diverticulitis, or some other infectious problem involving the digestive system from the pancreas to the rectum. When a patient presents with a classic liver abscess, a source should always be sought, reviewing the cross sectional imaging carefully for signs of diverticulitis or other infectious conditions that may require eventual treatment. Catheter drainage of a classic liver abscess may be prolonged and on some occasions operative drainage may be required. Infected bilomas (often referred to as liver abscesses) on the other hand typically occur in patients with a contaminated biliary tree, typically after a bilio-enteric bypass, with bile stasis, often secondary to obstruction from recurrent cancer, development of an anastomotic stricture, or even a stone. Treatment is also by catheter drainage of the "abscess" but, once again, the cause should be sought. Often the catheter will begin draining bile and a catheter study will identify the site of obstruction that can subsequently be treated by dilation, in the case of a benign anastomotic stricture, stent placement in the case of recurrent malignancy, or stone removal [see Part VII]. If the cause of the infected biloma is not treated, the abscess is likely to recur after catheter removal. The other "abscess" in the liver that can be treated percutaneously is a hydatid cyst. These are caused by the parasitic tapeworm Echinococcus and are very rare in the continental United States and unusual in Northern Europe. Endemic areas include the Mediterranean countries, the Middle East, southern parts of South America, Australia, New Zealand, and southern parts of Africa. Treatment is often medical with the administration of benzimidazole, but in some cases these are treated with the puncture, aspiration, injection, and re-aspiration (PAIR) technique. Special description of this technique is beyond the scope of this book and interested practitioners should seek information elsewhere.

Section Chapters

Core Biopsy of the Liver

32

Bedros Taslakian

INTRODUCTION

The primary intent of liver biopsy is diagnosing specific hepatic diseases, rejection following liver transplantation and differentiating primary malignancy from distant metastasis and benign lesions. Histopathologic grading of hepatic fibrosis offers prognostic information in hepatitis, cirrhosis, non-alcoholic fatty liver disease, and primary biliary cirrhosis, although non-invasive imaging techniques are being developed that may replace the need for biopsy to characterize and grade cirrhosis in the near future. Percutaneous needle biopsy, associated with low morbidity and mortality, provides sufficient sample for tissue diagnosis and cores can be obtained for research purposes and histology.

COMMON INDICATIONS

Targeted Liver Biopsy [1–4]

- Diagnosis of a suspicious hepatic lesion
- Hepatic lesion in cirrhotic liver without the typical imaging features of hepatocellular carcinoma on appropriately performed imaging tests
- Confirmation of suspected metastatic disease to the liver, for staging
- Core biopsy for markers, histopathology, molecular studies

Random Liver Biopsy [3–5]

- Diagnosis of specific hepatic diseases
- Grading and staging of infectious and non-infectious hepatitis
- Guidance regarding treatment of chronic hepatitis
- Evaluation in cases of autoimmune hepatitis
- Diagnosis of hemochromatosis, with quantitative analysis of iron levels
- Diagnosis of Wilson's disease, with quantitative analysis of copper levels
- Evaluation of abnormal liver function tests in case of negative or inconclusive serologic testing
- Evaluation of abnormal liver function tests and rejection following orthotopic liver transplantation
- Evaluation of abnormal liver function tests in patients status post stem cell transplant
- Evaluation of the donor liver before transplantation
- Obtaining tissue for culture in patients with fever of unknown origin
- Clinical presentation of acute liver failure

B. Taslakian (✉)
Department of Radiology, New York University Langone Medical Center, 660 First Ave, New York, NY 10016, USA
e-mail: btaslakian@gmail.com

B. Taslakian et al. (eds.), *Procedural Dictations in Image-Guided Intervention*,
DOI 10.1007/978-3-319-40845-3_32

COMMON CONTRAINDICATIONS [1–4, 6, 7]

- Uncooperative or unwilling patients
- Hemodynamic instability
- Lack of a safe route to the liver or target lesion
- Significant coagulopathy that cannot be adequately corrected
- Suspected hydatid cyst *(increased risk of anaphylactic shock)*
- Typical features of hepatocellular carcinoma on appropriately performed imaging tests
- Some consider ascites a relative contraindication

POSSIBLE COMPLICATIONS [2–4, 6, 7]

- Transient, localized discomfort, and pain at the biopsy site
- Vasovagal reaction
- Subcapsular or intrahepatic hematomas
- Major hemorrhage requiring embolization, *0.3–3.3 %*
- Pneumothorax requiring chest tube placement, *0.5 %*
- Unintended organ injury
- Bile duct injury leading to bile leak
- Malignant seeding along the needle tract, *extremely rare: 0–3.4 %*
- Mortality, *extremely rare*

PREPROCEDURAL ASSESSMENT AND PLANNING [8–10]

- History, indications, and physical examination *(Appendix 1* in Chap. 149*)*
- Evaluation of diagnostic imaging studies to determine the location of the lesion and relevant anatomy
- Periprocedural management of coagulation status *(Appendices 2* in Chap. 150 *and 3* in Chap. 151*)*
- Antibiotic prophylaxis: Not routinely recommended [8]
- Imaging modality for guidance: CT, CT fluoroscopy, ultrasound, MRI
- Positioning: Usually supine

PROCEDURE NOTE

Procedure: Percutaneous random liver biopsy/biopsy of hepatic lesion
Staff: [_]
Fellow: [_]
Resident: [_]
Clinical Information: Describe history and list indications
Allergies: None known/Allergic to [specify/type of allergy]
Anesthesia: Local anesthesia/conscious sedation
Medications: List any relevant medications used (sedation)
Field: Sterile
Procedure classification: Clean
Position: Supine/Left lateral decubitus/Right lateral decubitus/Oblique
Monitoring: Intravenous access line was secured and vital signs were continuously monitored by nursing staff/anesthesia team throughout the procedure
Cumulative radiation dose: (_) mGy

Description of Procedure *(Targeted Liver Biopsy):*
The risks, benefits, alternatives, and the procedure itself were explained to the patient/patient's Power of Attorney/patient's legal guardian, and informed written/verbal consent was obtained. Time out was performed to confirm the correct patient, procedure, and site.

The liver was evaluated using CT imaging after placement of a radiopaque [marker/grid]/ultrasound showing a (_) cm round/oval/irregular lesion in segment (_). The procedure was planned and the skin puncture site was marked using combined information from the location of the lesion and preliminary CT/ultrasound images. The angle of needle entry and the distance to the lesion were calculated from the planning images.

The skin was prepped and draped in the usual sterile fashion. Local anesthesia was administered. A small skin incision was made. Subsequently, using planning CT information/using CT fluoroscopy/under direct ultrasound visualization, a (_)-gauge [type] needle guide was advanced along the planned trajectory until the needle tip reached the target lesion, confirmed by imaging. (_) samples were obtained using the coaxial technique, placed in a formalin solution and sent for histopathological evaluation. The biopsy track was plugged using gelfoam pledgets while withdrawing the reference needle. Following this, immediate completion CT/ultrasound images were obtained at the level of the biopsy site.

The patient was transferred to the floor/recovery room following the procedure in a stable condition. Staff was present for the entire procedure.

Description of Procedure *(Random Liver Biopsy):*

The risks, benefits, alternatives, and the procedure itself were explained to the patient/patient's Power of Attorney/patient's legal guardian, and informed written/verbal consent was obtained. Time out was performed to confirm the correct patient, procedure, and site.

The liver was evaluated using CT imaging after placement of a radiopaque [marker/grid]/ultrasound. The procedure was planned and the skin puncture site was marked using combined information from the preliminary CT/ultrasound images and the location of the left/right hepatic lobe. The angle of needle entry and the distance to the liver parenchyma were calculated from the planning images.

The skin was prepped and draped in the usual sterile fashion. Local anesthesia was administered. A small skin incision was made. Subsequently, using planning CT information/under direct ultrasound visualization, a (_)-gauge [type] needle guide was advanced along the planned trajectory until the needle tip seen within the liver parenchyma, confirmed by imaging. (_) samples were obtained using the coaxial technique, placed in a formalin solution and sent for histopathological evaluation. The biopsy track was plugged using gelfoam pledgets while the reference needle was being withdrawn. Following this, immediate completion CT/ultrasound images were obtained at the level of the biopsy site.

The patient was transferred to the floor/recovery room/discharged home following the procedure in a stable condition. Staff was present for the entire procedure.

Intra-Procedure Findings: List all relevant findings.

Immediate Complications: None encountered during or directly after the procedure. List complications if any.

Post-Procedure Plan [2, 6]:

- Follow-up histopathology results.
- Obtain an upright chest X-ray to rule out pneumothorax if pleural space transgression is suspected.
- When post-biopsy images show no complications:
  - Observe the patient in the recovery room for 2–4 h.
  - Complete bed rest for 1–2 h; bathroom use with assistance.
  - Monitor vital signs in the recovery room every 15 min for 1 h, then every 30 min for 2 h, then every hour.
  - If the patient's condition deteriorates, or significant abdominal pain develops, obtain images of the abdomen/pelvis.
- Discharge instructions:
  - Abstain from strenuous activities for 3 days.
  - Visit the nearest emergency room promptly if any chest pain, shortness of breath, or severe abdominal pain develops.
  - Start clear liquid diet for the first hour, then regular diet thereafter if tolerated and no complications occur.

Impression:

- Percutaneous core biopsy of hepatic lesion/the liver, as described above.

- The patient tolerated the procedure well and left the interventional unit in a stable condition.
- The patient was unstable and the procedure was canceled/terminated prematurely.
- List any other relevant or important information/finding.

References

1. Purysko AS, Remer EM, Coppa CP, Leão Filho HM, Thupili CR, Veniero JC. LI-RADS: a case-based review of the new categorization of liver findings in patients with end-stage liver disease. Radiographics. 2012;32(7):1977–95.
2. Silverman SG, Segal D. Abdominal biopsies. In: Kandarpa K, Machan L, editors. Handbook of interventional radiologic procedures. 4th ed. Philadelphia: Lippincott Williams & Wilkins; 2011. p. 516–26.
3. Bravo AA, Sheth SG, Chopra S. Liver biopsy. N Engl J Med. 2001;344(7):495–500.
4. Thabet A. Liver biopsy. In: Gervais DA, Sabharwal T, editors. Interventional radiology procedures in biopsy and drainage. Heidelberg: Springer; 2011. p. 11–20.
5. Miraglia R, Luca A, Gruttadauria S, Minervini MI, Vizzini G, Arcadipane A, et al. Contribution of transjugular liver biopsy in patients with the clinical presentation of acute liver failure. Cardiovasc Intervent Radiol. 2006;29(6):1008–10.
6. Percutaneous biopsy. In: Burke CT, Dixon RG, Mauro MA, Murphy KPJ, Thomson KR, Venbrux AC, Zollikofer CL, editors. High yield imaging: interventional. Philadelphia: Saunders Elsevier; 2010. p. 384–5.
7. Gupta S, Wallace MJ, Cardella JF, Kundu S, Miller DL, Rose SC. Quality improvement guidelines for percutaneous needle biopsy. J Vasc Interv Radiol. 2010;21(7):969–75.
8. Venkatesan AM, Kundu S, Sacks D, Wallace MJ, Wojak JC, Rose SC, et al. Practice guidelines for adult antibiotic prophylaxis during vascular and interventional radiology procedures. J Vasc Interv Radiol. 2010;21(11):1611–30.
9. Taslakian B, Sebaaly MG, Al-Kutoubi A. Patient evaluation and preparation in vascular and interventional radiology: what every interventional radiologist should know (part 1: patient assessment and laboratory tests). Cardiovasc Intervent Radiol. 2016;39(3):325–33.
10. Taslakian B, Sebaaly MG, Al-Kutoubi A. Patient evaluation and preparation in vascular and interventional radiology: what every interventional radiologist should know (part 2: patient preparation and medications). Cardiovasc Intervent Radiol. 2016;39(4):489–99. doi: 10.1007/s00270-015-1239-4. [Epub 2015 Nov 25].

Hepatic Tumor Ablation

33

Nadim Muallem

Abbreviations

CT	Computed tomography
MWA	Microwave ablation
PCA	Patient-controlled anesthesia
PET	Positron emission tomography
RFA	Radiofrequency ablation

INTRODUCTION

Percutaneous image-guided ablation of liver tumors was one of the earliest practiced form of ablation and extensively reported upon in the literature. It has the largest body of evidence supporting its use, in some cases with outcomes approaching those from surgical resection [1, 2]. Radiofrequency ablation (RFA), microwave ablation (MWA), and cryoablation can be used with the choice depending on availability, operator preference, and experience. There is also the long existing option of chemical ablation using percutaneous ethanol (or acetic acid) injection via 20 or 22 gauge needle commonly used for primary hepatic tumors [3].

N. Muallem (✉)
Department of Radiology, Division of Interventional Radiology, Memorial Sloan Kettering Cancer Center, 1275 York Ave, New York, NY 10065, USA
e-mail: nadim.muallem@gmail.com; muallemn@mskcc.org

COMMON INDICATIONS [1–6]

Patient selection for ablation should be carefully performed by a multidisciplinary team.

- Primary liver disease: Very early or early stage hepatocellular carcinoma according to the Barcelona Clinic Liver Cancer (BCLC) classification in medically inoperable patients or in patients refusing surgical resection. Ideally, patients with primary liver disease should have either a single tumor less than 5 cm or no more than three tumors less than 3 cm each with no evidence of vascular invasion or extrahepatic spread, ECOG 0 and Child-Pugh class A or B. When used for solitary tumors in combination with hepatic arterial embolization these parameters can be expanded [5].
- Metastatic liver disease: *Predominantly from colorectal but also from other primary cancers including neuroendocrine and breast cancer,* limited to the liver or with limited extrahepatic metastases that are deemed

B. Taslakian et al. (eds.), *Procedural Dictations in Image-Guided Intervention*,
DOI 10.1007/978-3-319-40845-3_33

curable, in medically inoperable patients or in patients refusing surgical resection. Sometimes used as "test of time" in patients whose disease course or biology of disease is unclear at the time of presentation [6]. Number of lesions ideally less than 5. Tumor sizes less than 3 cm.

- Primary or secondary liver tumors with hepatic recurrence after previous resection, chemotherapy, or radiation therapy.
- Diffuse liver metastases *(number of lesions 5)* responding to systemic chemotherapy with a single lesion showing no response to systemic therapy is accepted by many but a survival benefits remains unproven.

COMMON CONTRAINDICATIONS [1–4]

Absolute contraindications:

- Significant coagulopathy that cannot be adequately corrected
- Tumors <1 cm from main biliary duct due to risk of thermal damage
- Pre-existing intrahepatic biliary ductal dilatation
- Bacteremia or active infections

Relative contraindications:

- Subcapsular tumors, initially thought to pose a risk of seeding [7], but later shown to be small if not similar to noncapsular lesions [3, 8]. The risk is minimized by use of cautery, approaching through normal liver parenchyma and extension of ablation zone to include capsule as long as protective measures are taken [3]. In addition the "no touch" technique described by Patel can be used [9].
- Bilioenteric anastomosis is a risk factor for hepatic abscess formation following ablation. This might be minimized by use of an antibiotic prophylaxis regimen that covers anaerobic bacteria beginning before and continuing for at least 10 days after the procedure [10, 11].
- Anatomic limitations with the target lesion adjacent to vital organs. If close to lung or gastrointestinal tract, consider using hydro/pneumodissection.
- Proximity to gallbladder and risk of iatrogenic cholecystitis

Depending on the ablation technique used:

- Patients with cardiac pacemakers and implantable defibrillators *(recommended to be deactivated during RFA, not applicable for cryoablation and chemical ablation, slightly better safety profile for MWA but precaution should also be taken*) [12].
- Metal implants *(small implants can potentially heat up due to the circuit created in RFA but are unlikely to be affected in MWA and certainly not affected in cryoablation and chemical ablation).*

POSSIBLE COMPLICATIONS [3, 4, 13, 14]

Minor complications:

- Post-ablation syndrome, *32–58 %*
- Asymptomatic pleural effusion and/or asymptomatic perihepatic fluid

Major Complications (overall rare 2.2–5.7 %):

- Hemorrhage, *most common <2 %;* Commonly intraperitoneal, but can be subcapsular or intralesional
- Liver abscess, *0.3–2 %;* Risk factors include prior biliary interventions including bilioenteric anastomosis, sphincterotomy, stent across sphincter, and presence of pneumobilia. Risk factors when present may be mitigated by use of prophylactic antibiotics.
- Injury to bile ducts leading to biliary strictures, bilomas, and cholecystitis - more common with central lesions
- Pleural complications from treatment of dome lesions *(pneumothorax, hemothorax, large effusion requiring drainage)*
- Injury to adjacent organs either from direct penetration or thermal injury, such as colonic perforation, *0.1–0.3 %.* Risk decreased by

maintaining minimum distance of 1 cm from ablation margin or by performing pneumodissection with air or CO_2 or hydrodissection with distilled water *(avoid saline in RFA since ionic solutions may conduct current)*. Risk is also less when procedures performed with CT rather than ultrasound guidance. Injury to lung can be avoided by inducing pneumothorax artificially and transiently during the ablation procedure. Ablation margins can also be monitored by use of temperature-sensing thermocouples placed near organs at risk.

- Skin burns, *<1 %;* typically at skin puncture site in all thermal ablation modalities or at grounding pad site in case of RFA
- Tumor seeding, *0.5–3 %;* believed by some to be minimized by cauterization of the ablation tract. If needle is suboptimally positioned, limited ablation could be performed to treat the immediate surrounding tissue prior to repositioning.
- Venous thrombosis: portal vein, *1.7 %;* hepatic vein, *1.4 %;* risk increased with reduced portal flow *(cirrhosis)*
- Hepatic infarction
- Arterio-venous fistulas, *rare*
- Cryoshock; rare systemic inflammatory response syndrome typically after large-volume liver cryoablation, mediated by cytokine production consisting of symptoms including hypotension, respiratory compromise, multi-organ failure, and disseminated intravascular coagulation.
- Liver failure, *rare*
- Mortality, *0–1.4 %;* secondary to intestinal perforation, portal vein thrombosis, liver failure, septic shock, or massive hepatic hemorrhage

PREPROCEDURAL ASSESSMENT AND PLANNING [1–4, 11]

- History, indications, and physical examination *(Appendix 1* in Chap. 149*)*
- Evaluation of diagnostic imaging studies *(Multiphase CT, PET-CT, MRI)* to assess indications and radiologically stage the tumor, and to determine the location of the lesion, the relevant anatomy, and develop trajectory route. This should be within 30 days of treatment and will serve as a baseline for follow-up.
- Histopathologic diagnosis of the lesion is often obtained before the ablation, unless the lesion fulfills clinical diagnostic criteria for hepatocellular carcinoma or the patient has a history of malignancy and develops a new liver lesion that is typical for a metastasis. If there is any doubt as to the nature of the lesion, biopsy should be performed. In selected cases when thought necessary, biopsy and ablation can be performed at the same setting, but in such cases immediate review of the biopsy specimen should be available. Baseline tumor markers in case of hepatocellular carcinoma can be helpful in assessing response and monitoring for recurrence.
- Periprocedural management of coagulation status *(Appendices 2* in Chap. 150 *and 3* in Chap. 151*)*
- Antibiotic prophylaxis: No consensus. However, in the presence of bilioenteric anastomosis where patients are at a significantly increased risk of intrahepatic abscess formation, prophylactic antibiotic use before and after the procedure for up to 10 days with coverage of enteric organisms is strongly advocated [10, 11].
- Imaging modality for guidance: CT, CT fluoroscopy, PET-CT, MRI, ultrasound
- Positioning: Most commonly supine; however, prone or lateral decubitus positioning can provide access to more difficult to reach lesions. Place appropriate supportive cushioning in areas with important neurovascular bundles *(to avoid injury)* and dispersive grounding pads in a well-prepared *(shaved)* area to allow good contact with the skin.

PROCEDURE NOTE [15]

Procedure: Radiofrequency/Microwave/Cryo/Alcohol/Acetic Acid ablation of segment [_] liver lesion
Staff: [_]
Fellow: [_]
Resident: [_]
Clinical Information: Specify existing diagnosis; describe history, and list indications
Allergies: No known allergic disorders/Allergic to [specify/type of allergy]
Anesthesia: Local anesthesia with conscious sedation/General anesthesia
Medications: List any relevant medications used (local anesthesia, sedation, antibiotics)
Field: Sterile
Procedure classification: Clean
Position: Supine/Prone/Left lateral decubitus/Right lateral decubitus/Oblique
Monitoring: Intravenous access line was secured and vital signs were continuously monitored by nursing staff/anesthesia team throughout the procedure.
Cumulative radiation dose: (_) mGy

Description of Procedure:

The risks, benefits, alternatives, and procedure itself were explained to the patient/patient's Power of Attorney/patient's legal guardian, and informed written consent was obtained. The site of the procedure was identified and marked. Time out was performed to confirm the correct patient, procedure and site.

Pre-procedure planning imaging (CT/ultrasound/MRI) was obtained and used to calculate the approach and distance to target lesion. One (or more) site of needle entry was/were determined and marked on the skin. The marked location(s) and surrounding skin area was/were prepped and draped in the usual sterile fashion.

Subcutaneous and liver capsular infiltration of local anesthetic was performed using a thin gauge needle.

A small skin incision was made at the marked site(s). Under image guidance, one (or more) applicator probe(s) was/were advanced along the planned trajectory and positioned into the target. No (one or more) repositioning was/were required. Ablation was performed by following the manufacturer's instructions until the target temperature was achieved and/or the perilesional edema was visualized/the iceball was visualized to encase the targeted lesion within an acceptable margin.

Probe positioning, repositioning, and ablation protocol are detailed below.

After completion, the tract of the liver parenchyma was cauterized using low-power application while withdrawing the radiofrequency electrode/microwave antenna from the liver.

After probe removal, immediate post-procedure CT images were obtained at the level of the lesion to evaluate the ablation zone, potential collateral damage, and detect complications.

The patient was transferred to the inpatient unit/recovery room/discharged home following the procedure in a stable condition.

Preprocedural Planning and Approach:
Target organ: Liver
Laterality: Right/Left
Reference scan/image for ablation target: CT dated [Month]/[Day]/[Year]. Series [series number] image [image number]
Target lesion size: Long axis: (_) cm, short axis: (_) cm
Specific target location: Specify liver segment (s), relationship to sensitive structures (diaphragm, vessels, nerves)
Target lesion appearance: Solid/Partial/Cavitary/Cystic
Patient position: Prone/Supine/Decubitus/Other
Approach: Posterior/Anterior/Lateral/Right/Left
Imaging guidance: Intra-procedural CT/CT-fluoroscopy/PET-CT/Ultrasound/MRI performed with/without multiplanar reconstruction confirming adequate positioning of the applicator within the target lesion.

Ablation Technique:
Ablation modality: Radiofrequency/Microwave/Cryoablation/Chemical
Ablation device: Specify device brand/model, type, length, gauge, active length, single, multiple, tined etc.…

Number of applicators: If more than one applicator, specify locations; if single applicator with more than one repositioning, also specify different locations

Number of ablations: (number) overlapping/nonoverlapping ablations *(list protocol details below)*

Protocol used: Device specific, but typically, power/wattage, duration, temperature achieved, and location if multiple probes or repositionings were needed

For RFA *(single applicator—in this case the Valleylab/Covidien Cool-tip RFA probe—with multiple repositioning and overlapping ablation)*

Ablation #1: Cooled, 3 min, 57 °C/Applicator #1 Posterior margin

Ablation #2: Cooled, 6 min, 58 °C/Applicator #1 Superior margin proximal

Ablation #3: …

For Cryoablation (with multiple applicators)

Ablation #1: 10 min freeze, 6 min active thaw, 10 min freeze, 8 min passive thaw, at 100 %, -() degrees Celsius/Applicator #1: superior margin

Ablation #2: 10 min freeze, 6 min active thaw, 10 min freeze, 8 min passive thaw, at 80 %, -() degrees Celsius/Applicator #2 inferior margin

Ablation #3: …

For Alcohol ablation

Ablation #1: 1–20 ml of anhydrous alcohol injected/22 g or 20 g needle, segment 5 lesion

Ablation #2: …

Post-Ablation Findings:

Post-ablation imaging: CT/MRI/ultrasound

Follow-up chest radiographs: (Immediate and) 2 h post-procedure chest radiographs *(if transpleural ablation was performed)*

Post-procedural imaging **(CT/MRI/PET-CT)** was performed at the level of the target lesion. The ablation zone could not be clearly delineated/was clearly outlined consisting of ice ball formation/decreased parenchymal attenuation encompassing the target tumor in its entirety with adequate margins extending (_) mm beyond the periphery of the lesion predictive of complete ablation/inadequate margins at the (_) border requiring additional targeted ablation *(complement with additional details as needed)*.

Immediate Complications: None encountered during or directly after the procedure. List complications if any.

Post-Procedure Plan [1, 2, 4, 10, 11, 16]

- Transfer patient to recovery unit.
- Observe in recovery unit for 2–4 h with continuous vital sign and pulse oximeter monitoring.
- Complete bedrest and NPO for the duration of observation. Maintain patient recumbent with the puncture site down.
- Post-procedure pain control as needed *(consider PCA, and admission for pain control if needed).*
- Administer supplemental nasal oxygen as needed *(O_2 saturation less than baseline/patient still sedated…)*
- If the patient's condition deteriorates during observation, suspect bleeding primarily and obtain cross sectional imaging of the abdomen immediately. Do not disregard other potential complications as well.
- If the patient underwent prior hepatic surgical intervention, bilioenteric anastomosis or biliary interventions: Prophylactic oral antibiotics for up to 10 days are recommended; however, the patient will still need to be followed closely in the post-operative setting even after finishing his antibiotic course.
- *Discharge Instructions:*
  - Abstain from strenuous activities for 3 days.
  - Visit the nearest emergency room promptly if any fevers, chills develop or worsening pain not controlled by oral medication.
  - Start clear liquid diet for the first hour after discharge from observation, then regular diet thereafter if tolerated and no complications occur.
  - Take prescribed pain medications as needed.
  - Take prescribed antibiotic medications as prescribed.

- *Follow-Up Imaging* [16]:
  - Obtain a new baseline multiphase contrast-enhanced CT scan or MRI within 4–6 weeks of the procedure.
  - PET-CT also helps in early detection of recurrence but should be performed after at least a 4 week interval to avoid false-positive results from inflammatory reaction. Most surveillance schedules suggest follow-up imaging every 3 months for the first 2 years.

Impression:

- Percutaneous radiofrequency/microwave/cryo/chemical ablation of segment (_) liver lesion, as described above.
- The patient tolerated the procedure well and left the interventional unit in a stable condition.
- List any other relevant or important information/finding/complications.
- The procedure was canceled/abandoned.
- The primary operator (specify name) was present for the entire/key parts of the procedure.

References

1. Lencioni R, Bozzi E, Crocetti L, Bartolozzi C. Energy-based ablation of hepatocellular cancer. In: Mauro M, Murphy K, Thomson K, Venbrux A, Morgan R, editors. Image-guided interventions. 2nd ed. Philadelphia: Saunders Elsevier; 2014. p. 1038–46e2.
2. Solbiati L. Energy-based ablation of other liver lesions. In: Mauro M, Murphy K, Thomson K, Venbrux A, Morgan R, editors. Image-guided interventions. 2nd ed. Philadelphia: Saunders Elsevier; 2014. p. 1047–54e2.
3. Ahmed M, Goldberg SN. Liver ablation. In: Hong K, Georgiades CS, editors. Percutaneous tumor ablation strategies and techniques. New York: Thieme Medical Publishers; 2010. p. 52–72.
4. Lencioni R, Crocetti L. Hepatic tumor ablation. In: Kandarpa K, Machan L, editors. Handbook of interventional radiologic procedures. 4th ed. Philadelphia: Lippincott Williams & Wilkins; 2011. p. 536–48.
5. Elnekave E, Erinjeri JP, Brown KT, Thornton RH, Petre EN, Maybody M, et al. Long-term outcomes comparing surgery to embolization-ablation for treatment of solitary HCC <7 cm. Ann Surg Oncol. 2013;20(9):2881–6.
6. Livraghi T, Solbiati L, Meloni F, Ierace T, Goldberg SN, Gazelle GS. Percutaneous radiofrequency ablation of liver metastases in potential candidates for resection: the "test-of-time approach.". Cancer. 2003;97(12):3027–35.
7. Llovet JM, Vilana R, Brú C, Bianchi L, Salmeron JM, Boix L, et al. Increased risk of tumor seeding after percutaneous radiofrequency ablation for single hepatocellular carcinoma. Hepatology. 2001;33(5): 1124–9.
8. Poon RT-P, Ng KK-C, Lam C-M, Ai V, Yuen J, Fan S-T. Radiofrequency ablation for subcapsular hepatocellular carcinoma. Ann Surg Oncol. 2004;11 (3):281–9.
9. Patel PA, Ingram L, Wilson ID, Breen DJ. No-touch wedge ablation technique of microwave ablation for the treatment of subcapsular tumors in the liver. J Vasc Interv Radiol. 2013;24(8):1257–62.
10. Venkatesan AM, Kundu S, Sacks D, Wallace MJ, Wojak JC, Rose SC, et al. Practice guideline for adult antibiotic prophylaxis during vascular and interventional radiology procedures. J Vasc Interv Radiol. 2010;21(11):1611–30.
11. Hoffmann R, Rempp H, Schmidt D, Pereira PL, Claussen CD, Clasen S. Prolonged antibiotic prophylaxis in patients with bilioenteric anastomosis undergoing percutaneous radiofrequency ablation. J Vasc Interv Radiol. 2012;23(4):545–51.
12. Skonieczki BD, Wells C, Wasser EJ, Dupuy DE. Radiofrequency and microwave tumor ablation in patients with implanted cardiac devices: Is it safe? Eur J Radiol. 2011;79(3):343–6.
13. Kim K, Thomas S. Complications of image-guided thermal ablation of liver and kidney neoplasms. Semin Intervent Radiol. 2014;31:138–48.
14. Erinjeri JP, Clark TWI. Cryoablation: mechanism of action and devices. J Vasc Interv Radiol. 2010;21(8 Suppl):S187–91.
15. Goldberg SN, Grassi CJ, Cardella JF, Charboneau JW, Dodd GD 3rd, Dupuy DE, et al. Image-guided tumor ablation: standardization of terminology and reporting criteria. J Vasc Interv Radiol. 2009;20(7 Suppl): S377–90.
16. Boas FE, Do B, Louie JD, Kothary N, Hwang GL, Kuo WT, et al. Optimal Imaging surveillance schedules after liver-directed therapy for hepatocellular carcinoma. J Vasc Interv Radiol. 2015;26 (1):69–73.

Liver Abscess Drainage

34

Bedros Taslakian

INTRODUCTION

Liver abscess may be caused by bacteria, fungi, or parasites. Pyogenic liver abscesses do not commonly arise spontaneously but rather occur as a result of ascending infection from sources such as diverticulitis or appendicitis. They can also be seen when there is contamination of the biliary tree with organisms and some degree of bile duct obstruction. Appropriate investigations should be carried out so that the underlying cause can be identified and treated. Pyogenic abscesses are the most common hepatic collections amenable to percutaneous drainage. It is usually performed under ultrasound or CT guidance. Fluoroscopy can be combined with ultrasound or CT to assist with catheter positioning in difficult cases.

COMMON INDICATIONS [1–9]

- Pyogenic liver abscess
- Infected hydatid cyst not responding to medical therapy >2 weeks
- Amebic abscess not responding to medical therapy
- Peripheral amebic abscess *(more prone to rupture)*
- Infected biloma

B. Taslakian (✉)
Department of Radiology, New York University Langone Medical Center, 660 First Ave, New York, NY 10016, USA
e-mail: Btaslakian@gmail.com

COMMON CONTRAINDICATIONS [1–3]

Most contraindications are relative.

- Significant coagulopathy that cannot be adequately corrected
- Sterile collections, such as hepatic hematoma *(risk of superimposed infection)*
- Lack of a safe pathway to access the collection
- Procedure requires transgression of pleura *(risk of pneumothorax, empyema, fistula, and pleural effusion)*
- Suspected hydatid (echinococcus) cyst *(increased risk of anaphylactic shock due to intra-peritoneal leakage; pre-treatment is required before drainage)*
- Malignant abscess requiring lifelong drainage
- Hemodynamic instability
- Inability of the patient to be adequately positioned for the procedure
- Pregnancy in cases when imaging guidance involves ionizing radiation

POSSIBLE COMPLICATIONS [1–3]

- Major hemorrhage, *1 %*; intraperitoneal hemorrhage, subcapsular, or parenchymal hematoma, hemobilia
- Bacteremia, *2–5 %*
- Septic shock, *1–2 %*
- Pleural transgression requiring intervention, *1 %*
- Bowel transgression with or without fistula formation or peritonitis, *1 %*

B. Taslakian et al. (eds.), *Procedural Dictations in Image-Guided Intervention*,
DOI 10.1007/978-3-319-40845-3_34

- Catheter malfunction, due to kinking, blockage, and dislodgment
- Pericatheter leak
- Mortality

PREPROCEDURAL ASSESSMENT AND PLANNING

- History, indications, and physical examination *(Appendix 1* in Chap. 149*)*
- Evaluation of diagnostic imaging studies to determine the location of the abscess, its size and relevant anatomy
- Periprocedural management of coagulation status *(Appendices 2* in Chap. 150 *and 3* in Chap. 151*)*
- Antibiotic prophylaxis: Routinely recommended [10]
- Imaging modality for guidance: CT, CT fluoroscopy, ultrasound, combined fluoroscopy with CT, or ultrasound [1, 3]
- Positioning: Oblique, lateral decubitus, or supine

PROCEDURE NOTE

Procedure: Percutaneous drainage of liver abscess
Staff: [_]
Fellow: [_]
Resident: [_]
Clinical Information: Describe history and list indications
Allergies: None known/Allergic to [specify/type of allergy]
Anesthesia: Local anesthesia/conscious sedation
Medications: List any relevant medications used (sedation, antibiotics)
Field: Sterile
Procedure classification: Dirty
Position: Supine/Left lateral decubitus/Right lateral decubitus/Oblique
Monitoring: Intravenous access line was secured and vital signs were continuously monitored by nursing staff/anesthesia team throughout the procedure
Cumulative radiation dose: (_) mGy

Description of Procedure:
The risks, benefits, alternatives and the procedure itself were explained to the patient/patient's Power of Attorney/legal guardian, and informed written/verbal consent was obtained. Time out was performed to confirm the correct patient, procedure, and site.

The abdomen was evaluated using CT imaging after placement of a radiopaque marker/grid/ultrasound and showed a (_) cm abscess cavity in segment (_) of the liver. The procedure was planned and the skin puncture site was marked using combined information from the location of the abscess and preliminary CT/ultrasound images. The angle of needle entry and the distance to the abscess were calculated from the planning images.

The skin was prepped and draped in the usual sterile fashion. Local anesthesia was administered. A small skin incision was made. Subsequently, a (_)-gauge [type] needle was advanced into the abscess cavity using planning CT information/direct ultrasound visualization. (_) mL of malodorous pus was aspirated, and sent for culture and gram stain. Then, a (_)-inch [type] guidewire was advanced through the needle into the abscess cavity and was positioned under fluoroscopy guidance. The tract was dilated up to the required size using (_)-French dilator(s). A (_)-French self-retaining [type/pigtail] catheter assembly with the stiffener was introduced over the guidewire to a satisfactory depth under fluoroscopy guidance. The stiffener of the catheter was left within the shaft until the catheter was advanced just beyond the wall of the abscess. The guidewire and stiffener were removed after advancing the catheter into the abscess cavity. The catheter was locked, anchored to the skin, and attached to a drainage system. Following this, completion CT/ultrasound images were obtained through the drainage area to confirm correct position of the catheter.

The patient was transferred to the floor/recovery room/intensive care unit following the procedure in a stable/critical condition. Staff was present for the entire procedure.

Intra-Procedure Findings: List all relevant findings.

Immediate Complications: None encountered during or directly after the procedure. List complications if any.

Post-Procedure Plan [1, 3, 11, 12]**:**

- Follow-up laboratory results and adjust/continue antibiotics treatment accordingly.
- Keep catheter under gravity drainage, as needed.
- Keep complete bed rest for 3–4 h and abstain from strenuous activities.
- Start clear liquid diet for the first hour, then regular diet thereafter if tolerated and otherwise not contraindicated.
- Check vital signs every 15 min for 1 h, every 30 min for 1 h and then every 60 min for 2 h.
- Inform interventional radiology team if systolic blood pressure <95 mm Hg, heart rate >100 beats per minute, or if any chest pain, shortness of breath or abdominal pain develops.
- If signs of peritonitis, bowel obstruction, or enteric fluid draining from the catheter are observed, perform catheter contrast injection (tubography) to check position, detect any fistula, and identify free peritoneal leak.
- Daily catheter care:
  - Inspect catheter and make sure that the 3-way stopcock is open to the drainage bag and the catheter has not been externally retracted.
  - Flush the catheter with 20 mL of bacteriostatic saline every 8 h; 10 mL toward the drainage bag and 10 mL towards the collection.
  - Record catheter outputs periodically.
- Inform interventional radiology team if the draining amount decreases, pericatheter leak or local skin complications occurs.
- In cases of persistent high output from the catheter (more than 50 mL per day) for 4–5 days after catheter insertion, perform catheter injection to determine the presence of a fistula to the biliary system or bowel loops.
- Catheter drainage is often prolonged, however, catheters can be removed safely when there is evidence of clinical improvement and imaging features that favor catheter removal:
  - Resolution of fever.
  - Absence of leukocytosis or other septic parameters.
  - Daily drainage via the catheter of less than 20 mL in the absence of catheter-related problems that might explain reduced output, such as catheter malposition, blockage, or kinking.
  - Demonstration of a small, well-drained cavity with no residual compartments at ultrasound, CT, or sinography.
  - No evidence of a fistula at sinography (tubography). If a fistula to the biliary tree is seen, and there is evidence of bile duct obstruction, the bile duct obstruction will need to be treated in order to maximize the chance of successful treatment of the liver abscess.
  - Perform tractography prior to removal of catheters draining by the transpleural or transperitoneal route to confirm the maturity of the tract.

Impression:

- Percutaneous drainage of liver abscess, as described above.
- The patient tolerated the procedure well and left the interventional unit in a stable condition.
- The patient was unstable and the procedure was canceled/terminated prematurely.
- List any other relevant or important information/finding.
- The primary operator (specify name) was present for the entire/key parts of the procedure.

References

1. Thabet A, Arellano RS. Catheter drainage of abdominal abscesses and fluid collections. In: Kandarpa K, Machan L, editors. Handbook of interventional radiologic procedures. 4th ed. Philadelphia: Lippincott Williams & Wilkins; 2011. p. 527–36.
2. Wallace MJ, Chin KW, Fletcher TB, Bakal CW, Cardella JF, Grassi CJ, et al. Quality improvement guidelines for percutaneous drainage/aspiration of abscess and fluid collections. J Vasc Interv Radiol. 2010;21(4):431–5.
3. Campbell JJ, Gervais DA. Percutaneous abscess drainage within the abdomen and pelvis. In: Murphy KPJ, Thomson KR, Venbrux AC, Morgan RA, editors. Image-guided interventions. 2nd ed. Philadelphia: Saunders Elsevier; 2014. p. 923.
4. D'Agostino HB, Hurvitz D, Nall L, et al. Transcatheter fluid drainage. In: Valji K, editor. Vascular and interventional radiology. 2nd ed. Philadelphia: Saunders Elsevier; 2006. p. 516–31.
5. Mueller PR, Dawson SL, Ferrucci JT Jr, Nardi GL. Hepatic echinococcal cyst: successful percutaneous drainage. Radiology. 1985;155:627–8.
6. Baijal SS, Agarwal DK, Roy S, Choudhuri G. Complex ruptured amebic liver abscesses: the role of percutaneous catheter drainage. Eur J Radiol. 1995;20:65–7.
7. El-Shamy M, Emara M, Attia A, Abd-Allah M, Said S. Huge amoebic liver abscess presented with massive right empyema: a case report. Iran J Parasitol. 2014;9(1):141–4.
8. Alsaif HS, Venkatesh SK, Chan DS, Archuleta S. CT appearance of pyogenic liver abscesses caused by Klebsiella pneumoniae. Radiology. 2011;260(1):129–38.
9. Mortelé KJ, Segatto E, Ros PR. The infected liver: radiologic-pathologic correlation. Radiographics. 2004;24(4):937–55.
10. Venkatesan AM, Kundu S, Sacks D, Wallace MJ, Wojak JC, Rose SC, et al. Practice guidelines for adult antibiotic prophylaxis during vascular and interventional radiology procedures. J Vasc Interv Radiol. 2010;21(11):1611–30.
11. Maher MM, Kealey S, McNamara A, O'Laoide R, Gibney RG, Malone DE. Management of visceral interventional radiology catheters: a troubleshooting guide for interventional radiologists. Radiographics. 2002;22(2):305–22.
12. Mezhir JJ, Fong Y, Jacks LM, Getrajdman GI, Brody LA, Covey AM, et al. Current management of pyogenic liver abscess: surgery is now second-line treatment. J Am Coll Surg. 2010;210(6):975–83.

Part VI
Non-vascular Interventional Procedures: Hepatobiliary-Gallbladder

Introduction by Aghiad Al-Kutoubi, Section Reviewer

With recent and ongoing improvements in imaging techniques, advances in ultrasound equipment, and an increasing spectrum of percutaneous biliary interventions, radiologists continue to play a pivotal role in the prompt diagnosis and percutaneous treatment of various hepatobiliary conditions. Percutaneous cholecystostomy is one image-guided procedure that has evolved and continues to serve a role in the management of gallbladder disease and its complications. It allows decompression of the inflamed gallbladder and provides a potential access for further intervention.

This section provides a comprehensive list of procedural reports that covers the vast majority of image-guided procedures for the management of gallbladder diseases with up-to-date explanatory notes, synopsis of the indications and contraindications, and potential complications in an organized and practical format.

Section Chapters

Percutaneous Cholecystolithotomy 35

Bedros Taslakian

INTRODUCTION

Cholelithiasis is a common condition and most patients will not experience symptoms or complications related to gallstones. Laparoscopic cholecystectomy is the treatment of choice for symptomatic gallstones. However, in certain group of patients who are poor surgical candidates, interventional radiologic procedures have emerged as an important alternative. Percutaneous image-guided stone extraction is usually performed in a staged fashion. When a patient presents for elective gallstone extraction, a percutaneous cholecystostomy drain is inserted first, and tract dilation and lithotomy can be performed on the next day. In acutely ill patients who present with acute cholecystitis, a cholecystostomy drain is inserted initially followed by a "cooling-off" period of several days until the patient is stable. Removing gallbladder calculi can be performed using Basket/electrohydraulic lithotripsy fragmentation through a choledochoscope. A route of entry at the end of the gallbladder fundus is the most appropriate access to reach calculi with the lithotripsy probe and facilitates clearance of the entire gallbladder lumen.

B. Taslakian (✉)
Department of Radiology, New York University Langone Medical Center, 660 First Ave, New York, NY 10016, USA
e-mail: Btaslakian@gmail.com

COMMON INDICATIONS [1, 2]

- Symptomatic cholecystolithiasis in patients who are not candidates for surgery

COMMON CONTRAINDICATIONS [1, 2]

- Significant coagulopathy that cannot be adequately corrected
- Hemodynamic instability
- Active infection *(cholangitis, cholecystitis)*
- Ascites *(consider drainage before the procedure)*
- Non-distensible gallbladder

POSSIBLE COMPLICATIONS [1–5]

Complications are related to cholecystostomy and subsequent tract dilatation.

- Hemorrhage, *2.2 %*
- Bacteremia and septic shock in cases of acute cholecystitis, *2.5 %*
- Abscess formation or peritonitis, *2.9 %*
- Transgression of adjacent structures, *1.6 %*
- Bile leak *(biloma, bile peritonitis)*
- Pleural transgression, mainly with right-sided punctures *(hemopneumothorax, empyema, pneumothorax, bilious effusion, fistula)*
- Pancreatitis

B. Taslakian et al. (eds.), *Procedural Dictations in Image-Guided Intervention*,
DOI 10.1007/978-3-319-40845-3_35

- Potential gallstone recurrence
- Gallbladder carcinoma related to chronic inflammation, *very rare*

PREPROCEDURAL ASSESSMENT AND PLANNING

- History, indications, and physical examination *(Appendix 1* in Chap. 149*)*
- Evaluation of diagnostic imaging studies to determine the stone burden and distribution as well as the relevant anatomy for planning
- Periprocedural management of coagulation status *(Appendices 2* in Chap. 150 *and 3* in Chap. 151*)*
- Antibiotic prophylaxis: Routine prophylaxis is recommended [1, 6] *(Appendices 4* in Chap. 152 *and 5* in Chap. 153*)*
- Imaging modality for guidance: Fluoroscopy; cholecystostomy access by any combination of CT, ultrasound, and fluoroscopy
- Positioning: Oblique or supine

PROCEDURE NOTE

Procedure: Percutaneous cholecystolithotomy
Staff: [_]
Fellow: [_]
Resident: [_]
Clinical Information: Describe history and list indications
Allergies: None known/Allergic to [specify/type of allergy]
Anesthesia: Local anesthesia/conscious sedation
Medications: List any relevant medications used (sedation, antibiotics)
Contrast Material: (_) mL of [type] contrast material was used for intra-biliary injection
Field: Sterile
Procedure classification: Clean-contaminated/Contaminated/Dirty
Position: Supine/Oblique
Monitoring: Intravenous access line was secured and vital signs were continuously monitored by nursing staff/anesthesia team throughout the procedure.
Total fluoroscopy time: (_) minutes
Cumulative radiation dose: (_) mGy

Description of Procedure *(the patient has an indwelling cholecystostomy drain):*
The risks, benefits, alternatives, and the procedure itself were explained to the patient/patient's Power of Attorney/legal guardian, and informed written/verbal consent was obtained. The site of the procedure was identified and marked. Time out was performed to confirm the correct patient, procedure, and site.

The skin and the indwelling cholecystostomy catheter were prepped and draped in the usual sterile fashion. (_) mL of contrast material was injected slowly through the catheter under fluoroscopy visualization to delineate the catheter, the gallbladder, and biliary tree. Local anesthesia was administered in the skin around the catheter. A (_)-inch [type] guidewire was then advanced through the catheter into the gallbladder. The tract was then dilated using series of dilators. The last dilator was then exchanged over the guidewire for a (_) French [type] sheath. Subsequently, another (_)-inch [type] guidewire was advanced through the sheath into the gallbladder cavity. The first guidewire was looped within the gallbladder and left as a safety wire outside the working access.

A (_)-French flexible choledochoscope was introduced through the sheath into the gallbladder and the stones were fragmented using a (_)-French intracorporeal electrohydraulic lithotripsy probe which was passed through the working channel of the choledochoscope to allow direct visualization during activation. The stone fragments were then removed using a basket. Choledochoscopy evaluation was performed to ensure that no residual stones remained in the gallbladder lumen. Then, cholangiography was performed through the sheath to evaluate the cystic and biliary ducts, showing no filling defects suggestive of impacted stones and documenting free passage of contrast into the duodenum.

At the end of the procedure, a large-bore (_)-French retention loop [type] catheter was inserted over the guidewire into the gallbladder to tamponade the tract used for endoscopy and allow drainage of any residual stone fragments. Spot fluoroscopy image was obtained after minimal contrast injection to confirm the catheter position and patency, for documentation and future reference. The catheter was locked, anchored to the skin, and attached to a gravity drainage system.

The patient was transferred to the floor/recovery room/intensive care unit following the procedure in a stable/critical condition. Staff was present for the entire procedure.

Intra-Procedure Findings: List all relevant findings.

Immediate Complications: None encountered during or directly after the procedure. List complications if any.

Post-Procedure Plan [1–3, 7]:

- Keep complete bed rest for 3–4 h and abstain from strenuous activities.
- Start clear liquid diet for the first hour, then regular diet thereafter if tolerated and otherwise not contraindicated.
- Check vital signs every 15 min for 1 h, every 30 min for 1 h, every 60 min for 2 h and then as needed.
- Inform interventional radiology team if systolic blood pressure <95 mm Hg, heart rate >100 beats per minute, or if any chest pain or shortness of breath develops.
- Replace bile loss with intravenous fluids as necessary during external drainage period.
- If signs of peritonitis, sepsis, bowel obstruction, hemorrhage, or enteric fluid draining from the catheter, abdominal pain, or pericatheter erythema are observed, take corrective measures as medically needed and inform interventional radiology team immediately.
- Check complete blood count, liver function tests, and blood cultures as needed.
- If the patient's condition worsens, image the catheter immediately preferably with CT scan or tube cholecystography.
- Daily catheter care:
  - Keep catheter under external gravity drainage.
  - Inspect catheter and make sure that the 3-way stopcock is open to the drainage bag and the catheter has not been externally retracted.
  - Flush the catheter slowly with 20 mL of bacteriostatic saline every 8 h; 10 mL toward the drainage bag and 10 mL toward the gallbladder.
  - Record the catheter outputs every 8 h and inform interventional radiology team if the draining amount decreases.
  - Inform the interventional radiology team if there is any suspicion of catheter dislodgment.
- Follow-up plan:
  - Once the patient has stabilized, perform a cholecystogram to assess the gallbladder, catheter position, and cystic duct patency.
  - Perform a cholangiography 2 weeks after the procedure to document patency of the cystic and common bile ducts.
  - If no residual stones are identified and the gallbladder drains appropriately into the central bile ducts, cap the catheter for 2 weeks to simulate internal drainage.
  - Once the patient tolerates internal drainage, remains asymptomatic with resolution of sepsis and documentation of clinical improvement, the catheter can be removed safely after documenting tract maturity by tractography.
  - The duration of antibiotic therapy after the procedure is to be determined by the clinical course of individual patients.
  - Follow-up patient in the interventional radiology clinic on an as-needed basis.
  - Change the catheter every 1–3 months if left in place.

Impression:

- Percutaneous cholecystolithotomy, as described above.
- The patient tolerated the procedure well and left the interventional unit in a stable condition.
- The patient was unstable and the procedure was canceled/terminated prematurely.
- List any other relevant or important information/finding.

References

1. Fahrbach TM, Wyse GM, Lawler LP, Kim HS. Percutaneous cholecystostomy. In: Mauro MA, Murphy KPJ, Thomson KR, Venbrux AC, Morgan RA, editors. Image-guided interventions. 2nd ed. Philadelphia: Saunders Elsevier; 2014. p. 1008–14.
2. Management of biliary calculi. In: Burke CT, Dixon RG, Mauro MA, Murphy KPJ, Thomson KR, Venbrux AC, Zollikofer CL, editors. High yield imaging: interventional. Philadelphia: Saunders Elsevier; 2010. p. 438–441.
3. Hunter DW. Percutaneous biliary interventions. In: Kandarpa K, Machan L, editors. Handbook of interventional radiologic procedures. 4th ed. Philadelphia: Lippincott Williams & Wilkins; 2011. p. 577–90.
4. Saad WE, Wallace MJ, Wojak JC, Kundu S, Cardella JF. Quality improvement guidelines for percutaneous transhepatic cholangiography, biliary drainage, and percutaneous cholecystostomy. J Vasc Interv Radiol. 2010;21(6):789–95.
5. Bortoff GA, Chen MY, Ott DJ, Wolfman NT, Routh WD. Gallbladder stones: imaging and intervention. Radiographics. 2000;20(3):751–66.
6. Venkatesan AM, Kundu S, Sacks D, Wallace MJ, Wojak JC, Rose SC, et al. Practice guidelines for adult antibiotic prophylaxis during vascular and interventional radiology procedures. J Vasc Interv Radiol. 2010;21(11):1611–30.
7. Maher MM, Kealey S, McNamara A, O'Laoide R, Gibney RG, Malone DE. Management of visceral interventional radiology catheters: a troubleshooting guide for interventional radiologists. Radiographics. 2002;22(2):305–22.

36 Percutaneous Cholecystostomy

Bedros Taslakian

INTRODUCTION

Acute cholecystitis is a common condition with significant morbidity and mortality. Although laparoscopic cholecystectomy is the treatment of choice, percutaneous cholecystostomy provides adequate decompression of the gallbladder for management of acute cholecystitis either definitively or as a temporizing measure before cholecystectomy. A transhepatic route is associated with lower risk of bile leakage, whereas a subhepatic or transperitoneal route is preferred for cholecystolithotomy through a larger tract.

COMMON INDICATIONS [1–4]

- Acute cholecystitis in patients who are poor surgical candidates
- Suspected acalculous cholecystitis in intensive care unit
- Empirical therapy in patients with unexplained fever or sepsis and suspected cholecystitis after excluding other sources
- Transcholecystic access for gallstones extraction
- Transcholecystic biliary tract access for therapeutic biliary interventions when other methods are contraindicated or have failed

COMMON CONTRAINDICATIONS [1–3]

Most contraindications are relative as cholecystostomy is frequently performed in severely ill and high-risk patients when alternative methods carry higher risk of morbidity and mortality.

- Absence of a safe route for needle placement *(e.g., Chilaiditi syndrome)*
- Gallbladder carcinoma *(risk of seeding)*
- Perforated decompressed gallbladder which prevents needle access and drainage tube formation
- Presence of numerous gallstones which prevent drainage tube formation/positioning
- Significant coagulopathy that cannot be adequately corrected
- Hemodynamic instability
- Large volume ascites *(consider drainage before the procedure)*

POSSIBLE COMPLICATIONS [1–3]

- Hemorrhage, *2.2 %*
- Septic shock, *2.5 %*
- Abscess formation, peritonitis, *2.9 %*
- Bile leak

B. Taslakian (✉)
Department of Radiology, New York University Langone Medical Center, 660 First Ave, New York, NY 10016, USA
e-mail: btaslakian@gmail.com

B. Taslakian et al. (eds.), *Procedural Dictations in Image-Guided Intervention*,
DOI 10.1007/978-3-319-40845-3_36

- Pleural transgression *(hemopneumothorax, empyema, pneumothorax, bile leak/fistula)*
- Transgression of adjacent structures, *1.6 %*
- Catheter malfunction *(kinking, blockage, dislodgment)*
- Pericatheter leak
- Infection at the catheter insertion site
- Vasovagal reaction during the procedure
- Mortality, *2.5 %*

PREPROCEDURAL ASSESSMENT AND PLANNING

- History, indications and physical examination *(Appendix 1* in Chap. 149*)*
- Evaluation of diagnostic imaging studies to determine the relevant anatomy
- Periprocedural management of coagulation status *(Appendices 2* in Chap. 150 *and 3* in Chap. 151*)*
- Antibiotic prophylaxis: Routine prophylaxis is recommended [5] *(Appendices 4* in Chap. 152 *and 5* in Chap. 153*)*
- Imaging modality for guidance: CT, CT fluoroscopy, ultrasound, combined ultrasound/CT, and fluoroscopy
- Positioning: Oblique or supine

PROCEDURE NOTE

Procedure: Percutaneous cholecystostomy
Staff: [_]
Fellow: [_]
Resident: [_]
Clinical Information: Describe history and list indications
Allergies: None known/Allergic to [specify/type of allergy]
Anesthesia: Local anesthesia/conscious sedation
Medications: List any relevant medications used (sedation, antibiotics)
Contrast Material: (_) mL of [type] contrast material was used for cholecystogram
Field: Sterile
Procedure classification: Dirty
Position: Supine/Oblique
Monitoring: Intravenous access line was secured and vital signs were continuously monitored by nursing staff/anesthesia team throughout the procedure
Cumulative radiation dose: (_) mGy

Description of Procedure:
The risks, benefits, alternatives, and the procedure itself were explained to the patient/patient's Power of Attorney/legal guardian, and informed written/verbal consent was obtained. The site of the procedure was identified and marked. Time out was performed to confirm the correct patient, procedure, and site.

The liver and gallbladder were evaluated using CT imaging after placement of a radiopaque marker/grid/ultrasound. The procedure was planned and the skin puncture site was marked using combined information from the location of the gallbladder and preliminary CT/ultrasound images. The angle of needle entry and the distance to the gallbladder were calculated from the planning images along the right (_) th intercostal/subcostal space anterior to midaxillary line. A transhepatic/transperitoneal approach was selected to access the gallbladder.

The skin was prepped and draped in the usual sterile fashion. Local anesthesia was administered. A small skin incision was made. Subsequently, using planning CT information/using CT fluoroscopy/under direct ultrasound visualization, a (_)-gauge [type] needle was advanced along the planned trajectory until the needle tip was within the gallbladder, confirmed by imaging. (_) mL of purulent/malodorous/clear bile/blood-tinged bile was aspirated to minimize the intracholecystic pressure and sent to laboratory for culture, Gram stain, and chemistry. A (_)-inch [type] guidewire was advanced through the needle into the gallbladder. The tract was dilated up to the required size using (_)-French dilator(s). Subsequently, a (_)-French self-retaining [type/pigtail] catheter assembly with the metal stiffener was introduced over the guidewire to a satisfactory depth under fluoroscopy guidance. The stiff trocar of the catheter was left within the shaft until the catheter was advanced just beyond the wall of the gallbladder.

The guidewire and stiffener were removed after advancing the catheter into the gallbladder cavity. The catheter was locked, anchored to the skin, and attached to a drainage system. Following this, completion CT/ultrasound/fluoroscopy images were obtained through the drainage area after injecting (_) mL of water-soluble contrast to confirm correct position of the catheter.

The patient was transferred to the floor/recovery room/intensive care unit following the procedure in a stable/critical condition. Staff was present for the entire procedure.

Intra-Procedure Findings: List all the relevant findings.

Immediate Complications: None were encountered during or directly after the procedure. List complications if any.

Post-Procedure Plan [1, 2, 6]**:**

- Follow-up laboratory results and adjust or continue antibiotics accordingly.
- Keep catheter under gravity drainage.
- Keep complete bed rest for 3–4 h and abstain from strenuous activities.
- Start clear liquid diet for the first hour, then regular diet thereafter if tolerated and otherwise not contraindicated.
- Check vital signs every 15 min for 1 h, every 30 min for 1 h, and then every 60 min for 2 h.
- Inform interventional radiology team if systolic blood pressure < 95 mm Hg, heart rate > 100 beats per minute, or if any chest pain, abdominal pain, or shortness of breath develops.
- If signs of peritonitis, bowel obstruction, or enteric fluid draining from the catheter are observed, perform catheter injection to check position, detect fistula, and identify free peritoneal leak.
- If the patient's condition worsens, image the catheter immediately preferably with CT scan or perform a cholecystogram.
- Daily catheter care:
  - Inspect catheter and make sure that the 3-way stopcock is open to the drainage bag and the catheter has not been externally retracted.
  - Flush the catheter slowly with 20 mL of bacteriostatic saline every 6–8 h; 10 mL toward the drainage bag and 10 mL toward the gallbladder.
  - Record the catheter outputs every 8 h.
  - Inform interventional radiology team if the draining amount decreases, or pericatheter leak or local skin complications occurs.
  - Inform the interventional radiology team if there is any suspicion of catheter dislodgment.
- Follow-up plan:
  - Once the patient has stabilized, perform a cholecystogram to assess the gallbladder, catheter position, and cystic duct patency.
  - Determine the suitability of the patient for elective cholecystectomy.
  - Removal of catheter is safe 3–4 weeks post-insertion and after clinical improvement is documented, with resolution of sepsis and documentation of cystic duct patency and tract maturity. Tract maturation may be prolonged in immunocompromised or critically ill patients.
  - The catheter should be clamped for 48 h before catheter removal to ensure the patient remains asymptomatic.
  - The duration of antibiotic therapy after the procedure is to be determined by the clinical course of individual patients.
  - Change the catheter every 1–3 months if left in place.

Impression:

- Percutaneous cholecystostomy, as described above.
- The patient tolerated the procedure well and left the interventional unit in a stable condition.
- The patient was unstable and the procedure was canceled/terminated prematurely.
- List any other relevant or important information/findings.

References

1. Fahrbach TM, Wyse GM, Lawler LP, Kim HS. Percutaneous cholecystostomy. In: Mauro MA,

Murphy KPJ, Thomson KR, Venbrux AC, Morgan RA, editors. Image-guided interventions. 2nd ed. Philadelphia: Saunders Elsevier; 2014. p. 1008–14.
2. Hunter DW. Percutaneous biliary interventions. In: Kandarpa K, Machan L, editors. Handbook of interventional radiologic procedures. 4th ed. Philadelphia: Lippincott Williams & Wilkins; 2011. p. 577–90.
3. Saad WE, Wallace MJ, Wojak JC, Kundu S, Cardella JF. Quality improvement guidelines for percutaneous transhepatic cholangiography, biliary drainage, and percutaneous cholecystostomy. J Vasc Interv Radiol. 2010;21(6):789–95.
4. Bortoff GA, Chen MY, Ott DJ, Wolfman NT, Routh WD. Gallbladder stones: imaging and intervention. Radiographics. 2000;20(3):751–66.
5. Venkatesan AM, Kundu S, Sacks D, Wallace MJ, Wojak JC, Rose SC, et al. Practice guidelines for adult antibiotic prophylaxis during vascular and interventional radiology procedures. J Vasc Interv Radiol. 2010;21(11):1611–30.
6. Maher MM, Kealey S, McNamara A, O'Laoide R, Gibney RG, Malone DE. Management of visceral interventional radiology catheters: a troubleshooting guide for interventional radiologists. Radiographics. 2002;22(2):305–22.

Percutaneous Diagnostic Cholecystocholangiography

37

Bedros Taslakian

INTRODUCTION

Percutaneous cholecystocholangiography is the image-guided injection of contrast media into the gallbladder using a fine needle or through an indwelling cholecystostomy catheter to visualize the gallbladder and the biliary tree. Diagnostic cholecystocholangiography may be performed instead of percutaneous transhepatic cholangiography. In patients with non-dilated intrahepatic bile ducts, who only require a diagnostic study, a gallbladder puncture with a 22-gauge needle can be used to delineate the biliary tree under fluoroscopy. To visualize the intrahepatic biliary tree, the patient may be tilted in Trendelenburg position.

COMMON INDICATIONS [1–4]

Tube cholecystocholangiogram

- Assess the patency of an indwelling cholecystostomy catheter
- Assess the position and integrity of an indwelling cholecystostomy catheter
- Determine the safety of cholecystostomy catheter removal by confirming the patency of the cystic and common bile ducts

Needle cholecystocholangiogram

- Assess the cystic and common bile ducts for residual calculi
- Evaluation of the biliary tract: biliary atresia, sclerosing cholangitis, biliary cirrhosis, and obstructive biliary diseases when other non-invasive imaging modalities fail to reach a diagnosis

COMMON CONTRAINDICATIONS

Tube cholecystocholangiogram: No absolute contraindications.

- Care should be taken during contrast injection in an infected system to avoid bacterial seeding and septicemia
- Pregnancy in cases when imaging guidance involves ionizing radiation

Needle cholecystocholangiogram:

- Significant coagulopathy that cannot be adequately corrected
- Hemodynamic instability
- Ascites
- Pregnancy

B. Taslakian (✉)
Department of Radiology, New York University Langone Medical Center, 660 First Ave, New York, NY 10016, USA
e-mail: btaslakian@gmail.com

B. Taslakian et al. (eds.), *Procedural Dictations in Image-Guided Intervention*,
DOI 10.1007/978-3-319-40845-3_37

POSSIBLE COMPLICATIONS [4, 5]

- Pain and discomfort
- Contrast extravasation
- Septic shock
- Catheter dislodgment
- Bile leak and bile peritonitis
- Gallbladder injury
- Bleeding

PREPROCEDURAL ASSESSMENT AND PLANNING

- History, indications, and physical examination *(Appendix 1* in Chap. 149*)*
- Evaluation of diagnostic imaging studies to determine the relevant anatomy
- Periprocedural management of coagulation status *(Appendices 2* in Chap. 150 *and 3* in Chap. 151*)*
- Antibiotic prophylaxis: Patients with cholecystostomy are usually on antibiotic therapy. Not routinely recommended for diagnostic needle cholecystocholangiography in a non-infected system. *(Appendices 4 in* Chap. 152 *and 5* in Chap. 153*)*
- Imaging modality for guidance: Fluoroscopy, combined ultrasound/CT and fluoroscopy for needle cholecystocholangiography
- Positioning: Oblique, supine

PROCEDURE NOTE

Procedure: Fluoroscopy-guided cholecystocholangiography
Staff: [_]
Fellow: [_]
Resident: [_]
Clinical Information: Describe history and list indications
Allergies: None known/Allergic to [specify/type of allergy]
Anesthesia: Local anesthesia/conscious sedation
Medications: List any relevant medications used (sedation, antibiotics)
Contrast Material: (_) mL of [type] contrast material was used for cholecystocholangiography
Field: Sterile
Procedure classification: Clean/Dirty (cholecystitis)
Position: Supine/Oblique
Monitoring: Intravenous access line was secured and vital signs were continuously monitored by nursing staff/anesthesia team throughout the procedure
Total fluoroscopy time: (_) minutes
Cumulative radiation dose: (_) mGy

Description of Procedure: *(tube cholecystocholangiogram):*
The risks, benefits, alternatives, and the procedure itself were explained to the patient/patient's Power of Attorney/legal guardian, and informed written/verbal consent was obtained. The site of the procedure was identified and marked. Time out was performed to confirm the correct patient, procedure, and site.

The skin and the indwelling cholecystostomy catheter were prepped and draped in the usual sterile fashion. (_) mL of contrast media was injected slowly through the catheter under fluoroscopy visualization to delineate the catheter, the gallbladder, and biliary tree.

The patient was transferred to the floor/recovery room/intensive care unit/discharged home following the procedure in a stable/critical condition. Staff was present for the entire procedure.

Description of Procedure: *(needle cholecystocholangiogram):*
The risks, benefits, alternatives, and the procedure itself were explained to the patient/patient's Power of Attorney/legal guardian, and informed written/verbal consent was obtained. The site of the procedure was identified and marked. Time out was performed to confirm the correct patient, procedure, and site.

The liver was evaluated using ultrasound/CT imaging after placement of a radiopaque marker/grid. The procedure was planned and the skin puncture site was marked using combined information from the planning images, the location of the gallbladder and the radiopaque marker/grid. The angle of needle entry and the distance to the gallbladder were calculated from planning images.

The skin was prepped and draped in the usual sterile fashion. Local anesthesia was administered. A small skin incision was made. Subsequently, a (_)-gauge [type] needle was advanced into the gallbladder using planning CT information/under direct ultrasound visualization. (_) mL of bile was aspirated, and sent to laboratory for evaluation.

(_) mL of contrast was slowly injected into the gallbladder, with the patient in Trendelenburg position, and the needle was withdrawn after adequate delineation of the gallbladder and the biliary tree. Completion spot images were obtained.

The patient was transferred to the floor/recovery room/discharged home following the procedure in a stable condition. Staff was present for the entire procedure.

Intra-Procedure Findings: List all the relevant findings.

Immediate Complications: None was encountered during or directly after the procedure. List the complications if any.

Post-Procedure Plan:

- Daily catheter care *(if cholecystostomy catheter is left in place):*
  - Keep the catheter under dependent drainage.
  - Record the catheter outputs daily.
  - Inspect catheter and make sure that the 3-way stopcock is open to the drainage bag and the catheter has not been externally retracted.
  - Flush the catheter slowly with 20 mL of bacteriostatic saline every 8 h; 10 mL toward the drainage bag and 10 mL toward the gallbladder.
- Follow-up plan:
  - Specify the plan according to the findings.
  - Removal of catheter is safe 3–4 weeks post-insertion and after clinical improvement is documented, with resolution of sepsis and documentation of tract maturity with tractography.
  - The catheter should be clamped for 24 h before catheter removal to ensure the patient remains asymptomatic.
  - The duration of antibiotic therapy after the procedure is to be determined by the clinical course of individual patients.
  - Replace the catheter every 1–3 months if left in place.

Impression:

1. Tube/needle cholecystocholangiography, as described above.
2. The patient tolerated the procedure well and left the interventional unit in a stable condition.
3. The patient was unstable and the procedure was canceled/terminated prematurely.
4. List any other relevant or important information/findings.

References

1. Lee SY, Kim GC, Choe BH, Ryeom HK, Jang YJ, Kim HJ, et al. Efficacy of US-guided percutaneous cholecystocholangiography for the early exclusion and type determination of biliary atresia. Radiology. 2011;261(3):916–22.
2. Maher MM, Kealey S, McNamara A, O'Laoide R, Gibney RG, Malone DE. Management of visceral interventional radiology catheters: a troubleshooting guide for interventional radiologists. Radiographics. 2002 Mar–Apr;22(2):305–22.
3. Fahrbach TM, Wyse GM, Lawler LP, Kim HS. Percutaneous cholecystostomy. In: Mauro MA, Murphy KPJ, Thomson KR, Venbrux AC, Morgan RA, editors. Image-guided interventions. 2nd ed. Philadelphia: Saunders Elsevier; 2014. p. 1008–14.
4. Hunter DW. Percutaneous biliary interventions. In: Kandarpa K, Machan L, editors. Handbook of interventional radiologic procedures. 4th ed. Philadelphia: Lippincott Williams & Wilkins; 2011. p. 577–90.
5. vanSonnenberg E, D'Agostino HB, Goodacre BW, Sanchez RB, Casola G. Percutaneous gallbladder puncture and cholecystostomy: results, complications, and caveats for safety. Radiology. 1992 Apr;183(1):167–70.

Part VII

Non-vascular Interventional Procedures: Hepatobiliary-Biliary Tract

Introduction by Karen T. Brown, Section Reviewer

Intervention in the biliary tree may be undertaken for many reasons but prior to any intervention a thorough understanding of the clinical situation, indication for the procedure, likelihood of success and relevant anatomical considerations must be sought. If the procedure is requested to decrease the bilirubin to allow for administration of chemotherapy and 75 % of the liver is replaced by tumor and the portal vein is occluded then a very frank discussion with the patient must precede the procedure, as the risk of an adverse event is higher than the chance of a successful outcome. Pruritus can almost always be palliated, even if only one sector of the liver is drained. In those cases, and many others, primary stent placement should be considered so that the patient does not have to live with an exteriorized catheter. In cases of high bile duct obstruction primary stent placement, keeping the stent above the Ampulla of Vater should be entertained in order to avoid contamination of the biliary tree with enteric contents; this may result in presentation with cholangitis if/when the stent occludes. Access to the biliary tree can be used to remove stones, either through a T-tube track left behind after cholecystectomy or via direct biliary puncture. Patients with benign bile duct strictures can be treated with balloon dilation. In all cases recent cross-sectional imaging should be reviewed to assess hepatic anatomy, status of the portal veins, presence of tumor, and ascites in order to plan a safe and efficient procedure.

This section provides a comprehensive list of procedural reports that covers the vast majority of percutaneous procedures performed in the biliary tract with up-to-date explanatory notes, synopsis of the indications and contraindications, and potential complications in an organized and practical format.

Section Chapters

Percutaneous Biliary Stone Extraction (Hepatolithotomy and Choledocolithotomy)

38

Bedros Taslakian

Abbreviation

ERCP Endoscopic retrograde cholangiopancreatography

INTRODUCTION

Percutaneous imaging-guided biliary drainage and biliary stone extraction is indicated in patients who are not candidate for surgery or when endoscopic retrograde cholangiopancreatography (ERCP) is not possible or has failed. The procedure is usually performed in a staged fashion. Removing ductal calculi can be performed using balloon dilation of the ampulla, followed by the use of balloons to dislodge calculi into the bowel or by Basket/electrohydraulic/laser lithotripsy fragmentation with or without a choledochoscope.

COMMON INDICATIONS [1–4]

- Symptomatic choledocolithiasis in patients who are not candidates for surgery or ERCP
- Retained biliary duct stones after surgery and failed ERCP
- Retained calculi following cholecystectomy with a surgical T-tube in place
- Intrahepatic biliary calculi peripheral to the hilum of the liver, rendering ERCP challenging and prone to failure
- Intrahepatic biliary calculi above a narrowed bilioenteric anastomosis

COMMON CONTRAINDICATIONS [1–3]

- Large volume ascites *(consider drainage before the procedure)*
- History of allergic contrast reaction *(contrast material may be introduced or absorbed into the vascular system during the procedure)*
- Active infection *(cholangitis, cholecystitis)*
- Acute pancreatitis

POSSIBLE COMPLICATIONS [1–5]

- Transient fever, pain, and hemobilia
- Hemorrhage *(subcapsular, peritoneal, or hemobilia)*
- Arterial injury *(e.g., pseudoaneurysm, focal arterial spasm, arterial–biliary, and arterial–venous fistulas)*

B. Taslakian (✉)
Department of Radiology, New York University Langone Medical Center, 660 First Ave, New York, NY 10016, USA
e-mail: btaslakian@gmail.com

B. Taslakian et al. (eds.), *Procedural Dictations in Image-Guided Intervention*,
DOI 10.1007/978-3-319-40845-3_38

- Bacteremia and septic shock
- Bile duct injury leading to bile leak and biliary peritonitis
- Cholangitis
- Pancreatitis
- Pleural transgression, mainly with right-sided punctures *(hemopneumothorax, empyema, pneumothorax, bilious effusion, fistula)*
- Transgression of adjacent abdominal structures *(colon, small bowel)*
- Death

PREPROCEDURAL ASSESSMENT AND PLANNING

- History, indications, and physical examination *(Appendix 1* in Chap. 149*)*
- Evaluation of diagnostic imaging studies to determine the extent of biliary dilatation, the stone burden, and distribution as well as the relevant anatomy for planning the access. MRCP is especially useful in these cases.
- Periprocedural management of coagulation status *(Appendices 2* in Chap. 150 *and 3* in Chap. 151*)*
- Antibiotic prophylaxis: Routine prophylaxis is recommended *(Appendices 4* in Chap. 152 *and 5* in Chap. 153*)* [1, 2, 6]
- Imaging modality for guidance: Fluoroscopy, combined ultrasound and fluoroscopy for biliary access
- Positioning: Supine

PROCEDURE NOTE

Procedure: Percutaneous hepatolithotomy/choledocolithotomy
Staff: [_]
Fellow: [_]
Resident: [_]
Clinical Information: Describe history and list indications
Allergies: None known/Allergic to [specify/type of allergy]
Anesthesia: Local anesthesia/conscious sedation/general anesthesia
Medications: List any relevant medications used (sedation, antibiotics)
Contrast Material: (_) mL of [type] contrast material
Field: Sterile
Procedure classification: Clean-contaminated/Contaminated
Position: Supine
Monitoring: Intravenous access line was secured and vital signs were continuously monitored by nursing staff/anesthesia team throughout the procedure
Total fluoroscopy time: (_) minutes
Cumulative radiation dose: (_) mGy

Description of Procedure *(staged procedure: the patient has internal–external biliary drain):* The risks, benefits, alternatives, and the procedure itself were explained to the patient/patient's Power of Attorney/legal guardian, and informed written/verbal consent was obtained. The site of the procedure was identified and marked. Time out was performed to confirm the correct patient, procedure, and site.

The skin and the previously inserted biliary drain were prepped and draped in the usual sterile fashion. Using fluoroscopy, a (0.035)-in. [type] guidewire was inserted through the drain and looped in the duodenum/intestine. The drain was then exchanged over the guidewire for a (_)-French [type] sheath. A second (0.035)-in. [stiff/type] guidewire was inserted and looped in the duodenum/intestine, leaving the first safety guidewire in place. Cholangiography was performed to confirm the location of the biliary obstruction and stone(s). A (10/12) mm [type] balloon was then advanced over the stiff guidewire and inflated across the Ampulla of Vater/bilioenteric anastomosis for (45–90) s to facilitate stone passage. Following this, a (_) mm [type] balloon was inflated to fragment the stone. It was then deflated, carefully withdrawn above the stone, reinflated, and then used to push the debris into the intestine. Cholangiography was performed through the sheath and showed clearing of the biliary tree of all stones with evidence of free passage of contrast through the common bile duct/bilioenteric anastamosis into the duodenum/intestine.

Subsequently, a (_)-French [internal–external self-retaining/type] biliary drainage catheter was inserted over the guidewire and its tip was formed in the duodenum/intestine. Spot fluoroscopy image was obtained after minimal contrast injection to confirm the catheter position and patency for documentation and future reference. The catheter was locked, anchored to the skin, and attached to a gravity drainage system.

The patient was transferred to the floor/recovery room following the procedure in a stable condition. Staff was present for the entire procedure.

Description of Procedure *(staged procedure, the patient has an external drain):*

The risks, benefits, alternatives, and the procedure itself were explained to the patient/patient's Power of Attorney/legal guardian, and informed written/verbal consent was obtained. The site of the procedure was identified and marked. Time out was performed to confirm the correct patient, procedure, and site.

The skin and the previously inserted external biliary drain were prepped and draped in the usual sterile fashion. Using fluoroscopy, a (0.035)-in. [type] guidewire was inserted through the drain and looped in the biliary tree. The drain was then exchanged over the guidewire for a (_)-French sheath. Cholangiography was performed to identify the site of stricture and confirm the intra-biliary position of the sheath. The first guidewire was left in place as a safety wire. Through the sheath, a (_) French [angiographic/biliary manipulation/type] catheter was inserted over a (0.035)-in. [hydrophilic/type] guidewire to navigate through the point of obstruction, which was successfully crossed. The catheter was advanced into the duodenum/intestine over the [hydrophilic/type] guidewire, which was then exchanged through the catheter for a (0.035)-in. [stiff/type] guidewire.

Cholangiography was performed to confirm the location of the biliary obstruction and stone(s). A (10/12) mm [type] balloon was then advanced over the stiff guidewire and inflated across the Ampulla of Vater/bilioenteric anastomosis for (45–90) s to facilitate stone passage. Following this, a (_) mm [type] balloon was inflated to fragment the stone(s). It was then deflated, carefully withdrawn above the stone(s), reinflated, and then used to push the debris into the intestine. Cholangiography was performed through the sheath and showed clearing of the biliary tree of all stones with evidence of free passage of contrast through the common bile duct/bilioenteric anastamosis into the duodenum/intestine.

Subsequently, a (_)-French [internal–external self-retaining/type] biliary drainage catheter was inserted over the guidewire and its tip was formed in the duodenum/intestine. Spot fluoroscopy image was obtained after minimal contrast injection to confirm the catheter position and patency for documentation and future reference. The catheter was locked, anchored to the skin, and attached to a gravity drainage system.

The patient was transferred to the floor/recovery room following the procedure in a stable condition. Staff was present for the entire procedure.

Description of Procedure *(access* via *a mature T-tube tract):*

The risks, benefits, alternatives, and the procedure itself were explained to the patient/patient's Power of Attorney/legal guardian, and informed written/verbal consent was obtained. The site of the procedure was identified and marked. Time out was performed to confirm the correct patient, procedure, and site.

The skin and the T-tube were prepped and draped in the usual sterile fashion. Local anesthesia was administered in the skin surrounding the T-tube. A small skin incision was made. T-tube cholangiography was performed, revealing a filling defect representing a stone in the [specify location]. Spot images of the biliary tree with dilute contrast were obtained in multiple projections for confirmation.

Subsequently, a (0.018)-in. [type] guidewire was advanced through the T-tube into the biliary tree. The tube was then exchanged over a (0.035)-in. [type] guidewire facilitating placement of a (_) French [type] sheath. Through the sheath, a (_) French [angiographic/biliary manipulation/type] catheter was inserted to navigate into the duodenum over a [hydrophilic/type] guidewire, which was then exchanged through the catheter for a (0.035)-in. [stiff/type] guidewire.

A (10/12) mm [type] balloon was then advanced over the stiff guidewire and inflated across the ampulla of Vater for (45–90) s to facilitate stone passage. Following this, a (_) mm [type] balloon was inflated to fragment the stone (s). It was then deflated, carefully withdrawn above the stone(s), reinflated, and then used to push the debris into the intestine. Cholangiography was performed through the sheath and showed clearing the biliary tree of all stones with evidence of free passage of contrast through the common bile duct into the duodenum.

Subsequently, a (_)-French [internal–external self-retaining/type] biliary drainage catheter was inserted over the guidewire and its tip was formed in the duodenum/intestine. Spot fluoroscopy image was obtained after minimal contrast injection to confirm the catheter position and patency for documentation and future reference. The catheter was locked, anchored to the skin, and attached to a gravity drainage system.

The patient was transferred to the floor/recovery room following the procedure in a stable condition. Staff was present for the entire procedure.

Intra-Procedure Findings: List all the relevant findings.

Immediate Complications: None was encountered during or directly after the procedure. List complications if any.

Post-Procedure Plan [1, 2, 7]:

- Follow-up laboratory results and adjust/continue antibiotics treatment accordingly.
- Replace bile loss with intravenous fluids as necessary during external drainage period.
- Keep complete bed rest for 3–4 h and abstain from strenuous activities.
- Start clear liquid diet for the first hour, then regular diet thereafter if tolerated and otherwise not contraindicated.
- Check vital signs every 15 min for 1 h, every 30 min for 1 h, every 60 min for 2 h and then as needed.
- Inform interventional radiology team if systolic blood pressure < 95 mm Hg, heart rate > 100 beats per minute, or if any chest pain or shortness of breath develops.
- If signs of peritonitis, sepsis or hemorrhage, chest or abdominal pain, pericatheter erythema are observed take corrective measures as medically needed and inform interventional radiology team immediately.
- Check complete blood count, liver function tests, and blood cultures as needed.
- Daily catheter care:
  - Inspect catheter and make sure that the 3-way stopcock is open to the drainage bag and the catheter has not been externally retracted.
  - Flush the catheter with 10 mL of bacteriostatic saline every 8 h during external drainage period and daily thereafter to prevent bile clogging.
  - Perform site cleaning and dressing change weekly or more frequently as needed.
  - Record the catheter outputs every 8 h during external drainage period.
- Follow-up plan:
  - Perform a cholangiography after 24 h and if no filling defects are present, cap the catheter and monitor the patient. The patient can be discharged home with instructions to return to the emergency department if any signs of cholangitis occurs.
  - Catheter can be safely removed after 2 weeks when there is evidence of clinical improvement, documentation of a mature duct, and imaging features that favor catheter removal *(cholangiography showing good flow through the ducts, with no evidence of obstruction or filling defects).*
  - Perform tractography prior to removal of catheters draining by the transpleural or transperitoneal route or if biliary–arterial communication is suspected to confirm tract maturity.

Impression:

- Percutaneous hepatolithotomy/choledocolithotomy, as described above.
- The patient tolerated the procedure well and left the interventional unit in a stable condition.
- The patient was unstable and the procedure was canceled/terminated prematurely.
- List any other relevant or important information/findings.

References

1. Brown DB, Picus DD. Management of Biliary Calculi. In: Mauro MA, Murphy KPJ, Thomson KR, Venbrux AC, Morgan RA, editors. Image-guided interventions. 2nd ed. Philadelphia: Saunders Elsevier; 2014. p. 1014–9.
2. Management of Biliary Calculi. In: Burke CT, Dixon RG, Mauro MA, Murphy KPJ, Thomson KR, Venbrux AC, Zollikofer CL, editors. High yield imaging: interventional. Philadelphia: Saunders Elsevier; 2010. p. 438–41.
3. Hoang JK, Little AF, Clarke A. Percutaneous intracorporeal lithotripsy of biliary calculi. Australas Radiol. 2007;51(Suppl):B324–7.
4. García-García L, Lanciego C. Percutaneous treatment of biliary stones: sphincteroplasty and occlusion balloon for the clearance of bile duct calculi. AJR Am J Roentgenol. 2004;182(3):663–70.
5. Winick AB, Waybill PN, Venbrux AC. Complications of percutaneous transhepatic biliary interventions. Tech Vasc Interv Radiol. 2001;4(3):200–6.
6. Venkatesan AM, Kundu S, Sacks D, Wallace MJ, Wojak JC, Rose SC, et al. Practice guidelines for adult antibiotic prophylaxis during vascular and interventional radiology procedures. J Vasc Interv Radiol. 2010;21(11):1611–30.
7. Maher MM, Kealey S, McNamara A, O'Laoide R, Gibney RG, Malone DE. Management of visceral interventional radiology catheters: a troubleshooting guide for interventional radiologists. Radiographics. 2002 Mar–Apr;22(2):305–22.

39 Percutaneous Transhepatic Biliary Balloon Dilation for Benign Biliary Strictures

Bedros Taslakian

INTRODUCTION

Cholestasis results from any obstruction, or relative obstruction, of the bile duct. It can be caused by benign or malignant conditions. Percutaneous balloon dilation of the duct is used alone, without stent placement, for treatment of benign strictures typically occurring at a surgical anastomosis. In general, self-expanding metallic stents should never be placed for benign strictures unless for some other reasons the patient's life expectancy is quite short since median stent patency is usually measured in months. The procedure is usually staged with a percutaneous transhepatic biliary drainage performed first. This allows for decompression of the biliary tree, resolution of cholangitis, and maturation of the transhepatic tract decreasing the risk of bacteremia and other associated complications.

COMMON INDICATIONS [1–3]

- Post-transplant anastomotic stricture
- Anastomotic stricture post choledochoenterostomy
- Iatrogenic proximal ductal stricture
- Iatrogenic distal biliary or common bile duct stricture after a failed endoscopic dilation
- Inflammatory, medication or radiation-induced and ischemic ductal strictures

COMMON CONTRAINDICATIONS [1–3]

- Asymptomatic patients
- Cholangitis or significant infection involving the percutaneous tract or entry site *(absolute contraindication)*
- Hemodynamic instability
- Diffuse process with the presence of multiple obstructed and isolated biliary segments *(the procedure is unlikely to succeed)*
- Worsening liver function despite adequate external biliary drainage
- Large volume ascites *(consider paracentesis before the procedure)*

POSSIBLE COMPLICATIONS [1–5]

Complications related to biliary access, manipulation, and dilatation:

- Hemorrhage, *2.5 %;* including subcapsular, peritoneal, or hemobilia
- Arterial injury *(e.g., pseudoaneurysm, focal arterial spasm, arterial–biliary, and arterial–venous fistulas)*
- Biliary sepsis, *2.5 %*
- Cholangitis

B. Taslakian (✉)
Department of Radiology, New York University Langone Medical Center, 660 First Ave, New York, NY 10016, USA
e-mail: Btaslakian@gmail.com

B. Taslakian et al. (eds.), *Procedural Dictations in Image-Guided Intervention*,
DOI 10.1007/978-3-319-40845-3_39

- Pleural transgression, *0.5 %;* mainly with right-sided punctures *(hemopneumothorax, empyema, pneumothorax, bilious effusion, fistula)*
- Transgression of adjacent abdominal structures *(colon, small bowel)*
- Recurrent stenosis after balloon dilatation of benign strictures
- Death, *1.7 %*

PREPROCEDURAL ASSESSMENT AND PLANNING

- History, indications, and physical examination *(Appendix 1* in Chap. 149*)*
- Evaluation of diagnostic imaging studies to determine the extent of biliary dilatation, level of obstruction, presence of isolation, status of portal vein, etiology, and the relevant anatomy for planning
- Periprocedural management of coagulation status *(Appendices 2* in Chap. 150 *and 3* in Chap. 151*)*
- Antibiotic prophylaxis: Routine prophylaxis is recommended *(Appendices 4* in Chap. 152 *and 5* in Chap. 153*)* [3, 6]
- Imaging modality for guidance: Fluoroscopy, combined with ultrasound for biliary access.
- Positioning: Supine

PROCEDURE NOTE

Procedure: Percutaneous biliary balloon dilation
Staff: [_]
Fellow: [_]
Resident: [_]
Clinical Information: Describe history and list indications
Allergies: None known/Allergic to [specify/type of allergy]
Anesthesia: Local anesthesia with conscious sedation/general anesthesia
Medications: List any relevant medications used (sedation, antibiotics)
Contrast Material: (_) mL of [type] contrast material
Field: Sterile
Procedure classification: Clean-contaminated/Contaminated
Position: Supine
Monitoring: Intravenous access line was secured and vital signs were continuously monitored by nursing staff/anesthesia team throughout the procedure
Total fluoroscopy time: (_) minutes
Cumulative radiation dose: (_) mGy

Description of Procedure *(the patient has an internal–external drain):*
The risks, benefits, alternatives, and the procedure itself were explained to the patient/patient's Power of Attorney/legal guardian, and informed written/verbal consent was obtained. The site of the procedure was identified and marked. Time out was performed to confirm the correct patient, procedure, and site.

The skin and the previously inserted biliary drain were prepped and draped in the usual sterile fashion. Using fluoroscopy, a (0.035)-in. [type] guidewire was inserted through the drain and looped in the duodenum/intestine. The drain was then exchanged over the guidewire for a (_)-French [type] sheath. A second (0.035)-in. [stiff/type] guidewire was inserted through the sheath and looped in the duodenum/intestine, leaving the first safety guidewire in place. Cholangiography was performed to identify the site of stricture. A (_) mm [noncompliant/type] high-pressure balloon catheter was inserted over the [stiff/type] guidewire to the level of the stricture. Dilation of the duct was performed by inflating the balloon manually with dilute contrast material using a (_)-mL syringe/inflating device, under fluoroscopy visualization until the "waist" at the stricture site disappeared. The balloon was left inflated for (1–3) min and the inflation was/was not repeated on (_) consecutive occasions.

[Additional dilation was performed using a bigger, (_) mm [type] balloon since post-dilatation cholangiography showed residual narrowing].

Subsequently, a (_)-French [internal–external/self-retaining/type] biliary drainage catheter was inserted over the guidewire and across the stricture. Spot fluoroscopy image was obtained after minimal contrast injection to confirm the catheter position and patency of the drainage catheter for documentation and future reference. The catheter was locked, anchored to the skin, and attached to a gravity drainage system.

The patient was transferred to the floor/recovery room following the procedure in a stable condition. Staff was present for the entire procedure.

Description of Procedure *(the patient has an external drain only):*
The risks, benefits, alternatives, and the procedure itself were explained to the patient/patient's Power of Attorney/legal guardian, and informed written/verbal consent was obtained. The site of the procedure was identified and marked. Time out was performed to confirm the correct patient, procedure and site.

The skin and the previously inserted external biliary drain were prepped and draped in the usual sterile fashion. Under fluoroscopy visualization, a (0.035)-in. [type] guidewire was inserted through the drain and looped in the biliary tree. The drain was then exchanged over the guidewire for a (_)-French sheath. Cholangiography was performed to identify the site of obstruction. The first guidewire was left in place as a safety wire. Through the sheath, a (_) French [angiographic/biliary manipulation/type] catheter was inserted over a (0.035)-in. [hydrophilic/type] guidewire to navigate through the point of stricture/obstruction, which was successfully crossed. The catheter was advanced into the duodenum/intestine over the [hydrophilic/type] guidewire, which was then exchanged through the catheter for a (0.035)-in. [stiff/type] guidewire. A (_) mm [noncompliant/type] high-pressure balloon catheter was inserted over the stiff guidewire to the level of the stricture. Dilation of the duct was performed by inflating the balloon manually with dilute contrast material using a (_)-mL syringe/inflating device, under fluoroscopy visualization until the "waist" at the stricture site disappeared. The balloon was left inflated for (1–3) min and the inflation was/was not repeated on (_) consecutive occasions.

[Additional dilation was performed using a bigger, (_) mm [type] balloon since post-dilatation cholangiography showed residual narrowing].

Subsequently, a (_)-French [internal–external/self-retaining/type] biliary drainage catheter was inserted over the guidewire and across the stricture. Spot fluoroscopy image was obtained after minimal contrast injection to confirm the catheter position and patency of the drainage catheter for documentation and future reference. The catheter was locked, anchored to the skin, and attached to a gravity drainage system.

The patient was transferred to the floor/recovery room following the procedure in a stable condition. Staff was present for the entire procedure.

Intra-Procedure Findings: List all the relevant findings.

Immediate Complications: None were encountered during or directly after the procedure. List complications if any.

Post-Procedure Plan [1–3, 7]:

- Follow-up laboratory results and adjust/continue antibiotics treatment as medically necessary.
- Keep complete bed rest for 3–4 h and abstain from strenuous activities.
- Start clear liquid diet for the first hour, then regular diet thereafter if tolerated and otherwise not contraindicated.
- Replace bile loss with intravenous fluids as necessary during external drainage period.
- Cap catheter when bile is clear and bilirubin has plateaued.
- Check vital signs every 15 min for 1 h, every 30 min for 1 h, every 60 min for 2 h and then as needed.
- Inform interventional radiology team if systolic blood pressure < 95 mm Hg, heart rate > 100 beats per minute, or if any chest pain or shortness of breath develops.
- If signs of peritonitis, sepsis or hemorrhage, chest/abdominal pain, or pericatheter

erythema are observed take corrective measures as medically needed and inform interventional radiology team immediately.

- Check complete blood count, liver function tests, and blood cultures as needed.
- Daily catheter care:
  - Inspect catheter and make sure that the 3-way stopcock is open to the drainage bag if not capped and the catheter has not been externally retracted.
  - Flush the catheter with 20 mL of bacteriostatic saline daily; 10 mL toward the drainage bag and 10 mL toward the liver. If a leak is present due to bile duct injury, the catheter can be flushed gently after 24 h of the procedure.
  - Perform site cleaning and dressing change weekly or more frequently as needed.
  - Record the catheter output every 8 h.
  - Inform interventional radiology team if the draining amount decreases or stops, or if pericatheter leak or local skin complications occur.
- Follow-up plan: *(balloon dilatation)*
  - Follow-up tube cholangiography after acute swelling has resolved in 2 weeks.
  - If repeat dilation is indicated, use progressively larger high-pressure balloon or a cutting balloon or both in each session.
  - Between sessions of balloon dilation, keep the internal–external biliary catheter in the duct under dependent drainage to prevent relapse.
  - After the stricture is visually resolved, keep the external–internal drain through the stricture for 3–4 weeks.
  - After a technically successful treatment and clinical follow-up, externalize and cap the biliary catheter *(place proximal to the site of previous stricture)* for 1 week. If the patient remains asymptomatic and laboratory test results are not suggestive of biliary obstruction, indicating good internal drainage, the catheter can be safely removed after cholangiography proofs adequate flow through the dilated duct segment.
  - Perform tractography prior to removal of catheters draining by the transpleural or transperitoneal route to confirm tract maturity or if biliary–arterial communication is suspected. Usually not necessary if catheter has been in place for a month or more.
  - Obtain liver function tests and clinical evaluation at 3 and 6 months after external catheter removal.

Impression:

- Imaging-guided percutaneous biliary dilation as described above.
- The patient tolerated the procedure well and left the interventional unit in a stable condition.
- The patient was unstable and the procedure was canceled/terminated prematurely.
- List any other relevant or important information/findings.

References

1. Hunter DW. Percutaneous biliary interventions. In: Kandarpa K, Machan L, editors. Handbook of interventional radiologic procedures. 4th ed. Philadelphia: Lippincott Williams & Wilkins; 2011. p. 577–90.
2. Saad WEA. Management of benign biliary strictures. In: Mauro MA, Murphy KPJ, Thomson KR, Venbrux AC, Morgan RA, editors. Image-guided interventions. 2nd ed. Philadelphia: Saunders Elsevier; 2014. p. 994–1001.
3. Management of benign biliary strictures. In: Burke CT, Dixon RG, Mauro MA, Murphy KPJ, Thomson KR, Venbrux AC, Zollikofer CL, editors. High yield imaging: interventional. Philadelphia: Saunders Elsevier; 2010:427–430.
4. Winick AB, Waybill PN, Venbrux AC. Complications of percutaneous transhepatic biliary interventions. Tech Vasc Interv Radiol. 2001;4(3):200–6.
5. Saad WE, Wallace MJ, Wojak JC, Kundu S, Cardella JF. Quality improvement guidelines for percutaneous transhepatic cholangiography, biliary drainage, and percutaneous cholecystostomy. J Vasc Interv Radiol. 2010;21(6):789–95.
6. Venkatesan AM, Kundu S, Sacks D, Wallace MJ, Wojak JC, Rose SC, et al. Practice guidelines for adult antibiotic prophylaxis during vascular and interventional radiology procedures. J Vasc Interv Radiol. 2010;21(11):1611–30.
7. Maher MM, Kealey S, McNamara A, O'Laoide R, Gibney RG, Malone DE. Management of visceral interventional radiology catheters: a troubleshooting guide for interventional radiologists. Radiographics. 2002 Mar–Apr;22(2):305–22.

Percutaneous Transhepatic Biliary Drainage

40

Bedros Taslakian

Abbreviations

ERCP Endoscopic retrograde cholangiopancreatography

INTRODUCTION

Endoscopic retrograde cholangiopancreatography (ERCP) and biliary drainage are often the first line therapy for low bile duct obstruction. Obstruction involving the confluence of left and right hepatic ducts is better managed percutaneously by interventional radiologists. The percutaneous approach also provides a portal of access to the biliary tract for percutaneous therapeutic interventions (e.g., balloon dilatation of benign biliary stricture, stenting of malignant bile duct stricture, extraction of bile duct stones, brachytherapy for cholangiocarcinoma, endoluminal tissue sampling, and foreign body retrieval).

COMMON INDICATIONS [1–6]

- Decompression of obstructed biliary tree to reduce serum bilirubin if needed for chemotherapy administration, intractable pruritus, or cholangitis
- Malignant or benign biliary obstruction with failed ERCP or any case of high bile duct obstruction as depicted on cross-sectional imaging
- Status post bilioenteric bypass where endoscopic approach unlikely to be successful
- Bile duct injury resulting in major biliary leakage, for diversion
- Provide a portal of access for percutaneous therapeutic interventions such as brachytherapy, or stone removal

COMMON CONTRAINDICATIONS [1–4, 6]

- Hemodynamic instability
- Large volume ascites *(consider drainage before the procedure)*
- History of allergic contrast reaction *(contrast material is often introduced into the vascular system during the procedure)*
- Presence of multiple obstructed and isolated biliary segments *(the procedure is unlikely to provide palliation and may introduce further complications)*

B. Taslakian (✉)
Department of Radiology, New York University Langone Medical Center, 660 First Ave, New York, NY 10016, USA
e-mail: Btaslakian@gmail.com

B. Taslakian et al. (eds.), *Procedural Dictations in Image-Guided Intervention*,
DOI 10.1007/978-3-319-40845-3_40

POSSIBLE COMPLICATIONS [1–7]

- Hemorrhage, *2.5 %*
- Transcatheter bleeding due to presence of catheter side holes near a transgressed portal or hepatic venous branch
- Arterial injury *(e.g., pseudoaneurysm, focal arterial spasm, arterial-biliary and arterial-venous fistulas)*
- Cholangitis, bacteremia, and septic shock, *2.5 %*
- Bile leak and biliary peritonitis
- Pancreatitis
- Pleural transgression, *0.5 %;* mainly with right-sided punctures *(hemopneumothorax, empyema, pneumothorax, bilious effusion, fistula)*
- Transgression of adjacent abdominal structures *(colon, small bowel)*
- Death, *1.7 %*

PREPROCEDURAL ASSESSMENT AND PLANNING

- History, indications, and physical examination *(Appendix 1* in Chap. 149*)*
- Recent cross-sectional imaging studies to determine the extent of biliary dilatation, level of obstruction, presence of isolation of parts of biliary tree from one another, status of portal veins, findings of hepatic atrophy, any anatomic considerations relevant for procedure planning (ascites, location of tumor, colon interposed between abdominal wall, and liver, etc.)
- Periprocedural management of coagulation status *(Appendices 2* in Chap. 150 *and 3* in Chap. 151*)*
- Antibiotic prophylaxis: Routine prophylaxis is recommended *(Appendices 4* in Chap. 152 *and 5* in Chap. 153*)* [1, 3, 5, 8]
- Imaging modality for guidance: Fluoroscopy, combined with ultrasound for biliary access
- Positioning: Supine

PROCEDURE NOTE

Procedure: Percutaneous transhepatic biliary drainage
Staff: [_]
Fellow: [_]
Resident: [_]
Clinical Information: Describe history and list indications
Allergies: None known/Allergic to [specify/type of allergy]
Anesthesia: Local anesthesia/conscious sedation/general anesthesia
Medications: List any relevant medications used (sedation, antibiotics)
Contrast Material: (_) mL of [type] contrast material
Field: Sterile
Procedure classification: Clean-contaminated/ Contaminated
Position: Supine
Monitoring: Intravenous access line was secured and vital signs were continuously monitored by nursing staff/anesthesia team throughout the procedure
Total fluoroscopy time: (_) minutes
Cumulative radiation dose: (_) mGy

Description of Procedure *(internal–external biliary drainage):*
The risks, benefits, alternatives and the procedure itself were explained to the patient/patient's Power of Attorney/legal guardian, and informed written/verbal consent was obtained. The site of the procedure was identified and marked. Time out was performed to confirm the correct patient, procedure and site.

The procedure was planned and the skin puncture site was marked using combined information from the preliminary ultrasound/fluoroscopy images along the epigastric area/right (_)th intercostal/subcostal space. The target duct of segment (_) was selected for optimal access to the biliary system.

The skin was prepped and draped in the usual sterile fashion. Local anesthesia was administered.

A small skin incision was made. The target duct was punctured with a (21)-gauge [Chiba/type] needle under ultrasound/fluoroscopy guidance through an epigastric/a right intercostal/a subcostal approach. After confirming the needle tip position with minimal contrast injection, a (0.018) in. guidewire was advanced into the biliary tree and used to place a (_)-French introducer. Bile was aspirated to decompress the system and to obtain a specimen for culture and sensitivity/cytology. Then, the biliary system was opacified with contrast under constant fluoroscopic control, demonstrating biliary obstruction/long/short-segment stricture/bile leak at [specify location]. Images of the biliary tree were obtained in multiple projections.

Subsequently, a (0.035)-in. [type] guidewire was advanced through the introducer system into the biliary tree, while keeping the (0.018)-in. safety guidewire in place. The introducer system was then exchanged over the (0.035)-in. [type] guidewire for a (_) French [type] sheath, with subsequent decompression of the biliary system. Through the sheath, a (_) French [angiographic/biliary manipulation/type] catheter was inserted over a (0.035)-in. [hydrophilic/type] guidewire to navigate through the point of stricture/obstruction/leak, which was successfully crossed. The catheter was advanced into the duodenum/intestine over the [hydrophilic/type] guidewire, which was then exchanged through the catheter for a (0.035)-in. [stiff/type] guidewire. Brush biopsy was performed at the site of obstruction/stricture using [specify type of instrument], with a (3-mm) brush at the end of a braided wire being advanced through the sheath to the level of the stricture. Biopsy of the stricture was obtained using (2 mm) alligator jaw forceps to grasp a specimen from the biliary tree at the point of stricture. Specimen was sent for cytopathology. Following this, a (_)-French internal–external [self-locking/type] biliary drainage catheter was inserted over the stiff guidewire and its tip was formed in the duodenum/intestine.

Images were obtained after contrast injection to confirm the catheter position and patency, for documentation and future reference. The catheter was locked, anchored to the skin, and attached to a gravity drainage system.

The patient was transferred to the floor/recovery room/intensive care unit following the procedure in a stable/critical condition. Staff was present for the entire procedure.

Description of Procedure *(external biliary drainage):*

The risks, benefits, alternatives, and the procedure itself were explained to the patient/patient's Power of Attorney/legal guardian, and informed written/verbal consent was obtained. The site of the procedure was identified and marked. Time out was performed to confirm the correct patient, procedure, and site.

The procedure was planned and the skin puncture site was marked using combined information from the preliminary ultrasound/fluoroscopy images along the epigastric area/right (_)th intercostal/subcostal space anterior to midaxillary line. The target duct of segment (_) was selected for optimal access to the biliary system.

The skin was prepped and draped in the usual sterile fashion. Local anesthesia was administered. A small skin incision was made. The target duct was punctured with a (21)-gauge [Chiba/type] needle under ultrasound/fluoroscopy guidance through an epigastric/a right intercostal/a subcostal approach. After confirming the needle tip position with minimal contrast injection, a (0.018) inch guidewire was advanced into the biliary tree and used to place a (_)-French introducer. Bile was aspirated to decompress the system and to obtain a specimen for culture and sensitivity/cytology. Then, the biliary system was opacified with contrast under constant fluoroscopic control, demonstrating biliary obstruction/long/short-segment stricture/bile leak at [specify location]. Images of the biliary tree were obtained in multiple projections. Subsequently, a (0.035)-in. [type] guidewire was advanced through the introducer system into the biliary tree, while keeping the (0.018)-in. safety guidewire in place.

Since the patient was unstable no attempt was made to cross the obstruction and a (_)-French external biliary drain was placed. OR The introducer system was then exchanged over the (0.035)-in. [type] guidewire for a (_) French

[type] sheath, with subsequent decompression of the biliary system. Through the sheath, a (_) French [angiographic/biliary manipulation/type] catheter was inserted over a (0.035)-in. [hydrophilic/type] guidewire to navigate through the point of stricture/obstruction/leak. This was not possible and consequently, a (_)-French external [self-locking/type] catheter was inserted over the guidewire proximally, for external drainage and to provide access for future interventions. Spot fluoroscopy image was obtained after minimal contrast injection to confirm the catheter position and patency, for documentation and future reference. The catheter was locked, anchored to the skin and attached to a gravity drainage system.

The patient was transferred to the floor/recovery room/intensive care unit following the procedure in a stable/critical condition. Staff was present for the entire procedure.

Intra-Procedure Findings: List all relevant findings.

Immediate Complications: None encountered during or directly after the procedure. List complications if any.

Post-Procedure Plan [1–3, 6, 9]:

- Follow-up laboratory results and adjust/continue antibiotics treatment accordingly.
- Keep catheter open to gravity drainage.
- Replace bile loss with intravenous fluids as necessary during external drainage period.
- Keep complete bed rest for 3–4 h and abstain from strenuous activities.
- Start clear liquid diet for the first hour, then regular diet thereafter if tolerated and otherwise not contraindicated.
- Check vital signs every 15 min for 1 h, every 30 min for 1 h, every 60 min for 2 h and then as needed.
- Inform interventional radiology team if systolic blood pressure < 95 mm Hg, heart rate > 110 beats per minute, or if any chest pain or shortness of breath develops.
- If signs of peritonitis, sepsis or hemorrhage; chest or abdominal pain; pericatheter erythema; and/or transcatheter bleeding are observed take corrective measures as medically needed and inform interventional radiology team immediately.
- Check complete blood count, liver function tests, and blood cultures as needed.
- Daily catheter care:
  - For internal/external catheters, the catheter can be capped after bile clears of any blood and bilirubin has normalized or plateaued. Check for catheter retraction.
  - For external catheters, inspect catheter and make sure that the 3-way stopcock is open to the drainage bag and the catheter has not been externally retracted.
  - Flush the catheter slowly with 5–10 mL of bacteriostatic saline every 8 h during external drainage period and daily thereafter to prevent bile clogging.
  - If the catheter is capped, flush it gently with 5–10 mL of normal saline at least every other day.
  - Perform site cleaning and dressing change weekly or more frequently as needed.
  - Record the catheter outputs every 8 h during external drainage period.
  - Inform interventional radiology team if the draining amount decreases or stops, pericatheter leak or local skin complications occur.
  - Avoid taking baths and swimming. Take showers with the tubes protected by plastic covering that is impervious to water.
- Follow-up plan *(biliary obstruction)*:
  - Internal/external catheters can be converted to stents when appropriate clinically.
  - If there is some reason the patient is not a candidate for stenting, then catheters should be routinely exchanged every 10–12 weeks.
  - When an external catheter has been placed a subsequent attempt at internalizing or converting to stent should be made in 1–2 weeks.

- Follow-up plan *(biliary leak)*:
  - The catheter can be internalized *(capped)* safely, when absence of biliary leak is confirmed.
  - If prolonged catheter drainage is anticipated, exchange the catheter for a larger softer multi-sidehole catheter.
  - Prolonged biliary drainage for several weeks to months may be necessary. Exchange the catheter over a guidewire during this period every 2 months.
  - Exchange the multi-sidehole catheter for a smaller one with no sideholes *(no draining function)* once the bile leak is sealed on repeat tube cholangiography, the clinical status of the patient improves, and resolution of associated biloma is confirmed on cross-sectional imaging and by significant decrease in the output of the catheter draining the biloma. The biliary catheter can be removed after a test period of 4–8 weeks.

Impression:

- Percutaneous transhepatic biliary drainage, as described above. The catheter placed drains the entire biliary tree/only the right/left side.
- The patient tolerated the procedure well and left the interventional unit in a stable condition.
- The patient was unstable and the procedure was canceled/terminated prematurely.
- List any other relevant or important information/finding.

References

1. Thornton RH, Covey AM. Management of malignant biliary tract obstruction. In: Mauro MA, Murphy KPJ, Thomson KR, Venbrux AC, Morgan RA, editors. Image-guided interventions. 2nd ed. Philadelphia: Saunders Elsevier; 2014. p. 981–93.
2. Portugaller RH, Hausegger KA. Management of biliary leaks. In: Mauro MA, Murphy KPJ, Thomson KR, Venbrux AC, Morgan RA, editors. Image-guided interventions. 2nd ed. Philadelphia: Saunders Elsevier; 2014. p. 1002–7.
3. Hunter DW. Percutaneous biliary interventions. In: Kandarpa K, Machan L, editors. Handbook of interventional radiologic procedures. 4th ed. Philadelphia: Lippincott Williams & Wilkins; 2011. p. 577–90.
4. Saad WE, Wallace MJ, Wojak JC, Kundu S, Cardella JF. Quality improvement guidelines for percutaneous transhepatic cholangiography, biliary drainage, and percutaneous cholecystostomy. J Vasc Interv Radiol. 2010;21(6):789–95.
5. Covey AM, Brown KT. Percutaneous transhepatic biliary drainage. Tech Vasc Interv Radiol. 2008;11: 14–20.
6. Percutaneous biliary drainage. In: Burke CT, Dixon RG, Mauro MA, Murphy KPJ, Thomson KR, Venbrux AC, Zollikofer CL, editors. High yield imaging: interventional. Philadelphia: Saunders Elsevier; 2010. p. 420–3.
7. Winick AB, Waybill PN, Venbrux AC. Complications of percutaneous transhepatic biliary interventions. Tech Vasc Interv Radiol. 2001;4(3):200–6.
8. Venkatesan AM, Kundu S, Sacks D, Wallace MJ, Wojak JC, Rose SC, et al. Practice guidelines for adult antibiotic prophylaxis during vascular and interventional radiology procedures. J Vasc Interv Radiol. 2010;21(11):1611–30.
9. Maher MM, Kealey S, McNamara A, O'Laoide R, Gibney RG, Malone DE. Management of visceral interventional radiology catheters: a troubleshooting guide for interventional radiologists. Radiographics. 2002;22(2):305–22.

Percutaneous Transhepatic Biliary Stent Placement

41

Bedros Taslakian

INTRODUCTION

Bile duct obstruction can be caused by benign or malignant conditions and patients can present with elevated liver function tests, jaundice, pruritus, cholangitis (when the biliary tree has been contaminated), or any combination of those signs/symptoms. Percutaneous biliary stent placement is used for symptomatic palliation of malignant biliary obstruction in patients who are not candidates for surgery. When patients have low bile duct obstruction, for instance from pancreatic cancer, this is often accomplished endoscopically and thus the patient never has an exteriorized catheter. Patients with high bile duct obstruction, and those who cannot be stented endoscopically, are stented percutaneously; the stent can be placed primarily, or the procedure staged with a percutaneous transhepatic biliary drainage performed first. Placement of a drainage catheter prior to stent placement is recommended for patients who present with cholangitis. This allows the transhepatic tract to mature and is associated with a lower complication rate.

B. Taslakian (✉)
Department of Radiology, New York University Langone Medical Center, 660 First Ave, New York, NY 10016, USA
e-mail: Btaslakian@gmail.com

COMMON INDICATIONS [1–4]

- Palliation of symptomatic malignant biliary obstruction in patients who are not candidates for surgical or endoscopic treatment
- Metal stents have very good patency rates and offer palliation without an exteriorized catheter. In addition, for high bile duct obstruction, a metal stent can be placed entirely above the Ampulla of Vater, avoiding contamination of the biliary tree.

COMMON CONTRAINDICATIONS [1–3]

- Asymptomatic patients
- Surgically resectable malignancy
- Cholangitis *(absolute contraindication)*
- Hemobilia with intra-ductal clot *(increased risk of stent occlusion)*
- Intra-ductal stones or debris *(increased risk of stent occlusion)*
- Hemodynamic instability
- Diffuse process with the presence of multiple obstructed and isolated biliary segments *(the procedure is unlikely to provide palliation)*
- Worsening liver function despite adequate external biliary drainage
- Large volume ascites *(consider drainage before the procedure)*

B. Taslakian et al. (eds.), *Procedural Dictations in Image-Guided Intervention*,
DOI 10.1007/978-3-319-40845-3_41

POSSIBLE COMPLICATIONS [1–6]

Complications related to biliary access and manipulation:

- Hemorrhage, *2.5 %;* including subcapsular, peritoneal, or hemobilia
- Arterial injury *(e.g., pseudoaneurysm, focal arterial spasm, arterial-biliary and arterial-venous fistulas)*
- Bile leak and biliary peritonitis
- Cholangitis, septic shock, *2.5 %*
- Pleural transgression, *0.5 %;* mainly with right-sided punctures *(hemopneumothorax, empyema, pneumothorax, bilious effusion, fistula)*
- Transgression of adjacent abdominal structures *(colon, small bowel)*
- Death, *1.7 %*

Complications related to stent placement:

- Stent misplacement
- Stent migration
- Pancreatitis and cholecystitis
- Stent malfunction due to tumor ingrowth and overgrowth
- Stent malfunction due to intraluminal debris, blood, or stones
- Stent occlusion leading to infection or jaundice
- Cholecystitis

PREPROCEDURAL ASSESSMENT AND PLANNING

- History, indications, and physical examination *(Appendix 1* in Chap. 149*)*
- Evaluation of diagnostic imaging studies to determine the extent of biliary dilatation, level of obstruction, the presence of isolation, status of portal vein, etiology, and the relevant anatomy for planning
- Periprocedural management of coagulation status *(Appendices 2* in Chap. 150 *and 3* in Chap. 151*)*
- Antibiotic prophylaxis: Routine prophylaxis is recommended *(Appendices 4* in Chap. 152 *and 5* in Chap. 153*)* [2, 7]
- Imaging modality for guidance: Fluoroscopy; combined with ultrasound for biliary access.
- Positioning: Supine

PROCEDURE NOTE

Procedure: Percutaneous biliary stent placement
Staff: [_]
Fellow: [_]
Resident: [_]
Clinical Information: Describe history and list indications
Allergies: None known/Allergic to [specify/type of allergy]
Anesthesia: Local anesthesia with conscious sedation/general anesthesia
Medications: List any relevant medications used (sedation, antibiotics)
Contrast Material: (_) mL of [type] contrast material was used for intra-biliary injection
Field: Sterile
Procedure classification: Clean-contaminated/Contaminated
Position: Supine
Monitoring: Intravenous access line was secured and vital signs were continuously monitored by nursing staff/anesthesia team throughout the procedure
Total fluoroscopy time: (_) minutes
Cumulative radiation dose: (_) mGy

Description of Procedure *(the patient has an internal-external drain):*
The risks, benefits, alternatives, and the procedure itself were explained to the patient/patient's Power of Attorney/legal guardian, and informed written/verbal consent was obtained. The site of the procedure was identified and marked. Time out was performed to confirm the correct patient, procedure, and site.

The skin and the previously inserted biliary drain were prepped and draped in the usual sterile fashion. Using fluoroscopy, a (0.035)-in. [type] guidewire was inserted through the drain and looped in the duodenum/intestine. The drain was then exchanged over the guidewire for a (_)-

French [type] sheath. Cholangiography was performed to identify the site of stricture.

[Due to poor contrast flow through the tight stricture, pre-dilation was performed using a (_) mm [non-compliant/type] high-pressure balloon catheter inserted over the [stiff/type] guidewire to the level of the stricture.] A (_) cm long, (_) mm diameter [type] stent was then advanced over the guidewire to the level of the stricture and was deployed. Once the stent was adequately placed through the stricture, cholangiography was performed to ensure that contrast material flowed freely into the bowel and the stent was flared at both ends. [Additional dilation was performed using a (_) mm [type] balloon since the stent was not well expanded and poor flow into bowel was noted.]

Subsequently, a (_)-French [external self-retaining/type] biliary drainage catheter was inserted over the guidewire and positioned above the stent. Spot fluoroscopy image was obtained after minimal contrast injection to confirm the catheter position and patency of the stent and drainage catheter, for documentation and future reference. The catheter was locked, anchored to the skin, and attached to a gravity drainage system.

The patient was transferred to the floor/recovery room following the procedure in a stable condition. Staff was present for the entire procedure.

Description of Procedure *(the patient has an external drain only):*

The risks, benefits, alternatives, and the procedure itself were explained to the patient/patient's Power of Attorney/legal guardian, and informed written/verbal consent was obtained. The site of the procedure was identified and marked. Time out was performed to confirm the correct patient, procedure, and site.

The skin and the previously inserted external biliary drain were prepped and draped in the usual sterile fashion. Under fluoroscopy visualization, a (0.035)-in. [type] guidewire was inserted through the drain and looped in the biliary tree. The drain was then exchanged over the guidewire for a (_)-French sheath. Cholangiography was performed to identify the site of obstruction. The first guidewire was left in place as a safety wire. Through the sheath, a (_) French [angiographic/biliary manipulation/type] catheter was inserted over a (0.035)-in. [hydrophilic/type] guidewire to navigate through the point of stricture/obstruction, which was successfully crossed. The catheter was advanced into the duodenum/intestine over the [hydrophilic/type] guidewire, which was then exchanged through the catheter for a (0.035)-in. [stiff/type] guidewire.

The safety guidewire was withdrawn. [Due to poor contrast flow through the tight stricture, pre-dilation was performed using a (_) mm [non-compliant/type] high-pressure balloon catheter inserted over the [stiff/type] guidewire to the level of the stricture.] A (_) cm long, (_) mm diameter [type] stent was then advanced over the guidewire to the level of the stricture and was deployed. Once the stent was adequately placed through the stricture, cholangiography was performed to ensure that contrast material flowed freely into the bowel and the stent was flared at both ends. [Additional dilation was performed using a (_) mm [type] balloon since the stent was not well expanded and poor flow into bowel was noted.]

Subsequently, a (_)-French [external self-retaining/type] biliary drainage catheter was inserted over the guidewire and positioned above the stent. Spot fluoroscopy image was obtained after minimal contrast injection to confirm the catheter position and patency of the stent and drainage catheter, for documentation and future reference. The catheter was locked, anchored to the skin, and attached to a gravity drainage system.

The patient was transferred to the floor/recovery room following the procedure in a stable condition. Staff was present for the entire procedure.

Intra-Procedure Findings: List all relevant findings.

Immediate Complications: None encountered during or directly after the procedure. List complications if any.

Post-Procedure Plan [1–3, 8]:

- Follow-up laboratory results and adjust/continue antibiotics treatment as medically necessary.
- Keep complete bed rest for 3–4 h and abstain from strenuous activities.
- Start clear liquid diet for the first hour, then regular diet thereafter if tolerated and otherwise not contraindicated.
- Replace bile loss with intravenous fluids as necessary during external drainage period.
- Cap catheter when bile is clear and bilirubin has plateaued.
- Check vital signs every 15 min for 1 h, every 30 min for 1 h, every 60 min for 2 h and then as needed.
- Inform interventional radiology team if systolic blood pressure <95 mm Hg, heart rate >100 beats per minute, or if any chest pain or shortness of breath develops.
- If signs of peritonitis, sepsis or hemorrhage; chest/abdominal pain; pericatheter erythema are observed, take corrective measures as medically needed and inform interventional radiology team immediately.
- Check complete blood count, liver function tests, and blood cultures as needed.
- Daily catheter care, until removed:
  - Inspect catheter and make sure that the three-way stopcock is open to the drainage bag if not capped and the catheter has not been externally retracted.
  - Flush the catheter with 20 mL of bacteriostatic saline daily; 10 mL towards the drainage bag and 10 mL towards the liver. If a leak is present due to bile duct injury, the catheter can be flushed gently after 24 h of the procedure.
  - Perform site cleaning and dressing change weekly or more frequently as needed.
  - Record the catheter output every 8 h.
  - Inform interventional radiology team if the draining amount decreases or stops, pericatheter leak or local skin complications occurs.
- Follow-up plan:
  - Keep biliary drainage catheter in place under dependent drainage for 24–48 h.
  - Follow a successful 24 h observation with cholangiography to document patency of the stent.
  - After a technically successful stenting and uneventful observation period (clearing of the bile, absence of symptoms, bilirubin trending down, or plateauing), the external drain can be capped and if the patient remains asymptomatic the drain can be safely removed.

Impression:

- Imaging-guided percutaneous metallic biliary stent placement, as described above.
- The patient tolerated the procedure well and left the interventional unit in a stable condition.
- The patient was unstable and the procedure was canceled/terminated prematurely.
- List any other relevant or important information/finding.

References

1. Thornton RH, Covey AM. Management of malignant biliary tract obstruction. In: Mauro MA, Murphy KPJ, Thomson KR, Venbrux AC, Morgan RA, editors. Image-guided interventions. 2nd ed. Philadelphia: Saunders Elsevier; 2014. p. 981–93.
2. Endobiliary stenting. In: Burke CT, Dixon RG, Mauro MA, Murphy KPJ, Thomson KR, Venbrux AC, Zollikofer CL, editors. High yield imaging: interventional. Philadelphia: Saunders Elsevier; 2010:416–9.
3. Hunter DW. Percutaneous biliary interventions. In: Kandarpa K, Machan L, editors. Handbook of interventional radiologic procedures. 4th ed. Philadelphia: Lippincott Williams & Wilkins; 2011. p. 577–90.
4. Krokidis M, Hatzidakis A. Percutaneous minimally invasive treatment of malignant biliary strictures: current status. Cardiovasc Intervent Radiol. 2014;37(2):316–23.
5. Winick AB, Waybill PN, Venbrux AC. Complications of percutaneous transhepatic biliary interventions. Tech Vasc Interv Radiol. 2001;4(3):200–6.
6. Saad WE, Wallace MJ, Wojak JC, Kundu S, Cardella JF. Quality improvement guidelines

for percutaneous transhepatic cholangiography, biliary drainage, and percutaneous cholecystostomy. J Vasc Interv Radiol. 2010;21(6):789–95.
7. Venkatesan AM, Kundu S, Sacks D, Wallace MJ, Wojak JC, Rose SC, et al. Practice guidelines for adult antibiotic prophylaxis during vascular and interventional radiology procedures. J Vasc Interv Radiol. 2010;21(11):1611–30.
8. Maher MM, Kealey S, McNamara A, O'Laoide R, Gibney RG, Malone DE. Management of visceral interventional radiology catheters: a troubleshooting guide for interventional radiologists. Radiographics. 2002;22(2):305–22.

Percutaneous Transhepatic Cholangiography

42

Bedros Taslakian

Abbreviations

ERCP	Endoscopic retrograde cholangiopancreatography
PTC	Percutaneous transhepatic cholangiography

INTRODUCTION

Percutaneous transhepatic cholangiography (PTC) is a safe and effective minimally invasive diagnostic procedure for evaluation of the biliary tree. PTC is rarely indicated and only in situations where non-invasive imaging modalities such as magnetic resonance cholangiopancreatography, ultrasound, or computed tomography provide insufficient information. PTC, of course, is performed as first step when biliary drainage is undertaken and images of diagnostic quality should be obtained in that circumstance before a catheter or stent is placed.

COMMON INDICATIONS [1–3]

- Evaluation of the biliary system prior to percutaneous biliary intervention
- Evaluation of tumor resectability in malignant biliary obstruction
- Evaluation for treatment planning in malignant biliary obstruction
- Patients status post biliary reconstruction with repeated episodes of cholangitis but without dilated ducts or obvious obstruction on cross sectional imaging
- Demonstrate site of bile leak
- Evaluate for the presence of suspected bile duct stones/intra-ductal tumor when other imaging modalities and ERCP fail
- Determine etiology of transplanted hepatic graft dysfunction

COMMON CONTRAINDICATIONS [1–3]

- Hemodynamic instability
- Large volume ascites *(consider drainage before the procedure)*
- History of allergic contrast reaction *(contrast material is often introduced into the vascular system during the procedure)*
- Absence of a safe route for needle placement (extremely rare)

B. Taslakian (✉)
Department of Radiology, New York University Langone Medical Center, 660 First Ave, New York, NY 10016, USA
e-mail: Btaslakian@gmail.com

B. Taslakian et al. (eds.), *Procedural Dictations in Image-Guided Intervention*,
DOI 10.1007/978-3-319-40845-3_42

POSSIBLE COMPLICATIONS [1–3]

- Hemorrhage *(subcapsular, peritoneal, or hemobilia)*
- Cholangitis with or without bacteremia and septic shock
- Pleural transgression, mainly with right-sided punctures *(hemopneumothorax, empyema, pneumothorax, bilious effusion, fistula)*
- Transgression of adjacent abdominal structures *(colon, small bowel)*
- Bile leak and secondary bile peritonitis

PREPROCEDURAL ASSESSMENT AND PLANNING [1, 3, 4–6]

- History, indications, and physical examination *(Appendix 1* in Chap. 149*)*
- Evaluation of diagnostic imaging studies to determine the extent of biliary dilatation, possible causes, and the relevant anatomy for planning
- Periprocedural management of coagulation status *(Appendices 2* in Chap. 150 *and 3* in Chap. 151*)*
- Antibiotic prophylaxis: Routine prophylaxis is recommended *(Appendices 4* in 152 *and 5* in Chap. 153*)* [1, 3, 4]
- Imaging modality for guidance: Fluoroscopy; combined with ultrasound for biliary access
- Positioning: Supine

PROCEDURE NOTE

Procedure: Percutaneous transhepatic cholangiography via left/right hepatic lobe
Staff: [_]
Fellow: [_]
Resident: [_]
Clinical Information: Describe history and list indications
Allergies: None known/Allergic to [specify/type of allergy]
Anesthesia: Local anesthesia/conscious sedation/general anesthesia
Medications: List any relevant medications used (sedation, antibiotics)
Contrast Material: (_) mL of [type] contrast material
Field: Sterile
Procedure classification: Clean-contaminated, contaminated *(in cases of biliary tree contamination—from ERCP or bilioenteric anastomosis for example)*
Position: Supine
Monitoring: Intravenous access line was secured and vital signs were continuously monitored by nursing staff/anesthesia team throughout the procedure
Total fluoroscopy time: (_) minutes
Cumulative radiation dose: (_) mGy

Description of Procedure:
The risks, benefits, alternatives, and the procedure itself were explained to the patient/patient's Power of Attorney/legal guardian, and informed written/verbal consent was obtained. The site of the procedure was identified and marked. Time out was performed to confirm the correct patient, procedure, and site.

The procedure was planned and the skin puncture site was marked using combined information from the preliminary ultrasound/fluoroscopy images along the epigastric area/right (_)th intercostal/subcostal space. The target duct of segment (_) was selected for optimal access to the biliary system.

The skin was prepped and draped in the usual sterile fashion. Local anesthesia was administered. A small skin incision was made. Segment (_) duct was punctured with a (21)-gauge [Chiba/type] needle under ultrasound/ fluoroscopy guidance through an epigastric/a right intercostal/a subcostal approach and was opacified. A (0.018) in. guidewire was advanced into the biliary tree and used to place a (_)-French introducer. The biliary system was then decompressed; aspirating as much bile as possible and sending a specimen for culture and sensitivity/cytology. The biliary system was opacified with contrast under constant fluoroscopic control. Spot images of the liver were obtained in multiple projections. Contrast and bile were then aspirated through the introducer which was subsequently removed. The patient was transferred to the floor/recovery room/discharged home following the procedure in a stable condition. Staff was scrubbed for the entire procedure.

Intra-Procedure Findings: List all relevant findings.

Immediate Complications: None encountered during or directly after the procedure. List complications if any.

Post-Procedure Plan [1, 3]:

1. Follow-up culture results and adjust antibiotics treatment accordingly.
2. Keep complete bed rest for 2–3 h and abstain from strenuous activities.
3. Start clear liquid diet for the first hour, then regular diet thereafter if tolerated and otherwise not contraindicated.
4. Check vital signs every 15 min for 1 h, every 30 min for 1 h and then every 60 min for 1 h.
5. Inform interventional radiology team if systolic blood pressure <95 mm Hg or heart rate >100 beats per minute.
6. Inform interventional radiology team if any new or worsening chest pain, shortness of breath or abdominal pain develops, or symptoms/signs of infection or melena are noted.
7. Outpatients: Instruct to seek medical attention if any new or worsening chest pain, shortness of breath, or abdominal pain develops or symptoms of infection or melena are noted.

Impression:

1. Diagnostic percutaneous transhepatic cholangiography via left/right liver, as described above.
2. The patient tolerated the procedure well and left the interventional unit in a stable condition.
3. The patient was unstable and the procedure was canceled/terminated prematurely.
4. List any other relevant or important information/finding.

References

1. Hunter DW. Percutaneous biliary interventions. In: Kandarpa K, Machan L, editors. Handbook of interventional radiologic procedures. 4th ed. Philadelphia: Lippincott Williams & Wilkins; 2011. p. 577–90.
2. Saad WE, Wallace MJ, Wojak JC, Kundu S, Cardella JF. Quality improvement guidelines for percutaneous transhepatic cholangiography, biliary drainage, and percutaneous cholecystostomy. J Vasc Interv Radiol. 2010;21(6):789–95.
3. Percutaneous transhepatic cholangiography. In: Burke CT, Dixon RG, Mauro MA, Murphy KPJ, Thomson KR, Venbrux AC, Zollikofer CL, editors. High yield imaging: interventional. Philadelphia: Saunders Elsevier; 2010. p. 424–6.
4. Venkatesan AM, Kundu S, Sacks D, Wallace MJ, Wojak JC, Rose SC, et al. Practice guidelines for adult antibiotic prophylaxis during vascular and interventional radiology procedures. J Vasc Interv Radiol. 2010;21(11):1611–30.
5. Taslakian B, Sebaaly MG, Al-Kutoubi A. Patient evaluation and preparation in vascular and interventional radiology: what every interventional radiologist should know (part 1: patient assessment and laboratory tests). Cardiovasc Intervent Radiol. 2016;39(3):325–33.
6. Taslakian B, Sebaaly MG, Al-Kutoubi A. Patient evaluation and preparation in vascular and interventional radiology: what every interventional radiologist should know (part 2: patient preparation and medications). Cardiovasc Intervent Radiol. 2016;39(4):489–99. doi: 10.1007/s00270-015-1239-4. [Epub 2015 Nov 25].

Part VIII

Non-vascular Interventional Procedures: Genitourinary-Kidneys

Introduction by Aghiad Al-Kutoubi, Section Reviewer

Interventional radiologists can play a pivotal role in the prompt diagnosis and percutaneous treatment of various genitourinary conditions by performing endovascular treatment, percutaneous urinary intervention, abscess or fluid drainage, and renal ablation and biopsy. These minimally invasive procedures can either obviate open surgery or stabilize the patient's condition prior to open surgery.

The commonest interventional emergency by far, nephrostomy procedures constitute a prominent item on every interventional radiologist worklist. Percutaneous nephrolithotomy procedures are now the mainstay in the treatment of large renal stones.

Advances in imaging and image guidance allowed the development of renal intervention particularly in the field of tumor ablation. Thermal tumor ablation techniques such as percutaneous radiofrequency ablation and cryoablation have assumed an important role in the management of renal tumors, particularly in patients who may be suboptimal candidates for open surgical techniques.

Complications of intervention on the kidney can be serious and management protocols of the possible complications should be formulated. Appropriate preprocedure antibiotics can reduce the septic complications substantially.

This section provides a comprehensive list of procedural reports that covers the vast majority of the currently performed image-guided, non-vascular renal procedures with up-to-date explanatory notes, synopsis of the indications and contraindications, and potential complications in an organized and practical format.

Section Chapters

Ablation of Renal Tumors

43

Nadim Muallem

Abbreviations

CT	Computed tomography
GFR	Glomerular filtration rate
MWA	Microwave ablation
PCA	Patient controlled anesthesia
PET	Positron emission tomography
RFA	Radiofrequency ablation

INTRODUCTION [1–3]

About 3.7 % of newly diagnosed cancer cases in 2015 in the United States involve the kidney and/or renal pelvis. With the refinement of nephron-sparing surgery, partial nephrectomy for early stage renal cell tumors has become the standard of care. Thermal ablation of both early stage solid renal cell carcinoma and complex cystic tumors smaller than 3 cm has shown high response and disease-free survival rates paralleling surgical results with support from at least two long-term studies. Thermal ablation has evolved to become incorporated in the treatment algorithm of renal malignancies in patients with major comorbidities, shortened life expectancy, or increased surgical risk.

N. Muallem (✉)
Department of Radiology, Division of Interventional Radiology, Memorial Sloan Kettering Cancer Center, 1275 York Ave, New York, NY 10065, USA
e-mail: nadim.muallem@gmail.com

COMMON INDICATIONS [2–6]

- T1a or T1b renal tumors or Bosniak type III and type IV cysts
- Less than 3 cm in size, eccentric tumor
- Comorbidities that preclude surgical intervention or general anesthesia
- Solitary kidney or renal insufficiency, recurrent disease following partial nephrectomy—thermal ablative modalities are superior to partial nephrectomy in preserving renal function and minimizing dialysis risk in the future
- Multiple tumors in the same kidney or conditions predisposing to multiple tumors such as Von Hippel–Lindau or Birt–Hogg–Dube are also ideal candidates for thermal ablation due to the inherent repeatability of the procedure
- Patient-instigated preference for minimally invasive technique

B. Taslakian et al. (eds.), *Procedural Dictations in Image-Guided Intervention*,
DOI 10.1007/978-3-319-40845-3_43

COMMON CONTRAINDICATIONS [2–6]

Absolute Contraindications:

- Uncorrectable coagulopathy

Relative Contraindications:

- Central tumors or tumors >3 cm—however with improvement of ablation techniques, the cutoff has been increased to tumors >5 cm. Large exophytic tumors can be more amenable to ablation than central or anteromedial small masses with no percutaneous access.
- Target lesion adjacent to vital organs/structures—protective measures such as hydro/pneumodissection or ureteral irrigation can be performed if ablation target is in close proximity with lung, adrenals, bowel, pancreas, gallbladder, ureter, or nerves. Liver involvement by the ablation zone is generally much better tolerated.
- Patients with metastatic disease or tumors involving renal or adjacent vasculature

Depending on the ablation technique used:

- Patients with cardiac pacemakers and implantable defibrillators *(recommended to be deactivated during RFA, not applicable for cryoablation, slightly better safety profile for MWA but precaution should also be taken* [7]*)*
- Metal implants *(small implants can potentially heat up due to the circuit created in RFA but are unlikely to be affected in MWA and certainly not affected in cryoablation)*

POSSIBLE COMPLICATIONS [4–6, 8]

- Hematuria, *20–40 %;* is typically self-limited and rarely requires intervention. In addition bladder clot formation is rare but could be managed by bladder irrigation.
- Hematoma whether subcapsular or extracapsular, *<5 %;* rarely requires intervention. Significant hemorrhage is more common with large central tumors and preliminary studies suggest some benefit from prophylactic embolization of large central tumors prior to ablation.
- Ureteral injury, *1–2 %;* is typically manifested by small urine leak or urinoma formation, generally from capsular disruption and injury to the collecting system. Treatment of lower pole lesions may lead to proximal ureteral injury and in some cases ureteral stricture and obstruction. The latter tend to be less common in cryoablation than with RFA or microwave and can be minimized by performing intra-procedural retrograde pyeloperfusion or ureteral irrigation.
- Infection is rare. Risk may be minimized by prophylactic antibiotic use.
- Pleural complications from treatment of superior pole lesions that may require a transpleural, transdiaphragmatic approach *(pneumothorax, hemothorax, large effusion requiring drainage).*
- Injury to adjacent organs, *rare;* either from direct penetration or thermal injury, such as colonic perforation. Risk decreased by maintaining minimum distance of 1 cm from ablation margin or by performing pneumodissection with air or CO_2 or hydrodissection with distilled water *(avoid saline in RFA since ionic solutions tend to conduct current).* Injury to lung could be avoided by inducing pneumothorax artificially and transiently during the ablation procedure. Ablation margins can also be monitored by use of temperature sensing thermocouples placed near organs at risk.
- Skin burns, *<1 %;* typically at skin puncture site in all thermal ablation modalities or at grounding pad site in case of RFA.
- Tumor seeding, *rare;* minimized by cauterization of the ablation tract, also by minimizing needle repositioning prior to ablation.
- Nerve injury, *<1 %;* the genitofemoral, iliohypogastric, and ilioinguinal nerves run over the anterior aspect of the psoas muscles and can be affected by thermal ablation of posteromedial lesions. This can result in pelvic, groin, or lower extremity paresthesias and/or weakness. Injury is less pronounced and recovery is more easily achieved following

cryoablation than after heat ablation modalities.

- Renal infarct is rare and of little clinical significance.
- Mortality, *rare*.

PREPROCEDURAL ASSESSMENT AND PLANNING [4–6, 9]

- History, indications, and physical examination *(Appendix 1* in Chap. 149*)*
- Evaluation of diagnostic imaging studies *(Contrast-enhanced CT urogram is ideal, but dynamic contrast enhanced MRI is a viable alternative)* to assess indications and radiological stage of the tumor, and to determine the location of the lesion, the relevant anatomy, and develop trajectory route. It also serves as a baseline for follow-up. Patients with glomerular filtration rate (GFR) of 30–60 mL/min/1.73 m^2 should undergo intravenous hydration prior to receiving iodinated contrast or should receive a decreased gadolinium contrast dose. Patients who have a GFR less than 30 should not receive any intravenous contrast. Time-of-flight MR imaging or non-enhanced CT imaging can be complemented by use of ultrasound imaging and by comparison to prior cross-sectional studies if available. Nuclear renal functional imaging can also be performed but is not essential.
- Histopathologic diagnosis of the lesion should ideally be obtained before the ablation, unless the lesion fulfills imaging diagnostic criteria of Bosniak type III and type IV cysts or the patient is considered to be at very high risk, in which case biopsy and ablation could be performed in one setting. Prior biopsy of solid tumors if achievable as well as prior detailed history and imaging is recommended in order to avoid unnecessary procedures in cases of extrarenal malignancy, suspected lymphoma, abscesses, or inflammatory masses.
- Periprocedural management of coagulation status *(Appendices 2* in Chap. 150 *and 3* in Chap. 151*)*
- Antibiotic prophylaxis: No consensus, but intravenous Cefazolin 1 g is usually given *(Appendices 4* in Chap. 152 *and 5* in Chap. 153*)*
- Imaging modality for guidance: CT, CT fluoroscopy, MRI, ultrasound
- Positioning: Most commonly prone; however, supine or lateral decubitus positioning can provide access to more difficult to reach lesions. Place appropriate supportive cushioning in areas with important neurovascular bundles *(to avoid injury)* and dispersive grounding pads in a well-prepared *(shaved)* area to allow good contact with the skin.

PROCEDURE NOTE [3]

Procedure:
Radiofrequency/Microwave/Cryoablation of [specify location] renal lesion
Staff: [_]
Fellow: [_]
Resident: [_]
Clinical Information: Specify existing diagnosis. Describe history and list indications
Allergies: No known allergic disorders/Allergic to [specify/type of allergy]
Anesthesia: Local anesthesia with conscious sedation/General anesthesia
Medications: List any relevant medications used (local anesthesia, sedation, antibiotics)
Field: Sterile
Position: Supine/Prone/Left lateral decubitus/Right lateral decubitus
Monitoring: Intravenous access line was secured and vital signs were continuously monitored by nursing staff/anesthesia team throughout the procedure
Cumulative radiation dose: (_) mGy

Description of Procedure:

The risks, benefits, alternatives, and procedure itself were explained to the patient/patient's

Power of Attorney/patient's legal guardian, and informed written consent was obtained. The site of the procedure was identified and marked. Time out was performed to confirm the correct patient, procedure and site.

Pre-procedure planning imaging [CT/ultrasound/MRI] was obtained and used to calculate the approach and distance to target lesion. One (or more) site of needle entry was determined and marked on the skin. The marked location(s) and surrounding skin area were prepped and draped in the usual sterile fashion. Subcutaneous infiltration of local anesthetic was performed using a thin gauge needle.

A small skin incision was made at the marked site(s). Under image guidance one (or more) applicator probe(s) was/were advanced along the planned trajectory and positioned into the target. No (one or more) repositioning was required. Ablation was performed by following the manufacturer's instructions until the target temperature was achieved and/or the perilesional edema was visualized/the ice ball was visualized to encase the targeted lesion within an acceptable margin.

Probe positioning, repositioning, and ablation protocol are detailed below.

After completion, the ablation tract was cauterized using low-power application while withdrawing the radiofrequency electrode/microwave antenna/probe from the lesion.

After probe removal, immediate post-procedure CT images were obtained at the level of the lesion to evaluate the ablation zone, potential collateral damage and detect complications.

The patient was transferred to the inpatient unit/recovery room following the procedure in a stable condition. Staff was present during the entire procedure.

Preprocedural Planning and Approach

Target organ: Kidney
Laterality: Right/left
Reference scan/image for ablation target: CT dated [Day]/[Month]/[Year]. Series [series number] image [image number]
Target lesion size: Long axis: [_] cm, short axis: [_] cm
Specific target location: Specify upper/middle/lower pole, anterior/posterior location and whether is an exophytic or endophytic lesion, relationship to sensitive structures (diaphragm, vessels, nerves, etc.)
Target lesion appearance: Solid/Partial/Cavitary/Cystic
Patient position: Prone/Supine/Decubitus/Other
Approach: Posterior/Anterior/Lateral/Right/Left
Imaging guidance: Intra-procedural CT/CT fluoroscopy/Ultrasound/MRI performed with/without multiplanar reconstruction confirming adequate positioning of the applicator within the target lesion

Ablation Technique:

Ablation modality: Radiofrequency/Microwave/Cryoablation/Other
Ablation device: Specify device brand/model, type, length, gauge, active length, single, multiple, tined, etc.…
Number of applicators: *If more than 1 applicator, specify locations, if single applicator with more than one repositioning, also specify different locations*
Number of ablations: *(number) overlapping/nonoverlapping ablations (list protocol details)*
Protocol used: Device specific, but typically, power/wattage, duration, temperature achieved, and location if multiple probes or repositionings were needed.

Eg. RFA (single applicator—in this case the Valleylab/Covidien Cool-tip RFA probe—with multiple repositioning and overlapping ablation)
Ablation #1: Cooled, 3 min, 57 °C/Applicator #1 Posterior margin
Ablation #2: Cooled, 6 min, 58 °C/Applicator #1 Superior margin proximal
Ablation #3: …

Eg. Cryoablation (with multiple applicators)
Ablation #1: 10 min freeze, 6 min active thaw, 10 min freeze, 8 min passive thaw, at 100 %, −160 °C/Applicator #1 superior margin
Ablation #2: 10 min freeze, 6 min active thaw, 10 min freeze, 8 min passive thaw, at 80 %, −140 °C/Applicator #2 inferior margin
Ablation #3: …

Post-Ablation Findings:

Post-ablation imaging: CT/MRI/Ultrasound

Follow-up chest radiographs: (Immediate and) 2 h post-procedure chest radiographs *(if transpleural ablation was performed)*

Post-procedural imaging (CT/MRI/PET-CT) was performed at the level of the target lesion. The ablation zone could not be clearly delineated/was clearly outlined consisting of ice ball formation/decreased parenchymal attenuation encompassing the target tumor in its entirety with adequate margins extending [_] mm beyond the periphery of the lesion predictive of complete ablation/inadequate margins at the [_] border requiring additional targeted ablation [complement with additional details as needed].

Immediate Complications: None encountered during or directly after the procedure. List complications if any.

Post-Procedure Plan [3–6]:

- Assuming successful procedure with no evidence of bleeding on post-procedural imaging:
  - Transfer patient to recovery unit.
  - Observe in recovery unit for 2–4 h with continuous vital sign and pulse oximeter monitoring.
  - Complete bed rest and NPO for the duration of observation. Maintain patient recumbent with the puncture site down.
  - Post-procedure pain control as needed *(consider PCA, and admission for pain control if needed).*
  - Administer supplemental nasal oxygen as needed *(O_2 saturation less than baseline/patient still sedated).*
  - If the patient's condition deteriorates during observation, suspect bleeding primarily and obtain cross-sectional imaging of the abdomen immediately. Do not disregard other potential complications as well.
- *Discharge Instructions:*
  - Abstain from strenuous activities for 3 days.
  - Visit the nearest emergency room promptly if any fever, chills, urinary retention develop, or worsening pain not controlled by oral medication.
  - Start clear liquid diet for the first hour after discharge from observation, then regular diet thereafter if tolerated and no complications occur.
  - Take prescribed pain medications as needed.
  - Take prescribed antibiotic medications as instructed.
- *Follow-Up Imaging:*
  - No consensus guidelines are available, but most reports recommend a baseline contrast enhanced CT or MRI one to three months following ablation in order to identify residual tumor from incomplete ablation.
  - Frequency of follow-up imaging also varies, and given the slow rate of growth of small renal cell carcinomas, some institutions advocate intervals of 6–12 months as cost-effective. However, some studies have shown that over 90 % of recurrences or incomplete treatments were detected within the first year and so more frequent (three to four) imaging studies are recommended within the first 12 months following the procedure.
  - Follow up should continue on a yearly basis for a minimum of 5 years in order to establish disease-free survival and parallel surgical standards.
  - Contrast enhanced CT and/or high resolution MRI are most sensitive at detecting the eccentric nodular enhancement characteristic of recurrent disease. PET-CT is currently not recommended due to decreased spatial resolution and masking of tracer uptake within the tumor secondary to adjacent intense tracer accumulation in the renal collecting system.

Impression:

- Percutaneous radiofrequency/microwave/cryoablation of [specify location] renal lesion, as described above.

- The patient tolerated the procedure well and left the interventional unit in a stable condition.
- List any other relevant or important information/findings.
- The primary operator (specify name) was present for the entire/key parts of the procedure.

References

1. Statistical summaries. Natl Cancer Inst SEER Database; 2015. http://seer.cancer.gov/statfacts/.
2. Gervais DA. Cryoablation versus radiofrequency ablation for renal tumor ablation: time to reassess? J Vasc Interv Radiol. 2013;24(8):1135–8.
3. Clark TW, Millward SF, Gervais DA, Goldberg SN, Grassi CJ, Kinney TB, et al. Reporting standards for percutaneous thermal ablation of renal cell carcinoma. J Vasc Interv Radiol. 2009;20(7 Suppl):S409–16.
4. Erinjeri JP, Clark TWI. Renal tumor ablation. In: Kandarpa K, Machan L, editors. Handbook of interventional radiologic procedures. Vol. 4th ed. Philadelphia: Lippincott Williams & Wilkins; 2011:548–55.
5. Ahrar K, Matin SF, Wallace MJ. Thermal ablation of renal cell carcinoma. In: Mauro M, Murphy K, Thomson K, Venbrux A, Morgan R, editors. Image-guided interventions. 2nd ed. Philadelphia: Saunders Elsevier; 2014. p. 1098–110.
6. Hinshaw JL, Lubner MG. Radiofrequency ablation, cryotherapy, and microwave ablation for renal tumors. In: Mueller PR, Adam A, editors. Interventional oncology: a practical guide for the interventional radiologist. Berlin: Springer; 2012:131–7.
7. Skonieczki BD, Wells C, Wasser EJ, Dupuy DE. Radiofrequency and microwave tumor ablation in patients with implanted cardiac devices: Is it safe? Eur J Radiol. 2011;79(3):343–6.
8. Kim K, Thomas S. Complications of image-guided thermal ablation of liver and kidney neoplasms. Semin Intervent Radiol. 2014;31:138–48.
9. Venkatesan AM, Kundu S, Sacks D, Wallace MJ, Wojak JC, Rose SC, et al. Practice guideline for adult antibiotic prophylaxis during vascular and interventional radiology procedures. J Vasc Interv Radiol. 2010;21(11):1611–30.

Alcohol Ablation of Renal Cyst

44

Bedros Taslakian

INTRODUCTION

Renal cysts are the most common benign lesions in the adult kidney. Only symptomatic or complicated cysts require treatment. The most effective treatment is percutaneous drainage followed by instillation of a sclerosing agent. Of all the proposed agents, alcohol sclerosis is easy, well tolerated, and widely available with excellent results. Pure ethanol rapidly inactivates the secreting epithelial cell lining and slowly penetrates the fibrous capsule of the cyst. Several treatment approaches have been proposed basically varying in relation to the number of sessions and period of retention of sclerosing agent. Multi-session injection may be required to achieve a prolonged ethanol-retention and ensure full ablation. However, single-session techniques were described in the literature with prolonged retention periods showing comparable outcome.

COMMON INDICATIONS [1–5]

Symptomatic benign renal cyst causing:

- Flank or back pain
- Compression of the urinary collecting system with mild to moderate hydronephrosis
- Hypertension after excluding other causes
- Pressure atrophy of the adjacent renal parenchyma

COMMON CONTRAINDICATIONS [2, 4]

- Significant coagulopathy that cannot be adequately corrected
- Lack of safe pathway to the cyst due to interposed viscera or vessels
- Inability of the patient to cooperate with, or to be positioned for, the procedure
- Pregnancy
- Peripelvic cysts *(relative contraindication because the risk of fibrosis of the ureteropelvic junction)*
- Communication with the collecting system

POSSIBLE COMPLICATIONS [1, 3–5]

- Hemorrhage
- Superinfection
- Pleural transgression
- Damage to adjacent organs
- Vascular injury
- Hematuria
- Ureteropelvic junction obstruction caused by sclerosis-induced fibrosis

B. Taslakian (✉)
Department of Radiology, New York University Langone Medical Center, 660 First Ave, New York, NY 10016, USA
e-mail: btaslakian@gmail.com

B. Taslakian et al. (eds.), *Procedural Dictations in Image-Guided Intervention*,
DOI 10.1007/978-3-319-40845-3_44

- Severe pain due to leakage of a small volume of the alcohol into the peritoneal cavity
- Minor, transient pain from the infusion of alcohol *(may be relieved by local instillation of lidocaine or intravenous analgesics)*
- Nausea, causalgia, or transient drunkenness due to intravasation and systemic alcohol absorption
- Recurrence of the ablated renal cysts

PREPROCEDURAL ASSESSMENT AND PLANNING [6, 7]

- History, indications, and physical examination *(Appendix 1* in Chap. 149*)*
- Evaluation of diagnostic imaging studies to determine the location of the renal cysts and the relevant anatomy
- Periprocedural management of coagulation status *(Appendices 2* in Chaps. 150 *and 3* in 151*)*
- Antibiotic prophylaxis: Not routinely recommended *(Appendices 4* in Chaps. 152 *and 5* in 153*)*
- Imaging modality for guidance: CT, CT fluoroscopy, combined ultrasound and fluoroscopy
- Positioning: Prone, prone oblique

PROCEDURE NOTE

Procedure: Alcohol ablation of renal cyst
Staff: [_]
Fellow: [_]
Resident: [_]
Clinical Information: Describe history and list indications
Allergies: None known/Allergic to [specify/type of allergy]
Anesthesia: Local anesthesia/conscious sedation
Medications: List any relevant medications used
Contrast Material: (_) mL of [type] contrast material was used for cystogram
Field: Sterile
Procedure classification: Clean
Position: Prone/Prone oblique
Monitoring: Intravenous access line was secured and vital signs were continuously monitored by nursing staff/anesthesia team throughout the procedure
Cumulative Radiation dose: (_) mGy

Description of Procedure *(CT-Guided Renal Cyst Ablation):*
The risks, benefits, alternatives, and the procedure itself were explained to the patient/patient's Power of Attorney/patient's legal guardian, and informed written consent was obtained. The site of the procedure was identified and marked. Time out was performed to confirm the correct patient, procedure, and site.

The procedure was planned and the skin puncture site was marked using combined information from the preliminary CT images, the location of the selected cyst and the radiopaque marker/grid. The angle of needle entry and the distance to the cyst were calculated from the preliminary CT images.

The skin was prepped and draped in the usual sterile fashion. The selected puncture site was infiltrated with lidocaine. A small skin incision was made. Subsequently, using planning CT information, an (18)-gauge [trocar/type] needle was advanced along the planned trajectory into the selected renal cyst. (_) mL of [specify color and viscosity] cystic fluid was aspirated, and collected for bacteriologic, cytologic, and biochemical tests. A (0.035)-in. [type] guidewire was advanced through the needle into the cyst and a (_)-French [pigtail/type] drainage catheter was inserted into the cyst after adequately dilating the percutaneous route. After confirming adequate positioning of the catheter tip with repeat imaging, the catheter was locked and anchored to the skin. The cyst was completely evacuated by aspirating (_) mL of cystic fluid. The shape of the cyst was evaluated and presence of a connection with the renal collecting system was excluded by injecting (_) mL of diluted contrast material.

The testing contrast material was aspirated and then a (_) mL of (95)% ethanol was injected slowly into the cyst. The catheter tip was capped and the injected ethanol was retained in the cyst for (_) minutes. The patient was rolled into supine, prone, and lateral decubitus positions at 10- to 15-minute intervals to increase contact between all surfaces of the cyst and ethanol. Afterwards, the residual fluid in the cyst was aspirated and the pigtail catheter was removed/left in place for continuous drainage and subsequent ablation sessions.

The patient was transferred to the floor/recovery room following the procedure in stable condition. Staff was present for the entire procedure.

Description of Procedure *(Ultrasound/Fluoroscopy-Guided Renal Cyst Ablation):* The risks, benefits, alternatives, and the procedure itself were explained to the patient/patient's Power of Attorney/patient's legal guardian, and informed written consent was obtained. The site of the procedure was identified and marked. Time out was performed to confirm the correct patient, procedure, and site.

The procedure was planned and the skin puncture site was marked using combined information from the preliminary ultrasound images and the location of the selected cyst. The skin was prepped and draped in the usual sterile fashion. The selected puncture site was infiltrated with lidocaine. A small skin incision was made. Subsequently, using direct ultrasound visualization, an (18)-gauge [trocar/type] needle was advanced into the selected renal cyst. (_) mL of [type] cystic fluid was aspirated, and collected for bacteriologic, cytologic, and biochemical tests. (_) mL of diluted contrast material was injected into the cyst under fluoroscopy to delineate the cyst and a (0.035)-inch [type] guidewire was advanced through the needle into the cyst. A (_)-French [pigtail/type] drainage catheter was inserted into the cyst after adequately dilating the percutaneous route. After confirming adequate positioning of the catheter tip with imaging, the catheter was locked and anchored to the skin. The cyst was completely evacuated by aspirating (_) mL of cystic fluid. Cystogram was performed by injecting (_) mL of diluted contrast material under fluoroscopy to evaluate the shape of the cyst and exclude the presence of a communication with the renal collecting system.

The testing contrast material was aspirated and then a (_) mL of (95) % ethanol was injected slowly into the cyst. The catheter tip was capped and the injected ethanol was retained in the cyst for (_) minutes. The patient was rolled into supine, prone, and lateral decubitus positions at 10- to 15-min intervals to increase contact between all surfaces of the cyst and ethanol. Afterwards, the residual fluid in the cyst was aspirated and the pigtail catheter was removed/left in place for continuous drainage and subsequent ablation sessions.

The patient was transferred to the floor/recovery room following the procedure in stable condition. Staff was present for the entire procedure.

Intra-Procedure Findings: List all relevant findings.

Immediate Complications: None encountered during or directly after the procedure. List complications if any.

Post-Procedure Plan:

- Follow-up laboratory and cytology results.
- Keep complete bed rest for 3–4 h and abstain from strenuous activities.
- Start clear liquid diet for the first hour, then regular diet thereafter if tolerated and otherwise not contraindicated.
- Check vital signs every 15 min for 1 h, every 30 min for 1 h, and then every 60 min for 2 h.
- Inform interventional radiology team if systolic blood pressure is <95 mm Hg, heart rate is >100 beats per minute, or if any chest pain or shortness of breath develops.
- Administer analgesics or antiemetics, if necessary, for 1–3 days.
- Follow the residual size of the ablated cysts by ultrasound, CT, or both at 3- to 6-month intervals for at least 1 year.
- Check biochemical renal function tests at 3 months after the procedure.
- A second aspiration and sclerosis may be required, especially with larger cysts.

Impression:

- Percutaneous aspiration and alcohol ablation of right/left renal cyst, as described above.
- The patient tolerated the procedure well and left the interventional unit in a stable condition.
- The injection was discontinued and the procedure was terminated prematurely due to intolerable pain during ethanol instillation.
- List any other relevant or important information/finding.

References

1. Lin YH, Pan HB, Liang HL, Chung HM, Chen CY, Huang JS, et al. Single-session alcohol-retention sclerotherapy for simple renal cysts: comparison of 2- and 4-hr retention techniques. AJR Am J Roentgenol. 2005;185(4):860–6.
2. Lucey BC, Kuligowska E. Radiologic management of cysts in the abdomen and pelvis. AJR Am J Roentgenol. 2006;186(2):562–73.
3. Mohsen T, Gomha MA. Treatment of symptomatic simple renal cysts by percutaneous aspiration and ethanol sclerotherapy. BJU Int. 2005;96(9):1369–72.
4. Akinci D, Akhan O, Ozmen M, Gumus B, Ozkan O, Karcaaltincaba M, et al. Long-term results of single-session percutaneous drainage and ethanol sclerotherapy in simple renal cysts. Eur J Radiol. 2005;54(2):298–302.
5. Lee J, Darcy M. Renal cysts and urinomas. Semin Intervent Radiol. 2011;28(4):380–91.
6. Taslakian B, Sebaaly MG, Al-Kutoubi A. Patient evaluation and preparation in vascular and interventional radiology: what every interventional radiologist should know (part 1: patient assessment and laboratory tests). Cardiovasc Intervent Radiol. 2016;39(3):325–33.
7. Taslakian B, Sebaaly MG, Al-Kutoubi A. Patient evaluation and preparation in vascular and interventional radiology: what every interventional radiologist should know (part 2: patient preparation and medications). Cardiovasc Intervent Radiol. 2016;39(4):489–99. doi: 10.1007/s00270-015-1239-4. [Epub 2015 Nov 25].

Antegrade Nephrostogram

45

Bedros Taslakian

INTRODUCTION

Percutaneous antegrade nephrostogram is fluoroscopic-guided injection of contrast media into the indwelling nephrostomy catheter to delineate and assess the catheter, the renal collecting system, ureters and ureteric stents. This will confirm the position and patency of the catheter and assess the drainage route of the kidney.

COMMON INDICATIONS [1–4]

- Assess ureteric stent patency through the safety nephrostomy catheter before removal
- Assess the position, patency, and integrity of the nephrostomy catheter
- Assess the urinary tract after placement of nephrostomy catheter for treatment of obstructive lesions
- Assess the urinary tract in cases of urinary tract injury or fistula *(i.e., delineation of the fistula)*
- Assess for residual stone fragments following percutaneous nephrolithotomy
- Assess response to therapy after instillation of medications into the collecting system *(e.g., treatment of fungal ball)*

B. Taslakian (✉)
Department of Radiology, New York University Langone Medical Center, 660 First Ave, New York, NY 10016, USA
e-mail: btaslakian@gmail.com

COMMON CONTRAINDICATIONS [4]

- Care should be taken during injection of contrast in an infected system to avoid bacterial seeding *(delay for 24–48 h)*
- Pregnancy

POSSIBLE COMPLICATIONS [4]

- Catheter dislodgment
- Pain
- Contrast extravasation
- Respiratory insufficiency due to prone position
- Bacteremia and septic shock *(fever, chills with hypotension)*

PREPROCEDURAL ASSESSMENT AND PLANNING [5, 6]

- History, indications, and physical examination *(Appendix 1* in Chap. 149*)*
- Evaluation of diagnostic imaging studies to evaluate for the presence of hydronephrosis, assess the location of the existing nephrostomy tube, and determine the relevant anatomy *(anatomic variants, cysts, tumors, stones, and perinephric urinoma)*
- Periprocedural management of coagulation status: Not applicable
- Antibiotic prophylaxis: Patients with urinary tract infection should be receiving antibiotic

B. Taslakian et al. (eds.), *Procedural Dictations in Image-Guided Intervention*,
DOI 10.1007/978-3-319-40845-3_45

treatment *(Appendices 4* in Chaps. 152 *and 5* in 153*)*

- Imaging modality for guidance: Fluoroscopy
- Positioning: Prone, prone oblique

Procedure Note

Procedure: Fluoroscopy-guided antegrade nephrostogram
Staff: [_]
Fellow: [_]
Resident: [_]
Clinical Information: Describe history and list indications
Allergies: None known/Allergic to [specify/type of allergy]
Anesthesia: None
Medications: List any relevant medications used
Contrast Material: (_) mL of [type] contrast material was used for nephrostogram
Field: Sterile
Position: Prone/Prone oblique
Monitoring: Intravenous access line was secured and vital signs were continuously monitored by nursing staff/anesthesia team throughout the procedure
Total fluoroscopy time: (_) minutes
Cumulative radiation dose: (_) mGy

Description of Procedure:

The risks, benefits, alternatives, and the procedure itself were explained to the patient/patient's Power of Attorney/patient's legal guardian, and informed written/verbal consent was obtained. The site of the procedure was identified and marked. Time out was performed to confirm the correct patient, procedure, and site.

The skin and previously inserted left/right nephrostomy catheter were prepped and draped in the usual sterile fashion. (_) mL of diluted contrast material was slowly injected through the nephrostomy catheter under fluoroscopy visualization to delineate the catheter and urinary tract.

The nephrostomy catheter was removed after confirmation of clinical improvement and patency of the urinary tract/double J ureteric stent/resolution of the fistula.

The nephrostomy catheter was left in place and repeat nephrostogram/insertion of double J catheter was scheduled.

The patient was transferred to the floor/discharged home following the procedure in a stable condition. Staff was present for the entire procedure.

Intra-Procedure Findings: List all relevant findings.
Immediate Complications: None encountered during or directly after the procedure. List complications if any.

Post-Procedure Plan:

- Follow-up plan: *(specify the plan according to the findings).*
- Daily catheter care *(if the nephrostomy catheter left in place):*
  - Inspect catheter and make sure that the 3-way stopcock is open to the drainage bag and the catheter has not been externally retracted.
  - Flush the catheter slowly with 20 mL of bacteriostatic saline and aspirate every 4 h if clots are persistent and obstructing the system *(10 mL toward the drainage bag and 10 mL toward the urinary system).*

Impression:

- Left/Right antegrade nephrostogram, as described above.
- The patient tolerated the procedure well and left the interventional unit in a stable condition.
- List any other relevant or important information/finding.

References

1. Stokes LA, Meranze SG. Percutaneous nephrostomy, cystostomy, and nephroureteral Stenting. In: Mauro MA, Murphy KPJ, Thomson KR, Venbrux AC, Morgan RA, editors. Image-guided interventions. 2nd ed. Philadelphia: Saunders Elsevier; 2014. p. 1076–88.

2. Punamiya S. Percutaneous nephrostomy and antegrade ureteric stenting. In: Gervais DA, Sabharwal T, editors. Interventional radiology procedures in biopsy and drainage. Heidelberg: Springer; 2011. p. 165–77.
3. Maher MM, Kealey S, McNamara A, O'Laoide R, Gibney RG, Malone DE. Management of visceral interventional radiology catheters: a troubleshooting guide for interventional radiologists. Radiographics. 2002;22(2):305–22.
4. Dyer RB, Regan JD, Kavanagh PV, Khatod EG, Chen MY, Zagoria RJ. Percutaneous nephrostomy with extensions of the technique: step by step. Radiographics. 2002;22(3):503–25.
5. Taslakian B, Sebaaly MG, Al-Kutoubi A. Patient evaluation and preparation in vascular and interventional radiology: what every interventional radiologist should know (part 1: patient assessment and laboratory tests). Cardiovasc Intervent Radiol. 2016;39(3):325–33.
6. Taslakian B, Sebaaly MG, Al-Kutoubi A. Patient evaluation and preparation in vascular and interventional radiology: what every interventional radiologist should know (part 2: patient preparation and medications). Cardiovasc Intervent Radiol. 2016;39(4):489–99. doi: 10.1007/s00270-015-1239-4. [Epub 2015 Nov 25].

Core Biopsy of the Kidney

46

Bedros Taslakian

INTRODUCTION

Image-guided percutaneous needle biopsy of the kidney with CT or ultrasound guidance has minimal associated morbidity and mortality. A combination of core biopsy and fine needle aspiration produces the greatest diagnostic yield, particularly for solid masses. A non-focal "random" biopsy of the kidney samples any portion of the renal cortex. Usually, the safest trajectory is chosen, passing from the midpole renal cortex to the lower pole cortex, avoiding the central hilum.

COMMON INDICATIONS

Focal Renal Biopsy *[1–4]*

- Focal solid renal lesion in patients with known extra-renal primary malignancy
- Focal suspicious unrespectable solid renal lesion on imaging
- Focal suspicious solid renal lesion in patients with multiple surgical comorbidities
- Focal renal lesion suspicious for infectious process rather than malignancy
- Histologic confirmation of malignancy before percutaneous renal ablation therapy
- Suspicious cystic renal lesion to rule out cystic renal cell carcinoma

Random Renal Biopsy *[3–5]*

- Evaluation for nephropathies
- Renal failure of unknown etiology
- Workup in patient presenting with a renal transplant rejection
- Evaluation of systemic diseases affecting the kidneys *(e.g., systemic lupus erythematosus, HIV-associated nephropathy)*

COMMON CONTRAINDICATIONS [1–3, 5]

- Uncooperative or unwilling patients
- Hemodynamic instability
- Significant coagulopathy that cannot be adequately corrected *(use transjugular approach for random biopsy)*
- Pregnancy in cases when imaging guidance involves ionizing radiation

POSSIBLE COMPLICATIONS [1–6]

- *Perinephric hematoma, 44–65 %*
- *Bleeding into the collecting system causing hematuria, 45 % of non-focal renal biopsies*
- Hemorrhage requiring transfusion or intervention, *0.5–2.7 %*
- Pneumothorax, *0.5 %*

B. Taslakian (✉)
Department of Radiology, New York University Langone Medical Center, 660 First Ave, New York, NY 10016, USA
e-mail: btaslakian@gmail.com

B. Taslakian et al. (eds.), *Procedural Dictations in Image-Guided Intervention*,
DOI 10.1007/978-3-319-40845-3_46

- Vasovagal reaction
- Unintended adjacent organ injury *(e.g., liver, spleen, colon)*
- Arteriovenous fistula, arteriocaliceal fistula, pseudoaneurysm
- Infection, *rare*
- Renal loss, *extremely rare-0.1 %*
- Malignant seeding of the needle tract, *extremely rare*

PREPROCEDURAL ASSESSMENT AND PLANNING [7–9]

- History, indications, and physical examination *(Appendix 1* in Chap. 149*)*
- Evaluation of diagnostic imaging studies to determine the location of the lesion and relevant anatomy
- Periprocedural management of coagulation status *(Appendices 2* in Chaps. 150 *and 3* in 151*)*
- Antibiotic prophylaxis: Not routinely recommended [7] *(Appendices 4* in Chaps. 152 *and 5* in 153*)*
- Imaging modality for guidance: CT, CT fluoroscopy, ultrasound, MRI [3]
- Positioning:
  - *Ipsilateral side down*—better for focal biopsies to splint the normal kidney motion, with the needle inserted from a posterior approach
  - *Prone*—easy position for focal and non-focal biopsy of the native kidneys, especially when the lesion is along the lateral edge of the kidney which makes the access via an ipsilateral side down approach not accessible
  - *Supine*—transplant kidney

PROCEDURE NOTE

Procedure: Percutaneous fine needle aspiration/and core biopsy of left/right renal lesion/random renal biopsy
Staff: [_]
Fellow: [_]
Resident: [_]
Clinical Information: Describe history and list indications
Allergies: None known/Allergic to [specify/type of allergy]
Anesthesia: Local anesthesia/conscious sedation
Medications: List any relevant medications used (sedation)
Field: Sterile
Procedure classification: Clean
Position: Prone/Supine/Left lateral decubitus/Right lateral decubitus
Monitoring: Intravenous access line was secured and vital signs were continuously monitored by nursing staff/anesthesia team throughout the procedure
Cumulative radiation dose: (_) mGy

Description of Procedure *(Targeted Renal Biopsy):*

The risks, benefits, alternatives, and the procedure itself were explained to the patient/patient's Power of Attorney/patient's legal guardian, and informed written consent was obtained. The site of the procedure was identified and marked. Time out was performed to confirm the correct patient, procedure, and site.

The left/right kidney was evaluated using CT imaging after placement of a radiopaque marker/grid/ultrasound showing a (_) cm lesion in [specify location]. The procedure was planned and the skin puncture site was marked using combined information from the location of the lesion and preliminary CT/ultrasound images. The angle of needle entry and the distance to the lesion were calculated from the planning images. The skin was prepped and draped in the usual sterile fashion. Local anesthesia was administered. A small skin incision was made. Subsequently, using planning CT information/using CT fluoroscopy/under direct ultrasound visualization, a (_)-gauge [type] needle guide was advanced along the planned trajectory until the needle tip reached the target lesion, confirmed by imaging.

Fine needle aspiration was performed using a (_)-gauge [type] longer needle placed coaxially through the reference needle (*coaxial technique*). Suction was generated using the syringe attached to the needle, which was passed through the target lesion using to-and-fro motion to obtain cells. The suction was then released and the needle was withdrawn. One or two drops of the aspirated fluid were smeared on glass slides for on-site cytological assessment/fixed in a preservative solution and the remainder were washed into a solution of formalin/saline.

Then, (_) core biopsy samples were obtained using the coaxial technique, placed in a formalin/saline solution and sent for histopathological evaluation. The biopsy track was plugged using gelfoam pledgets while withdrawing the reference needle. Following this, immediate completion CT/ultrasound images were obtained at the level of the biopsy site.

The patient was transferred to the floor/recovery room following the procedure in a stable condition. Staff was present for the entire procedure.

Description of Procedure *(Random Renal Biopsy):*

The risks, benefits, alternatives, and the procedure itself were explained to the patient/patient's Power of Attorney/patient's legal guardian, and informed written consent was obtained. The site of the procedure was identified and marked. Time out was performed to confirm the correct patient, procedure, and site.

The left/right/transplant kidney was evaluated using CT imaging after placement of a radio-paque marker/grid/ultrasound. The procedure was planned and the skin puncture site was marked using combined information from the location of the lesion and preliminary CT/ultrasound images. The angle of needle entry and the distance to the renal cortex were calculated from the planning images.

The skin was prepped and draped in the usual sterile fashion. Local anesthesia was administered. A small skin incision was made. Subsequently, using planning CT information/using CT fluoroscopy/under direct ultrasound visualization, a (_)-gauge [type] needle guide was advanced along the planned trajectory until the needle tip reached the outer aspect of the renal cortex, confirmed by imaging. Then, (_) core biopsy samples were obtained from the cortex using the coaxial technique, placed in an ice cold saline solution and sent for histopathological evaluation. Following this, immediate completion CT/ultrasound images were obtained at the level of the biopsy site.

The patient was transferred to the floor/recovery room following the procedure in a stable condition. Staff was present for the entire procedure.

Intra-Procedure Findings: List all relevant findings.

Immediate Complications: None encountered during or directly after the procedure. List complications if any.

Post-Procedure Plan [2, 3]**:**

- Follow-up cytology and histopathology results.
- Obtain chest x-ray or CT scan to rule out pneumothorax if pleural space transgression is suspected.
- When post-biopsy CT/ultrasound images show no complications
  - Observe the patient in the recovery room following the procedure for 2–4 h.
  - Complete bed rest for 1–2 h, bathroom use with assistance.
  - Place a sand bag under the site where the biopsy was taken for 2 h.
  - Administer supplemental nasal oxygen *(if a small pneumothorax develops).*
  - Monitor vital signs in recovery area every 15 min for 1 h, then every 30 min for 2 h, then every hour.
  - If the patient's condition deteriorates during observation, obtain images of the abdomen immediately.
- Discharge instructions:
  - Abstain from strenuous activities for 3 days.
  - Visit the nearest emergency room promptly if any abdominal, chest or flank pain; significant hematuria or shortness of breath develops.
  - Start clear liquid diet for the first hour, then regular diet thereafter if tolerated and no complications occur.

Impression:

- Percutaneous needle biopsy of left/right renal lesion/kidney/renal transplant, as described above.
- The patient tolerated the procedure well and left the interventional unit in a stable condition.
- The patient was unstable and the procedure was canceled/terminated prematurely.
- List any other relevant or important information/finding.

References

1. Desai SB, Lewandowski RJ, Nemcek AA Jr. Percutaneous biopsy. In: Mauro MA, Murphy KPJ, Thomson KR, Venbrux AC, Morgan RA, editors. Image-guided interventions. 2nd ed. Philadelphia: Saunders Elsevier; 2014. p. 918–23.
2. Silverman SG, Segal D. Abdominal biopsies. In: Kandarpa K, Machan L, editors. Handbook of interventional radiologic procedures. 4th ed. Philadelphia: Lippincott Williams & Wilkins; 2011. p. 516–26.
3. Catalano OA, Samir AE. Renal biopsy. In: Gervais DA, Sabharwal T, editors. Interventional radiology procedures in biopsy and drainage. Heidelberg: Springer; 2011. p. 59–65.
4. Uppot RN, Harisinghani MG, Gervais DA. Imaging-guided percutaneous renal biopsy: rationale and approach. AJR Am J Roentgenol. 2010;194(6):1443–9.
5. Kobayashi K, Censullo ML, Rossman LL, Kyriakides PN, Kahan BD, Cohen AM. Interventional radiologic management of renal transplant dysfunction: indications, limitations, and technical considerations. Radiographics. 2007;27(4):1109–30.
6. Gupta S, Wallace MJ, Cardella JF, Kundu S, Miller DL, Rose SC. Quality improvement guidelines for percutaneous needle biopsy. J Vasc Interv Radiol. 2010;21(7):969–75.
7. Venkatesan AM, Kundu S, Sacks D, Wallace MJ, Wojak JC, Rose SC, et al. Practice guidelines for adult antibiotic prophylaxis during vascular and interventional radiology procedures. J Vasc Interv Radiol. 2010;21(11):1611–30.
8. Taslakian B, Sebaaly MG, Al-Kutoubi A. Patient evaluation and preparation in vascular and interventional radiology: what every interventional radiologist should know (part 1: patient assessment and laboratory tests). Cardiovasc Intervent Radiol. 2016;39(3):325–33.
9. Taslakian B, Sebaaly MG, Al-Kutoubi A. Patient evaluation and preparation in vascular and interventional radiology: what every interventional radiologist should know (part 2: patient preparation and medications). Cardiovasc Intervent Radiol. 2016;39(4):489–99. doi: 10.1007/s00270-015-1239-4. [Epub 2015 Nov 25].

Nephrostomy

47

Bedros Taslakian

INTRODUCTION

Percutaneous nephrostomy is defined as the imaging-guided placement of a catheter of sufficient size into the renal collecting system to provide adequate drainage or an access for subsequent minimally invasive endourologic interventional procedures. Bleeding complications can be minimized by entering the kidney in a relatively avascular zone created by branching of the renal artery, just posterior to the lateral convex border of the kidney. The specific site of renal entry depends on the indication for access and the anatomic constraints, with the lower pole posterior calix accessed via a subcostal approach being the best for simple urinary drainage. On the other hand, a posterior calix of the upper or middle collecting system offers the easiest access to the ureteropelvic junction for potential endoureteral interventions.

COMMON INDICATIONS [1–6]

- Urosepsis secondary to pyonephrosis or infected hydronephrosis
- Supravesical urinary tract obstruction causing intractable pain or acute renal failure
- Urinary diversion for management of hemorrhagic cystitis, urinary leak or fistula
- Access for interventional procedures:
  - Removal of renal and ureteral stones
  - Balloon dilatation of ureteric or ureteropelvic junction stricture *(endopyelotomy)*
  - Antegrade ureteric stent placement
  - Instillation of medications into the collecting system *(fungal balls, upper tract transitional cell carcinomas, dissolution of calculi)*
  - Foreign body retrieval
  - Nephroscopy and ureteroscopy *(e.g., diagnostic evaluation, endoscopic biopsy, endoscopic resection of upper tract transitional cell carcinomas)*

COMMON CONTRAINDICATIONS [1–3, 6]

- Unwilling or uncooperative patients
- Severely compromised cardiopulmonary function or hemodynamic instability
- Uncorrectable coagulopathy
- Severe uncorrected metabolic imbalance such as hyperkalemia or metabolic acidosis *(correction is necessary to decrease the risk of complications such as arrhythmias or cardioplegia)*
- Absence of safe route to the kidney *(e.g., retro-renal colon)*
- History of allergic contrast reaction

B. Taslakian (✉)
Department of Radiology, New York University Langone Medical Center, 660 First Ave, New York, NY 10016, USA
e-mail: btaslakian@gmail.com

B. Taslakian et al. (eds.), *Procedural Dictations in Image-Guided Intervention*,
DOI 10.1007/978-3-319-40845-3_47

- Pregnancy in cases when imaging guidance involves ionizing radiation

POSSIBLE COMPLICATIONS [1–6]

Minor complications:

- Pain and discomfort
- Microscopic hematuria *(clears within 12–24 h)*
- Macroscopic hematuria *(clears within 24–48 h)*
- Catheter malfunction *(dislodgment, blockage)*
- Urine extravasation
- Respiratory insufficiency due to prone position

Major complications:

- Septic shock *(fever, chills with hypotension), 1–3 % (in setting of pyonephrosis 7–9 %)*
- Hemorrhage requiring transfusion, *1–4 %*
- Vascular injury requiring nephrectomy or embolization, *0.1–1 %; e.g., intercostal vessel injury, arteriovenous fistula, pseudoaneurysm, arterial–calyceal fistula*
- Bowel transgression, *0.2 %;* nephrocolic fistula and peritonitis
- Pleural transgression, *0.1–0.2 %; e.g., pneumothorax, empyema, hydrothorax, hemothorax*
- Respiratory distress due to air embolism during complex endourologic procedures
- Renal pelvis injury

PREPROCEDURAL ASSESSMENT AND PLANNING

- History, indications, and physical examination *(Appendix 1* in Chap. 149*)*
- Evaluation of diagnostic imaging studies to determine the degree of hydronephrosis, possible causes of obstruction and determine the relevant anatomy *(anatomic variants, cysts, tumors, stones, and perinephric urinoma)*
- Periprocedural management of coagulation status *(Appendices 2* in Chaps. 150 *and 3* in 151*)*
- Antibiotic prophylaxis: Routine prophylaxis is recommended, except for routine nephrostomy tube replacement in noninfected system [7] *(Appendices 4* in Chaps. 152 *and 5* in 153*)*
- Imaging modality for guidance: Fluoroscopy, combined CT or combined ultrasound/fluoroscopy-based technique for puncture in difficult cases
- Positioning: Prone, prone oblique *(with the puncture side elevated 45°)*

PROCEDURE NOTE

Procedure: Percutaneous nephrostomy tube insertion
Staff: [_]
Fellow: [_]
Resident: [_]
Clinical Information: Describe history and list indications
Allergies: None known/Allergic to [specify/type of allergy]
Anesthesia: Local anesthesia/Conscious sedation/General anesthesia
Medications: List any relevant medications used (sedation, antibiotics)
Contrast Material: (_) mL of [type] contrast material
Field: Sterile
Procedure classification: Clean-contaminated/Contaminated/Dirty
Position: Prone/Prone oblique
Monitoring: Intravenous access line was secured and vital signs were continuously monitored by nursing staff/anesthesia team throughout the procedure
Total fluoroscopy time: (_) minutes
Cumulative radiation dose: (_) mGy

Description of Procedure *(Double-Stick Nephrostomy Tube Insertion):*
The risks, benefits, alternatives, and the procedure itself were explained to the patient/patient's Power of Attorney/patient's legal guardian, and informed written consent was obtained. The site of the procedure was identified and marked. Time out was performed to confirm the correct patient, procedure, and site.

The procedure was planned and the skin puncture site was marked using combined information from the preliminary ultrasound/ fluoroscopy images along the right/left posterior axillary line, (_) cm below the 12th rib/at the (_)th intercostal space. The skin was prepped and draped in the usual sterile fashion. Local anesthesia was administered. A small skin incision was made. After sonographic localization, the collecting system was punctured with a (21/22)-gauge [Chiba/type] needle under ultrasound/ fluoroscopy guidance. The fine needle was advanced perpendicularly from the back, directly into the most dilated part of the collecting system. The stylet was removed and the tip of the needle was pulled back until urine was observed. Urine sample was sent for culture and urine analysis/ cytology. After confirming the needle tip position with minimal contrast injection, the urinary system was mildly decompressed to minimize bacterial seeding during manipulation. Then, the urinary system was gently opacified with iodinated contrast and air/carbon dioxide under constant fluoroscopic control for caliceal definition.

Following that, under fluoroscopy guidance, a (_)-gauge needle was advanced toward the intended posterior calyx of the upper/middle/ lower pole from a dorsolateral position at an angle of approximately (50–60°) from the horizontal plane. Free urine drainage was noted/ Urine was aspirated from the needle and the urinary collecting system was gently opacified to confirm the needle position. Subsequently, the needle was exchanged over a (0.018)-in. [type] guidewire for an upsizing introducer system. The internal stiffener was removed and urine was aspirated. A (0.038/0.035)-in. [type] guidewire was then advanced through the introducer system into the renal pelvis. The introducer system was exchanged for a (_)-French [self-retaining/type] nephrostomy catheter assembly. The stiff trocar of the pigtail was left within the shaft of the catheter until the catheter traversed the renal cortex. The catheter was advanced into the renal pelvis/pyeloureteric junction/proximal ureter and its tip was reformed. Spot fluoroscopy image was obtained after minimal contrast injection to confirm the catheter tip position, for documentation and future reference. The catheter was locked, anchored to the skin and attached to a gravity drainage system.

The patient was transferred to the floor/ recovery room/intensive care unit following the procedure in a stable/critical condition. Staff was present for the entire procedure.

Description of Procedure *(Single-Stick Nephrostomy Tube Insertion):*

The risks, benefits, alternatives, and the procedure itself were explained to the patient/patient's Power of Attorney/patient's legal guardian, and informed written consent was obtained. The site of the procedure was identified and marked. Time out was performed to confirm the correct patient, procedure, and site.

The procedure was planned and the skin puncture site was marked using combined information from the preliminary ultrasound/fluoroscopy images along the right/left posterior axillary line, (_) cm below the 12th rib/at the (_)th intercostal space. The skin was prepped and draped in the usual sterile fashion. Local anesthesia was administered. A small skin incision was made. Using direct ultrasound visualization/fluoroscopy guidance, a (21/22)-gauge [Chiba/type] needle was advanced toward the intended posterior calyx of the upper/ middle/lower pole. The stylet was removed and the tip of the needle was gently pulled back. Free urine drainage was noted/Urine was aspirated from the needle and sent for culture and urine analysis/cytology. After confirming the needle tip position with minimal contrast injection, the urinary system was mildly decompressed to minimize bacterial seeding during manipulation. The urinary system was gently opacified with contrast under constant fluoroscopic control.

Subsequently, the needle was exchanged over a (0.018)-in. [type] guidewire for an upsizing introducer system. The internal stiffener was removed and urine was aspirated. A (0.038/0.035)-in. [type] guidewire was then advanced through the introducer system into the renal pelvis. The introducer system was exchanged for a (_)-French [self-retaining/type] nephrostomy catheter assembly. The stiff trocar of the pigtail was left within the shaft of the catheter until the catheter traversed the renal cortex. The catheter was advanced into the renal pelvis/pyeloureteric junction/proximal ureter and its tip was reformed. Spot fluoroscopy image was obtained after minimal contrast injection to confirm the catheter tip position, for documentation and future reference. The catheter was locked, anchored to the skin and attached to a gravity drainage system.

The patient was transferred to the floor/ recovery room/intensive care unit following the procedure in a stable/critical condition. Staff was present for the entire procedure.

Description of Procedure *(Nephrostomy Tube Exchange):*
The risks, benefits, alternatives, and the procedure itself were explained to the patient/patient's Power of Attorney/patient's legal guardian, and informed written consent was obtained. The site of the procedure was identified and marked. Time out was performed to confirm the correct patient, procedure, and site.

The skin and the nephrostomy catheter were prepared by using standard sterile procedures. A scout radiograph was obtained to document the site of catheter entry through the patient's skin by placing a metal forceps at the site of skin entry. A small amount of dilute contrast material was injected through the catheter to assess catheter patency and the position of the catheter within the left/right renal pelvis/ proximal ureter. The catheter was then unlocked by releasing the locking mechanism/cut. A (0.035)-in. [type] guidewire was advanced through the catheter. Once there was a sufficient length of guidewire within the urinary collecting system, the old catheter was removed over the guidewire. A (_)-French [self-retaining/ type] catheter assembly with the stiffener was introduced over the guidewire. The stiff/plastic trocar of the pigtail was left within the shaft of the catheter until the catheter traversed the renal cortex. The catheter was advanced into the renal pelvis/pyeloureteric junction/proximal ureter and its tip was reformed after removing the stiffener. The catheter was locked, anchored to the skin and attached to a gravity drainage system. Following this, contrast material was injected through the catheter at the end of the procedure to confirm optimal catheter position and ensure that all side holes were placed within the urinary system.

The patient was transferred to the floor/ recovery room/intensive care unit following the procedure in a stable/critical condition. Staff was present for the entire procedure.

Intra-Procedure Findings: List all relevant findings.

Immediate Complications: None encountered during or directly after the procedure. List complications if any.

Post-Procedure Plan [1–3, 8]:

- Follow-up urine analysis/culture/cytology results and adjust antibiotics treatment as per sensitivity profile.
- Complete bed rest for 4 h or until hematuria begins to clear.
- Abstain from strenuous activities for 3 days.
- Administer supplemental nasal oxygen *(if a small pneumothorax develops).*
- Monitor vital signs every 15 min for 1 h, then every 30 min for 3 h, then every hour for 4 h.
- Inform interventional radiology unit if systolic blood pressure <95 mm Hg, heart rate >100 beats per minute, or if any chest pain or shortness of breath develops.
- If the patient's condition deteriorates during observation, hemoglobin drop is noted without gross hematuria, or significant hematuria is noted, inform interventional radiology unit immediately.
- Monitor fluid input/output and adjust intravenous volume replacement as needed.
- Start clear liquid diet for the first hour, then resume preprocedural diet thereafter if tolerated and no complications occur.
- Treat pain and fever symptomatically as necessary.
- Daily catheter care:
  - Inspect catheter and make sure that the 3-way stopcock is open to the drainage bag and the catheter has not been externally retracted.

  - Flush the catheter gently with 20 mL of bacteriostatic saline and aspirate every 4 h if clots are persistent and obstructing the system *(10 mL toward the drainage bottle and 10 mL toward the urinary system).*
- Follow-up instructions:
  - Continue drainage until adequate decompression is achieved or infection resolves, after restoring antegrade flow.
  - Nephrostomy tubes placed for subsequent endourologic intervention can be capped or attached to dependent drainage as needed.
  - Nephrostomy tubes placed for subsequent antegrade ureteric stent placement should be left under dependent drainage for 1 week and until the urine is clear from blood/blood clots.
  - Inform interventional radiology team if the draining amount decreases, pericatheter leak or local skin complications occurs.
  - The patient can be discharged home 24 h after tube placement if no complications occur or hospitalization is not indicated for other reasons.
  - Catheter exchange is recommended every 3 months to prevent bacterial/fungal colonization and occlusion from debris.

Impression:

- Left/right percutaneous nephrostomy tube insertion, as described above.
- The patient tolerated the procedure well and left the interventional unit in a stable condition.
- The patient was unstable and the procedure was canceled/terminated prematurely.
- List any other relevant or important information/finding.

References

1. Stokes LA, Meranze SG. Percutaneous nephrostomy, cystostomy, and nephroureteral Stenting. In: Mauro MA, Murphy KPJ, Thomson KR, Venbrux AC, Morgan RA, editors. Image-guided interventions. 2nd ed. Philadelphia: Saunders Elsevier; 2014. p. 1076–88.
2. Covey AM, Aruny JE, Kandarpa K. Percutaneous nephrostomy and antegrade ureteral stenting. In: Kandarpa K, Machan L, editors. Handbook of interventional radiologic procedures. 4th ed. Philadelphia: Lippincott Williams & Wilkins; 2011. p. 590–606.
3. Punamiya S. Percutaneous nephrostomy and antegrade ureteric stenting. In: Gervais DA, Sabharwal T, editors. Interventional radiology procedures in biopsy and drainage. Heidelberg: Springer; 2011. p. 165–77.
4. Hausegger KA, Portugaller HR. Percutaneous nephrostomy and antegrade ureteral stenting: technique-indications-complications. Eur Radiol. 2006;16(9):2016–30.
5. Dyer RB, Regan JD, Kavanagh PV, Khatod EG, Chen MY, Zagoria RJ. Percutaneous nephrostomy with extensions of the technique: step by step. Radiographics. 2002;22(3):503–25.
6. Ramchandani P, Cardella JF, Grassi CJ, Roberts AC, Sacks D, Schwartzberg MS, et al. Quality improvement guidelines for percutaneous nephrostomy. J Vasc Interv Radiol. 2003;14(9 Pt 2):S277–81.
7. Venkatesan AM, Kundu S, Sacks D, Wallace MJ, Wojak JC, Rose SC, et al. Practice guidelines for adult antibiotic prophylaxis during vascular and interventional radiology procedures. J Vasc Interv Radiol. 2010;21(11):1611–30.
8. Maher MM, Kealey S, McNamara A, O'Laoide R, Gibney RG, Malone DE. Management of visceral interventional radiology catheters: a troubleshooting guide for interventional radiologists. Radiographics. 2002;22(2):305–22.

Part IX

Non-vascular Interventional Procedures: Genitourinary-Ureters and Urinary Bladder

Introduction by Aghiad Al-Kutoubi, Section Reviewer

Interventional radiologists can play a pivotal role in the prompt diagnosis and percutaneous treatment of various genitourinary conditions. These minimally invasive procedures can either obviate open surgery or stabilize the patient's condition prior to open surgery.

The interventionalist is frequently called upon to perform percutaneous insertion of ureteric stents as a bail out procedure in cases where transvesical insertion fails or if there is no access. It is also possible to preform transurethral stent exchange under imaging guidance avoiding the need for cystoscopy and anesthesia. In many cases, imaging-guided interventions play a crucial role in the management of urine leaks. Percutaneous urinary diversion is often required to facilitate healing within the genitourinary system. "Rendezvous procedures" have been described in the treatment of traumatic ureteric transection.

This section provides a comprehensive list of procedural reports that covers the vast majority of the currently performed image-guided procedures in the ureters and urinary bladder with up-to-date explanatory notes, synopsis of the indications and contraindications, and potential complications in an organized and practical format.

Section Chapters

Antegrade Ureteral Stenting

48

Bedros Taslakian

INTRODUCTION

Ureteral "double J" stents facilitate drainage from the renal pelvis to the bladder in patients with normal urinary bladder function who have urinary tract obstruction secondary to ureteral pathology. Antegrade insertion of ureteral stent has become an established alternative when retrograde approach fails especially in patients with pelvic, bladder, or prostate malignancy. The procedure is performed either in one stage or more commonly in two stages with a nephrostomy access established first and antegrade stent insertion performed a few days later.

COMMON INDICATIONS [1–5]

- Obstructive uropathy caused by intrinsic or extrinsic ureteral obstruction related to inflammatory, neoplastic, or iatrogenic causes
- Urinary diversion for urinary leak or fistulae

B. Taslakian (✉)
Department of Radiology, New York University Langone Medical Center, 660 First Ave, New York, NY 10016, USA
e-mail: Btaslakian@gmail.com

COMMON CONTRAINDICATIONS [1–4]

In addition to the contraindications of nephrostomy (see Chap. 47), the prerequisite for antegrade ureteric stenting, the contraindications for ureteral stent insertion include the following:

- Significant bleeding after nephrostomy *(higher rate of stent occlusion, defer the procedure until after the urine is clear from blood clots)*
- Active or suspected urinary infection
- Untreated infra-vesical urinary obstruction
- Lower urinary tract fistulae
- Urinary bladder tumors *(relative contraindication; results recurrent bleeding due to mechanical irritation of the tumor)*
- Irritable or neurogenic bladder *(increased pressure in the bladder resulting in urinary reflux)*
- Urinary incontinence
- Pregnancy

POSSIBLE COMPLICATIONS [1–4]

Complications related to access: Refer to complications of nephrostomy (see Chap. 47).

Specific complications related to ureteric stenting:

- Iatrogenic perforation of the renal collecting system or ureter
- Encrustation, resulting in stent malfunction and fracture

B. Taslakian et al. (eds.), *Procedural Dictations in Image-Guided Intervention*,
DOI 10.1007/978-3-319-40845-3_48

- Loss of stent patency from obstructing blood clots
- Loss of the stent patency from a transient severe mucosal edema
- Malpositioning or migration of the stent
- Bladder irritative symptoms
- Ascending urinary tract infection
- Mild hematuria *(common, clears spontaneously, and is caused by irritation of the urothelium)*
- Persistent hematuria *(can be secondary to tumor erosion by the stent)*
- Erosion of the stent through the renal pelvis causing urinoma, vascular injury, or retroperitoneal abscess formation
- Erosion of the stent into the iliac artery causing intermittent or massive hematuria

PREPROCEDURAL ASSESSMENT AND PLANNING

- History, indications, and physical examination *(Appendix 1* in Chap. 149*)*
- Evaluation of diagnostic imaging studies to determine the degree of hydronephrosis and possible causes as well as the relevant anatomy *(anatomic variants, cysts, tumors, stones, and perinephric urinoma)*
- Periprocedural management of coagulation status *(Appendices 2* in Chap. 150 *and 3* in Chap. 151*)*
- Antibiotic prophylaxis: Routine prophylaxis is recommended [6] *(Appendices 4* in Chap. 152 *and 5* in Chap. 153*)*
- Imaging modality for guidance: Fluoroscopy
- Positioning: Prone, prone oblique

PROCEDURE NOTE

Procedure: Antegrade ureteric stent insertion and balloon angioplasty of ureteral stricture
Staff: [_]
Fellow: [_]
Resident: [_]
Clinical Information: Describe history and list indications
Allergies: None known/Allergic to [specify/type of allergy]
Anesthesia: Local anesthesia with conscious sedation/general anesthesia
Medications: List any relevant medications used (sedation, antibiotics)
Contrast Material: (_) mL of [type] contrast material was used for injection
Field: Sterile
Procedure classification: Clean-contaminated/Contaminated
Position: Prone/Prone oblique
Monitoring: Intravenous access line was secured and vital signs were continuously monitored by nursing staff/anesthesia team throughout the procedure
Total fluoroscopy time: (_) minutes
Cumulative radiation dose: (_) mGy

Description of Procedure:
The risks, benefits, alternatives, and the procedure itself were explained to the patient/patient's Power of Attorney/patient's legal guardian, and informed written consent was obtained. The site of the procedure was identified and marked. Time out was performed to confirm the correct patient, procedure, and site.

The skin and the previously inserted nephrostomy catheter were prepped and draped in the usual sterile fashion. A scout radiograph was obtained to document the site of catheter entry through the patient's skin by placing a metal forceps at the site of skin entry. A small amount of dilute contrast material was injected through the catheter to assess catheter patency and position within the collecting system. The catheter was then unlocked by releasing the locking mechanism/cut.

Under fluoroscopy visualization, a (0.035)-in. [type] guidewire was inserted through the drain and looped in the renal pelvis. The drain was then exchanged over the guidewire for a (_)-French peel-away sheath. The urinary system was gently opacified with contrast under constant fluoroscopic control. Through the introducer system, a (_) French [angiographic/type] catheter was inserted over a (0.035)-in. [hydrophilic/type] guidewire to navigate through the point of stricture/obstruction/leak, which was successfully crossed. The catheter was advanced into the urinary bladder over the [hydrophilic/type] guidewire, which was then exchanged through the catheter for a (0.035)-in. [stiff/type] guidewire. Pre-dilation of the stricture was performed using a (4) mm [non-compliant/type] balloon catheter inserted over the [stiff/type] guidewire to the level of the stricture. Progressive dilation was performed by inflating the balloon manually with iodinated contrast material using a (_)-mL syringe/inflation device, under direct fluoroscopy visualization until the "waist" at the stricture site disappeared.

A (_)-French, (_) cm long, [type] ureteral stent was then mounted on the guidewire and advanced through the sheath down the ureter into the bladder. After adequately positioning of the tip beyond the ureteral orifice of the bladder (ureterovesicular junction), the guidewire was retracted to reform the distal loop of the stent. The sheath and guidewire were then further withdrawn and the proximal loop of the stent was reformed within the renal pelvis. The stent was adjusted using the suture material placed through the proximal side whole of the stent. A safety (_)-French [self-retaining/pigtail/type] nephrostomy tube was placed through the sheath, after removing the string, and its tip was reformed in the renal pelvis. The peel-away sheath was then divided and removed, as well as the guidewire. The nephrostomy tube was attached to a gravity drainage bag. The catheter was locked, anchored to the skin and attached to a gravity drainage system. Following this, contrast material was injected through the catheter at the end of the procedure to confirm optimal catheter position and ensure that all side holes were placed within the urinary system and the ureteral stent is functioning.

The patient was transferred to the floor/recovery room/intensive care unit following the procedure in a stable/critical condition. Staff was present for the entire procedure.

Intra-Procedure Findings: List all relevant findings.

Immediate Complications: None encountered during or directly after the procedure. List complications if any.

Post-Procedure Plan [1–5, 7]:

- Complete bed rest for 4 h or until hematuria begins to clear.
- Abstain from strenuous activities for 3 days.
- Monitor vital signs every 15 min for 1 h, then every 30 min for 3 h, then every hour for 4 h.
- Inform interventional radiology unit if systolic blood pressure <95 mm Hg or heart rate >100 beats per minute.
- If the patient's condition deteriorates during observation, hemoglobin drop is noted without gross hematuria, or significant hematuria is noted, inform interventional radiology team immediately.
- Monitor fluid input/output and adjust intravenous volume replacement as needed.
- Start clear liquid diet for the first hour, then resume preprocedural diet thereafter if tolerated and no complications occur.
- Treat pain and fever symptomatically as necessary.
- Instructions regarding the safety nephrostomy catheter:
  - Keep the safety nephrostomy catheter under gravity drainage for 24–48 h after the procedure or until the urine is clear from blood/blood clots.
  - Flush the catheter with 20 mL of bacteriostatic saline and aspirate every 4 h if clots are persistent and obstructing the system *(10 mL toward the drainage bag and 10 mL toward the urinary system).*
  - Thereafter, cap the nephrostomy catheter for 24 h to allow for physiologic trial of internal drainage, while monitoring the patient's clinical status, vital signs, creatinine, and white count closely.
  - The nephrostomy tube can be removed safely, however over a guidewire and under fluoroscopy guidance, if all the following are documented during a satisfactory 24 h period of capping:

1. The patient remains asymptomatic, with no pain or clinical signs of infection/sepsis.
2. The patient is able to void normally, with adequate urine output.
3. No pericatheter leak is noted.
4. Stable or decreasing creatinine and white blood cell count.
5. Nephrostogram shows no blood clots in the urinary system or hydronephrosis, and a functioning ureteral stent with contrast reaching the urinary bladder.

- Ureteral stents should be routinely exchanged every 3–6 months to prevent encrustation, secondary to deposition of crystalline urine components on the outer or inner surface of the stent, resulting in stent malfunction and fractures.

Impression:

- Left/right ureteric stent placement/and balloon angioplasty of ureteral stricture, with placement of a temporary safety nephrostomy tube, as described above.
- The patient tolerated the procedure well and left the interventional unit in a stable condition.
- The patient was unstable and the procedure was canceled/terminated prematurely.
- List any other relevant or important information/finding.

References

1. Stokes LA, Meranze SG. Percutaneous nephrostomy, cystostomy, and nephroureteral stenting. In: Mauro MA, Murphy KPJ, Thomson KR, Venbrux AC, Morgan RA, editors. Image-guided interventions. 2nd ed. Philadelphia: Saunders Elsevier; 2014. p. 1076–88.
2. Covey AM, Aruny JE, Kandarpa K. Percutaneous nephrostomy and antegrade ureteral stenting. In: Kandarpa K, Machan L, editors. Handbook of interventional radiologic procedures. 4th ed. Philadelphia: Lippincott Williams & Wilkins; 2011. p. 590–606.
3. Punamiya S. Percutaneous nephrostomy and antegrade ureteric stenting. In: Gervais DA, Sabharwal T, editors. Interventional radiology procedures in biopsy and drainage. Heidelberg: Springer; 2011. p. 165–77.
4. Hausegger KA, Portugaller HR. Percutaneous nephrostomy and antegrade ureteral stenting: technique-indications-complications. Eur Radiol. 2006;16(9):2016–30.
5. Dyer RB, Regan JD, Kavanagh PV, Khatod EG, Chen MY, Zagoria RJ. Percutaneous nephrostomy with extensions of the technique: step by step. Radiographics. 2002;22(3):503–25.
6. Venkatesan AM, Kundu S, Sacks D, Wallace MJ, Wojak JC, Rose SC, et al. Practice guidelines for adult antibiotic prophylaxis during vascular and interventional radiology procedures. J Vasc Interv Radiol. 2010;21(11):1611–30.
7. Maher MM, Kealey S, McNamara A, O'Laoide R, Gibney RG, Malone DE. Management of visceral interventional radiology catheters: a troubleshooting guide for interventional radiologists. Radiographics. 2002;22(2):305–22.

Nephroureterostomy

49

Bedros Taslakian

INTRODUCTION

Percutaneous nephroureterostomy is the imaging-guided placement of a catheter of sufficient size into the renal collecting system, with the catheter extending down the ureter terminating in the urinary bladder or ileal conduit. The nephroureteral catheters provide internal and external drainage and are less prone to dislodgment when compared to nephrostomy tubes. When treating urinary leak, urinoma or fistula, the holes of the catheter should be only in the renal pelvis and bladder, rather than along the entire course of the catheter to allow healing.

COMMON INDICATIONS [1–3]

- Obstructive uropathy caused by intrinsic or extrinsic ureteral obstruction related to stones, malignancies, or iatrogenic causes
- Urinary diversion for urinary leak, urinoma, or fistulae

B. Taslakian (✉)
Department of Radiology, New York University Langone Medical Center, 660 First Ave, New York, NY 10016, USA
e-mail: btaslakian@gmail.com

COMMON CONTRAINDICATIONS [1, 2]

In addition to the contraindications of nephrostomy (see Chap. 47), the contraindications for nephroureterostomy include

- Significant bleeding after nephrostomy access *(higher rate of stent occlusion)*
- Active or suspected urinary infection
- Untreated infravesical urinary obstruction
- Urinary bladder tumors *(relative contraindication; results recurrent bleeding due to mechanical irritation of the tumor)*
- Irritable or neurogenic bladder
- Urinary incontinence
- Pregnancy

POSSIBLE COMPLICATIONS [1, 2]

Complications related to access: Refer to complications of nephrostomy (see Chap. 47).

Specific complications related to nephroureterostomy tube:

- Iatrogenic perforation of the renal collecting system or ureter
- Encrustation, resulting in tube malfunction and fracture
- Loss of tube patency from obstructing blood clots
- Dislodgment and malpositioning
- Bladder irritative symptoms
- Mild hematuria
- Ascending urinary tract infection

B. Taslakian et al. (eds.), *Procedural Dictations in Image-Guided Intervention*,
DOI 10.1007/978-3-319-40845-3_49

- Erosion of the stent through the renal pelvis causing urinoma, vascular injury, or retroperitoneal abscess formation
- Erosion of the stent into the iliac artery causing intermittent or massive hematuria

PREPROCEDURAL ASSESSMENT AND PLANNING

- History, indications, and physical examination *(Appendix 1* in Chap. 149*)*
- Evaluation of diagnostic imaging studies to determine the degree of hydronephrosis, possible causes of obstruction and determine the relevant anatomy *(anatomic variants, cysts, tumors, stones, and perinephric urinoma)*
- Periprocedural management of coagulation status *(Appendices 2* in Chap. 150 *and 3* in Chap. 151*)*
- Antibiotic prophylaxis: Routine prophylaxis is recommended, except for routine tube replacement in noninfected system [4] *(Appendices 4* in Chap. 152 *and 5* in Chap. 153*)*
- Imaging modality for guidance: Fluoroscopy, combined CT or ultrasound/fluoroscopy-based technique for puncture in difficult cases
- Positioning: Prone, prone oblique *(with the puncture side elevated 45 degrees)*

PROCEDURE NOTE [5, 6]

Procedure: Percutaneous nephroureterostomy tube insertion
Staff: [_]
Fellow: [_]
Resident: [_]
Clinical Information: Describe history and list indications
Allergies: None known/Allergic to [specify/type of allergy]
Anesthesia: Local anesthesia with conscious sedation/General anesthesia
Medications: List any relevant medications used (sedation, antibiotics)
Contrast Material: (_) mL of [type] contrast material
Field: Sterile
Procedure classification: Clean-contaminated/contaminated
Position: Prone/Prone oblique
Monitoring: Intravenous access line was secured and vital signs were continuously monitored by nursing staff/anesthesia team throughout the procedure
Total fluoroscopy time: (_) minutes
Cumulative radiation dose: (_) mGy

Description of Procedure *(Single-Stick Nephroureterostomy Tube Insertion):*
The risks, benefits, alternatives, and the procedure itself were explained to the patient/patient's Power of Attorney/patient's legal guardian, and informed written consent was obtained. The site of the procedure was identified and marked. Time out was performed to confirm the correct patient, procedure, and site.

The procedure was planned and the skin puncture site was marked using combined information from the preliminary ultrasound/fluoroscopy images along the right/left posterior axillary line, (_) cm below the 12th rib/at the (_) th intercostal space. The skin was prepped and draped in the usual sterile fashion. Local anesthesia was administered. A small skin incision was made. Using direct ultrasound visualization/fluoroscopy guidance a (21/22)-gauge [Chiba/type] needle was advanced toward the intended posterior calyx of the upper/middle pole. The stylet was removed and the tip of the needle was gently pulled back. Free urine drainage was noted/Urine was aspirated from the needle. Urine sample was sent for culture and urine analysis/cytology. After confirming the needle tip position with minimal contrast injection, the urinary system was mildly decompressed to minimize bacterial seeding during manipulation.

Subsequently, the needle was exchanged over a (0.018)-in. [type] guidewire for an upsizing introducer system. The internal stiffener was removed and urine was aspirated. The urinary system was gently opacified with contrast under constant fluoroscopic control. Through the introducer system, a (_) French [angiographic/type] catheter was inserted over a (0.035)-in. [hydrophilic/type] guidewire to navigate through the point of stricture/obstruction/leak, which was successfully crossed. The catheter was advanced into the urinary bladder/ileal conduit over the [hydrophilic/type] guidewire, which was then exchanged through the catheter for a (0.035)-in. [stiff/type] guidewire. A (_) mm [non-compliant/type] balloon catheter was inserted over the [stiff/type] guidewire to the level of the stricture. Progressive dilation was performed by inflating the balloon manually with iodinated contrast material using a (_)-mL syringe/inflation device, under fluoroscopy visualization until the "waist" at the stricture site disappeared.

Subsequently, the introducer system was exchanged for a (_)-French [self-retaining/type] nephroureterostomy catheter assembly. The stiffener was left within the shaft of the catheter until the tip traversed the renal cortex. The catheter was advanced into the urinary bladder/ileal conduit over the guidewire and its tip was reformed. Spot fluoroscopy image was obtained after minimal contrast injection to confirm the catheter position, for documentation and future reference. The proximal loop of the catheter was then formed in the renal pelvis. The catheter was locked, anchored to the skin and attached to a gravity drainage system.

The patient was transferred to the floor/recovery room/intensive care unit following the procedure in a stable/critical condition. Staff was present for the entire procedure.

Description of Procedure *(Conversion of Nephrostomy to Nephroureterostomy):*
The risks, benefits, alternatives, and the procedure itself were explained to the patient/patient's Power of Attorney/patient's legal guardian, and informed written consent was obtained. The site of the procedure was identified and marked. Time out was performed to confirm the correct patient, procedure, and site.

The skin and the previously inserted nephrostomy drain were prepped and draped in the usual sterile fashion. A scout radiograph was obtained to document the site of catheter entry through the patient's skin by placing a metal forceps at the site of skin entry. A small amount of dilute contrast material was injected through the catheter to assess catheter patency and position within the collecting system. The catheter was then unlocked by releasing the locking mechanism/cut.

Under fluoroscopy visualization, a (0.035)-in. [type] guidewire was inserted through the catheter and looped in the renal pelvis. The drain was then exchanged over the guidewire for a (_)-French peel-away sheath. The urinary system was gently opacified with contrast under constant fluoroscopic control. Through the sheath, a (_) French [angiographic/type] catheter was inserted over a (0.035)-in. [hydrophilic/type] guidewire to navigate through the point of stricture/obstruction/leak, which was successfully crossed. The catheter was advanced into the urinary bladder/ileal conduit over the [hydrophilic/type] guidewire, which was then exchanged through the catheter for a (0.035)-in. [stiff/type] guidewire. A (_) mm [non-compliant/type] balloon catheter was inserted over the [stiff/type] guidewire to the level of the stricture. Progressive dilation was performed by inflating the balloon manually with iodinated contrast material using a (_)-mL syringe/inflating device, under fluoroscopy visualization until the "waist" at the stricture site disappeared.

Subsequently, a (_)-French [self-retaining/type] nephroureterostomy catheter was advanced through the sheath into the urinary bladder/ileal conduit over the guidewire and its tip was reformed. The sheath was removed. Spot fluoroscopy image was obtained after minimal contrast injection to confirm the catheter position, for documentation and future reference. The proximal loop of the catheter was then formed in the renal pelvis. The catheter was locked, anchored to the skin and attached to a gravity drainage system.

The patient was transferred to the floor/recovery room/intensive care unit following the procedure in a stable/critical condition. Staff was present for the entire procedure.

Description of Procedure *(Nephroureterostomy Tube Replacement):*
The risks, benefits, alternatives, and the procedure itself were explained to the patient/patient's Power of Attorney/patient's legal guardian, and informed written consent was obtained. The site of the procedure was identified and marked.

Time out was performed to confirm the correct patient, procedure, and site.

The skin and the previously inserted nephrostomy drain were prepped and draped in the usual sterile fashion. A scout radiograph was obtained to document the site of catheter entry through the patient's skin by placing a metal forceps at the site of skin entry. A small amount of dilute contrast material was injected through the catheter to assess catheter patency and position within the urinary bladder/ileal conduit. The catheter was then unlocked by releasing the locking mechanism/cut. A (0.035)-in. [stiff/type] guidewire was advanced through the catheter. Once there was a sufficient length of guidewire within the urinary bladder/ileal conduit, the old catheter was withdrawn over the guidewire under fluoroscopic guidance. A new (_)-French [self-retaining/type] catheter was advanced over the guidewire and its distal tip was reformed in the urinary bladder. The guidewire was pulled and the proximal loop of the catheter was formed in the renal pelvis. The catheter was locked, anchored to the skin and attached to a gravity drainage system. Following this, contrast material was injected through the catheter at the end of the procedure to confirm optimal catheter position and ensure that all side holes were placed within the urinary system.

The patient was transferred to the floor/recovery room following the procedure in a stable condition. Staff was present for the entire procedure.

Intra-Procedure Findings: List all relevant findings.

Immediate Complications: None encountered during or directly after the procedure. List complications if any.

Post-Procedure Plan [1, 2]**:**

- Follow-up urine analysis/culture/cytology results and adjust antibiotics treatment as per sensitivity profile.
- Complete bed rest for 4 h or until hematuria begins to clear.
- Abstain from strenuous activities for 3 days.
- Administer supplemental nasal oxygen *(if a small pneumothorax develops).*
- Monitor vital signs every 15 min for 1 h, then every 30 min for 3 h, then every hour for 4 h.
- Inform interventional radiology team if systolic blood pressure <95 mm Hg, heart rate >100 beats per minute, or if any chest pain or shortness of breath develops.
- If the patient's condition deteriorates during observation, hemoglobin drop is noted without gross hematuria, significant hematuria is noted, inform interventional radiology team immediately.
- Monitor fluid input/output and adjust intravenous volume replacement as needed.
- Start clear liquid diet for the first hour, then resume preprocedural diet thereafter if tolerated and no complications occur.
- Treat pain and fever symptomatically as necessary.
- Daily catheter care:
  - Inspect catheter and make sure that the 3-way stopcock is open to the drainage bag and the catheter has not been externally retracted.
  - Flush the catheter with 20 mL of bacteriostatic saline and aspirate every 4 h if clots are persistent and obstructing the system *(10 mL toward the drainage bag and 10 mL toward the urinary system).*
- Further instructions:
  - Continue drainage until adequate decompression is achieved and infection/blood clots resolve.
  - Inform interventional radiology team if the draining amount decreases, pericatheter leak or local skin complications occurs.
  - The catheter can be capped to allow internal drainage after confirming resolution of hematuria and tube patency along its length with a nephrostogram.
  - Catheter exchange is recommended every 3 months to prevent bacterial/fungal colonization and occlusion from debris and encrustation
  - Return to external gravity drainage if the patient experiences fever, chills, flank pain, or leakage around the drain at any time while the drain is capped.

Impression:

- Left/right nephroureterostomy tube insertion/exchange, as described above.
- The patient tolerated the procedure well and left the interventional unit in a stable condition.
- The patient was unstable and the procedure was canceled/terminated prematurely.
- List any other relevant or important information/finding.

References

1. Stokes LA, Meranze SG. Percutaneous nephrostomy, cystostomy, and nephroureteral stenting. In: Mauro MA, Murphy KPJ, Thomson KR, Venbrux AC, Morgan RA, editors. Image-guided interventions. 2nd ed. Philadelphia: Saunders Elsevier; 2014. p. 1076–88.
2. Covey AM, Aruny JE, Kandarpa K. Percutaneous nephrostomy and antegrade ureteral stenting. In: Kandarpa K, Machan L, editors. Handbook of interventional radiologic procedures. 4th ed. Philadelphia: Lippincott Williams & Wilkins; 2011. p. 590–606.
3. Dyer RB, Regan JD, Kavanagh PV, Khatod EG, Chen MY, Zagoria RJ. Percutaneous nephrostomy with extensions of the technique: step by step. Radiographics. 2002;22(3):503–25.
4. Venkatesan AM, Kundu S, Sacks D, Wallace MJ, Wojak JC, Rose SC, et al. Practice guidelines for adult antibiotic prophylaxis during vascular and interventional radiology procedures. J Vasc Interv Radiol. 2010;21(11):1611–30.
5. Taslakian B, Sebaaly MG, Al-Kutoubi A. Patient evaluation and preparation in vascular and interventional radiology: what every interventional radiologist should know (part 1: patient assessment and laboratory tests). Cardiovasc Intervent Radiol. 2016;39(3):325–33.
6. Taslakian B, Sebaaly MG, Al-Kutoubi A. Patient evaluation and preparation in vascular and interventional radiology: what every interventional radiologist should know (part 2: patient preparation and medications). Cardiovasc Intervent Radiol. 2016;39(4):489–99. doi: 10.1007/s00270-015-1239-4. [Epub 2015 Nov 25].

Suprapubic Cystostomy

50

Bedros Taslakian

INTRODUCTION

A percutaneous suprapubic cystostomy *(vesicostomy or epicystostomy)* is the image-guided insertion of a urinary catheter to drain urine from the bladder in individuals with obstruction of normal urinary flow. It can provide rapid relief of acute urinary retention when transurethral catheterization of the bladder is contraindicated or not possible. In addition, suprapubic cystostomy can be used for imaging-guided insertion of antegrade transurethral Foley catheter in patients who have suffered a traumatic or iatrogenic injury to the urethra. The urinary bladder is accessed approximately 2–3 cm above the pubic symphysis or at the junction of the mid and lower thirds of the anterior bladder wall, avoiding the area of the trigone and subsequent bladder spasm. As the inferior epigastric artery lies along the lateral edge of the rectus sheath, the vertical midline or slight paramedian approach helps to avoid arterial injury.

COMMON INDICATIONS [1–4]

Acute urinary retention when transurethral catheterization of the bladder is not possible or contraindicated

- Bladder outlet obstruction secondary to benign prostatic hypertrophy
- Bladder outlet obstruction secondary to prostate cancer
- Bladder outlet obstruction secondary to neurogenic bladder dysfunction
- Scrotal or penile infection or abscess
- Penile or perineal ulceration
- Vulvar vestibulitis
- Patients with urethral trauma
- Radiation-induced cystitis
- Vesicocolonic, vesicouterine, and vesicovaginal fistulae
- Provide access for image-guided antegrade transurethral Foley catheter insertion

B. Taslakian (✉)
Department of Radiology, New York University Langone Medical Center, 660 First Ave, New York, NY 10016, USA
e-mail: Btaslakian@gmail.com

B. Taslakian et al. (eds.), *Procedural Dictations in Image-Guided Intervention*,
DOI 10.1007/978-3-319-40845-3_50

COMMON CONTRAINDICATIONS [1]

- Unwilling patients
- Uncorrectable coagulopathy
- Absence of safe route due to inability to adequately distend the bladder
- Multiple previous abdominopelvic surgeries with extensive scar tissue
- Urinary bladder tumor
- Morbid obesity

POSSIBLE COMPLICATIONS [1, 2, 4]

Minor complications:
- Hematuria
- Catheter dislodgment and blockage
- Pain
- Urine extravasation/leak
- Increased risk for infection and stone formation *(chronically indwelling catheters)*

Major complications:
- Sepsis
- Hemorrhage requiring transfusion
- Vascular injury
- Bowel transgression, fistula, and peritonitis

PREPROCEDURAL ASSESSMENT AND PLANNING

- History, indications, and physical examination *(Appendix 1* in Chap. 149*)*
- Evaluation of diagnostic imaging studies to determine the relevant anatomy *(anatomic variants, urinary bladder distention, stones, adhesions, and urinoma)*
- Periprocedural management of coagulation status *(Appendices 2* in Chap. 150 *and 3* in Chap. 151*)*
- Antibiotic prophylaxis: Routine prophylaxis is recommended [1, 2, 4]
- Imaging modality for guidance: Ultrasound *(trocar technique)*, combined ultrasound/fluoroscopy-based technique for puncture in difficult cases using modified Seldinger technique
- Positioning: Supine

PROCEDURE NOTE [5, 6]

Procedure: Percutaneous suprapubic cystostomy
Staff: [_]
Fellow: [_]
Resident: [_]
Clinical Information: Describe history and list indications
Allergies: None known/Allergic to [specify/type of allergy]
Anesthesia: Local anesthesia/conscious sedation
Medications: List any relevant medications used (sedation, antibiotics)
Contrast Material: (_) mL of [type] contrast material
Field: Sterile
Procedure classification: Clean-contaminated/Contaminated/Dirty
Position: Supine
Monitoring: Intravenous access line was secured and vital signs were continuously monitored by nursing staff/anesthesia team throughout the procedure.
Total fluoroscopy time: (_) minutes
Cumulative radiation dose: (_) mGy

Description of Procedure *(bladder is adequately distended → ultrasound guided, trocar technique):*
The risks, benefits, alternatives, and the procedure itself were explained to the patient/patient's Power of Attorney/patient's legal guardian, and informed written/verbal consent was obtained. The site of the procedure was identified and marked. Time out was performed to confirm the correct patient, procedure, and site.

The procedure was planned and the skin puncture site was marked (2–3) cm above the pubic symphysis at the midline, using combined information from the preliminary ultrasound images.

The skin was prepped and draped in the usual sterile fashion. Local anesthesia was administered. A small skin incision was made. Ultrasound examination showed an adequately distended urinary bladder.

Subsequently, a (_)-French [type] catheter was loaded on a trocar delivery system. The tip of the catheter with the delivery system was placed in the skin incision and was then advanced under direct ultrasound guidance to enter the urinary bladder. Once the catheter was optimally placed, the inner stylet was removed and urine was aspirated through the metal stiffener. The catheter was then unlocked from the stiffening cannula and advanced to coil within the bladder while holding the stiffener steady. The stiffening cannula was removed. The catheter was locked, anchored to the skin and attached to a drainage system. Following this, completion ultrasound images were obtained through the suprapubic area to confirm correct position of the catheter for future reference and screen for complications.

The patient was transferred to the floor/recovery room/intensive care unit following the procedure in a stable/critical condition. Staff was present for the entire procedure.

Description of Procedure *(bladder is under-distended, combined ultrasound/fluoroscopy-guided Seldinger technique):*
The risks, benefits, alternatives, and the procedure itself were explained to the patient/patient's Power of Attorney/patient's legal guardian, and informed written/verbal consent was obtained. The site of the procedure was identified and marked. Time out was performed to confirm the correct patient, procedure, and site.

The procedure was planned and the skin puncture site was marked (2–3) cm above the pubic symphysis at the midline, using combined information from the preliminary ultrasound images.

The skin was prepped and draped in the usual sterile fashion. Local anesthesia was administered. A small skin incision was made. Ultrasound examination showed an under-distended urinary bladder, with inability to insert a Foley catheter for distention.

Under direct ultrasound visualization, a (_)-gauge [type] needle was inserted and the bladder was distended by injecting (_) mL of dilute contrast. Once the bladder was fully distended, a (0.035)-in. [stiff Amplatz/type] guidewire was advanced through the needle and coiled within the urinary bladder under fluoroscopic guidance*. The tract was dilated with sequential (_)-French fascial dilators. A (_)-French peel-away sheath was advanced over the guidewire. An end hole was created at the tip of a (_)-French Foley catheter, which was then advanced over the guidewire through the peel-away sheath. The wire and peel-away sheath were removed; and the Foley balloon was inflated with sterile saline and pulled up against the anterior wall of the bladder.

The patient was transferred to the floor/recovery room/intensive care unit following the procedure in a stable/critical condition. Staff was present for the entire procedure.

* Note: Placement of a large catheter may be difficult in patients with extensive scar tissue related to previous surgeries or in patients who are obese, in which case a two-step procedure may be necessary, with initial placement of a small pigtail drain that can be upsized after the tract has formed. A 10- or 12-Fr locking pigtail drain is usually adequate for urgent decompression of the bladder. However, subsequent placement of a Foley catheter that is at least 16 Fr in diameter is required for effective long-term bladder drainage.

Description of Procedure *(Small pigtail insertion for urgent decompression and in cases of extensive scaring/obesity)*
The risks, benefits, alternatives, and the procedure itself were explained to the patient/patient's Power of Attorney/patient's legal guardian, and informed written/verbal consent was obtained. The site of the procedure was identified and marked. Time out was performed to confirm the correct patient, procedure, and site.

The procedure was planned and the skin puncture site was marked (2–3) cm above the pubic symphysis at the midline, using combined information from the preliminary ultrasound images.

The skin was prepped and draped in the usual sterile fashion. Local anesthesia was administered. A small skin incision was made. Ultrasound examination showed an under-distended urinary bladder, with inability to insert a Foley catheter for distention.

Under direct ultrasound visualization, a (_)-gauge [type] needle was inserted and the bladder was distended by injecting (_) mL of dilute contrast. Once the bladder was fully distended, a (0.035)-in. [stiff Amplatz/type] guidewire was advanced through the needle and coiled within the urinary bladder under fluoroscopic guidance.

Subsequently, a (_)-French [self-retaining pigtail/type] catheter assembly with the metal stiffener was introduced over the guidewire to a satisfactory depth. The stiff trocar of the pigtail was left within the shaft of the catheter until the catheter traversed the anterior wall of the bladder. The guidewire and metal stiffener were removed, after advancing the catheter into the urinary bladder. The catheter was locked, anchored to the skin and attached to a drainage system.

Following this, completion spot fluoroscopy image was obtained after minimal contrast injection to confirm correct position of the catheter for documentation and future reference.

The patient was transferred to the floor/recovery room/intensive care unit following the procedure in a stable/critical condition. Staff was present for the entire procedure.

Intra-Procedure Findings: List all relevant findings.

Immediate Complications: None encountered during or directly after the procedure. List complications if any.

Post-Procedure Plan [1]:

1. Follow-up urine analysis/culture/cytology results and adjust antibiotics treatment as per sensitivity profile.
2. Complete bed rest for 4 h or until hematuria begins to clear.
3. Abstain from strenuous activities for 3 days.
4. Monitor vital signs every 15 min for 1 h, then every 30 min for 3 h, then every hour for 4 h.
5. Inform interventional radiology unit if systolic blood pressure <95 mm Hg, heart rate >100 beats per minute.
6. Monitor fluid input/output and adjust intravenous volume replacement as indicated.
7. Treat pain and fever symptomatically as necessary.
8. Daily catheter care:
   - Inspect catheter and make sure that the catheter has not been externally retracted.
   - Flush the catheter with 20 mL of bacteriostatic saline and aspirate every 4 h if clots are persistent and obstructing the system *(10 mL toward the drainage bag and 10 mL toward the urinary system).*
   - Flush the catheter with 20 mL of bacteriostatic saline and aspirate daily, after bleeding and clots are resolved.
9. Inform interventional radiology team if the draining amount decreases, pericatheter leak or local skin complications occurs.
10. Catheter exchange is recommended every 2–3 months to prevent bacterial/fungal colonization and occlusion from debris and encrustation.

Impression:

- Percutaneous suprapubic cystostomy tube insertion, as described above.
- The patient tolerated the procedure well and left the interventional unit in a stable condition.
- The patient was unstable and the procedure was canceled/terminated prematurely.
- List any other relevant or important information/finding.

References

1. Stokes LA, Meranze SG. Percutaneous nephrostomy, cystostomy, and nephroureteral stenting. In: Mauro MA, Murphy KPJ, Thomson KR, Venbrux AC, Morgan RA, editors. Image-guided interventions. 2nd ed. Philadelphia: Saunders Elsevier; 2014. p. 1076–88.
2. Lee MJ, Papanicolaou N, Nocks BN, Valdez JA, Yoder IC. Fluoroscopically guided percutaneous

suprapubic cystostomy for long-term bladder drainage: an alternative to surgical cystostomy. Radiology. 1993;188(3):787–9.
3. Thabet A, Kalva SP, Liu B, Mueller PR, Lee SI. Interventional radiology in pregnancy complications: indications, technique, and methods for minimizing radiation exposure. Radiographics. 2012;32(1):255–74.
4. Cronin CG, Prakash P, Gervais DA, Hahn PF, Arellano R, Guimares A, et al. Imaging-guided suprapubic bladder tube insertion: experience in the care of 549 patients. AJR Am J Roentgenol. 2011;196(1):182–8.
5. Taslakian B, Sebaaly MG, Al-Kutoubi A. Patient evaluation and preparation in vascular and interventional radiology: what every interventional radiologist should know (part 1: patient assessment and laboratory tests). Cardiovasc Intervent Radiol. 2016;39(3):325–33.
6. Taslakian B, Sebaaly MG, Al-Kutoubi A. Patient evaluation and preparation in vascular and interventional radiology: what every interventional radiologist should know (part 2: patient preparation and medications). Cardiovasc Intervent Radiol. 2016;39(4):489–99. doi: 10.1007/s00270-015-1239-4. [Epub 2015 Nov 25].

Part X

Non-vascular Interventional Procedures: Musculoskeletal

Introduction by Aghiad Al-Kutoubi, Section Reviewer

The field of interventional musculoskeletal radiology is constantly undergoing a change. With advances in imaging technology, there has been a significant increase in the number and range of interventional musculoskeletal image-guided procedures. Percutaneous musculoskeletal intervention encompasses a wide range of diagnostic and therapeutic procedures ranging from simple aspiration to post-traumatic applications and tumor management using a variety of tools. The applications of ablation methodology is expanding rapidly in benign and malignant conditions. The ongoing development of percutaneous instrumentation is opening the door for more involvement of interventionalists in the management of spinal diseases and pelvic fractures. Pain management in the spine and various joints is now becoming more dependent on imaging with potential expansion of the role of interventionalists in these common ailments.

These minimally invasive procedures may be performed under ultrasound, fluoroscopic, computed tomography, or magnetic resonance imaging guidance based on the location, type of pathology, patient characteristics, and operator preference.

This section provides a comprehensive list of procedural reports that covers the vast majority of the currently performed musculoskeletal procedures with up-to-date explanatory notes, synopsis of the indications and contraindications, and potential complications in an organized and practical format.

Section Chapters

Bone Biopsy

51

Jad Chokr

INTRODUCTION

Biopsy of bone and marrow for analysis has been recognized for centuries; however, image-guided bone biopsy is a relatively recent development. It has become an important part of managing skeletal lesions, including primary and secondary bone tumors and infections. Percutaneous needle biopsies have a very low complication rate (1.1 %), whereas open biopsy has a complication rate of up to 16 %.

COMMON INDICATIONS [1–3]

- Establish whether a skeletal lesion is benign or malignant with nonspecific imaging findings
- Confirm or exclude skeletal metastasis in a patient who has a known primary tumor
- Exclude malignancy in vertebral body compression, particularly metastases or myeloma
- Evaluation for tumor recurrence
- Investigate and confirm diagnosis of musculoskeletal infection and to obtain sample for microbiological analysis
- Investigate the cause of a pathologic fracture

J. Chokr (✉)
Department of Diagnostic Radiology, Neuroradiology Division, Banner University Medical Center, Tucson, AZ, USA
e-mail: Jad_1986@hotmail.com

COMMON CONTRAINDICATIONS [1, 2]

- Bleeding diathesis
- Decreased platelet count
- Suspected hypervascular lesion in the thoracic or cervical vertebrae
- Infection in the surrounding soft tissues
- Uncooperative patient
- Inaccessible sites
- Pregnancy in cases when imaging guidance involves ionizing radiation

POSSIBLE COMPLICATIONS [1–3]

- Needle breakage
- Bleeding
- Infection
- Neurologic injury including paralysis and cord compression (*e.g., bleeding from vertebral hemangioma or metastatic renal cell carcinoma*)
- Pneumothorax
- Tumor seeding along the needle track; minimized further by careful planning of the biopsy track in conjunction with the surgeon and excision of the biopsy track during definitive surgery; it can be facilitated by tattooing the skin with indelible ink
- Diagnostic errors are possible related to sampling factors, tumor type, sample

B. Taslakian et al. (eds.), *Procedural Dictations in Image-Guided Intervention*,
DOI 10.1007/978-3-319-40845-3_51

fixation/handling methods, and pathologist experience

- Mortality from a biopsy procedure is extremely low (0.02 %), related to meningitis leading to death after a spinal biopsy

PREOPERATIVE ASSESSMENT AND PLANNING [4–6]

- History, indications, and physical examination *(Appendix 1* in Chap. 149*)*
- Evaluation of diagnostic imaging studies to determine the location of the lesion, its extent and relevant anatomy (*major neuro-vascular bundles*)
- Periprocedural management of coagulation status *(Appendices 2* in Chap. 150 *and 3* in Chap. 151*)*
- Antibiotic prophylaxis: Not routinely recommended [4] *(Appendices 4* in Chap. 152 *and 5* in Chap. 153*)*
- Imaging modality for guidance: CT, MRI or fluoroscopy
- Positioning: Patient is placed supine or prone, depending on the location of the lesion and the trajectory route

PROCEDURE NOTE

Procedure: CT/MRI/Fluoroscopic-guided percutaneous biopsy of [name the bone] bone lesion
Staff: [_]
Fellow: [_]
Resident: [_]
Clinical Information: Describe history and list indications
Allergies: None known/Allergic to [specify/type of allergy]
Anesthesia: Local anesthesia/conscious sedation/none
Medications: List any relevant medications used (sedation, antibiotics)
Field: Sterile
Procedure classification: Clean/dirty (if infection is suspected)
Position: Supine/sitting position/left lateral decubitus/right lateral decubitus/prone
Monitoring: Intravenous access line was secured and vital signs were continuously monitored by nursing staff/anesthesia team throughout the procedure.
Cumulative radiation dose: (_) mGy/not applicable

Description of Procedure:

The risks, benefits, alternatives and the procedure itself were explained to the patient/patient's Power of Attorney/legal guardian, and informed written/verbal consent was obtained. The site of the procedure was identified and marked. Time out was performed to confirm the correct patient, procedure and site.

The bone lesion was evaluated using CT scan/MRI/fluoroscopy after placement of a radiopaque marker/grid. The angle of needle entry and the distance to the lesion were calculated from the planning images in accordance with the presumed surgical approach.

The skin was prepped and draped in the usual sterile fashion. Local anesthesia was administered. A small skin incision was made. Subsequently, a (_)-gauge spinal needle was advanced to the bone cortex with subsequent injection of lidocaine to permeate the periosteum. Reimaging of the lesion was performed to ensure proper needle location and trajectory. A (_)-gauge cutting/trephine needle was then burrowed through the cortex to create a tract through the periosteum. The coaxial outer sheath of the cannula was secured in the cortex and (_) cores were obtained from the lesion. Specimens were divided for histopathology, cytology, and culture. Direct compression to the puncture site was performed for approximately 10 min, followed by dressing covering the area around the skin puncture.

The patient was transferred to the floor/recovery room following the procedure in a stable condition. Staff was present for the entire procedure.

Intra-Procedure Findings: List any additional findings if relevant.

Immediate Complications: None encountered during or directly after the procedure. List the complication if any.

Post-Procedure Plan [1]:

- Obtain chest imaging after thoracic spine biopsy to rule out a possible pneumothorax.
- Patient observation during recovery for 2–4 h to monitor analgesic control; check for dizziness, pain, weakness, ability to ambulate, bleeding, and general condition.
- Follow-up correlation of the imaging study with the pathology results.

Impression:

- Percutaneous biopsy of [name the bone] bone, as described above.
- The patient tolerated the procedure well and left the interventional unit in a stable condition.
- The patient was unstable and the procedure was canceled/terminated prematurely.
- List any other relevant or important information/finding.

References

1. Percutaneous Bone Biopsy. In: Burke CT, Dixon RG, Mauro MA, Murphy KPJ, Thomson KR, Venbrux AC, Zollikofer CL, editors. High yield imaging: interventional. Philadelphia: Saunders Elsevier; 2010. p. 506–9.
2. Gogna A, Peh WC, Munk PL. Image-guided musculoskeletal biopsy. Radiol Clin North Am. 2008;46(3):455–73.
3. Gandi A, Guth S, Dietemann JL, Roy C. Musculoskeletal intervention. In: Kaufman JA, Lee MJ, editors. The requisites: vascular and interventional radiology. Philadelphia: Mosby; 2004. p. 648–70.
4. Venkatesan AM, Kundu S, Sacks D, Wallace MJ, Wojak JC, Rose SC, et al. Practice guidelines for adult antibiotic prophylaxis during vascular and interventional radiology procedures. J Vasc Interv Radiol. 2010;21(11):1611–30.
5. Taslakian B, Sebaaly MG, Al-Kutoubi A. Patient evaluation and preparation in vascular and interventional radiology: what every interventional radiologist should know (part 1: patient assessment and laboratory tests). Cardiovasc Intervent Radiol. 2016;39(3):325–33.
6. Taslakian B, Sebaaly MG, Al-Kutoubi A. Patient evaluation and preparation in vascular and interventional radiology: what every interventional radiologist should know (part 2: patient preparation and medications). Cardiovasc Intervent Radiol. 2016;39(4):489–99. doi: 10.1007/s00270-015-1239-4. [Epub 2015 Nov 25].

Discography

52

Serine Baydoun

INTRODUCTION

Discography is a fluoroscopic guided procedure whereby contrast is injected into the intervertebral disc in order to reproduce the patient's symptomatology. Historically, it was performed for diagnosing degenerative disc disease and herniation of the nucleus pulposus. Nowadays, in an era with cross sectional imaging, discography is a complementary diagnostic procedure to aid physicians in identifying the culprit discogenic level inciting the patient's pain in the setting of equivocal/non-diagnostic imaging. It also serves to aid the neurosurgeon in pre-operative planning.

COMMON INDICATIONS [1–4]

- Evaluate persistent radicular (cervical or lumbar) pain in the setting of normal cross sectional imaging.
- Determine disc level causing pain in the setting of equivocal cross sectional imaging.
- Evaluate specific disc level when there is discordance between imaging and clinical findings.
- Pre-operative planning for spinal fusion in patients with multilevel disc disease *(i.e., determine most symptomatic level).*
- Differentiate recurrent disc disease from scar tissue.
- Evaluate previously operated disc in patients with recurrent pain

COMMON CONTRAINDICATIONS [1, 4]

- Uncorrectable bleeding diathesis
- Sepsis or overlying skin infection at puncture site
- Severe contrast allergy
- Pregnancy
- Posterior bone fusion obviating disc access
- Severe central canal stenosis

POSSIBLE COMPLICATIONS [1, 3, 5]

- Disc infection
- Meningitis, arachnoiditis
- Subdural or epidural abscess
- Intrathecal hemorrhage
- Disc damage
- Cerebrospinal fluid leak
- Nausea/vomiting
- Headache
- Retroperitoneal hemorrhage or injury *(ureters/kidneys)*

S. Baydoun (✉)
Department of Radiology,
University of Iowa Hospitals and Clinics,
Iowa City, IA, USA
e-mail: serine-baydoun@uiowa.edu

B. Taslakian et al. (eds.), *Procedural Dictations in Image-Guided Intervention*,
DOI 10.1007/978-3-319-40845-3_52

PREPROCEDURAL ASSESSMENT AND PLANNING [6, 7]

- History, indications, and physical examination *(Appendix 1* in Chap. 149)
- Evaluation of diagnostic imaging studies (CT and/or MRI) to assess for presence/severity of degenerative disc disease, potential postoperative change and correlate clinical symptoms with imaging
- Periprocedural management of coagulation status: (*Appendices 2* in Chap. 150 *and 3* in Chap. 151)
- Antibiotic prophylaxis: Routinely recommended [4]
- Imaging modality for guidance: Fluoroscopy
- Positioning: Prone/lateral/prone oblique

PROCEDURE NOTE

Procedure: Fluoroscopic guided cervical/thoracic/lumbar discography
Staff: [_]
Fellow: [_]
Resident: [_]
Clinical Information: Describe history and list indications
Allergies: None known/Allergies to [specify/type of allergy]
Anesthesia: Local anesthesia/conscious sedation/none
Medications: List any relevant medications used (sedation, antibiotics)
Contrast Used: (_) mL of [type] contrast media was used for disc injection
Field: Sterile
Procedure Classification: Clean
Position: Prone/Lateral/Prone Oblique
Monitoring: Intravenous access line was secured and vital signs were continuously monitored by nursing staff/anesthesia team throughout the procedure
Total fluoroscopy time: (_) minutes
Cumulative radiation dose: (_) mGy

Description of Procedure:
The risks, benefits, alternatives, and the procedure itself were explained to the patient/patient's Power of Attorney/patient's legal guardian, and informed written/verbal consent was obtained. The site of the procedure was identified and marked. Time out was performed to confirm the correct patient, procedure and site.

The spine was evaluated using fluoroscopy to identify the symptomatic discogenic level and align the endplates. A hemostat was placed as an external marker to identify the level of entry, and the skin was then marked at the specific disc level [specify disc levels]. Skin puncture point was 8–10 cm from the midline.

The skin was prepped and draped in the usual sterile fashion. Local anesthesia was administered. The outer (_)-gauge needle was advanced through the soft tissues. Once adequate positioning was ensured using serial anteroposterior and lateral fluoroscopic imaging, the inner (_)-gauge needle was advanced into the (_) disc space, and lodged in the center of the nucleus pulposus. Appropriate placement of the needle was then confirmed in the anteroposterior and lateral projections. The stylet was removed and the needle was attached to a (_) mL syringe filled with nonionic contrast. (_) mL of contrast was injected to confirm the needle's position. The same procedure was performed at [specify disc level] disc spaces.

The designated disc levels were injected with contrast. The volume injected, endpoint (hard/soft) and concordance versus discordance of intra-procedural pain with preprocedural symptoms were recorded. Anteroposterior and lateral spot views were obtained after each disc injection to assess the disc's morphology.

The needles were then removed, and the patient's back was cleansed. Bandages were placed at the puncture sites. The patient was then transferred to the floor/recovery room/discharged home following the procedure in a stable condition. Staff was present for the entire procedure.

Intra-Procedure Findings: List all relevant findings.

Immediate Complications: None encountered during or directly after the procedure. List complications if any.

Post-Procedure Plan [4]:

- Complete bed rest for 2 h post-procedure.
- Check vital signs immediately after the procedure. If stable, recheck prior to discharge. If abnormal, check vital signs every 30 min until they normalize.
- Start clear liquid diet for the first hour, then regular diet thereafter if tolerated and otherwise not contraindicated.
- Abstain from strenuous activities for the next 24–48 h.
- Resume regular pain medication as prescribed.
- Expect pain exacerbation over the next few days. However, if persistent or new symptoms develop, contact interventional radiologist who performed the procedure.
- In case of fever, contact interventional radiologist and go to the nearest emergency department.

Impression:

- Fluoroscopic guided cervical/thoracic/lumbar discography, as described above.
- The patient tolerated the procedure well and left the interventional unit in stable condition.
- The patient was unstable/unable to tolerate the pain and the procedure was canceled/terminated prematurely.
- List any other relevant or important information/finding.

References

1. McGraw JK. Chapter 12, Discography. In: Interventional radiology of the spine: image-guided pain therapy. New York: Springer; 2010. p. 149–66.
2. Ray CE. Chapter 9, Discography. In: Pain management in interventional radiology. Cambridge: Cambridge University Press; 2008. p. 131–50.
3. Schweitzer ME, Laredo JD. Chapter 20, Discography. In: New techniques in interventional musculoskeletal radiology. New York: Informa Healthcare USA; 2007. p. 223–42.
4. Gangi A, Guth S, Guermazi A. Chapter 7, Provocative Discography. In: Imaging in percutaneous musculoskeletal interventions. New York: Springer; 2009. p. 119–37.
5. Tehranzadeh J. Discography 2000. Radiol Clin North Am. 1998;36(3):463–95.
6. Taslakian B, Sebaaly MG, Al-Kutoubi A. Patient evaluation and preparation in vascular and interventional radiology: what every interventional radiologist should know (part 1: patient assessment and laboratory tests). Cardiovasc Intervent Radiol. 2016;39(3):325–33.
7. Taslakian B, Sebaaly MG, Al-Kutoubi A. Patient evaluation and preparation in vascular and interventional radiology: what every interventional radiologist should know (part 2: patient preparation and medications). Cardiovasc Intervent Radiol. 2016;39(4):489–99. doi: 10.1007/s00270-015-1239-4. [Epub 2015 Nov 25].

53 Intra-articular Facet Joint Injection

Karim Masrouha

INTRODUCTION

Facet syndrome is a common cause of back pain, however, it can pose a significant diagnostic and therapeutic challenge. Imaging is rarely of any help in arriving at the diagnosis, which is made after excluding other causes of back pain. The typical signs include pain with rotation, side bending, and hyperextension of the spine, as well as localized tenderness and a positive straight leg raise test [1]. Infiltration of the joint with saline can reproduce the pain while injection of local anesthetic relieves the pain, thus achieving the diagnosis of facet syndrome. The diagnostic value of this procedure when performed correctly can be very high, although false-positive rates may be high with single blocks. The therapeutic outcome is variable with good short-term outcome and limited evidence regarding medium- to long-term outcome.

COMMON INDICATIONS

Indications can be broadly divided into two groups depending on the desired results—Diagnostic or Therapeutic [2].

Diagnostic:

- A strong clinical suspicion of facet syndrome by history and physical exam
- Long-standing cervical or lumbar pain not responding to conservative therapy including NSAIDs and physiotherapy with normal imaging
- Persistent low back pain following posterolateral fusion or post-laminectomy with no evidence of recurrence

Therapeutic:

- Confirmed facet syndrome with strong response to diagnostic facet injection
- Inability to continue oral or parenteral drug therapy
- Adjacent segment disease following posterolateral fusion
- Attrition across spondylolytic defects causing pain

COMMON CONTRAINDICATIONS [2]

- Traumatic injury that can lead to pain with movement
- Presence of necrotic tissue requiring surgical debridement
- Significant coagulopathy that cannot be adequately corrected
- Severely compromised cardiopulmonary function or hemodynamic instability
- Inability of the patient to cooperate with, or to be positioned for, the procedure

K. Masrouha (✉)
Division of Orthopedic Surgery, Department of Surgery, American University of Beirut Medical Center, Riad Elsolh, Beirut 1107 2020, Lebanon
e-mail: km34@aub.edu.lb

B. Taslakian et al. (eds.), *Procedural Dictations in Image-Guided Intervention*,
DOI 10.1007/978-3-319-40845-3_53

- Pregnancy in cases when imaging guidance involves ionizing radiation

POSSIBLE COMPLICATIONS

- Infection
- Hematoma
- Transient increase in pain
- Transient paresthesia or paralysis

PREOPERATIVE ASSESSMENT AND PLANNING [3, 4]

- History, indications, and physical examination *(Appendix 1* in Chap. 149*)*
- Evaluation of diagnostic imaging studies
- Periprocedural management of coagulation status *(Appendices 2* in Chap. 150 *and 3* in Chap. 151*)*
- Antibiotic prophylaxis: Not routinely recommended.
- Imaging modality for guidance: Fluoroscopy *(alternatively computed tomography for thoracic cases with extensive degenerative changes and/or deformities).*
- Positioning: Prone with or without elevation of the side to be injected

PROCEDURE NOTE

Procedure: Fluoroscopy/CT-guided intra-articular facet joint injection of cervical/thoracic/lumbar spine
Staff: [_]
Fellow: [_]
Resident: [_]
Clinical Information: Describe history and list indications
Allergies: None known/Allergic to [specify/type of allergy]
Anesthesia: Local anesthesia *(Avoid sedation as it may interfere with assessment after facet injection)*
Medications: List any relevant medications used (sedation, antibiotics, Depo-Medrol, lidocaine)
Contrast Material: (_) mL of non-ionic contrast [Specify type]
Field: Sterile
Procedure classification: Clean
Position: Prone
Monitoring: Intravenous access line was secured and vital signs were continuously monitored by nursing staff/anesthesia team throughout the procedure.
Total fluoroscopy time: (_) minutes
Cumulative radiation dose: (_) mGy

Description of Procedure:

The risks, benefits, alternatives, and procedure itself were explained to the patient/patient's Power of Attorney/patient's legal guardian, and informed written consent was obtained. The site of the procedure was identified and marked. Time out was performed to confirm the correct patient, procedure, and site.

The skin was prepped and draped in the usual sterile fashion. Local anesthesia was administered. The most posterior portion of the facet was visualized by moving the fluoroscopy tube from AP to oblique/CT image. A (22)-gauge (3.5)-in. spinal needle was used to enter the joint, aiming for its midportion. The needle was moved around slightly until it was felt to fall into the joint. Intra-articular placement of the needle was confirmed by injecting 0.5 mL of non-ionic contrast material [specify type] and obtaining a fluoroscopic/CT image. After confirmation, a (1) mL mix of (0.5) mL [(20) mg] methylprednisolone/triamcinolone with (0.5) mL of 0.5 % Bupivacaine/1 % lidocaine was injected into the space. The needle was then retrieved and a small sterile adherent dressing was applied.

The patient was transferred to the floor/recovery room/discharged home following the procedure in a stable condition. Staff was present for the entire procedure.

Intra-Procedure Findings: List all the relevant findings.

Immediate Complications: None were encountered during or directly after the procedure. List complications if any.

Post-Procedure Plan:

- Observe for 15 min to confirm that no major hematoma had developed.
- Instruct the patient to be aware of the possible complications such as infection, hematoma, or transient paresthesia.
- Inform the patient that it is preferred that someone drives them home.

Impression:

- Infiltration of the cervical/lumbar/sacral facet joint(s), as described above.
- The patient tolerated the procedure well and left the interventional unit in a stable condition.
- The patient was unable to tolerate the procedure which was canceled/terminated prematurely.
- List any other relevant or important information/findings.

References

1. Silbergleit R, Mehta BA, Sanders WP, Talati SJ. Imaging-guided injection techniques with fluoroscopy and CT for spinal pain management. Radiographics Rev Publ Radiol Soc North Am, Inc. 2001;21(4):927–939 (discussion 940–922).
2. Peh W. Image-guided facet joint injection. Biomed Imaging Interv J. 2011;7(1):e4.
3. Taslakian B, Sebaaly MG, Al-Kutoubi A. Patient evaluation and preparation in vascular and interventional radiology: what every interventional radiologist should know (part 1: patient assessment and laboratory tests). Cardiovasc Intervent Radiol. 2016;39(3):325–33.
4. Taslakian B, Sebaaly MG, Al-Kutoubi A. Patient evaluation and preparation in vascular and interventional radiology: what every interventional radiologist should know (part 2: patient preparation and medications). Cardiovasc Intervent Radiol. 2016;39(4):489–99. doi: 10.1007/s00270-015-1239-4. [Epub 2015 Nov 25].

Kyphoplasty

54

Jad Chokr

INTRODUCTION

Vertebroplasty and kyphoplasty are minimally invasive surgical procedures for treating vertebral compression fractures where a surgical cement is injected into the fractured bone. This stabilizes the fracture and provides immediate pain relief in the majority of cases. In kyphoplasty, a special balloon is inserted and gently inflated inside the fractured vertebrae prior to cement injection. This step will help to restore height to the bone thus reducing deformity of the spine. It will also make it possible to use high viscosity cement therefore reducing the risk of leak.

COMMON INDICATIONS [1–4]

- Recent vertebral compression fracture with intractable pain and no neurological symptoms due to:
  - Tumors *(metastases, multiple myeloma)*
  - Osteoporosis
  - Vertebral hemangiomas

COMMON CONTRAINDICATIONS [1–3, 5]

- Systemic or spinal infection
- Hemorrhagic diathesis
- Allergy to cement or opacification materials
- Lesions with epidural extension, substantial canal narrowing, or disruption of the posterior cortex *(relative)*
- Unstable fracture or complete vertebral collapse *(>70 % loss of height)*

POSSIBLE COMPLICATIONS [1–3, 5]

- Cement leaks *(epidural/paravertebral veins, epidural space, or neural foramina)*
- Nerve or spinal cord damage
- Pulmonary embolism
- Pneumothorax
- Worsened pain or failure to treat
- Infection
- Bleeding
- Death (1 in 50,000); the etiology includes severe allergy and pulmonary emboli

PREOPERATIVE ASSESSMENT AND PLANNING [6–8]

- History, indications, and physical examination *(Appendix 1* in Chap. 149*)*

J. Chokr (✉)
Department of Diagnostic Radiology, Neuroradiology Division, Banner University Medical Center, Tucson, AZ, USA
e-mail: Jad_1986@hotmail.com

B. Taslakian et al. (eds.), *Procedural Dictations in Image-Guided Intervention*,
DOI 10.1007/978-3-319-40845-3_54

- Evaluation of diagnostic imaging studies to determine the affected vertebral body, the underlying cause, estimate the loss of height and the extension to posterior elements or spinal canal
- Periprocedural management of coagulation status *(Appendices 2* in Chap. 150 *and 3* in Chap. 151*)*
- Antibiotic prophylaxis: Routinely recommended *(1 g cefazolin IV 30 min before the procedure. If the patient is allergic to penicillin or cephalosporins, vancomycin may be administrated)* [6] *(Appendices 4* in Chap. 152 *and 5* in Chap. 153*)*
- Imaging modality for guidance: CT or fluoroscopy
- Positioning: Prone or supine

PROCEDURE NOTE

Procedure: Fluoroscopic/CT-guided kyphoplasty of [name the level] vertebral body/bodies
Staff: [_]
Fellow: [_]
Resident: [_]
Clinical Information: Describe history and list indications
Allergies: None known/Allergic to [specify/type of allergy]
Anesthesia: Local anesthesia/conscious sedation
Medications: List any relevant medications used (sedation, antibiotics)
Field: Sterile
Procedure classification: Clean
Position: Prone/Supine
Monitoring: Intravenous access line was secured and vital signs were continuously monitored by nursing staff/anesthesia team throughout the procedure.
Total fluoroscopy time: (_) minutes
Cumulative radiation dose: (_) mGy

Description of Procedure:

The risks, benefits, alternatives, and the procedure itself were explained to the patient/patient's Power of Attorney/legal guardian, and informed written/verbal consent was obtained. The site of the procedure was identified and marked. Time out was performed to confirm the correct patient, procedure, and site. Conscious sedation was administered with continuous hemodynamic monitoring.

The skin was prepped and draped in the usual sterile fashion. The levels of the compression fractures were determined under fluoroscopic/CT guidance and the pedicles were identified and marked with a skin marker. A transpedicular/parapedicular approach to the vertebral body was selected. An (_)-gauge needle was advanced through the [_] pedicle to the junction of the pedicle and vertebral body on the right/left/bilaterally. Positioning was confirmed with biplane fluoroscopy/CT. Following satisfactory placement of the needle, the stylet was removed. A guide pin was inserted through the needle to a (_) mm from the anterior cortex. Images were taken to verify position and trajectory. Alongside of the guide pin a paramedian incision was made. The needle was then removed leaving the guide pin in place. The osteointroducer was placed over the guide pin and advanced through the pedicle. At the junction of the pedicle and the vertebral body, images were taken to insure that the cannula was correctly positioned. Through the cannula, a drill was advanced into the vertebral body under fluoroscopic/CT guidance toward the anterior cortex, creating a channel. The anterior cortex was probed with the guide pin to ensure no perforations in the anterior cortex. After completing the entry into the vertebral body, a (_) mm inflatable bone tamp was inserted through the cannula and advanced under guidance into the vertebral body near the anterior cortex. The radiopaque marker bands on the bone tamp were identified. The above sequence of instrument placement was then repeated on the right/left/bilaterally of the [_] vertebral body. Once both bone tamps were in position, they were inflated to (_) cc and (_) psi. Expansion of the bone tamps was done sequentially in increments of (_) cc of contrast, with careful attention being paid to the inflation pressures and balloon position. The inflation was monitored under imaging guidance. The final balloon volume was

(_) cc on the right/left side and (_) cc on the right/left. There was no breach of the lateral wall or anterior cortex of the vertebral body. Direct reduction of the fracture was achieved, end plate movement was noted and approximately (_) mm of height restoration was achieved. Under fluoroscopic/CT imaging, and the use of the bone void fillers, internal fixation was achieved through a low-pressure injection of bone cement. The cavity was filled with a total volume of (_) cc on the right/left side and (_) cc on the right/left side. No cement leakage into the epidural space/veins was identified. The needle systems were withdrawn with no cement spikes identified. Manual compression was applied over the access sites for 5 min to promote clotting and prevent bleeding. The patient was kept in a prone/supine position for approximately 10 min post cement injection, turned supine, and monitored briefly. Throughout the procedure, there were no intraoperative complications and the patient was moving both lower extremities at the end of the procedure.

The patient was transferred to the floor/recovery room following the procedure in a stable condition. Staff was present for the entire procedure.

Intra-Procedure Findings: List any additional findings if relevant.

Immediate Complications: None were encountered during or directly after the procedure. List the complications if any.

Post-procedure Plan [1–3]:

- Keep complete bed rest for 2 h after the procedure.
- Give patient 15–30 mg of ketorolac intravenously, in case of immediate post-procedural pain *(unless renal insufficiency is an issue)*.
- Monitor vital signs and perform neurologic examinations every 15 min for the first hour, then every 30 min for the second hour.
- Record pain level at the end of procedure and at 2 h post procedure. Compare with baseline values and notify physician if pain increases above baseline.
- Allow liquids by mouth if not nauseated.
- Discontinue intravenous drips later on the same day if recovery is otherwise uneventful.
- Discharge patient home with adult companion the next day or later the same day.
- Patient instruction:
  - Return home; remain at bed rest and keep to minimal activity for 24 h.
  - Keep operative site covered for 24 h. Bandages may then be removed and site washed with a damp cloth. Do not soak.
  - Notify physician/facility if you have increasing pain, redness, swelling, or drainage from the operative site.
  - Notify physician/facility if you have difficulty with walking, changes in sensation in your hips or legs, new pain, or problems with bowel or bladder function.

Impression:

- Kyphoplasty of [_] vertebral body/bodies, as described above.
- The patient tolerated the procedure well and left the interventional unit in a stable condition.
- The patient was unable to tolerate the procedure which was canceled/terminated prematurely.
- List any other relevant or important information/findings.

References

1. Kyphoplasty. In: Burke CT, Dixon RG, Mauro MA, Murphy KPJ, Thomson KR, Venbrux AC, Zollikofer CL, editors. High yield imaging: interventional. Philadelphia: Saunders Elsevier; 2010. P. 514–8.
2. Gandi A, Guth S, Dietemann JL, Roy C. Musculoskeletal intervention. In: Kaufman JA, Lee MJ, editors. The requisites: vascular and interventional radiology. Philadelphia: Mosby; 2004. p. 648–70.
3. Yoo AJ, Eskey CJ, Hirsch JA. Vertebral height restoration. In: Matthew AM, Kieran PJM, Kenneth RT, Anthony CV, Christoph LZ, editors. Image-guided

interventions. Philadelphia: Saunders Elsevier; 2008. p. 1683–95.
4. Theodorou DJ, Theodorou SJ, Duncan TD, Garfin SR, Wong WH. Percutaneous balloon kyphoplasty for the correction of spinal deformity in painful vertebral body compression fractures. J Clin Imaging. 2002;26:1–5.
5. McGraw JK, Cardella J, Barr JD, Mathis JM, Sanchez O, Schwartzberg MS, et al. Society of interventional radiology quality improvement guidelines for percutaneous vertebroplasty. J Vasc Interv Radiol. 2003;14(7):827–31.
6. Venkatesan AM, Kundu S, Sacks D, Wallace MJ, Wojak JC, Rose SC, et al. Practice guidelines for adult antibiotic prophylaxis during vascular and interventional radiology procedures. J Vasc Interv Radiol. 2010;21(11):1611–30.
7. Taslakian B, Sebaaly MG, Al-Kutoubi A. Patient evaluation and preparation in vascular and interventional radiology: what every interventional radiologist should know (part 1: patient assessment and laboratory tests). Cardiovasc Intervent Radiol. 2016;39(3):25–33.
8. Taslakian B, Sebaaly MG, Al-Kutoubi A. Patient evaluation and preparation in vascular and interventional radiology: what every interventional radiologist should know (part 2: patient preparation and medications). Cardiovasc Intervent Radiol. 2016; 39(4):489–99. doi: 10.1007/s00270-015-1239-4. [Epub 2015 Nov 25].

Percutaneous Epidural and Nerve Root Block

55

Serine Baydoun

INTRODUCTION

Axial spinal pain, usually secondary to disc herniation, is one of the most frequently encountered complaints in outpatient clinics and a leading cause of disability. Management of sciatica and radiculopathy includes conventional medical therapy, minimally invasive spinal injections, and surgical intervention. In the setting of gnawing radicular pain not responding to oral medication, percutaneous epidural injections are an effective and relatively conservative option for symptom relief. Local anesthetic agents are used to provide analgesia. Steroids, either solely or in addition to the analgesic, may be instilled to counteract the inflammatory response occurring in the nerve roots.

COMMON INDICATIONS [1–5]

- Irritative radiculopathy not responding to medical therapy
- Post-discectomy syndrome
- Diagnosis of discogenic level causing pain

COMMON CONTRAINDICATIONS [3–5]

- Uncorrectable bleeding diathesis
- Local or systemic infection
- Pregnancy
- Cauda equina syndrome/severe spinal stenosis
- Pilonidal cysts
- Diabetes mellitus *(relative contraindication if giving steroids)*
- Gastric ulcers *(relative contraindication if giving steroids)*

POSSIBLE COMPLICATIONS [2–5]

- Meningitis, arachnoiditis, discitis
- Epidural abscess
- Epidural hemorrhage
- Inadvertent nerve puncture or injury to spinal artery
- Pneumothorax *(in thoracic injections)*
- Insomnia, flushing, nausea *(secondary to steroids)*
- Epidural lipomatosis *(secondary to steroids)*
- Postural hypotension/vasovagal reaction
- Transient increase in pain *(secondary to the osmotic effect of long acting steroids)*

S. Baydoun (✉)
Department of Radiology, University
of Iowa Hospitals and Clinics, Iowa City, IA, USA
e-mail: serine-baydoun@uiowa.edu

B. Taslakian et al. (eds.), *Procedural Dictations in Image-Guided Intervention*,
DOI 10.1007/978-3-319-40845-3_55

PREPROCEDURAL ASSESSMENT AND PLANNING [6, 7]

- History, indications, and physical examination (*Appendix 1* in Chap. 149)
- Evaluation of diagnostic imaging studies (radiographs, CT, and/or MRI) to assess for normal anatomy of the spine, evaluate for and identify the symptomatic discogenic level
- Periprocedural management of coagulation status (*Appendices 2* in Chap. 150 *and 3* in Chap. 151)
- Antibiotic prophylaxis: Not routinely recommended
- Imaging modality for guidance: CT
- Positioning: Prone/lateral decubitus

PROCEDURE NOTE

Procedure: CT-guided cervical/thoracic/lumbar epidural steroid/anesthetic injection
Staff: [_]
Fellow: [_]
Resident: [_]
Clinical Information: Describe history and list indications
Allergies: None known/Allergies to [specify/type of allergy]
Anesthesia: Local anesthesia/conscious sedation
Medications: List any relevant medications used (sedation, antibiotics)
Contrast Used: (_) mL of [type] contrast media was used for confirmation of epidural positioning
Field: Sterile
Procedure Classification: Clean
Position: Prone/Lateral decubitus
Monitoring: Intravenous access line was secured and vital signs were continuously monitored by nursing staff/anesthesia team throughout the procedure
Total fluoroscopy time: (_) minutes
Cumulative radiation dose: (_) mGy

Description of Procedure:

The risks, benefits, alternatives, and the procedure itself were explained to the patient/patient's Power of Attorney/patient's legal guardian, and informed written consent was obtained. The site of the procedure was identified and marked. Time out was performed to confirm the correct patient, procedure, and site.

Serial axial CT images were obtained in order to identify the level and point of disc entry. The skin was prepped and draped in the usual sterile fashion. Local anesthesia was administered.

Using CT-guidance, a ()-gauge spinal needle was advanced to the level of the symptomatic nerve root [specify nerve root level]. Back aspiration through the needle was performed to ensure there was no blood or cerebrospinal fluid return. (_) mL of contrast was injected and further imaging was performed to ensure epidural positioning. (_) mL of corticosteroid/anesthetic was then injected. The same procedure was performed at [specify nerve root level] nerve root.

The needle was removed, and the patient's back was cleansed. Sterile dressings were placed at the entry sites. The patient was then transferred to the floor/discharged home following the procedure in a stable condition. Staff was present for the entire procedure.

Intra-Procedure Findings: List all relevant findings.
Immediate Complications: None encountered during or directly after the procedure. List complications if any.

Post-Procedure Plan [1, 3, 5]**:**
- Monitor patient for 30 min post-procedure to ensure stability.
- Avoid strenuous activity for 24–48 h post-procedure.
- Remove sterile dressings in 36 h.
- Limit salt intake for 1 week post-procedure (if given steroids)

Impression:
- CT-guided percutaneous epidural steroid/anesthetic injection of the [specify level] nerve root.
- The patient tolerated the procedure well and left the interventional unit in stable condition.

- The patient was unable to tolerate the procedure which was canceled/terminated prematurely.
- List any other relevant or important information/finding.

References

1. Kaufman A, Lee MJ. Chapter 24, Musculoskeletal intervention. In: Vascular and interventional radiology: the requisites, 2nd ed. Philadelphia: Saunders Elsevier; 2013. p. 527–44.
2. Link SC, El-Khoury GY, Guilford WB. Percutaneous epidural and nerve root block and percutaneous lumbar sympatholysis. Radiol Clin North Am. 1998;36 (3):509–21.
3. Gangi A, Guth S, Guermazi A. Chapter 6, Percutaneous treatment of disc herniation. In: Imaging in percutaneous musculoskeletal interventions. New York: Springer; 2009. p. 93–116.
4. Schweitzer ME, Laredo JD. Chapter 8, Epidural steroids. In: New techniques in interventional musculoskeletal radiology. New York: Informa Healthcare USA; 2007. p. 89–108.
5. Dean LM. Chapter 163, Selective nerve root block. In: Image-guided interventions, 2nd ed. Philadelphia: Saunders; 2014. p. 1217–1232.
6. Taslakian B, Sebaaly MG, Al-Kutoubi A. Patient evaluation and preparation in vascular and interventional radiology: what every interventional radiologist should know (part 1: patient assessment and laboratory tests). Cardiovasc Intervent Radiol. 2016;39(3): 325–33.
7. Taslakian B, Sebaaly MG, Al-Kutoubi A. Patient evaluation and preparation in vascular and interventional radiology: what every interventional radiologist should know (part 2: patient preparation and medications). Cardiovasc Intervent Radiol. 2016;39(4):489–99. doi: 10.1007/s00270-015-1239-4. [Epub 2015 Nov 25].

Percutaneous Management of Malignant Bone Tumors

56

Serine Baydoun

INTRODUCTION

Nowadays, percutaneous interventional techniques play a major role in the management of malignant bone tumors, whether primary osseous lesions or metastatic. These techniques include alcohol ablation, radiofrequency ablation, cementoplasty, laser photocoagulation as well as cryoablation. Alcohol causes cellular dehydration and vascular thrombosis. Laser photocoagulation and radiofrequency ablation utilize heating/friction for tissue destruction, whereas cryoablation utilizes extreme cold temperatures to induce necrosis. Some therapies are directed for pain control and palliation, whereas others are curative in nature. Deciding on the technique of choice is largely based on the number and size of the lesions. A curative approach is used for slow-growing tumors, smaller than 3 cm in size and usually less than 3 total lesions. Otherwise, pain control and tumor debulking are usually the ultimate goal of therapy.

COMMON INDICATIONS [1–7]

- Palliative care in patients with diffuse osseous tumor burden
- Pain control in case of resistance to conventional pain management/requiring high opiate dosing
- Tumor debulking prior to or after chemoradiation
- Extensive soft tissue involvement (particularly for alcohol ablation)
- Tumor recurrence
- Less frequently, curative purpose for poor surgical candidates with less than 3 malignant lesions

COMMON CONTRAINDICATIONS [1–4]

- Associated infection or sepsis
- Adjacent surgical metallic equipment (in case of radiofrequency ablation)
- Close proximity to vital organs or neurologic structures *(require thermal insulation in case of thermal ablation)*
- Cord compression (requires surgical decompression)
- Uncontrollable bleeding diathesis
- Risk of fracture—will require additional consolidative therapy (cementoplasty)

POSSIBLE COMPLICATIONS [3–5]

- Septic osteitis
- Fever

S. Baydoun (✉)
Department of Radiology, University of Iowa Hospitals and Clinics, Iowa City, IA, USA
e-mail: serine-baydoun@uiowa.edu

B. Taslakian et al. (eds.), *Procedural Dictations in Image-Guided Intervention*,
DOI 10.1007/978-3-319-40845-3_56

- Hematomas/bleeding
- Reflex sympathetic dystrophy/worsening pain, particularly in the first two days following the ablation (25 % of patients who underwent alcohol ablation)
- Vascular injury
- Neurologic injury
- Alcohol leak—leading to skin or muscle necrosis
- Tumor seeding along needle tract

PREPROCEDURAL ASSESSMENT AND PLANNING [6, 8–10]

- History, indications, and physical examination (*Appendix 1* in Chap. 149)
- Evaluation of diagnostic imaging studies (CT and/or MRI) to evaluate the location and extent of the tumor, to determine ablative method of choice and decide if consolidative therapy is also needed
- Periprocedural management of coagulation status (*Appendices 2* in Chap. 150 *and 3* in Chap. 151)
- Antibiotic prophylaxis: Recommended, usually cefazolin particularly if cementoplasty/vertebroplasty will also be necessary [6, 8] *(Appendices 4* in Chap. 152 *and 5* in Chap. 153*)*
- Imaging modality for guidance: CT
- Positioning: Prone/Prone Oblique/Supine

PROCEDURE NOTE

Procedure: CT-guided alcohol/radiofrequency ablation of bone tumor
Staff: [_]
Fellow: [_]
Resident: [_]
Clinical Information: Describe history and list indications
Allergies: None known/Allergies to [specify/type of allergy]
Anesthesia: General sedation/conscious sedation
Medications: List any relevant medications used (sedation, antibiotics)
Field: Sterile
Procedure Classification: Clean
Position: Prone/Prone Oblique/Supine
Monitoring: Intravenous access line was secured and vital signs were continuously monitored by nursing staff/anesthesia team throughout the procedure
Cumulative radiation dose: (_) mGy

Description of Procedure:
The risks, benefits, alternatives, and the procedure itself were explained to the patient/patient's Power of Attorney/patient's legal guardian, and informed written/verbal consent was obtained. The site of the procedure was identified and marked. Time out was performed to confirm the correct patient, procedure, and site.

The tumor was evaluated using CT scan after placement of a radiopaque marker/grid showing its complete extent, soft tissue involvement, and distance from vital organs and neurologic structures. The skin was then marked at the site of entry.

The skin was prepped and draped in the usual sterile fashion. Local anesthesia was administered. A (_)-gauge coaxial needle was advanced through the soft tissues to the level of the tumor.

For Alcohol Ablation: (_) mixture of lidocaine and contrast was injected to evaluate the expected infiltration route of the alcohol solution and assess for any potential leak. After adequate positioning was attained, (_) 95 % ethanol solution was injected slowly. Using CT-guidance, the needle was repositioned into a different part of the lesion. (_) total injections were performed.

For Radiofrequency Ablation: The inner stylet was removed and the radiofrequency probe [type] was introduced through the (_)-gauge needle into the tumor. Appropriate needle placement was confirmed using serial CT images. (_) watts were provided for (_) minutes to generate a temperature of (_) degrees Celsius. Continuous saline infusion was given at a rate of (_) mL/hr. (Thermal insulation was necessary using hydrodissection/CO_2 insufflation/balloon interposition). (_) total ablations were performed.

Serial CT images were provided to ensure adequate tumor ablation and assess for any potential direct complication.

The needles were then removed, the access site was cleansed and covered with sterile dressing. The patient was then transferred to the floor/recovery room/discharged home following the procedure in a stable condition. Staff was present for the entire procedure.

Intra-Procedure Findings: List all relevant findings.

Immediate Complications: None encountered during or directly after the procedure. List complications if any.

Post-Procedure Plan [7]:

- Monitor for 3 h after the procedure if ablation site is adjacent to vital organs.
- Check vitals at the end of the procedure and prior to discharge.
- Start fluid diet for the first hour, then regular diet thereafter if tolerated and not contraindicated.
- Prescribe analgesics, muscle relaxants, and anti-inflammatory medication for pain control.
- Follow-up MRI with Gadolinium 1 week post procedure to evaluate tumor response.
- Depending on the location of the procedure, physical therapy may be necessary.

Impression:

- CT-guided percutaneous alcohol/radiofrequency ablation of [specify location] osseous lesion.
- The patient tolerated the procedure well and left the interventional unit in stable condition.
- The patient was unable to tolerate the procedure which was canceled/terminated prematurely.
- List any other relevant or important information/finding

References

1. Gangi A, Buy X. Percutaneous bone tumor management. Semin Interv Radiol. 2010;27(2):124–36.
2. Mueller P, Andreas A. Chapter 17, Percutaneous bone tumor management. In: Interventional oncology. New York: Springer; 2012. p. 169–72.
3. Schweitzer ME, Laredo JD. Chapter 28, Percutaneous alcohol injection for the treatment of metastatic disease. In: New techniques in interventional musculoskeletal radiology. New York: Informa Healthcare USA; 2007. p. 303–5.
4. Schweitzer ME, Laredo JD. Chapter 29, Radiofrequency ablation of osseous metastatic disease. In: New techniques in interventional musculoskeletal radiology. New York: Informa Healthcare USA; 2007. p. 307–14.
5. Kaufman A, Lee MJ. Chapter 24, Musculoskeletal intervention. In: Vascular and interventional radiology: the requisites. 2nd ed. Philadelphia: Saunders Elsevier; 2013. p. 659–61.
6. Filippiadis D, Tutton S, Mazioti A, Kelekis A. Percutaneous image-guided ablation of bone and soft tissue tumors: a review of available techniques and protective measures. Insights Imaging. 2014;5 (3):339–46.
7. Ward E, Munk PL, Rashid F, Torreggiani WC. Musculoskeletal interventional radiology: radiofrequency ablation. Radiol Clin North Am. 2008;46 (3):599–610.
8. Venkatesan AM, Kundu S, Sacks D, Wallace MJ, Wojak JC, Rose SC, et al. Practice guidelines for adult antibiotic prophylaxis during vascular and interventional radiology procedures. J Vasc Interv Radiol. 2010;21(11):1611–30.
9. Taslakian B, Georges Sebaaly M, Al-Kutoubi A. Patient evaluation and preparation in vascular and interventional radiology: what every interventional radiologist should know (part 1: patient assessment and laboratory tests). Cardiovasc Intervent Radiol. 2016;39(3):325–33.
10. Taslakian B, Sebaaly MG, Al-Kutoubi A. Patient evaluation and preparation in vascular and interventional radiology: what every interventional radiologist should know (part 2: patient preparation and medications). Cardiovasc Intervent Radiol. 2016;39 (4):489–99. doi:10.1007/s00270-015-1239-4. [Epub 2015 Nov 25].

57 Percutaneous Nucleotomy

Serine Baydoun

INTRODUCTION

Herniation of the nucleus pulposus is most commonly secondary to age-related degenerative change of the annulus fibrosis. Patients will complain of severe neck or back pain even in the absence of nerve root compression. In case of resistance to conservative routes of therapy, percutaneous disc decompression is used to target patients with contained disc herniation (by the annulus fibrosis or posterior longitudinal ligament). This may be achieved mechanically, chemically (using alcohol or ozone), or thermally (using laser or radiofrequency). By removing part of the central nucleus pulposus, intradiscal pressure is decreased and symptom control is attained.

COMMON INDICATIONS [1–3]

- Sciatica resistant to oral therapy or percutaneous injections for 6 weeks
- Contained disc herniation
- Recurrence of disc herniation at previously operated disc level
- Laterally-oriented disc herniation
- Infectious discitis

S. Baydoun (✉)
Department of Radiology, University of Iowa Hospitals and Clinics, Iowa City, IA, USA
e-mail: serine-baydoun@uiowa.edu

COMMON CONTRAINDICATIONS [1, 2]

- Migrated disc fragments
- Cauda equina syndrome
- Severe spinal stenosis
- Uncontrolled bleeding diathesis
- Pregnancy
- Arachnoiditis
- Extensive posterior osteophytes preventing disc entry
- Fracture
- Severe spondylolisthesis

POSSIBLE COMPLICATIONS [1, 2, 4]

- Septic discitis/Osteomyelitis
- Thermal aseptic discitis
- Hemorrhage
- Dural puncture
- Injury of the annulus fibrosis
- Endplate injury
- Recurrent disc herniation or extrusion

PREPROCEDURAL ASSESSMENT AND PLANNING

- History, indications, and physical examination (*Appendix 1* in Chap. 149)
- Evaluation of diagnostic imaging studies (CT and/or MRI) to evaluate the level of herniated

B. Taslakian et al. (eds.), *Procedural Dictations in Image-Guided Intervention*,
DOI 10.1007/978-3-319-40845-3_57

nucleus pulposus and procedural plan for route of entry
- Periprocedural management of coagulation status (*Appendices* 2 in Chap. 150 *and 3 in* Chap. 151)
- Imaging modality for guidance: Fluoroscopy
- Positioning: Prone/Prone Oblique

PROCEDURE NOTE

Procedure: CT-guided cervical/thoracic/lumbar percutaneous nucleotomy
Staff: [_]
Fellow: [_]
Resident: [_]
Clinical Information: Describe history and list indications
Allergies: None known/Allergies to [specify/type of allergy]
Anesthesia: Local anesthesia/conscious sedation/none
Medications: List any relevant medications used
Field: Sterile
Procedure Classification: Clean
Position: Prone/Prone Oblique
Monitoring: Intravenous access line was secured and vital signs were continuously monitored by nursing staff/anesthesia team throughout the procedure
Total fluoroscopy time: (_) minutes
Cumulative radiation dose: (_) mGy

Description of Procedure

The risks, benefits, alternatives, and the procedure itself were explained to the patient/patient's Power of Attorney/patient's legal guardian, and informed written/verbal consent was obtained. The site of the procedure was identified and marked. Time out was performed to confirm the correct patient, procedure, and site.

The spine was evaluated using CT scan after placement of a radiopaque marker/grid showing the symptomatic disc level. The skin was then marked at the [specify disc level].

The skin was prepped and draped in the usual sterile fashion. Local anesthesia was administered. A (_)-gauge needle was advanced through the soft tissues to the level of the posterior annulus. The stylet was removed and the optical fiber/radiofrequency probe [type] was introduced through a (_)-gauge needle to the level of the junction of the annulus and nucleus pulposus posteriorly. Appropriate needle placement was confirmed using serial CT images.

For Percutaneous Laser Disc Decompression: After confirming adequate needle placement, the laser was turned on to produce 15–20 W with (_) second pulses at (_) second intervals. This was repeated to reach the predetermined recommended laser dose. CT images were obtained every (_) Joules to monitor disc vaporization.

For Percutaneous Radiofrequency Decompression: After confirming adequate needle placement, the radiofrequency probe was withdrawn back to starting position with the coagulation mode turned on. Once at starting position, it was turned clockwise and re-advanced, each time in a different direction in order to form different channels and attain maximal heat-induced tissue reduction. CT scan was then obtained to exclude any potential direct complications.

The needles were then removed; the skin at the entry site was cleaned and covered with sterile dressing. The patient was then transferred to the floor/recovery room/discharged home following the procedure in a stable condition. Staff were present for the entire procedure.
Intra-Procedure Findings: List all relevant findings.
Immediate Complications: None encountered during or directly after the procedure. List complications if any.

Post-Procedure Plan [2, 4, 5]:
- Complete bed rest for 3 h post-procedure.
- Check vitals at the end of the procedure and prior to discharge.
- Start fluid diet for the first hour, then regular diet thereafter if tolerated and not contraindicated.
- Prescribe analgesics, muscle relaxants, and anti-inflammatory medication for pain control.

- Avoid bending, sitting, or extreme flexion/extension for 2 weeks after the procedure.
- Avoid strenuous activity or physical exercise for 6 weeks after the procedure.
- Avoid water reaching the wound until full skin healing has been achieved.
- Begin physical therapy 3 weeks after the procedure.
- Follow up with primary physician 6 weeks after the procedure to assess neurologic function.

Impression:

- CT-guided percutaneous nucleotomy of the [specify level] disc using laser/radiofrequency.
- The patient tolerated the procedure well and left the interventional unit in stable condition.
- The patient was unable to tolerate the procedure which was canceled/terminated prematurely.
- List any other relevant or important information/finding

References

1. Slipman CW, Derby R, Simeone F, Mayer T. Chapter 85, Percutaneous disc decompression. In: Interventional spine: an algorithmic approach. Philadelphia: Saunders; 2007. p. 927–37.
2. Gangi A, Guth S, Guermazi A. Chapter 6, Percutaneous treatment of disc herniation. In: Imaging in percutaneous musculoskeletal interventions. New York: Springer; 2009. p. 93–116.
3. Kastler B, BArral FG, Fergane B, Pereira OP. Chapter 19, Interventional MRI in pain therapy. In: Interventional radiology in pain treatment. New York: Springer; 2007. p. 187.
4. Schweitzer ME, Laredo JD. Chapter 22, Percutaneous laser and radiofrequency disc decompression. In: New techniques in interventional musculoskeletal radiology. New York: Informa Healthcare USA; 2007. p. 251–7.
5. Buy X, Gangi A. Percutaneous treatment of intervertebral disc herniation. Semin Interv Radiol. 2010;27 (2):148–59.

Radiofrequency Ablation of Osteoid Osteoma

58

Mohamad Nasser Eddine

INTRODUCTION

Osteoid osteoma is a painful benign bone tumor with no malignant potential. It represents about 10 % of benign bone tumors and 5 % of all tumors with male predominance involving mainly younger patients. Lesions are characterized radiographically by a nidus within a dense, reactive bone of variable thickness. Percutaneous radiofrequency ablation is lately replacing the surgical approach; it works by using thermal coagulation to induce necrosis in the nidus in a minimally invasive manner.

COMMON INDICATIONS [1–3]

- Pain control using NSAIDS is not adequate
- Contraindication for use of NSAIDS
- Contraindication for surgical procedure
- Lesions that are surgically demanding or involve anatomic places that needs dissecting major organs to reach
- Patient preference
- Patients with skin problems or prone to scar formation

COMMON CONTRAINDICATIONS [1, 3]

- Bleeding diathesis
- Infection in the surrounding soft tissues
- Infection in the surrounding soft tissues
- Uncooperative patient
- Pregnancy
- Inability to rule out malignancy

Possible Complications [1, 2, 4, 5]

Usually radiofrequency ablation of osteoid osteoma is a very safe procedure and complication rate is very rare

- Fractures that usually involve only one cortex *(the nature of sclerotic bone helps avoid any progression of the fracture)*
- Skin burns with subcutaneous tissue necrosis
- Neural injury
- Infection
- Breakage of needle or probe
- Bleeding
- Transient paresthesia
- Erythema
- Hyperthermia

M. Nasser Eddine (✉)
Department of Surgery, Division of Orthopedic Surgery, American University of Beirut Medical Center, Riad Elsolh, Beirut 1107 2020, Lebanon
e-mail: mn103@aub.edu.lb

B. Taslakian et al. (eds.), *Procedural Dictations in Image-Guided Intervention*,
DOI 10.1007/978-3-319-40845-3_58

PREOPERATIVE ASSESSMENT AND PLANNING

- History, indications and physical examination *(Appendix 1* in Chap. 149*)*
- Evaluation of diagnostic imaging studies to determine the location of the lesion, its extent and relevant anatomy (*major neurovascular bundles*)
- Periprocedural management of coagulation status *(Appendices 2* in Chap. 150 *and 3 in* Chap. 151*)*
- Antibiotic prophylaxis: Not routinely recommended or use first generation cephalosporin if possible breakage of sterility is anticipated [6]
- Imaging modality for guidance: CT or fluoroscopy
- Positioning: Patient is placed supine or prone, depending on the location of the lesion and the planned route

PROCEDURE NOTE

Procedure: CT/Fluoroscopy-guided biopsy and radiofrequency ablation of [name the bone/location] osteoid osteoma
Staff: [_]
Fellow: [_]
Resident: [_]
Clinical Information: Describe history and list indications
Allergies: None known/Allergic to [specify/type of allergy]
Anesthesia: General anesthesia/deep sedation with local anesthesia
Medications: List any relevant medications used (sedation, antibiotics)
Field: Sterile
Procedure classification: Clean
Position: Supine/left lateral decubitus/right lateral decubitus/oblique/prone
Monitoring: Intravenous access line was secured and vital signs were continuously monitored by nursing staff/anesthesia team throughout the procedure
Cumulative radiation dose: (_) mGy

Description of Procedure [2–5, 7]:
The risks, benefits, alternatives, and the procedure itself were explained to the patient/patient's Power of Attorney/legal guardian, and informed written consent was obtained. The site of the procedure was identified and marked. Time out was performed to confirm the correct patient, procedure, and site.

The [name the bone] lesion was evaluated using CT scan/fluoroscopy after placement of a radiopaque marker/grid. The procedure was planned and the skin puncture site was marked using combined information from the location of the lesion and preliminary CT images. The angle of needle entry and the distance to the nidus of the lesion away from the neurovascular bundle were calculated from the planning images. Dispersive grounding pads were applied to patient back.

The skin was prepped and draped in the usual sterile fashion. Local anesthesia was administered. A small skin incision was made. Subsequently, an (11)-gauge bone biopsy needle was advanced to the bone lesion and repeat CT imaging confirmed adequate position of the needle tip. Bone biopsy was performed. Then, a (14) gauge [type] side deployment electrode was advanced deep into the nidus. To ensure proper location and trajectory of the probe, repeat imaging was performed confirming location. The electrode was heated to (90 °C) for (5–6 min) according to manufacturer protocol, using a [type] radiofrequency generator.

Following the procedure, the probe and biopsy needle guide were removed. A sterile pressure dressing was applied to the puncture site.

The patient was transferred to the floor/recovery room following the procedure in a stable condition. Staff was present for the entire procedure.

Intra-Procedure Findings: List any additional findings if relevant.
Immediate Complications: None encountered during or directly after the procedure. List the complication if any.

Post-Procedure Plan:

- Monitor the patient in the recovery room for 2–4 h for pain control; check for skin burns, bleeding, motor, and sensory power in the affected limb.

- Ensure adequate pain control on discharge.
- Advise patient to avoid excessive physical activity for 1 month after the procedure *(if the lesion was in a weight bearing bone).*
- Follow-up in 7 days to assess patient and to get pathology results if biopsy was taken and ensure adequate relief of pain related to osteoid osteoma.
- Perform an MRI or CT scan 1 month after the procedure *(coagulation necrosis of the lesion and decrease of bone edema suggests a successful procedure).*

Impression:

- Radiofrequency ablation of [name the bone] osteoid osteoma, as described above.
- The patient tolerated the procedure well and left the interventional unit in a stable condition.
- The patient was unable to tolerate the procedure which was canceled/terminated prematurely.
- List any other relevant or important information/finding.

References

1. Martin R, Kiere M. Radiofrequency ablation of osteoid osteoma. In: Handbook of interventional radiology. Philadelphia: Lippincott Williams & Wilkins; 2010. p. 623–30.
2. Torriani M, Rosenthal D. Percutaneous radiofrequency treatment of osteoid osteoma. Ped Radiol. 2002;32 (8):615–8.
3. Jankharia B, Burute N. Percutaneous radiofrequency ablation for osteoid osteoma: how we do it. Indian J Radiol Imaging. 2009;19(1):36.
4. Çakar M, Esenyel C, Seyran M, Tekin A, Adaş M, Bayraktar M, et al. Osteoid osteoma treated with radiofrequency ablation. Adv Orthop. 2015;2015:1–5.
5. Motamedi D, Learch T, Ishimitsu D, Motamedi K, Katz M, Brien E, et al. Thermal ablation of osteoid osteoma: overview and step-by-step guide 1. Radiographics. 2009;29(7):2127–41.
6. Venkatesan A, Kundu S, Sacks D, Wallace M, Wojak J, Rose S, et al. Practice guideline for adult antibiotic prophylaxis during vascular and interventional radiology procedures. J Vasc Interv Radiol. 2010;21(11):1611–30.
7. Busser W, Hoogeveen Y, Veth R, Schreuder H, Balguid A, Renema W, et al. Percutaneous radiofrequency ablation of osteoid osteomas with use of real-time needle guidance for accurate needle placement: a pilot study. Cardiovasc Interv Radiol. 2010;34 (1):180–3.

Sacroiliac Joint Injection

59

Karim Masrouha

INTRODUCTION

Like other joints, the sacroiliac (SI) joint may develop degenerative or traumatic arthritis, which can lead to significant pain and disability. Lower back pain from the SI joint can be a diagnostic challenge, and is usually a diagnosis of exclusion. Injection of anesthetic with or without corticosteroids into the SI joint under fluoroscopic or CT guidance can confirm the diagnosis and provide the patient with pain relief [1].

COMMON INDICATIONS

- Sacroiliitis due to spondyloarthropathies
- Sacroiliac joint osteoarthritis not responding to non-steroidal anti-inflammatory drugs
- Diagnosis of sacroiliac joint arthritis when it is unclear

COMMON CONTRAINDICATIONS [1]

- Known bleeding disorder or currently on anticoagulation/antiplatelet
- Allergies to local anesthetic agents or corticosteroids
- Ongoing systemic infection
- Infection or loss of integrity of skin around injection site
- Uncontrolled hypertension, diabetes, coronary artery disease, or congestive heart failure
- Inability to lay in the prone position

POSSIBLE COMPLICATIONS

- Infection
- Hematoma
- Neurapraxia

PREOPERATIVE ASSESSMENT AND PLANNING [2–5]

- History, indications, and physical examination *(Appendix 1* in Chap. 149*)*
- Evaluation of diagnostic imaging studies
- Periprocedural management of coagulation status *(Appendices 2* in Chap. 150 *and 3* in Chap. 151*)*
- Antibiotic prophylaxis: Not routinely recommended
- Imaging modality for guidance: Fluoroscopy, CT or Ultrasound [2, 3]
- Positioning: Prone

K. Masrouha (✉)
Department of Surgery, Division of Orthopedic Surgery, American University of Beirut Medical Center, Riad Elsolh, Beirut 1107 2020, Lebanon
e-mail: km34@aub.edu.lb

B. Taslakian et al. (eds.), *Procedural Dictations in Image-Guided Intervention*,
DOI 10.1007/978-3-319-40845-3_59

PROCEDURE NOTE

Procedure: Image-guided left/right sacroiliac joint infiltration
Staff: [_]
Fellow: [_]
Resident: [_]
Clinical Information: Describe history and list indications
Allergies: None known/Allergic to [specify/type of allergy]
Anesthesia: Local anesthesia/conscious sedation
Medications: List any relevant medications used (sedation, local anesthesia, corticosteroids)
Contrast Material: (0.5 mL) of [type] contrast media for intra-articular injection
Field: Sterile
Procedure classification: Clean
Position: Prone
Monitoring: Intravenous access line was secured and vital signs were continuously monitored by nursing staff/anesthesia team throughout the procedure
Total fluoroscopy time: (_) minutes
Cumulative radiation dose: (_) mGy

Description of Procedure

The risks, benefits, alternatives, and procedure itself were explained to the patient/patient's Power of Attorney/patient's legal guardian, and informed written consent was obtained. The site of the procedure was identified and marked. Time out was performed to confirm the correct patient, procedure and site.

The distal 1 cm of the sacroiliac joint was identified under fluoroscopy/after obtaining planning CT images and marked. The skin was then prepped and draped in a sterile manner. The previously marked skin site was anesthetized. A 22-gauge (straight/10° curved) spinal needle was advanced perpendicular to the fluoroscopic table/using planning CT information. The fluoroscopy tube was angled approximately 20° cephalad to line up the anterior and posterior ends of the joint. The needle was then directed toward the posterior sacroiliac joint. After aspirating to confirm that there was no intravascular placement, the intra-articular position was confirmed by injecting (0.5) mL of [type] contrast material through the needle. Once contrast material was seen spreading within the joint and no vascular run-off was observed, a solution of (4) mL of [name the local anesthesia agent] and (40) mg methylprednisolone acetate were injected slowly.

The patient was transferred to the floor/recovery room/discharged home following the procedure in a stable condition. Staff was present for the entire procedure.

Intra-Procedure Findings: List all relevant findings.
Immediate Complications: None encountered during or directly after the procedure. List complications if any.

Post-Procedure Plan:

- Observe for 15 min to confirm absence of major hematoma.
- Instruct the patient to be aware of the possible complications such as infection, hematoma, or neurapraxia.

Impression:

- Infiltration of the left/right sacroiliac joint, as described above.
- The patient tolerated the procedure well and left the interventional unit in a stable condition.
- The patient was unable to tolerate the procedure which was canceled/terminated prematurely.
- List any other relevant or important information/finding.

References

1. Stone JA, Bartynski WS. Treatment of facet and sacroiliac joint arthropathy: steroid injections and radiofrequency ablation. Techn vasc interv radiol. 2009;12(1):22–32.
2. Soneji N, Bhatia A, Seib R, Tumber P, Dissanayake M, Peng PW. Comparison of fluoroscopy and ultrasound

guidance for sacroiliac joint injection in patients with chronic low back pain. Pain Pract Off J World Inst Pain. 2015. doi:10.1111/papr.12304 (Epub ahead of print).
3. Althoff CE, Bollow M, Feist E, Marticorena-Garcia SR, Eshed I, Diekhoff T. CT-guided corticosteroid injection of the sacroiliac joints: quality assurance and standardized prospective evaluation of long-term effectiveness over six months. Clin Rheumatol. 2015;34 (6):1079–84.
4. Taslakian B, Sebaaly MG, Al-Kutoubi A. Patient evaluation and preparation in vascular and interventional radiology: what every interventional radiologist should know (part 1: patient assessment and laboratory tests). Cardiovasc Intervent Radiol. 2016;39(3):325–33.
5. Taslakian B, Sebaaly MG, Al-Kutoubi A. Patient evaluation and preparation in vascular and interventional radiology: what every interventional radiologist should know (part 2: patient preparation and medications). Cardiovasc Intervent Radiol. 2016;39(4):489–99. doi: 10.1007/s00270-015-1239-4. [Epub 2015 Nov 25].

Sacroplasty

60

Karim Masrouha

INTRODUCTION

Insufficiency fractures of the sacrum are not uncommon, with multiple risk factors including osteoporosis, metastasis, chronic steroid use, irradiation, and rheumatoid arthritis [1]. Osteoporotic fractures occur in the weakest segment of the sacrum where applied stress overcomes the biomechanical strength of the bone. This area is typically the segment between the sacroiliac joint and neural foramina, which also bears the greatest shear stress from the downward force of the torso centrally and the upward force of the hips laterally. Percutaneous sacroplasty by stabilizing the fracture with polymethylmethacrylate (PMMA) is a relatively safe, reliable, and effective treatment of pain related to these fractures [2].

COMMON INDICATIONS [2]

- The diagnosis of unilateral or bilateral sacral insufficiency fractures seen on bone scintigraphy or CT/MRI

COMMON CONTRAINDICATIONS

- Known bleeding disorder or currently on anticoagulation/antiplatelet
- Ongoing systemic infection
- Infection or loss of integrity of skin around injection site
- Uncontrolled hypertension, diabetes, coronary artery disease, or congestive heart failure
- Inability to lay in the prone position

POSSIBLE COMPLICATIONS

- Infection
- Hematoma
- Injury to sacral nerves
- Pulmonary emboli
- Leakage or extrusion into the neural foramina

PREOPERATIVE ASSESSMENT AND PLANNING

- History, indications and physical examination *(Appendix 1* in Chap. 149*)*
- Evaluation of diagnostic imaging studies
- Periprocedural management of coagulation status *(Appendices 2* in Chap. 150 *and 3* in Chap. 151*)*
- Antibiotic prophylaxis: Not routinely recommended

K. Masrouha (✉)
Department of Surgery, Division of Orthopedic Surgery, American University of Beirut Medical Center, Riad Elsolh, Beirut 1107 2020, Lebanon
e-mail: km34@aub.edu.lb

B. Taslakian et al. (eds.), *Procedural Dictations in Image-Guided Intervention*,
DOI 10.1007/978-3-319-40845-3_60

- Imaging modality for guidance: Fluoroscopy or CT
- Positioning: Prone

Procedure Note

Procedure: Fluoroscopy/CT-guided left/right/bilateral sacroplasty
Staff: [_]
Fellow: [_]
Resident: [_]
Clinical Information: Describe history and list indications
Allergies: None known/Allergic to [specify/type of allergy]
Anesthesia: Local anesthesia with conscious sedation
Medications: List any relevant medications used
Contrast Material: None
Field: Sterile
Procedure classification: Clean
Position: Prone
Monitoring: Intravenous access line was secured and vital signs were continuously monitored by nursing staff/anesthesia team throughout the procedure.
Total fluoroscopy time: (_) minutes
Cumulative radiation dose: (_) mGy

Description of Procedure [3]:

The risks, benefits, alternatives and procedure itself were explained to the patient/patient's Power of Attorney/patient's legal guardian, and informed written consent was obtained. The site of the procedure was identified and marked. Time out was performed to confirm the correct patient, procedure, and site.

Under conscious sedation the patient was placed in the prone position. Using a CT scanner with CT fluoroscopy capability, the entire sacrum was imaged. Based on the CT images, the location, path, and number of the needles were determined. It was decided that (X) needles would be necessary for adequate distribution of the cement.

Small metallic markers were placed on the skin at the proposed entry site of each of the needles. Limited CT sections at the level of the markers were obtained to confirm the correct location and these sites were marked using a sterile skin marker. Local anesthetic (1 % lidocaine) was then infiltrated at these levels into the skin and subcutaneous tissues. The periosteum was anesthetized at the level of S1 with 0.25 % Marcaine.

Using CT/fluoroscopy, (11)-gauge bone biopsy needles were inserted at the level of S1. The needles were advanced to the ventral aspect of the sacrum and polymethylmethacrylate cement was intermittently injected as the needle was progressively positioned more posteriorly. With each repositioning, the needle was depressurized to avoid unintentional cement leakage or flow into veins. A limited series of CT/fluoroscopy images were taken after every (0.25) mL of cement injection to confirm contained and controlled distribution. A total of (2) ml was injected at each level. After injection of the cement, the needles were withdrawn and a complete CT of the sacrum was performed, confirming adequate location and amount of cement. A sterile adherent dressing was then applied over the wounds.

The patient was transferred to the floor/recovery room/discharged home following the procedure in a stable condition. Staff was present for the entire procedure.

Intra-Procedure Findings: List all relevant findings.
Immediate Complications: None encountered during or directly after the procedure. List complications if any.

Post-Procedure Plan:

- Observe for 15 min to confirm that no major hematoma had developed.
- Instruct the patient to be aware of the possible complications such as infection, hematoma, or nerve injury.
- Inform the patient that it is preferred that someone drives them home.

Impression:

- Left/right/bilateral sacroplasty, as described above.
- The patient tolerated the procedure well and left the interventional unit in a stable condition.
- The patient was unable to tolerate the procedure which was canceled/terminated prematurely.
- List any other relevant or important information/finding.

References

1. Gjertsen O, Schellhorn T, Nakstad PH. Fluoroscopy-guided sacroplasty: special focus on preoperative planning from three-dimensional computed tomography. Acta Radiol. 2008;49(9):1042–8.
2. Pommersheim W, Huang-Hellinger F, Baker M, Morris P. Sacroplasty: a treatment for sacral insufficiency fractures. AJNR Am J Neuroradiol. 2003;24 (5):1003–7.
3. Layton KF, Thielen KR, Wald JT. Percutaneous sacroplasty using CT fluoroscopy. AJNR Am J Neuroradiol. 2006;27(2):356–8.

Shoulder Arthrography

61

Naji S. Madi

INTRODUCTION

Shoulder arthrography is performed typically to evaluate the rotator cuff, especially if followed by MRI. Depending on the purpose of the injection, the definitive contrast material is injected.

COMMON INDICATIONS [1–3]

Indications can be largely divided into groups; diagnostic or therapeutic.

- Diagnostic:
  - Rotator cuff tear—mainly for complete tears
  - Adhesive capsulitis
  - Rotator interval tear
  - Glenoid labrum tear
  - Septic arthritis
  - Prosthetic loosening or infection
  - Part of MR arthrogram
  - Biceps tendon injury
- Therapeutic:
  - Adhesive capsulitis
  - Impingement syndrome refractory to non-surgical treatment in patients older than 40 years

COMMON CONTRAINDICATIONS [2]

- Allergy to contrast media
- Allergy to local anesthetic drugs
- Pregnancy
- Uncorrectable coagulopathy
- Specific contraindications to MRI in case of MR arthrogram
- Skin infection overlying the shoulder area

POSSIBLE COMPLICATIONS [4]

This procedure is classified as low risk and safe intervention; rare complications, however, might occur:

- Joint infection
- Hematoma
- Joint damage
- Joint pain
- Allergic reaction to contrast media

PREOPERATIVE ASSESSMENT AND PLANNING

- History, indications and physical examination *(Appendix 1* in Chap. 149*)*
- Evaluation of diagnostic imaging studies; review radiographs of the shoulder, AP with internal and external rotations views, obtained to identify rotator cuff calcifications

N.S. Madi (✉)
Division of Orthopedic Surgery, Department of Surgery, American University of Beirut Medical Center, Riad El Solh, 1107 2020 Beirut, Lebanon
e-mail: nm88@aub.edu.lb

B. Taslakian et al. (eds.), *Procedural Dictations in Image-Guided Intervention*,
DOI 10.1007/978-3-319-40845-3_61

- Periprocedural management of coagulation status *(Appendices 2* in Chap. 150 *and 3* in Chap. 151*)*
- Antibiotic prophylaxis: Not routinely recommended
- Imaging modality for guidance: Fluoroscopy
- Positioning: Supine

PROCEDURE NOTE

Procedure: Left/right shoulder arthrography
Staff: [_]
Fellow: [_]
Resident: [_]
Clinical information: Describe history and list indications
Allergies: None known/Allergic to [specify/type of allergy]
Anesthesia: Local anesthesia/conscious sedation
Medications: List any relevant medications used
Contrast used: (_) mL of [type] contrast material was used for intra-articular injection
Field: Sterile
Procedure classification: Clean
Position: Supine
Monitoring: Intravenous access line was secured and vital signs were continuously monitored by nursing staff throughout the procedure
Total fluoroscopy time: (_) minutes
Cumulative radiation dose: (_) mGy

Description of Procedure:
The risks, benefits, alternatives and the procedure itself were explained to the patient/patient's Power of Attorney/patient's legal guardian, and informed written consent was obtained. The site of the procedure was identified and marked. Time out was performed to confirm the correct patient, procedure and site.

The shoulder was evaluated using plain radiographs (anteroposterior, external and internal rotations) to identify rotator cuff calcifications, before starting the procedure.

The skin was prepped and draped in the usual sterile fashion. Local anesthesia was administered. The shoulder was placed in minimal external rotation to expose the glenohumeral joint anteriorly and facilitate needle insertion. A mark was placed over the humeral head; fluoroscopy was used to ensure the correct placement, lateral to the medial cortex of the humeral head.

Subsequently, a (20/22)-gauge [spinal] needle was inserted anteroposteriorly, perpendicular to the fluoroscopic beam, and advanced until it hits the humeral head. Proper position was verified by fluoroscopy, the stylet was removed then a "test injection" of (1–2) mL of iodinated contrast media was made, and contrast flow was observed between the glenoid and humeral head confirming the intra-articular location of the tip. At this stage, (10–15) mL of [type] contrast media was injected.

The patient was transferred to the floor/recovery room/CT unit/MR unit/discharged home following the procedure in a stable condition. Staff was present for the entire procedure.
Intra-Procedure Findings: List all relevant findings
Immediate Complications: None encountered during or directly after the procedure. List complications if any.

Post-Procedure Plan [5]:
- Observe the patient for any allergic reaction or vasovagal syncope for 15–30 min.
- Prescribe pain medications to patient before discharge *(pain is the most frequent complaint after shoulder arthrography).*

Impression:
- Arthrography of *right/left* shoulder, as described above.
- The patient tolerated the procedure well and left the interventional unit in stable condition.
- The patient was unable to tolerate the procedure which was canceled/terminated prematurely.

- List any other relevant or important information/finding.

References

1. Jacobson JA, Lin J, Hayes CW. Aids to successful shoulder arthrography performed with a fluoroscopically guided anterior approach. Radiographics. 2003;23 (2):373–8.
2. Uberoi R. Musculoskeletal intervention. In: Interventional radiology. Oxford specialist handbooks in radiology. Oxford: Oxford University Press; 2009. p. 432–33.
3. Dépelteau H, Bureau NJ, Cardinal E, Aubin B, Brassard P. Arthrography of the shoulder: a simple fluoroscopically guided approach for targeting the rotator cuff interval. AJR Am J Roentgenol. 2004;182(2):329–32.
4. Saupe N, Zanetti M, Pfirrmann CW, Wels T, Schwenke C, Hodler J. Pain and other side effects after MR arthrography: prospective evaluation in 1085 patients. Radiology. 2009;250(3):830–8.
5. Giaconi JC, Link TM, Vail TP. Morbidity of direct MR arthrography. AJR Am J Roentgenol. 2011;196(4): 868–74.

Soft Tissue Biopsy

62

Karim Masrouha

Abbreviations

CT	Computed tomography
MRI	Magnetic resonance imaging

INTRODUCTION

Image-guided percutaneous soft tissue biopsies are safe procedures with very high sensitivity, specificity, and diagnostic accuracy [1]. They are performed under ultrasound, but may be done under computed tomography (CT) or magnetic resonance imaging (MRI) guidance.

COMMON INDICATIONS [2]

- Diagnosis of a soft tissue lesion
- To exclude metastasis in patients with a known primary malignancy
- To isolate organisms in suspected infections

COMMON CONTRAINDICATIONS [2]

- Uncooperative patient
- Bleeding disorders
- Inaccessible site
- Ongoing systemic infection

POSSIBLE COMPLICATIONS [2, 3]

- Infection
- Hematoma
- Neuropraxia

PREOPERATIVE ASSESSMENT AND PLANNING

- History, indications, and physical examination *(Appendix 1* in Chap. 149*)*
- Evaluation of diagnostic imaging studies to determine the location and extent of the lesion, as well as the location of surrounding neurovascular structures [2, 3]
- Coordination with the oncologic surgeon regarding surgical implications of the biopsy site [2, 3]
- Periprocedural management of coagulation status *(Appendices 2* in Chap. 150 *and 3* in Chap. 151*)*
- Antibiotic prophylaxis: Not routinely recommended *(Appendices 4* in Chap. 152 *and 5* in Chap. 153*)*

K. Masrouha (✉)
Department of Surgery, Division of Orthopedic Surgery, American University of Beirut Medical Center, Riad Elsolh, 1107 2020 Beirut, Lebanon
e-mail: km34@aub.edu.lb

B. Taslakian et al. (eds.), *Procedural Dictations in Image-Guided Intervention*,
DOI 10.1007/978-3-319-40845-3_62

- Imaging modality for guidance: Ultrasound *(alternatively, CT or MRI)*
- Positioning: Oblique, lateral decubitus, prone, or supine

PROCEDURE NOTE

Procedure: Ultrasound-guided percutaneous soft tissue biopsy [list site of biopsy]
Staff: [_]
Fellow: [_]
Resident: [_]
Clinical information: Describe history and list indications
Allergies: None known/Allergic to [specify/type of allergy]
Anesthesia: Local anesthesia/conscious sedation
Medications: List any relevant medications used (sedation, antibiotics)
Field: Sterile
Procedure classification: Clean/Dirty
Position: Supine/Left lateral decubitus/Right lateral decubitus/Oblique/Prone
Monitoring: Intravenous access line was secured and vital signs were continuously monitored by nursing staff/anesthesia team throughout the procedure

Description of Procedure:

The risks, benefits, alternatives, and procedure itself were explained to the patient/patient's Power of Attorney/patient's legal guardian, and informed written consent was obtained. The site of the procedure was identified and marked. Time out was performed to confirm the correct patient, procedure, and site.

The skin at the area of the biopsy was prepped and draped in a sterile manner. The approach with the shortest path to access the lesion was selected along the line of the proposed surgical incision. The skin was then infiltrated with local anesthetic. A 5 mm longitudinal skin incision was made to introduce the core needle. The biopsy needle was then inserted into the lesion under direct ultrasound visualization. Three cores were taken and placed in containers with 10 % formalin, which were then sent for pathology/inserted in a container for culture. Areas showing vascularity on Doppler were targeted.

After removal of the core needle, an ultrasound of the area was performed to rule out a hematoma.

The wound was cleaned and a sterile dressing was applied. The patient was transferred to the floor/recovery room/discharged home following the procedure in a stable condition. Staff was present for the entire procedure.

Intra-Procedure Findings: List all relevant findings.
Immediate Complications: None encountered during or directly after the procedure. List complications if any.

Post-Procedure Plan:

- Observe for 15 min to confirm that no major hematoma had developed.
- Instruct the patient to be aware of the possible complications such as infection, hematoma, or neurapraxia.

Impression:

- Soft tissue biopsy from the [specify anatomic location], as described above.
- The patient tolerated the procedure well and left the interventional unit in a stable condition.
- The patient was unable to tolerate the procedure which was canceled/terminated prematurely.
- List any other relevant or important information/finding.

References

1. Pohlig F, Kirchhoff C, Lenze U, Schauwecker J, Burgkart R, Rechl H, et al. Percutaneous core needle biopsy versus open biopsy in diagnostics of bone and soft tissue sarcoma: a retrospective study. Eur J Med Res. 2012;17:29.
2. Le HB, Lee ST, Munk PL. Image-guided musculoskeletal biopsies. Semin Intervent Radiol. 2010;27(2):191–8.
3. Errani C, Traina F, Perna F, Calamelli C, Faldini C. Current concepts in the biopsy of musculoskeletal tumors. Sci World J. 2013;2013:538152.

Steroid Injection in the Shoulder

63

Naji S. Madi

INTRODUCTION [1, 2]

Shoulder pain is a common symptom, caused by a wide spectrum of diseases; the rotator cuff and the subacromial bursa are frequently involved. Intra-articular corticosteroid injection has been shown to improve pain and function in chronic shoulder pain. Depending on the location of inflammation/disease, the site of injection is determined. Ultrasound-guided injection has been found to be superior to blind injection. It is a safe procedure with rare complications.

COMMON INDICATIONS [1, 3]

- Rotator cuff arthropathy
- Adhesive capsulitis
- Glenohumeral joint osteoarthritis
- Subacromial bursitis
- Tear of the long head of the biceps tendon
- Acromioclavicular joint pain

COMMON CONTRAINDICATIONS [4]

- Allergy to corticosteroids drugs
- Local cellulitis
- Shoulder septic arthritis
- Uncorrectable coagulopathy

POSSIBLE COMPLICATIONS [4, 5]

Intra-articular corticosteroids injection is a low risk and safe procedure; rare complications might occur:

- Shoulder infection/septic arthritis
- Localized erythema
- Tendon weakening or rupture
- Synovitis
- Skin atrophy and depigmentation
- Systemic corticosteroids effects (especially in diabetics)

PREOPERATIVE ASSESSMENT AND PLANNING

- History, indications, and physical examination *(Appendix 1* in Chap. 149*)*
- Evaluation of diagnostic imaging studies such as radiographs, ultrasound, or MRI shoulder
- Periprocedural management of coagulation status *(Appendices 2* in Chap. 150 *and 3* in Chap. 151*)*
- Antibiotic prophylaxis: Not routinely recommended
- Imaging modality for guidance: Ultrasound
- Positioning: Sitting with back supported or supine

N.S. Madi (✉)
Division of Orthopedic Surgery, Department of Surgery, American University of Beirut Medical Center, Riad Elsolh, 1107 2020 Beirut, Lebanon
e-mail: nm88@aub.edu.lb

B. Taslakian et al. (eds.), *Procedural Dictations in Image-Guided Intervention*,
DOI 10.1007/978-3-319-40845-3_63

PROCEDURE NOTE

Procedure: Ultrasound-guided left/right shoulder corticosteroids injection
Staff: [_]
Fellow: [_]
Resident: [_]
Clinical information: Describe history and list indications
Allergies: None known/Allergic to [specify/type of allergy]
Anesthesia: Local anesthesia/conscious sedation
Medications: List any relevant medications used
Field: Sterile
Procedure classification: Clean
Position: Sitting with back supported or supine, arm in neutral position
Monitoring: Intravenous access line was secured and vital signs were continuously monitored by nursing staff throughout the procedure

Description of Procedure *(Subacromial/Subdeltoid bursa injection):*
The risks, benefits, alternatives, and the procedure itself were explained to the patient/patient's Power of Attorney/patient's legal guardian, and informed written consent was obtained. The site of the procedure was identified and marked. Time out was performed to confirm the correct patient, procedure, and site.

The shoulder was evaluated using real-time ultrasound images. The skin was prepped and draped in the usual sterile fashion. The ultrasound probe was covered with a sterile drape, and sterile gel was used.

The probe was oriented in the scapular plane and placed over the tip of the acromion. The supraspinatus tendon was identified as a hyperechoic structure passing beneath the acromion. Above the tendon, the bursa was identified as an anechoic structure. Subsequently, a (22)-gauge needle was introduced lateral to the acromion and advanced to enter the bursa and a (3) mL mix of (40) mg/1 mL Methylprednisolone acetate with (2) mL of 1 % Lidocaine was injected.

The patient was transferred to the floor/recovery room/discharged home following the procedure in a stable condition. Staff was present for the entire procedure.

Description of Procedure *(Glenohumeral joint injection):*
The risks, benefits, alternatives, and the procedure itself were explained to the patient/patient's Power of Attorney/patient's legal guardian, and informed written consent was obtained. The site of the procedure was identified and marked. Time out was performed to confirm the correct patient, procedure, and site.

The shoulder was evaluated using real-time ultrasound images. The skin was prepped and draped in the usual sterile fashion. The ultrasound probe was covered with a sterile drape, and sterile gel was used.

The patient was asked to pull back his shoulders. The probe was placed posteriorly, parallel to the spine of the scapula. The humeral head, glenoid, and labrum were identified. Subsequently, 2 cm lateral to the probe, behind the humeral head, a (3–4 inch) (_) gauge needle was introduced longitudinally, with 30° inclination of the tip. Then, the needle was rotated to direct the tip point anteriorly. The needle was advanced till it entered the joint and a (3) mL mix of (40) mg/1 mL Methylprednisolone acetate with (2) ml of 1 % Lidocaine was injected.

The patient was transferred to the floor/recovery room/discharged home following the procedure in a stable condition. Staff was present for the entire procedure.

Intra-Procedure Findings: List all relevant findings.
Immediate Complications: None encountered during or directly after the procedure. List complications if any.

Post-Procedure Plan [6]:

- Monitor the patient for 30 min after the intervention.
- Instruct patient to limit the range of motion of the injected shoulder for few hours and to expect relief of pain within 24–72 h post procedure.

Impression:

- Corticosteroids injection of right/left shoulder, as described above.
- The patient tolerated the procedure well and left the interventional unit in stable condition.
- The patient was unable to tolerate the procedure which was canceled/terminated prematurely.
- List any other relevant or important information/finding.

References

1. Schaefer MP, Fox K. Ultrasound-guided shoulder joint and bursa injections. In: Narouze SN, editor. Atlas of ultrasound-guided procedures in interventional pain management. New York: Springer; 2011. p. 293–306.
2. Soh E, Li W, Ong KO, Chen W, Bautista D. Image-guided versus blind corticosteroid injections in adults with shoulder pain: a systematic review. BMC Musculoskelet Disord. 2011;12:137.
3. Wittich CM, Ficalora RD, Mason TG, Beckman TJ. Musculoskeletal injection. Mayo Clin Proc. 2009;84(9):831–7.
4. Uberoi R. Musculoskeletal intervention. In: Radiology Interventional, editor. Oxford specialist handbooks in radiology. Oxford: Oxford University Press; 2009. p. 432–3.
5. Nichols AW. Complications associated with the use of corticosteroids in the treatment of athletic injuries. Clin J Sport Med. 2005;5:370–5.
6. Kennedy DJ, Schneider B, Casey E, Rittenberg J, Conrad B, Smuck M, et al. Vasovagal rates in flouroscopically guided interventional procedures: a study of over 8,000 injections. Pain Med. 2013;14(12):1854–9.

Vertebroplasty

64

Jad Chokr

INTRODUCTION

Percutaneous vertebroplasty is an intervention with a goal to prevent vertebral body collapse and pain in patients with pathologic vertebral bodies. The first case was performed by Deramond and colleagues, who originated the method in 1984. Vertebroplasty dramatically improves back pain within hours of the procedure, provides long-term pain relief and has a low complication rate, as demonstrated in multiple studies.

COMMON INDICATIONS [1–5]

- Symptomatic vertebral hemangiomas
- Symptomatic vertebral body compression fractures related to tumors *(e.g., multiple myeloma, metastases)*
- Painful compression fracture related to osteoporosis

COMMON CONTRAINDICATIONS [1–3]

- Systemic or spinal infection
- Hemorrhagic diathesis
- Allergy to cement or opacification materials
- Lesions with epidural extension, substantial canal narrowing, or disruption of the posterior cortex *(relative)*
- Unstable fracture or complete vertebral collapse *(>70 % loss of height)*

POSSIBLE COMPLICATIONS [1, 3, 4]

- Cement leak into the epidural/paravertebral veins, epidural space, or neural foramina
- Nerve or spinal cord damage
- Pulmonary embolism
- Pneumothorax
- Worsened pain or failure to treat
- Infection
- Bleeding
- Death (1 in 50,000); the etiology includes severe allergy and pulmonary emboli

PREOPERATIVE ASSESSMENT AND PLANNING [6–8]

- History, indications, and physical examination *(Appendix 1* in Chap. 149*)*
- Evaluation of diagnostic imaging studies to determine the affected vertebral body and the underlying cause, and to estimate the loss of height and the extension to posterior elements or spinal canal

J. Chokr (✉)
Department of Diagnostic Radiology, Neuroradiology Division, Banner University Medical Center, Tucson, AZ, USA
e-mail: Jad_1986@hotmail.com

B. Taslakian et al. (eds.), *Procedural Dictations in Image-Guided Intervention*,
DOI 10.1007/978-3-319-40845-3_64

- Periprocedural management of coagulation status *(Appendices 2* in Chap. 150 *and 3* in Chap. 151*)*
- Antibiotic prophylaxis: Routinely recommended *(1 g intravenous cefazolin 30 min before the procedure; if the patient is allergic to penicillin or cephalosporins, vancomycin may be administrated)* [6] *(Appendices 4* in Chap. 152 *and 5* in Chap. 153*)*
- Imaging modality for guidance: CT or fluoroscopy
- Positioning: Prone or supine

PROCEDURE NOTE

Procedure: Fluoroscopic/CT-guided vertebroplasty of [_] vertebral body/bodies
Staff: [_]
Fellow: [_]
Resident: [_]
Clinical Information: Describe history and list indications
Allergies: None known/Allergic to [specify/type of allergy]
Anesthesia: Local anesthesia/Conscious sedation/General anesthesia
Medications: List any relevant medications used
Field: Sterile
Procedure classification: Clean
Position: Prone/Supine
Monitoring: Intravenous access line was secured and vital signs were continuously monitored by nursing staff/anesthesia team throughout the procedure.
Total fluoroscopy time: (_) minutes
Cumulative radiation dose: (_) mGy

Description of Procedure:

The risks, benefits, alternatives, and the procedure itself were explained to the patient/patient's Power of Attorney/legal guardian, and informed written consent was obtained. The site of the procedure was identified and marked. Time out was performed to confirm the correct patient, procedure, and site.

Conscious sedation/general anesthesia was administered with continuous hemodynamic monitoring. The skin was prepped and draped in the usual sterile fashion. The site of entry was determined by imaging and using a radiopaque marker. The skin and periosteum were anesthetized with local anesthetic along the planned trajectory. A small nick was made in the skin. Under fluoroscopic biplane/CT guidance, two (_)-gauge cannulas were introduced via transpedicular/parapedicular/transcostovertebral/anterolateral/posterolateral approach into the anterior portion of the [_] vertebra/vertebrae. Using a low-pressure injection system, the methacrylate cement was then gently injected into the [_] vertebra/vertebrae with filling of the vertebral bodies anteriorly. No cement leakage into the epidural space was identified. The needle systems were withdrawn with no cement spikes identified. Hemostasis was achieved by compression and sterile dressing was applied. The patient was kept in the prone/supine position for approximately 15 min post cement injection, turned supine, and monitored briefly. Throughout the procedure, there were no intraoperative complications and the patient was moving both lower extremities at the end of the procedure.

The patient was then transferred to the floor/recovery room following the procedure in a stable condition. Staff was present for the entire procedure.

Intra-Procedure Findings: List any additional findings if relevant.
Immediate Complications: None encountered during or directly after the procedure. List the complication if any.

Post-Procedure Plan [1–3]:

- Keep at bed rest for 1 h after the procedure *(may roll side to side).*
- Allow sitting with assistance after 1 h.

- Monitor vital signs and perform neurologic examinations every 15 min for the first hour, then every 30 min for the second hour.
- Record pain level at the end of procedure and at 2 h post procedure. Compare with baseline values and notify physician if pain increases above baseline.
- Allow liquids by mouth if not nauseated or otherwise contraindicated.
- Discontinue intravenous drips after 1 h if recovery is otherwise uneventful.
- Discharge patient home with adult companion after 2 h if recovery is uneventful.
- Patient instruction:
  - Return home; remain at bed rest, and keep to minimal activity for 24 h
  - Keep operative site covered for 24 h. Bandages may then be removed and site washed with a damp cloth. Do not soak.
  - Notify physician/facility if you have increasing pain, redness, swelling, or drainage from the operative site.
  - Notify physician/facility if you have difficulty with walking, changes in sensation in your hips or legs, new pain, or problems with bowel or bladder function.

Impression:

- Vertebroplasty of [_] vertebral body/bodies, as described above.
- The patient tolerated the procedure well and left the interventional unit in a stable condition.
- The patient was unable to tolerate the procedure which was canceled/terminated prematurely.
- List any other relevant or important information/finding.

References

1. Vertebroplasty (Interventional). In: Burke CT, Dixon RG, Mauro MA, Murphy KPJ, Thomson KR, Venbrux AC, Zollikofer CL, editors. High yield imaging: interventional. Philadelphia: Saunders Elsevier; 2010. P. 510–513.
2. Gandi A, Guth S, Dietemann JL, Roy C. Musculoskeletal intervention. In: Kaufman JA, Lee MJ, editors. The requisites: vascular and interventional radiology. Philadelphia: Mosby; 2004. p. 648–70.
3. Pastel DA, Yoo AJ, Eskey CJ, Hirsch JA. Vertebroplasty and kyphoplasty. In: Mauro MA, Murphy KPJ, Thomson KR, Venbrux AC, Morgan RA, editors. Image-guided interventions. 2nd ed. Philadelphia: Saunders Elsevier; 2014. p. 1188–96.
4. Mathis JM, Barr JD, Belkoff SM, Barr MS, Jensen ME, Deramond H. Percutaneous vertebroplasty: a developing standard of care for vertebral compression fractures. AJNR Am J Neuroradiol. 2001;22(2):373–81.
5. Peh WC, Gilula LA, Peck DD. Percutaneous vertebroplasty for severe osteoporotic vertebral body compression fractures. Radiology. 2002;223(1):121–6.
6. Venkatesan AM, Kundu S, Sacks D, Wallace MJ, Wojak JC, Rose SC, et al. Practice guidelines for adult antibiotic prophylaxis during vascular and interventional radiology procedures. J Vasc Interv Radiol. 2010;21(11):1611–30.
7. Taslakian B, Sebaaly MG, Al-Kutoubi A. Patient evaluation and preparation in vascular and interventional radiology: what every interventional radiologist should know (part 1: patient assessment and laboratory tests). Cardiovasc Intervent Radiol. 2016;39(3):325–33.
8. Taslakian B, Sebaaly MG, Al-Kutoubi A. Patient evaluation and preparation in vascular and interventional radiology: what every interventional radiologist should know (part 2: patient preparation and medications). Cardiovasc Intervent Radiol. 2016;39(4):489–99. doi: 10.1007/s00270-015-1239-4. [Epub 2015 Nov 25].

Part XI

Non-vascular Interventional Procedures: Miscellaneous

Introduction by Aghiad Al-Kutoubi, Section Reviewer

Since Dr. Charles Dotter, the father of interventional radiology, performed the first angioplasty on January 16, 1964, interventional radiologists have been responsible for much of the medical innovation and development of the minimally invasive procedures. With the recent and ongoing improvements in imaging techniques, advances in ultrasound equipment, and an increasing spectrum of image-guided interventions, radiologists continue to play a pivotal role in modern medicine.

This section provides a comprehensive list of procedural reports that covers a vast majority of non-vascular interventional procedures not included in the previous system-based sections, with up-to-date explanatory notes, synopsis of the indications and contraindications, and potential complications in an organized and practical format.

Section Chapters

Aspiration of Abdominopelvic Fluid Collection

65

Bedros Taslakian

INTRODUCTION

Percutaneous image-guided aspiration of fluid collection is the therapeutic evacuation or diagnostic sampling of fluid collection during a single imaging session.

COMMON INDICATIONS [1–4]

- Fluid characterization
- Evacuation of symptomatic fluid collection

COMMON CONTRAINDICATIONS [1–4]

- Significant coagulopathy that cannot be adequately corrected
- Hemodynamic instability
- Lack of safe pathway to the collection
- Inability of the patient to be positioned for the procedure
- Procedure requires transgression of pleura *(risk of pneumothorax, empyema, and pleural effusion)*
- Hydatid cyst *(risk of anaphylaxis due to intraperitoneal leakage of content)*

POSSIBLE COMPLICATIONS [1–4]

- Hemorrhage
- Septic shock and bacteremia
- Peritonitis
- Pleural transgression *(hemothorax, empyema, pneumothorax)*
- Unintended organ injury
- Mortality

PREPROCEDURAL ASSESSMENT AND PLANNING [5–7]

- History, indications, and physical examination *(Appendix 1* in Chap. 149*)*
- Evaluation of diagnostic imaging studies to determine the location of the collection, its size, and relevant anatomy
- Periprocedural management of coagulation status *(Appendices 2* in Chap. 150 *and 3* in Chap. 151*)*
- Antibiotic prophylaxis: Routinely recommended if infection is suspected [5] *(Appendices 4* in Chap. 152 *and 5* in Chap. 153*)*
- Imaging modality for guidance: CT, ultrasound
- Positioning: Oblique, lateral decubitus, prone, supine

B. Taslakian (✉)
Department of Radiology, New York University Langone Medical Center, 660 First Ave, New York, NY 10016, USA
e-mail: btaslakian@gmail.com

B. Taslakian et al. (eds.), *Procedural Dictations in Image-Guided Intervention*,
DOI 10.1007/978-3-319-40845-3_65

PROCEDURE NOTE

Procedure: Percutaneous aspiration of abdominal/pelvic fluid collection
Staff: [_]
Fellow: [_]
Resident: [_]
Clinical Information: Describe history and list indications
Allergies: None known/Allergic to [specify/type of allergy
Anesthesia: Local anesthesia/conscious sedation
Medications: List any relevant medications used
Field: Sterile
Procedure classification: Clean/Clean-contaminated/Contaminated/Dirty
Position: Supine/Prone/Left lateral decubitus/Right lateral decubitus/Oblique
Monitoring: Intravenous access line was secured and vital signs were continuously monitored by nursing staff/anesthesia team throughout the procedure
Cumulative radiation dose: (_) mGy

Description of Procedure:

The risks, benefits, alternatives, and the procedure itself were explained to the patient/patient's Power of Attorney/legal guardian, and informed written/verbal consent was obtained. The site of the procedure was identified and marked. Time out was performed to confirm the correct patient, procedure, and site.

The abdomen/pelvis was evaluated using ultrasound/CT imaging after placement of a radiopaque marker/grid. The procedure was planned and the skin puncture site was marked using combined information from the location of the fluid collection and preliminary CT/ultrasound images. The angle of needle entry and the distance to the collection were calculated from the planning images.

The skin was prepped and draped in the usual sterile fashion. Local anesthesia was administered. A small skin incision was made. Subsequently, a (_)-gauge [type] needle was advanced into the collection using planning CT information/under direct ultrasound visualization. (_) mL of clear fluid/serosanguineous fluid/malodorous pus was aspirated, and sent to laboratory for culture/gram stain/cytology/chemistry. (_) mL of fluid was drained for symptomatic relief after insertion of a (_)-French catheter over a (_)-inch [type] guidewire. The catheter/needle was removed and completion ultrasound/CT images were obtained.

The patient was transferred to the floor/recovery room/discharged home following the procedure in a stable condition. Staff was present for the entire procedure.

Intra-Procedure Findings: List all relevant findings.
Immediate Complications: None encountered during or directly after the procedure. List complications if any.

Post-Procedure Plan:

- Follow-up laboratory results and adjust antibiotics treatment accordingly.
- Keep complete bed rest for 3–4 h and abstain from strenuous activities.
- Start clear liquid diet for the first hour, then regular diet thereafter if tolerated and otherwise not contraindicated.
- Check vital signs every 15 min for 1 h, every 30 min for 1 h and then every 60 min for 2 h.
- Inform interventional radiology team if systolic blood pressure <95 mm Hg, heart rate >100 beats per minute, or if any chest pain, abdominal pain, or shortness of breath develops.

Impression:

- Percutaneous aspiration of abdominal/pelvic fluid collection, as described above.
- The patient tolerated the procedure well and left the interventional unit in a stable condition.
- List any other relevant or important information/finding.

References

1. Thabet A, Arellano RS. Catheter drainage of abdominal abscesses and fluid collections. In: Kandarpa K, Machan L, editors. Handbook of interventional radiologic procedures. 4th ed. Philadelphia: Lippincott Williams & Wilkins; 2011. p. 527–36.
2. Wallace MJ, Chin KW, Fletcher TB, Bakal CW, Cardella JF, Grassi CJ, et al. Quality improvement guidelines for percutaneous drainage/aspiration of abscess and fluid collections. J Vasc Interv Radiol. 2010;21(4):431–5.
3. Campbell JJ, Gervais DA. Percutaneous abscess drainage within the abdomen and pelvis. In: Murphy KPJ, Thomson KR, Venbrux AC, Morgan RA, editors. Image-guided interventions. 2nd ed. Philadelphia: Saunders Elsevier; 2014. p. 923–31.
4. Bakal CW, Sacks D, Burke DR, Cardella JF, Chopra PS, Dawson SL, et al. Quality improvement guidelines for adult percutaneous abscess and fluid drainage. J Vasc Interv Radiol. 2003;14(9 Pt 2):S223–5.
5. Venkatesan AM, Kundu S, Sacks D, Wallace MJ, Wojak JC, Rose SC, et al. Practice guidelines for adult antibiotic prophylaxis during vascular and interventional radiology procedures. J Vasc Interv Radiol. 2010;21(11):1611–30.
6. Taslakian B, Sebaaly MG, Al-Kutoubi A. Patient evaluation and preparation in vascular and interventional radiology: what every interventional radiologist should know (part 1: patient assessment and laboratory tests). Cardiovasc Intervent Radiol. 2016;39(3):325–33.
7. Taslakian B, Sebaaly MG, Al-Kutoubi A. Patient evaluation and preparation in vascular and interventional radiology: what every interventional radiologist should know (part 2: patient preparation and medications). Cardiovasc Intervent Radiol. 2016;39(4):489–99. doi: 10.1007/s00270-015-1239-4. [Epub 2015 Nov 25].

Catheter Drainage of Abdominopelvic Abscess

66

Bedros Taslakian

INTRODUCTION

Percutaneous drainage is the placement of a catheter using image guidance to provide continuous drainage of a fluid collection. The appropriate imaging modality for guidance and the optimal route for catheter drainage should be selected based on the available imaging studies. Intravenous and/or oral contrast administration might be required in selected cases to distinguish the collection from, and avoid transgression, of surrounding normal and vital structures. In the pelvis, alternative routes might be considered instead of the usual approach, such as transvaginal, transgluteal, or transrectal approaches, to avoid transgression of vital structures.

COMMON INDICATIONS [1–4]

- Fluid characterization
- Drainage of symptomatic fluid collection
- Suspicion that the collection is infected
- Treatment of sepsis in patients with complex collections
- Curative drainage in patients with simple collection
- Obliteration of recurring cysts or collections with sclerosing agents

COMMON CONTRAINDICATIONS [1–4]

- Significant coagulopathy that cannot be adequately corrected
- Presence of necrotic tissue that needs surgical debridement
- Hemodynamic instability
- Lack of safe pathway to the collection
- Inability of the patient to be positioned for the procedure
- Procedure requires transgression of pleura *(risk of pneumothorax, empyema, and pleural effusion)*
- Hydatid cyst *(risk of anaphylaxis due to intraperitoneal leakage of contents)*
- Malignant abscess requiring prolonged drainage

POSSIBLE COMPLICATIONS [1–4]

- Hemorrhage requiring transfusion, *1 %*
- Septic shock, *1–2 %*
- Significant bacteremia, *2–5 %*
- Enteric fistula
- Peritonitis

B. Taslakian (✉)
Department of Radiology, New York University Langone Medical Center, 660 First Ave, New York, NY 10016, USA
e-mail: btaslakian@gmail.com

B. Taslakian et al. (eds.), *Procedural Dictations in Image-Guided Intervention*,
DOI 10.1007/978-3-319-40845-3_66

- Pleural transgression *(hemothorax, empyema, pneumothorax, hemopneumothorax)* requiring intervention, *1 %*
- Unintended organ injury
- Superinfection of a sterile collection, *1 %*
- Infection at the catheter insertion site
- Catheter malfunction *(kinking, blockage, dislodgment)*
- Pericatheter leak
- Mortality

PREPROCEDURAL ASSESSMENT AND PLANNING

- History, indications, and physical examination *(Appendix 1* in Chap. 149*)*
- Evaluation of diagnostic imaging studies to determine the location of the collection, its size, and relevant anatomy
- Periprocedural management of coagulation status *(Appendices 2* in Chap. 150 *and 3* in Chap. 151*)*
- Antibiotic prophylaxis: Routinely recommended if infection is suspected [1, 5] *(Appendices 4* in Chap. 152 *and 5* in Chap. 153*)*
- Imaging modality for guidance: CT, ultrasound, combined fluoroscopy with CT or ultrasound
- Positioning: Oblique, lateral decubitus, prone, supine

PROCEDURE NOTE

Procedure: Percutaneous drainage of abdominal/pelvic collection
Staff: [_]
Fellow: [_]
Resident: [_]
Clinical Information: Describe history and list indications
Allergies: None known/Allergic to [specify/type of allergy]
Anesthesia: Local anesthesia/conscious sedation
Medications: List any relevant medications used (sedation, antibiotics)
Field: Sterile
Procedure classification: Dirty
Position: Supine/Prone/Left lateral decubitus/Right lateral decubitus/Oblique
Monitoring: Intravenous access line was secured and vital signs were continuously monitored by nursing staff/anesthesia team throughout the procedure
Cumulative radiation dose: (_) mGy

Description of Procedure
(Seldinger technique):
The risks, benefits, alternatives, and the procedure itself were explained to the patient/patient's Power of Attorney/legal guardian, and informed written/verbal consent was obtained. The site of the procedure was identified and marked. Time out was performed to confirm the correct patient, procedure, and site.

The abdomen/pelvis was evaluated using ultrasound/CT imaging after placement of a radiopaque marker/grid. The procedure was planned and the skin puncture site was marked using combined information from the location of the collection and preliminary CT/ultrasound images. The angle of needle entry and the distance to the collection were calculated from the planning images.

The skin was prepped and draped in the usual sterile fashion. Local anesthesia was administered. A small skin incision was made. Subsequently, a (_)-gauge [type] needle was advanced into the collection using planning CT information/under direct ultrasound visualization. (_) mL of malodorous pus was aspirated, and sent for culture and gram stain. Then, a (_)-inch [type] guidewire was advanced through the needle into the collection and was positioned under fluoroscopy guidance. The tract was dilated up to the required size using (_)-French dilator(s). A (_)-French self-retaining [type/pigtail] catheter assembly with the metal stiffener was introduced over the guidewire to a satisfactory depth under fluoroscopy guidance. The stiff trocar of the catheter was left within the shaft until the catheter was advanced just beyond the wall of the collection. The guidewire and stiffener were removed after advancing the catheter into the collection cavity. The catheter was locked, anchored to the skin and attached to a drainage system. The collection content was aspirated and the cavity was irrigated using (_) mL of normal saline until the aspirate became clear. Following this, completion CT/ultrasound images were obtained through the drainage area to confirm correct position of the catheter for future reference, to ensure that the cavity is completely emptied, detect any undrained separate collections and screen for complications.

The patient was transferred to the floor/recovery room/intensive care unit following the procedure in a stable/critical condition. Staff was present for the entire procedure.

Description of Procedure *(trocar technique):*
The risks, benefits, alternatives, and the procedure itself were explained to the patient/patient's Power of Attorney/legal guardian, and informed written/verbal consent was obtained. The site of the procedure was identified and marked. Time out was performed to confirm the correct patient, procedure, and site.

The abdomen/pelvis was evaluated using ultrasound/CT imaging after placement of a radiopaque marker/grid. The procedure was planned and the skin puncture site was marked using combined information from the location of the collection and preliminary CT/ultrasound images. The angle of entry and the distance to the collection were calculated from the planning images.

The skin was prepped and draped in the usual sterile fashion. Local anesthesia was administered. A small skin incision was made. Subsequently, using planning CT information/under direct ultrasound visualization, a (_)-gauge [type] diagnostic needle was advanced through the abdominal wall/back/through a transgluteal approach into the collection. (_) mL of malodorous pus was aspirated, and sent to laboratory for culture, gram stain, and chemistry.

Once the needle was in optimal position, confirmed by imaging, a (_)-French [type] catheter was loaded on a trocar delivery system. The delivery system was placed in the skin incision while holding the shaft parallel to the diagnostic needle. The catheter was then advanced in tandem to the needle to the predetermined depth calculated from planning CT images/under direct ultrasound visualization to enter the cavity. Once the catheter was optimally placed within the cavity, the inner stylet was removed and fluid was aspirated through the metal stiffener. The catheter was then unlocked from the stiffening cannula and advanced to coil within the collection while holding the stiffener steady. The stiffening cannula was removed. The catheter was locked, anchored to the skin and attached to a drainage system.

The collection content was aspirated and the cavity was irrigated using (_) mL of normal saline until the aspirate became clear. Following this, completion CT/ultrasound images were obtained through the drainage area to confirm correct position of the catheter for future reference, to ensure that the cavity is completely emptied, detect any undrained separate collections and screen for complications.

The patient was transferred to the floor/recovery room/intensive care unit following the procedure in a stable/critical condition. Staff was present for the entire procedure.

Intra-Procedure Findings: List all relevant findings.
Immediate Complications: None encountered during or directly after the procedure. List complications if any.

Post-Procedure Plan [1, 6]:
- Follow-up laboratory results and adjust antibiotics treatment accordingly.
- Keep catheter under gravity drainage/continuous suction, as needed.
- Keep complete bed rest for 3–4 h and abstain from strenuous activities.
- Start clear liquid diet for the first hour, then regular diet thereafter if tolerated and otherwise not contraindicated.
- Check vital signs every 15 min for 1 h, every 30 min for 1 h, and then every 60 min for 2 h.
- Inform interventional radiology team if systolic blood pressure <95 mm Hg, heart rate >100 beats per minute, or if any chest pain,

abdominal pain, or shortness of breath develops.

- If signs of peritonitis, bowel obstruction, or enteric fluid draining from the catheter are observed, perform catheter injection to check position, detect any fistula and identify free peritoneal leak.
- In case of persistent high output from the catheter *(more than 50 mL per day)* for 4–5 days after catheter insertion, perform catheter injection to determine the presence of a fistula to the biliary system, pancreatic duct, or bowel loops.
- Daily catheter care:
  - Inspect catheter and make sure that the 3-way stopcock is open to the drainage bag and the catheter has not been externally retracted.
  - Flush the catheter with 20 mL of bacteriostatic saline every 8 h; 10 mL toward the drainage bag and 10 mL toward the collection.
  - Record the catheter output every 8 h.
  - Inform interventional radiology team if the draining amount decreases, pericatheter leak, or local skin complications occurs.
- Catheter can be removed safely when there is evidence of clinical improvement and imaging features that favor catheter removal
  - Resolution of fever.
  - Absence of leukocytosis or other septic parameters.
  - Daily drainage via the catheter of less than 20 mL in the absence of catheter-related problems that might explain reduced output, such as catheter malposition, blockage, or kinking.
  - Demonstration of a well-drained cavity with no residual compartments at ultrasonography, computed tomography, or sinography *(tubography)*.
  - No evidence of a fistula at sinography *(tubography)*.
- Perform tractography prior to removal of catheters draining by the transpleural or transperitoneal route to confirm the maturity of the tract.

Impression:

- Percutaneous drainage of abdominal/pelvic collection, as described above.
- The patient tolerated the procedure well and left the interventional unit in a stable condition.
- The patient was unstable and the procedure was canceled/terminated prematurely.
- List any other relevant or important information/finding.

References

1. Thabet A, Arellano RS. Catheter drainage of abdominal abscesses and fluid collections. In: Kandarpa K, Machan L, editors. Handbook of interventional radiologic procedures. 4th ed. Philadelphia: Lippincott Williams & Wilkins; 2011. p. 527–36.
2. Wallace MJ, Chin KW, Fletcher TB, Bakal CW, Cardella JF, Grassi CJ, et al. Quality improvement guidelines for percutaneous drainage/aspiration of abscess and fluid collections. J Vasc Interv Radiol. 2010;21(4):431–5.
3. Campbell JJ, Gervais DA. Percutaneous abscess drainage within the abdomen and pelvis. In: Murphy KPJ, Thomson KR, Venbrux AC, Morgan RA, editors. Image-guided interventions. 2nd ed. Philadelphia: Saunders Elsevier; 2014. p. 923–31.
4. Bakal CW, Sacks D, Burke DR, Cardella JF, Chopra PS, Dawson SL, et al. Quality improvement guidelines for adult percutaneous abscess and fluid drainage. J Vasc Interv Radiol. 2003;14(9 Pt 2):S223–5.
5. Venkatesan AM, Kundu S, Sacks D, Wallace MJ, Wojak JC, Rose SC, et al. Practice guidelines for adult antibiotic prophylaxis during vascular and interventional radiology procedures. J Vasc Interv Radiol. 2010;21(11):1611–30.
6. Maher MM, Kealey S, McNamara A, O'Laoide R, Gibney RG, Malone DE. Management of visceral interventional radiology catheters: a troubleshooting guide for interventional radiologists. Radiographics. 2002;22(2):305–22.

Catheter Drainage of Ascites

67

Bedros Taslakian

INTRODUCTION

The development of large-volume ascites can cause significant morbidity, markedly decreasing the patient's quality of life. The goal of management is the effective relief of symptoms in the safest, most convenient manner for the patient. Paracentesis or placement of a drainage catheter is often necessary.

COMMON INDICATIONS [1–5]

- Fluid characterization
- Treatment of sepsis in patients with infected ascites
- Symptomatic ascites that warrant drainage
- Ascites drainage prior to abdominal interventions to decrease the risk of uncontrolled bleeding *(e.g., liver biopsy, percutaneous biliary interventions, gastrostomy)*

COMMON CONTRAINDICATIONS [2, 4, 5]

- Significant coagulopathy that cannot be adequately corrected
- Hemodynamic instability
- Lack of safe pathway
- Inability of the patient to be positioned for the procedure

POSSIBLE COMPLICATIONS [2, 4, 5]

- Hemorrhage
- Enteric fistulas
- Peritonitis
- Bowel perforation
- Superinfection
- Injury of adjacent organs or vessels
- Catheter malfunction *(kinking, blockage, dislodgment)*
- Pericatheter leak
- Infection at the catheter insertion site
- Mortality

PREPROCEDURAL ASSESSMENT AND PLANNING

- History, indications, and physical examination *(Appendix 1* in Chap. 149*)*
- Evaluation of diagnostic imaging studies to determine the severity of the ascites, its possible causes, and the relevant anatomy
- Periprocedural management of coagulation status *(Appendices 2* in Chap. 150 *and 3* in Chap. 151*)*
- Antibiotic prophylaxis: Not routinely recommended unless infection is suspected *(i.e.,*

B. Taslakian (✉)
Department of Radiology, New York University Langone Medical Center, 660 First Ave, New York, NY 10016, USA
e-mail: btaslakian@gmail.com

B. Taslakian et al. (eds.), *Procedural Dictations in Image-Guided Intervention*,
DOI 10.1007/978-3-319-40845-3_67

primary bacterial peritonitis) (Appendices 4 in Chap. 152 *and 5* in Chap. 153*)*
- Imaging modality for guidance: CT, ultrasound
- Positioning: Oblique, supine

PROCEDURE NOTE

Procedure: Percutaneous drainage of ascites
Staff: [_]
Fellow: [_]
Resident: [_]
Clinical Information: Describe history and list indications
Allergies: None known/Allergic to [specify/type of allergy]
Anesthesia: Local anesthesia/conscious sedation
Medications: List any relevant medications used (sedation, antibiotics)
Field: Sterile
Procedure classification: Clean/Dirty (primary bacterial peritonitis)
Position: Supine/Oblique
Monitoring: Intravenous access line was secured and vital signs were continuously monitored by nursing staff/anesthesia team throughout the procedure
Cumulative radiation dose: (_) mGy

Description of Procedure:

The risks, benefits, alternatives, and the procedure itself were explained to the patient/patient's Power of Attorney/legal guardian, and informed written/verbal consent was obtained. The site of the procedure was identified and marked. Time out was performed to confirm the correct patient, procedure, and site.

The abdomen was evaluated using ultrasound/CT imaging after placement of a radiopaque marker/grid and showed a small/moderate/large amount of ascites. The procedure was planned and the skin puncture site was marked using combined information from the preliminary CT/ultrasound images. The angle of needle entry and the distance to the peritoneal cavity were calculated from the planning images.

The skin was prepped and draped in the usual sterile fashion. Local anesthesia was administered. A small skin incision was made. Subsequently, a (_)-gauge [type] needle was advanced through the abdominal wall of the right/left lower quadrant into the peritoneal cavity under direct ultrasound visualization/using planning CT information. (_) mL of clear fluid/serosanguineous fluid/blood/malodorous pus was aspirated, and sent for culture/gram stain/cytology/chemistry. A (_)-inch [type] guide wire was advanced through the needle into the peritoneal cavity and the tract was dilated up to the required size using (_)-French dilator(s). A (_)-French self-retaining [type/pigtail] catheter assembly with the metal stiffener was introduced over the guide wire to a satisfactory depth. The stiff trocar of the catheter was left within the shaft until the catheter traversed the skin abdominal wall. The guide wire and metal stiffener were removed, after advancing the catheter into the peritoneal cavity. The catheter was locked, anchored to the skin, and attached to a drainage system. Following this, ultrasound/CT images were obtained through the drainage area to confirm the position of the tube.

The patient was transferred to the floor/recovery room/discharged home following the procedure in a stable condition. Staff was present for the entire procedure.

Intra-Procedure Findings: List all the relevant findings.
Immediate Complications: None were encountered during or directly after the procedure. List the complications if any.

Post-Procedure Plan [2, 6]:

- Follow-up laboratory results and adjust antibiotics treatment accordingly.
- Keep catheter under gravity drainage.
- Keep complete bed rest for 3–4 h and abstain from strenuous activities.
- Start clear liquid diet for the first hour, then regular diet thereafter if tolerated and otherwise not contraindicated.
- Check vital signs every 15 min for 1 h, then every 30 min for 1 h.
- Inform interventional radiology team if systolic blood pressure <95 mm Hg, heart rate >100 beats per minute, or if any chest pain,

abdominal pain, or shortness of breath develops.
- If signs of peritonitis, bowel obstruction, or enteric fluid draining from the catheter are observed, perform catheter injection to check position and detect any fistula.
- Daily catheter care:
  - Inspect catheter and make sure that the 3-way stopcock is open to the drainage bag and the catheter has not been externally retracted.
  - Flush the catheter with 20 mL of bacteriostatic saline every 8 h; 10 mL toward the drainage bag and 10 mL toward the peritoneal cavity.
  - Record the catheter output every 8 h.
  - Inform interventional radiology team if the draining amount decreases, pericatheter leak or local skin complications occurs.
- Catheters draining an infected ascites can be removed safely when there is evidence of clinical improvement and imaging features that favor catheter removal:
  - Resolution of fever.
  - Absence of leukocytosis or other septic parameters.
  - Daily drainage via the catheter of less than 20 mL in the absence of catheter-related problems that might explain reduced output, such as catheter malposition, blockage, or kinking.
  - Demonstration of resolution of the ascites on imaging studies.

Impression:
- Percutaneous catheter drainage of ascites, as described above.
- The patient tolerated the procedure well and left the interventional unit in a stable condition.
- The patient was unstable and the procedure was canceled/terminated prematurely.
- List any other relevant or important information/finding.

References

1. Yu H, Stavas JM. The role of interventional radiology in management of benign and malignant gynecologic diseases. Obstet Gynecol Surv. 2013;68(10):691–701.
2. Thabet A, Arellano RS. Catheter drainage of abdominal abscesses and fluid collections. In: Kandarpa K, Machan L, editors. Handbook of interventional radiologic procedures. 4th ed. Philadelphia: Lippincott Williams & Wilkins; 2011. p. 527–36.
3. Hunter DW. Percutaneous biliary interventions. In: Kandarpa K, Machan L, editors. Handbook of interventional radiologic procedures. 4th ed. Philadelphia: Lippincott Williams & Wilkins; 2011. p. 577–90.
4. Wallace MJ, Chin KW, Fletcher TB, Bakal CW, Cardella JF, Grassi CJ, et al. Quality improvement guidelines for percutaneous drainage/aspiration of abscess and fluid collections. J Vasc Interv Radiol. 2010;21(4):431–5.
5. Bakal CW, Sacks D, Burke DR, Cardella JF, Chopra PS, Dawson SL, et al. Quality improvement guidelines for adult percutaneous abscess and fluid drainage. J Vasc Interv Radiol. 2003;14(9 Pt 2):S223–5.
6. Maher MM, Kealey S, McNamara A, O'Laoide R, Gibney RG, Malone DE. Management of visceral interventional radiology catheters: a troubleshooting guide for interventional radiologists. Radiographics. 2002;22(2):305–22.

Celiac Plexus Neurolysis and Block

68

Bedros Taslakian

INTRODUCTION

Chronic refractory abdominal pain is a common problem in patients with chronic pancreatitis and upper abdominal malignancies, significantly affecting the quality of life. The celiac plexus, which is the largest visceral plexus, is a network of ganglia serving as a relay center for nociceptive impulses that originate from upper abdominal viscera. It is located deep in the retroperitoneum, around the origin of the celiac trunk over the anterolateral surface of the aorta between T12-L1 and L2. Refractory visceral abdominal pain can be effectively diminished by percutaneous celiac plexus neurolysis or block, which helps reducing opioid requirements. Celiac plexus block is accomplished by injecting corticosteroids or long-acting local anesthetics to temporary disrupt pain transmission via the celiac plexus. On the other hand, celiac plexus neurolysis with ethanol or phenol is the permanent destruction of the ganglia used for long-term pain relief. Percutaneous celiac plexus neurolysis and block may be performed using various imaging modalities for guidance, through an anterior or posterior approach. Computed tomography allows direct visualization of the spread of the neurolytic agent in the antecrural space and has superseded other modalities for imaging guidance.

COMMON INDICATIONS [1–3]

- Persistent and intractable abdominal pain caused by pancreatic, gastric, esophageal, or biliary malignancy
- Persistent and intractable abdominal pain caused by metastatic liver disease and retroperitoneal lymph node disease
- Severe nausea and vomiting in patients with pancreatic cancer
- Chronic refractory abdominal pain in patients with chronic pancreatitis

COMMON CONTRAINDICATIONS [1–3]

- Uncooperative or unwilling patients
- Lack of a safe pathway to the anatomic location
- Significant coagulopathy and thrombocytopenia that cannot be adequately corrected
- Local or intra-abdominal infection and sepsis
- Bowel obstruction
- Presence of large soft-tissue masses obscuring the retroperitoneal fat planes
- Significant direct tumor invasion of the celiac plexus

B. Taslakian (✉)
Department of Radiology, New York University Langone Medical Center, 660 First Ave, New York, NY 10016, USA
e-mail: btaslakian@gmail.com

B. Taslakian et al. (eds.), *Procedural Dictations in Image-Guided Intervention*,
DOI 10.1007/978-3-319-40845-3_68

- Hypotension
- Pain caused by diffuse or multifocal metastasis to the skeleton and muscle

POSSIBLE COMPLICATIONS [1–3]

- Procedure-related back pain, *96 %*; often radiating to the shoulder *(can persist for up to 72 h)*
- Infection *(e.g., retroperitoneal abscess)*
- Orthostatic hypotension, *10–52 %*
- Transient diarrhea, *44 %*
- Chronic diarrhea, *rare*
- Pleural transgression *(e.g., pneumothorax, hemothorax, pleuritis)*
- Organ injury *(e.g., gastric perforation, pancreatic fistula, and subcapsular liver hematoma)*
- Neurologic injuries, < *0.15 %*; *(e.g., monoplegia and anal and bladder sphincter dysfunction)*
- Arterial injury *(e.g., dissection)*
- Local hematoma
- Retroperitoneal hemorrhage *(transaortic approach)*
- Transient hematuria
- Pericarditis
- Intervertebral disk injury *(trans-intervertebral approach)*
- Urinoma formation *(when traversing renal parenchyma)*
- Chemical peritonitis
- Mortality, *rare*

PREPROCEDURAL ASSESSMENT AND PLANNING [1–5]

- History, indications and physical examination *(Appendix 1* in Chap. 149*)*
  - Complete preprocedure neurologic examination as a baseline for assessing possible neurologic complications
  - Record the patient's baseline pain intensity on a subjective scale, to assess the effectiveness of treatment
- Evaluation of diagnostic imaging studies to determine the relevant anatomy and thus the patient position, imaging approach and site of neurolytic agent injection
- Periprocedural management of coagulation status *(Appendices 2* in Chap. 150 and *3* in Chap. 151*)*
- Antibiotic prophylaxis: Not routinely recommended
- Imaging modality for guidance: CT, CT fluoroscopy, ultrasound, fluoroscopy, MRI [3]
- Positioning: select the position that allows the shortest and least complicated route to the celiac plexus [1–3]
  - *Prone:* Used most frequently as it facilitates a bilateral posterior antecrural approach
  - *Lateral Decubitus:* often used with a posterior approach in patients who are unable to lie prone
  - *Supine:* the most comfortable position for patients and is used with an anterior antecrural or a lateral approach
  - *Oblique:* used with a bilateral posterior antecrural approach

PROCEDURE NOTE

Procedure: Celiac plexus neurolysis/block
Staff: [_]
Fellow: [_]
Resident: [_]
Clinical Information: Describe history and list indications
Allergies: None known/Allergic to [specify/type of allergy]
Anesthesia: Local anesthesia/conscious sedation
Medications: List any relevant medications used (sedation, antibiotics, blocking and neurolytic agents)
Field: Sterile
Procedure classification: Clean
Position: Supine/Prone/Left lateral decubitus/Right lateral decubitus/Oblique
Monitoring: Intravenous access line was secured and vital signs were continuously monitored by nursing staff/anesthesia team throughout the procedure
Cumulative radiation dose: (_) mGy

Description of Procedure *(Bilateral posterior para-vertebral antecrural approach):*

The risks, benefits, alternatives and the procedure itself were explained to the patient/patient's Power of Attorney/patient's legal guardian, and informed written consent was obtained. The site of the procedure was identified and marked. Time out was performed to confirm the correct patient, procedure and site.

Bilateral posterior para-vertebral antecrural approach was selected and the patient was positioned. Planning unenhanced CT examination was performed to localize the celiac artery and plexus, select the puncture site, determine the angle and depth of needle entry, identify the needle path, and determine the site of injection.

The skin was prepped and draped in the usual sterile fashion. Local anesthesia was administered. Subsequently, using planning CT information, a (20/24)-gauge [Chiba/type] needle was advanced alongside the vertebral bodies on each side into the antecrural space. After the position of the needle tip was confirmed, aspiration was performed, no blood return was observed and (5) mL of dilute iodinated contrast material was injected into the antecrural space. After confirming free diffusion of contrast material in the antecrural space and absence of numbness or motor dysfunction in the lower extremities, approximately (_) mL of Marcaine solution was injected followed by injection of (_) mL of neurolytic/blocking agent through the needle and into the antecrural space on each side. Completion CT images showed diffuse spread of the solution in the preaortic space. Before the needle was withdrawn, (5) mL of normal saline solution was injected to minimize the risk of spreading any neurolytic/blocking agent that remains in the needle and prevent the burning pain that results from leakage into the puncture route.

The patient was transferred to the floor/recovery room following the procedure in a stable condition. Staff was present for the entire procedure.

Description of Procedure *(Anterior approach):*

The risks, benefits, alternatives and the procedure itself were explained to the patient/patient's Power of Attorney/patient's legal guardian, and informed written consent was obtained. The site of the procedure was identified and marked. Time out was performed to confirm the correct patient, procedure and site.

Anterior approach was selected and the patient was positioned in a supine position. Planning unenhanced CT examination was performed to localize the celiac artery and celiac plexus, select the puncture site, determine the angle and depth of needle entry, identify the needle path to the celiac plexus, and determine the site of neurolytic/blocking agent injection.

The skin was prepped and draped in the usual sterile fashion. Local anesthesia was administered. Subsequently, using planning CT information, a (20/24)-gauge [Chiba/type] needle was advanced through the anterior abdominal wall and the liver, along the planned trajectory into the antecrural space on each side. After the position of the needle tip was confirmed, aspiration was performed, no blood return was observed and (5) mL of diluted iodinated contrast material was injected into the antecrural space. After confirming free diffusion of contrast material and absence of numbness or motor dysfunction in the lower extremities, approximately (_) mL Marcaine solution was injected, followed by injection of (_) mL of neurolytic/blocking agent through the needle into the antecrural space on each side. Completion CT images showed diffuse spread of the solution in the preaortic space. Before the needle was withdrawn, (5) mL of normal saline solution was injected to minimize the risk of spreading any neurolytic/blocking agent that remains in the needle and prevent the burning pain that results from leakage into the puncture route.

The patient was transferred to the floor/recovery room following the procedure in a stable condition. Staff was present for the entire procedure.

Description of Procedure *(Posterior trans-intervertebral disk approach):*

The risks, benefits, alternatives and the procedure itself were explained to the patient/patient's Power of Attorney/patient's legal guardian, and informed written consent was obtained. The site of the procedure was identified and marked. Time out was performed to confirm the correct patient, procedure and site.

Posterior trans-intervertebral disk approach was selected and the patient was positioned in a prone position. Planning unenhanced CT examination was performed to localize the celiac artery and celiac plexus, select the puncture site, determine the angle and depth of needle entry, identify the percutaneous needle path, and determine the site of neurolytic/blocking agent injection.

The skin was prepped and draped in the usual sterile fashion. Local anesthesia was administered. Subsequently, using planning CT information, a (20/24)-gauge [Chiba/type] needle was advanced through the posterior abdominal wall, traversing T12-L1/L1-L2 intervertebral disk to reach the antecrural, paraaortic space. After confirming the position of the needle tip, aspiration was performed, no blood return was observed and (5) mL of diluted iodinated contrast material was injected into the antecrural space. After confirming free diffusion of contrast material and absence of numbness or motor dysfunction in the lower extremities, approximately (_) mL of Marcaine solution was injected, followed by injection of (_) mL of neurolytic/blocking agent through the needle and into the antecrural space on each side. Completion CT images showed diffuse spread of the solution in the preaortic space. Before the needle was withdrawn, (5) mL of normal saline solution was injected to minimize the risk of spreading any neurolytic/blocking agent that remains in the needle and prevent the burning pain that results from leakage into the puncture route.

The patient was transferred to the floor/recovery room following the procedure in a stable condition. Staff was present for the entire procedure.

Intra-Procedure Findings: List all relevant findings.

Immediate Complications: None encountered during or directly after the procedure. List complications if any.

Post-Procedure Physical Examination: Neurological examination directly after the procedure showed no evidence of neurologic deficit, or loss of bladder and bowel function. List all relevant findings.

Post-Procedure Plan [1–3]

- Obtain chest X-ray or CT scan to rule out pneumothorax if pleural space transgression is suspected.
- Complete bed rest for 12 h, bathroom use with assistance.
- Administer supplemental nasal oxygen *(if a small pneumothorax develops).*
- Monitor vital signs in recovery area every 15 min for 1 h, then every 30 min for 2 h, then every hour.
- Inform interventional radiology team if systolic blood pressure <95 mm Hg, heart rate >100 beats per minute, or if any chest pain or shortness of breath develops.
- Adequate fluid replacement in the form of intravenous fluids as needed.
- Perform a focused motor and sensory neurologic examination of the lower extremities every 8 h, to detect neurologic complications.

Impression:

- Percutaneous celiac plexus neurolysis/block, as described above.
- The patient tolerated the procedure well and left the interventional unit in a stable condition.
- The patient was unstable and the procedure was canceled/terminated prematurely.
- List any other relevant or important information/finding.

References

1. Nitschke AM, Ray CE Jr. Percutaneous neurolytic celiac plexus block. Semin Interv Radiol. 2013;30 (3):318–21.
2. Wang PJ, Shang MY, Qian Z, Shao CW, Wang JH, Zhao XH. CT-guided percutaneous neurolytic celiac plexus block technique. Abdom Imaging. 2006;31 (6):710–8.
3. Kambadakone A, Thabet A, Gervais DA, Mueller PR, Arellano RS. CT-guided celiac plexus neurolysis: a review of anatomy, indications, technique, and tips for successful treatment. Radiographics. 2011;31 (6):1599–621.
4. Taslakian B, Sebaaly MG, Al-Kutoubi A. Patient evaluation and preparation in vascular and interventional radiology: what every interventional radiologist should know (part 1: patient assessment and laboratory tests). Cardiovasc Intervent Radiol. 2016;39(3): 325–33.
5. Taslakian B, Sebaaly MG, Al-Kutoubi A. Patient evaluation and preparation in vascular and interventional radiology: what every interventional radiologist should know (part 2: patient preparation and medications). Cardiovasc Intervent Radiol. 2016;39(4):489–99. doi: 10.1007/s00270-015-1239-4. [Epub 2015 Nov 25].

Core Biopsy of Abdominopelvic Lesions

69

Bedros Taslakian

INTRODUCTION

Image-guided percutaneous needle biopsy is an established, safe, and effective procedure for selected patients with suspected pathologic processes and associated with low morbidity and mortality. The key to these procedures has been the use of imaging guidance, which allows for the safe passage of a needle into a lesion. Knowing that, access route planning for percutaneous biopsy of deep abdominal and pelvic masses may be challenging because vital structures often obstruct the projected needle path and various alternative approaches can be used.

COMMON INDICATIONS [1–4]

- Diagnosis of primary malignancy
- Diagnosis of benign lesions
- Confirmation of suspected metastatic disease for staging
- Monitoring response to treatment in patients with known malignancy
- To obtain material for microbiologic analysis in patients with suspected or known infections refractory to antimicrobial therapy

COMMON CONTRAINDICATIONS [1–4]

- Uncooperative patients
- Lack of a safe pathway to the lesion
- Unsafe target for biopsy, such as highly vascular tumors
- Significant coagulopathy that cannot be adequately corrected
- Hemodynamic instability
- Pregnancy in cases when imaging guidance involves ionizing radiation
- Suspected hydatid cysts *(increased risk of anaphylactic shock)*
- Large volume ascites *(consider drainage before the procedure)*

POSSIBLE COMPLICATIONS [1–5]

- Pain and discomfort
- Vasovagal reaction
- Major hemorrhage requiring transfusion or intervention, *0.1–3 %*
- Infection
- Pleural transgression requiring intervention, *0.5 %*
- Unintended organ injury *(primary or adjacent organ)*
- Malignant seeding of the needle tract, *0–3.4 %*
- Mortality, *rare*

B. Taslakian (✉)
Department of Radiology, New York University Langone Medical Center, 660 First Ave, New York, NY 10016, USA
e-mail: btaslakian@gmail.com

B. Taslakian et al. (eds.), *Procedural Dictations in Image-Guided Intervention*,
DOI 10.1007/978-3-319-40845-3_69

PREPROCEDURAL ASSESSMENT AND PLANNING [6–8]

- History, indications, and physical examination *(Appendix 1* in Chap. 149*)*
- Evaluation of diagnostic imaging studies to determine the location of the lesion and relevant anatomy
- Periprocedural management of coagulation status *(Appendices 2* in Chap. 150 and *3* in Chap. 151*)*
- Antibiotic prophylaxis: Not routinely recommended [6] *(Appendices 4* in Chap. 152 and *5* in Chap. 153*)*
- Imaging modality for guidance: CT, CT fluoroscopy, ultrasound, PET
- Positioning: Oblique, lateral decubitus, supine, prone

PROCEDURE NOTE

Procedure: Core biopsy of [specify organ/location]
Staff: [_]
Fellow: [_]
Resident: [_]
Clinical Information: Describe history and list indications
Allergies: None known/Allergic to [specify/type of allergy]
Anesthesia: Local anesthesia/conscious sedation
Medications: List any relevant medications used (sedation, antibiotics)
Field: Sterile
Procedure classification: Clean
Position: Supine/Prone/Left lateral decubitus/Right lateral decubitus/Oblique
Monitoring: Intravenous access line was secured and vital signs were continuously monitored by nursing staff/anesthesia team throughout the procedure
Cumulative radiation dose: (_) mGy

Description of Procedure:

The risks, benefits, alternatives, and the procedure itself were explained to the patient/patient's Power of Attorney/patient's legal guardian, and informed written consent was obtained. The site of the procedure was identified and marked. Time out was performed to confirm the correct patient, procedure, and site.

The abdomen/pelvis was evaluated using CT imaging after placement of a radiopaque marker/grid/ultrasound showing a (_) cm round/oval/irregular lesion in [specify organ/location]. The procedure was planned and the skin puncture site was marked using combined information from the location of the lesion and preliminary CT/ultrasound images. The angle of needle entry and the distance to the lesion were calculated from the planning images.

The skin was prepped and draped in the usual sterile fashion. Local anesthesia was administered. A small skin incision was made. Subsequently, using planning CT information/using CT fluoroscopy/under direct ultrasound visualization, a (_)-gauge [type] needle guide was advanced along the planned trajectory until the needle tip reached the target lesion, confirmed by imaging. (_) samples were obtained using the coaxial technique, placed in a formalin solution and sent for histopathological evaluation. Following this, immediate completion CT/ultrasound images were obtained at the level of the biopsy site.

The patient was transferred to the floor/recovery room following the procedure in a stable condition. Staff was present for the entire procedure.

Intra-Procedure Findings: List all relevant findings.
Immediate Complications: None encountered during or directly after the procedure. List complications if any.

Post-Procedure Plan [1–3]

- Follow-up histopathology results.
- Obtain an upright chest X-ray or chest CT scan to rule out pneumothorax if pleural transgression is suspected.
- When post-biopsy images show no complications
  - Observe the patient in the recovery room following the procedure for 2 h.

- Complete bed rest for 1–2 h, bathroom use with assistance.
- Administer supplemental nasal oxygen *(if a small pneumothorax develops).*
- Monitor vital signs in recovery area every 15 min for 1 h, then every 30 min for 2 h, then every hour.
- If the patient's condition deteriorates during observation, obtain images of the abdomen immediately.
- Discharge patient after 2 h if vital signs are stable and no complications are noted.
  Discharge Instructions:
  Abstain from strenuous activities for 3 days.
  Visit the nearest emergency room promptly if any chest pain, abdominal pain or shortness of breath develops.
  Start clear liquid diet for the first hour, then regular diet thereafter if tolerated and no complications occur.

Impression:

- Percutaneous needle biopsy of [specify organ/location] lesion, as described above.
- The patient tolerated the procedure well and left the interventional unit in a stable condition.
- The patient was unstable and the procedure was canceled/terminated prematurely.
- List any other relevant or important information/finding.

References

1. Percutaneous biopsy. In: Burke CT, Dixon RG, Mauro MA, Murphy KPJ, Thomson KR, Venbrux AC, Zollikofer CL, editors. High yield imaging: interventional. Philadelphia: Saunders Elsevier; 2010. p. 384–5.
2. Silverman SG, Segal D. Abdominal biopsies. In: Kandarpa K, Machan L, editors. Handbook of interventional radiologic procedures. 4th ed. Philadelphia: Lippincott Williams & Wilkins; 2011. p. 516–26.
3. Desai SB, Lewandowski RJ, Nemcek AA Jr. Percutaneous biopsy. In: Murphy KPJ, Thomson KR, Venbrux AC, Morgan RA, editors. Image-guided interventions. 2nd ed. Philadelphia: Saunders Elsevier; 2014. p. 918–22.
4. Gupta S, Wallace MJ, Cardella JF, Kundu S, Miller DL, Rose SC. Quality improvement guidelines for percutaneous needle biopsy. J Vasc Interv Radiol. 2010;21(7):969–75.
5. Gupta S, Nguyen HL, Morello FA Jr, Ahrar K, Wallace MJ, Madoff DC, et al. Various approaches for CT-guided percutaneous biopsy of deep pelvic lesions: anatomic and technical considerations. Radiographics. 2004;24(1):175–89.
6. Venkatesan AM, Kundu S, Sacks D, Wallace MJ, Wojak JC, Rose SC, et al. Practice guidelines for adult antibiotic prophylaxis during vascular and interventional radiology procedures. J Vasc Interv Radiol. 2010;21(11):1611–30.
7. Taslakian B, Sebaaly MG, Al-Kutoubi A. Patient evaluation and preparation in vascular and interventional radiology: what every interventional radiologist should know (part 1: patient assessment and laboratory tests). Cardiovasc Intervent Radiol. 2016;39(3):325–33.
8. Taslakian B, Sebaaly MG, Al-Kutoubi A. Patient evaluation and preparation in vascular and interventional radiology: what every interventional radiologist should know (part 2: patient preparation and medications). Cardiovasc Intervent Radiol. 2016;39(4):489–99. doi: 10.1007/s00270-015-1239-4. [Epub 2015 Nov 25].

Exchange of Drainage Catheter 70

Bedros Taslakian

INTRODUCTION

Image-guided exchange of a drain, usually performed under fluoroscopy guidance, is a simple and safe procedure used in cases of blockage or malposition of, or to upsize, an existing catheter without the need for de novo puncture.

COMMON INDICATIONS [1, 2]

- Tube malfunction *(malposition, dislodgement, kinking, clotting)*
- Exchange of a previously inserted catheter for a larger catheter

COMMON CONTRAINDICATIONS [2, 3]

- Uncooperative patients
- Hemodynamic instability
- Pregnancy
- Complete dislodgment of the catheter *(access can be regained depending on tract maturity)*

POSSIBLE COMPLICATIONS [2]

- Migration of the string ahead of the guidewire during exchange
- Snaring of adjacent internal stent by the pigtail during exchange
- Catheter fracture
- Superinfection of a sterile fluid collection
- Catheter malfunction *(malposition, dislodgement, kinking, clotting)*

PREPROCEDURAL ASSESSMENT AND PLANNING [4–7]

- History, indications and physical examination *(Appendix 1* in Chap. 149*)*
- Evaluation of diagnostic imaging studies to determine the location of the collection, its size, the relevant anatomy and the position of the indwelling catheter
- Periprocedural management of coagulation status *(Appendices 2* in Chap. 150 and *3* in Chap. 151*)*
- Antibiotic prophylaxis: Required when draining abscess or potentially infected collection [4, 5]
- Imaging modality for guidance: Fluoroscopy [5]
- Positioning: Oblique, lateral decubitus, prone, supine

B. Taslakian (✉)
Department of Radiology, New York University Langone Medical Center, 660 First Ave, New York, NY 10016, USA
e-mail: btaslakian@gmail.com

B. Taslakian et al. (eds.), *Procedural Dictations in Image-Guided Intervention*,
DOI 10.1007/978-3-319-40845-3_70

PROCEDURE NOTE

Procedure: Fluoroscopy-guided exchange of abdominal/pelvic drainage catheter
Staff: [_]
Fellow: [_]
Resident: [_]
Clinical Information: Describe history and list indications
Allergies: None known/Allergic to [specify/type of allergy]
Anesthesia: Local anesthesia/conscious sedation
Medications: List any relevant medications used (sedation, antibiotics)
Contrast Material: (_) mL of [type] contrast material was used for tubogram/Not required
Field: Sterile
Procedure classification: Clean/Dirty
Position: Supine/Prone/Left lateral decubitus/Right lateral decubitus/Oblique
Monitoring: Intravenous access line was secured and vital signs were continuously monitored by nursing staff/anesthesia team throughout the procedure
Cumulative radiation dose: (_) mGy

Description of Procedure:
The risks, benefits, alternatives and procedure itself were explained to the patient/patient's Power of Attorney/patient's legal guardian, and informed written consent was obtained. The site of the procedure was identified and marked. Time out was performed to confirm the correct patient, procedure and site.

The skin and the existing catheter were prepared by using standard sterile procedures. A plain radiograph was obtained to document the site of catheter entry through the patient's skin by placing a metal forceps over the site of the skin entry. A small amount of diluted contrast material was injected through the catheter to assess catheter patency, the size of the cavity and the position of the catheter within the cavity. The catheter was then cut/unlocked by releasing the self-locking mechanism. A (_)-inch [type] guidewire was advanced through the existing catheter and coiled in the cavity, under fluoroscopy guidance. Once there was a sufficient length of guidewire within the cavity, the old catheter was withdrawn over the guidewire. A new (_)-French self-retaining [type/pigtail] catheter assembly with the metal/plastic stiffener was advanced over the guidewire to a satisfactory depth. The guidewire and stiffener were removed after advancing the catheter into the cavity. Following this, contrast material was injected through the catheter at the end of the procedure to confirm optimal catheter position and ensure that all side holes were placed within the cavity. The catheter was locked, anchored to the skin and attached to a drainage system.

The patient was transferred to the floor/recovery room/discharged home following the procedure in a stable condition. Staff were present for the entire procedure.
Intra-Procedure Findings: List all relevant findings.
Immediate Complications: None encountered during or directly after the procedure. List complications if any.

Post-Procedure Plan [2, 5]**:**
- Follow-up laboratory results if applicable.
- Keep catheter under dependent drainage or low continuous suction (20–30 cm water) as needed.
- Daily catheter care:
  - Inspect catheter and make sure that the three-way stopcock is open to the drainage bag and the catheter has not been externally retracted.
  - Flush the catheter with 20 mL of bacteriostatic saline every 8 h; 10 mL towards the drainage system and 10 mL towards the cavity.
  - Record the catheter output every 8 h.
  - Inform interventional radiology team if the draining amount decreases, peri-catheter leak or local skin complications occurs.
- Catheter can be removed safely when there is evidence of clinical improvement and imaging features that favor catheter removal:
  - Resolution of fever.
  - Absence of leukocytosis or other septic parameters.

- Daily drainage via the catheter of less than 20 mL in the absence of catheter-related problems that might explain reduced output, such as catheter malposition, blockage, or kinking.
- Demonstrations of a well-drained cavity with no residual compartments or loculi on cross sectional imaging or sinography.
- No evidence of a fistula at sinography *(tubography)*.
- Perform tractography prior to removal of catheters draining by the transpleural or transperitoneal route to confirm tract maturity.

Impression:

- Exchange of abdominal/pelvic drainage catheter, as described above.
- The patient tolerated the procedure well and left the interventional unit in a stable condition.
- The patient was unstable and the procedure was canceled/terminated prematurely.
- List any other relevant or important information/finding.

References

1. Nair AV, D'Agostino HR. Transcatheter fluid drainage. In: Valji K, editor. The practice of interventional radiology. Philadelphia: Saunders Elsevier; 2010. p. 106–25.
2. Maher MM, Kealey S, McNamara A, O'Laoide R, Gibney RG, Malone DE. Management of visceral interventional radiology catheters: a troubleshooting guide for interventional radiologists. Radiographics. 2002;22(2):305–22.
3. Wallace MJ, Chin KW, Fletcher TB, Bakal CW, Cardella JF, Grassi CJ, et al. Quality improvement guidelines for percutaneous drainage/aspiration of abscess and fluid collections. J Vasc Interv Radiol. 2010;21(4):431–5.
4. Venkatesan AM, Kundu S, Sacks D, Wallace MJ, Wojak JC, Rose SC, et al. Practice guidelines for adult antibiotic prophylaxis during vascular and interventional radiology procedures. J Vasc Interv Radiol. 2010;21(11):1611–30.
5. Thabet A, Arellano RS. Catheter drainage of abdominal abscesses and fluid collections. In: Kandarpa K, Machan L, editors. Handbook of interventional radiologic procedures. 4th ed. Philadelphia: Lippincott Williams & Wilkins; 2011. p. 527–36.
6. Taslakian B, Sebaaly MG, Al-Kutoubi A. Patient evaluation and preparation in vascular and interventional radiology: what every interventional radiologist should know (part 1: patient assessment and laboratory tests). Cardiovasc Intervent Radiol. 2016;39(3):325–33.
7. Taslakian B, Sebaaly MG, Al-Kutoubi A. Patient evaluation and preparation in vascular and interventional radiology: what every interventional radiologist should know (part 2: patient preparation and medications). Cardiovasc Intervent Radiol. 2016;39(4):489–99. doi: 10.1007/s00270-015-1239-4. [Epub 2015 Nov 25].

Fluoroscopy-Guided Lumbar Puncture

71

Roula Hourani

Abbreviations

CSF Cerebrospinal fluid

INTRODUCTION

Fluoroscopy-guided lumbar puncture is a commonly requested radiologic procedure, usually in the setting of a difficult or failed bedside lumbar puncture attempt. Compared with the conventional bedside approach, there is a higher success rate of obtaining cerebrospinal fluid (CSF) with fluoroscopic guidance because of the ability to visualize important bony landmarks and to avoid any adjacent obstructing degenerative bony changes.

COMMON INDICATIONS [1, 2]

- Suspicion of meningitis
- Suspicion of subarachnoid hemorrhage with negative CT scan of the brain
- Suspicion of central nervous system diseases such as Guillain–Barré syndrome, demyelinating disease, and carcinomatous meningitis
- Therapeutic relief of pseudotumor cerebri
- Measurement of CSF opening pressure
- Injection of anesthetic medications or chemotherapy drugs into the CSF

COMMON CONTRAINDICATIONS [1, 2]

- Findings suggestive of increased intracranial pressure seen on CT such as midline shift, loss of suprachiasmatic and basilar cisterns, posterior fossa mass, loss of the superior cerebellar cistern, or loss of the quadrigeminal plate cistern
- Coagulopathy
- Hemodynamically unstable patient
- Infection at the entry site

POSSIBLE COMPLICATIONS

- Headache, low back pain, injection site soreness
- Nerve root injury
- Nausea, vomiting
- Seizure
- Meningitis

R. Hourani (✉)
Department of Diagnostic Radiology, American University of Beirut Medical Center, Riad El Solh, Beirut 1107 2020, Lebanon
e-mail: rh64@aub.edu.lb

B. Taslakian et al. (eds.), *Procedural Dictations in Image-Guided Intervention*,
DOI 10.1007/978-3-319-40845-3_71

PREPROCEDURAL ASSESSMENT AND PLANNING [3, 4]

- History, indications, and physical examination *(Appendix 1* in Chap. 149*)*
- Evaluation of diagnostic imaging studies
- Periprocedural management of coagulation status *(Appendices 2* in Chap. 150 and *3* in Chap. 151*)*
- Antibiotics prophylaxis: No consensus. Prophylaxis not routinely recommended, although meticulous sterile technique and appropriate preprocedural preparation is mandatory.
- Imaging modality for guidance: Fluoroscopy
- Positioning: Prone, oblique

PROCEDURE NOTE

Procedure: Fluoroscopy-guided lumbar puncture
Staff: [_]
Fellow: [_]
Resident: [_]
Clinical Information: Describe history and list indications
Allergies: None known/Allergic to [specify/type of allergy]
Anesthesia: Local anesthesia/conscious sedation
Medications: List any relevant medications used (sedation, antibiotics)
Field: Sterile
Procedure classification: Clean
Position: Supine/Left lateral decubitus/Right lateral decubitus/Oblique
Monitoring: Intravenous access line was secured and vital signs were continuously monitored by nursing staff/anesthesia team throughout the procedure
Total fluoroscopy time: (_) minutes
Cumulative radiation dose: (_) mGy

Description of Procedure:

The risks, benefits, alternatives, and procedure itself were explained to the patient/patient's Power of Attorney/patient's legal guardian, and informed written consent was obtained. The site of the procedure was identified and marked. Time out was performed to confirm the correct patient, procedure, and site.

The patient was placed on the fluoroscopic table, and the lower back was prepped and draped in the usual sterile fashion. Under fluoroscopic guidance, the interlaminar space was localized, and overlying skin and subcutaneous tissue were infiltrated with Lidocaine. A (_) gauge, [_] inch styletted spinal needle was then inserted into the subarachnoid space, with free return of clear cerebrospinal fluid. CSF opening pressure was measured and documented (pressure cm H_2O). CSF samples were collected and sent to laboratory/( ) mL of CSF was drained/( ) mL of [name the medication and concentration] was injected slowly in the CSF space. At the end of procedure, the stylet was reinserted and the needle was removed. The skin was cleaned and sterile dressing was applied.

The patient was transferred to the floor/recovery room/discharged home following the procedure in a stable condition. Staff was present for the entire procedure.

Intra-Procedure Findings: List all relevant findings.

Immediate Complications: None encountered during or directly after the procedure. List complications if any.

Impression:

- Lumbar puncture, as described above.
- The patient tolerated the procedure well and left the interventional unit in stable condition.
- List any other relevant or important information/findings.

References

1. Farley A, McLafferty E. Lumbar puncture. Nurs Stand. 2008;22(22):46–8.
2. Cooper N. Lumbar puncture. Acute Med. 2011;10 (4):188–93.
3. Taslakian B, Sebaaly MG, Al-Kutoubi A. Patient evaluation and preparation in vascular and interventional radiology: what every interventional radiologist should know (part 1: patient assessment and laboratory tests). Cardiovasc Intervent Radiol. 2016;39(3):325–33.
4. Taslakian B, Sebaaly MG, Al-Kutoubi A. Patient evaluation and preparation in vascular and interventional radiology: what every interventional radiologist should know (part 2: patient preparation and medications). Cardiovasc Intervent Radiol. 2016;39(4):489–99. doi: 10.1007/s00270-015-1239-4. [Epub 2015 Nov 25].

Myelography

72

Roula Hourani

INTRODUCTION

Several imaging diagnostic tests exist for spinal disorders. Myelography is the fluoroscopically monitored intrathecal administration of a nonionic water-soluble iodinated contrast medium and has its own strengths and weaknesses. It is now mainly used when magnetic resonance imaging is not possible or inconclusive.

COMMON INDICATIONS [1, 2]

- Demonstration of the site of cerebrospinal fluid leak
- Evaluate spinal canal stenosis and nerve root impingement
- Diagnosis of lumbar disc herniation and presurgical assessment, when magnetic resonance imaging is contraindicated
- Diagnostic evaluation of spinal or basal cisternal disease or arachnoid cyst
- Postsurgical fusion assessment

COMMON CONTRAINDICATIONS [1, 2]

- Increased intracranial pressure
- Coagulation disorder

COMPLICATIONS [2–4]

- Headache, low back pain, injection site soreness
- Nerve roots injury
- Nausea, vomiting
- Seizure
- Meningitis

PREPROCEDURAL ASSESSMENT AND PLANNING [5, 6]

- History, indications, and physical examination *(Appendix 1* in Chap. 149*)*
- Evaluation of diagnostic imaging studies
- Periprocedural management of coagulation status *(Appendices 2* in Chap. 150 *and 3* in Chap. 151*)*
- Antibiotics prophylaxis: Prophylaxis not routinely recommended, although meticulous sterile technique and appropriate preprocedural preparation is mandatory
- Positioning: Prone, oblique

R. Hourani (✉)
Department of Diagnostic Radiology, American University of Beirut Medical Center, Riad El Solh, Beirut 1107 2020, Lebanon
e-mail: rh64@aub.edu.lb

B. Taslakian et al. (eds.), *Procedural Dictations in Image-Guided Intervention*,
DOI 10.1007/978-3-319-40845-3_72

PROCEDURE NOTE

Procedure: Myelography
Staff: [_]
Fellow: [_]
Resident: [_]
Clinical Information: Describe history and list indications
Allergies: None known/Allergic to [specify/type of allergy]
Anesthesia: Local anesthesia/conscious sedation
Medications: List any relevant medications used
Contrast Material: (_) mL of [type] contrast material was used for intrathecal injection
Field: Sterile
Procedure classification: Clean
Position: Prone/Oblique
Monitoring: Vital signs were continuously monitored by nursing staff/anesthesia team throughout the procedure
Total fluoroscopy time: (_) minutes
Cumulative radiation dose: (_) mGy

Description of Procedure:
The risks, benefits, alternatives, and procedure itself were explained to the patient/patient's Power of Attorney/patient's legal guardian, and informed written consent was obtained. The site of the procedure was identified and marked. Time out was performed to confirm the correct patient, procedure, and site.

The patient was placed on the fluoroscopic table, and the lower back was prepped and draped in the usual sterile fashion. Under fluoroscopic guidance, the interlaminar space was localized, and the overlying skin and subcutaneous tissue were infiltrated with local anesthesia. A (_) gauge, (_) inch styletted spinal needle was then inserted into the subarachnoid space, with free return of clear cerebrospinal fluid. (_) mL of [type/concentration] contrast material was then injected into the subarachnoid space under fluoroscopic guidance. The X-ray table was tilted slowly, allowing the contrast material to reach different levels in the spinal canal. At the end of procedure, the stylet was reinserted and the needle was removed. The flow was observed under fluoroscopy, and spot images were obtained with the table tilted at various angles. The patient was secured to the table top by a support device prior to being tilted into Trendelenburg/reverse Trendelenburg position. After the completion of the procedure, the patient was transferred to the CT suite for performance of CT myelography of the concerned anatomical area.
Intra-Procedure Findings: List all relevant findings.
Immediate Complications: None encountered during or directly after the procedure. List complications if any.
Post-Procedure Plan: Keep patient in bed rest for 2 h.

Impression:
- Myelography, as described above.
- The patient tolerated the procedure well and left the interventional unit in stable condition.
- List any other relevant or important information/findings.

References

1. Naderi S, Sonntag V. The current role of CT myelography and myelography in neurosurgical practice. Crit Rev Neurosurg. 1997;7:24–8.
2. Mathis JM, Johnson BA, Staats PS, Wetzel FT, editors. Image-guided spine interventions. New York: Springer; 2004.
3. Kennedy DJ, Dreyfuss P, Aprill CN, Bogduk N. Paraplegia following image guided transforaminal lumbar spine epidural steroid injection: two case reports. Pain Med. 2009;10(8):1389–94.
4. Karaman H, Kavak GO, Tüfek A, Yldrm ZB. The complications of transforaminal lumbar epidural steroid injections. Spine (Phila Pa 1976). 2011;36(13):E819–24.
5. Taslakian B, Sebaaly MG, Al-Kutoubi A. Patient evaluation and preparation in vascular and interventional radiology: what every interventional radiologist should know (part 1: patient assessment and laboratory tests). Cardiovasc Intervent Radiol. 2016;39(3):325–33.
6. Taslakian B, Sebaaly MG, Al-Kutoubi A. Patient evaluation and preparation in vascular and interventional radiology: what every interventional radiologist should know (part 2: patient preparation and medications). Cardiovasc Intervent Radiol. 2016;39(4):489–99. doi: 10.1007/s00270-015-1239-4. [Epub 2015 Nov 25].

Tractography (Pull-Out Tractography)

73

Bedros Taslakian

INTRODUCTION

It is essential to have a mature tract before removing catheters inserted into the biliary tract or an infected collection by the transpleural or transperitoneal route, to avoid leakage of bile or infected fluid. It usually takes around 3–6 weeks for the catheter tract to mature. However, tract formation can be significantly delayed due to immunosuppression or steroid therapy. Tractography can be performed prior to the removal of any catheter that requires a mature tract, to confirm adequate tract formation and to exclude a communication between the biliary tree and the arterial or portal venous system before removal of biliary catheters. It is performed under fluoroscopy guidance with injection of contrast media through the side port of a hemostatic sheath inserted over a guidewire.

COMMON INDICATIONS [1–3]

- Assess the tract prior to removal of catheters that require a mature tract:
  - Cholecystostomy catheters
  - Transpleural or transperitoneal catheters inserted into an infected collection or the biliary tract
  - Catheters inserted in critically ill or immunosuppressed patients or patients receiving steroids
- Exclude a biliary-arterial or biliary-portal communication before removal of biliary catheters

COMMON CONTRAINDICATIONS

- Presence of active infection
- Pregnancy

POSSIBLE COMPLICATIONS

- Loss of access into the system
- Pain
- Contrast extravasation
- Septic shock if contrast is injected into an infected cavity or system

PREPROCEDURAL ASSESSMENT AND PLANNING [4, 5]

- History, indications, and physical examination *(Appendix 1* in Chap. 149*)*
- Evaluation of diagnostic imaging studies to determine the position of the indwelling

B. Taslakian (✉)
Department of Radiology, New York University Langone Medical Center, 660 First Ave, New York, NY 10016, USA
e-mail: btaslakian@gmail.com

B. Taslakian et al. (eds.), *Procedural Dictations in Image-Guided Intervention*,
DOI 10.1007/978-3-319-40845-3_73

catheter, resolution of the abscess, and the relevant anatomy

- Periprocedural management of coagulation status *(Appendices 2* in Chap. 150 *and 3* in Chap. 151*)*
- Antibiotic prophylaxis: Not routinely recommended
- Imaging modality for guidance: Fluoroscopy [1]
- Positioning: Supine

PROCEDURE NOTE

Procedure: Fluoroscopy-guided tractography (Pull-Out Tractography)
Staff: [_]
Fellow: [_]
Resident: [_]
Clinical Information: Describe history and list indications
Allergies: None known/Allergic to [specify/type of allergy]
Anesthesia: Local anesthesia/conscious sedation
Medications: List any relevant medications used (sedation, antibiotics)
Contrast Material: (_) mL of [type] contrast material was used for injection
Field: Sterile
Procedure classification: Clean-contaminated, contaminated
Position: Supine
Monitoring: Intravenous access line was secured and vital signs were continuously monitored by nursing staff/anesthesia team throughout the procedure
Total fluoroscopy time: (_) minutes
Cumulative radiation dose: (_) mGy

Description of Procedure:

The risks, benefits, alternatives, and the procedure itself were explained to the patient/patient's Power of Attorney/legal guardian, and informed written consent was obtained. The site of the procedure was identified and marked. Time out was performed to confirm the correct patient, procedure, and site.

The skin and the previously inserted catheter were prepped and draped in the usual sterile fashion. Under fluoroscopy visualization, a (0.035)-inch [type] guidewire was inserted through the drain and looped in the duodenum/intestine/abscess cavity/biliary duct/gallbladder. The drain was then exchanged over the guidewire for a (_)-French [type] vascular sheath. A second (0.035)-inch [stiff/type] guidewire was inserted, leaving the first safety guidewire in place. The dilator component of the sheath was withdrawn over the guidewire. Once the sheath was within the system with sufficient guidewire to secure access, the sheath was then quickly withdrawn along the tract, with simultaneous injection of (_) mL of contrast material via the side port and acquisition of a series of digital images. The area was examined fluoroscopically for free flow of contrast material into the peritoneal/pleural cavity.

Images showed a mature tract, with the contrast material outlining the tract without free flow of contrast material into the peritoneal/pleural cavity. After confirming the clinical improvement of the patient, resolution of the cavity, and the presence of a mature tract, the sheath and guidewire were removed. Sterile dressing was applied and the patient was transferred to the floor/discharged home following the procedure in a stable condition. Staff was present and scrubbed for the entire procedure.

Intra-Procedure Findings: List all relevant findings.
Immediate Complications: None encountered during or directly after the procedure. List complications if any.

Post-Procedure Plan:

- Specify the plan if any.

Impression:

- Tractography, as described above.
- The indwelling catheter was removed safely without complications.
- The patient tolerated the procedure well and left the interventional unit in stable condition.
- List any other relevant or important information/finding.

References

1. Maher MM, Kealey S, McNamara A, O'Laoide R, Gibney RG, Malone DE. Management of visceral interventional radiology catheters: a troubleshooting guide for interventional radiologists. Radiographics. 2002;22(2):305–22.
2. Hunter DW. Percutaneous biliary interventions. In: Kandarpa K, Machan L, editors. Handbook of interventional radiologic procedures. 4th ed. Philadelphia: Lippincott Williams & Wilkins; 2011. p. 577–90.
3. Management of biliary calculi. In: Burke CT, Dixon RG, Mauro MA, Murphy KPJ, Thomson KR, Venbrux AC, Zollikofer CL, editors. High yield imaging: interventional. Philadelphia: Saunders Elsevier; 2010. p. 438–41.
4. Taslakian B, Sebaaly MG, Al-Kutoubi A. Patient evaluation and preparation in vascular and interventional radiology: what every interventional radiologist should know (part 1: patient assessment and laboratory tests). Cardiovasc Intervent Radiol. 2016;39(3):325–33.
5. Taslakian B, Sebaaly MG, Al-Kutoubi A. Patient evaluation and preparation in vascular and interventional radiology: what every interventional radiologist should know (part 2: patient preparation and medications). Cardiovasc Intervent Radiol. 2016;39(4):489–99. doi: 10.1007/s00270-015-1239-4. [Epub 2015 Nov 25].

Tubography (Sinography) 74

Bedros Taslakian

INTRODUCTION

Tubography or sinography is a useful study to assess the patency and position of indwelling drainage catheters, confirm the reduction in size of the drained abscess cavity, and exclude fistulous communication prior to the removal of any drainage catheter. It is performed under fluoroscopy guidance with the injection of contrast media through the catheter.

COMMON INDICATIONS [1]

- Exclude communication with the intestine, biliary tract, urinary tract, or pancreatic duct prior to catheter removal, to avoid re-accumulation of the collection
- Demonstrate a small, well-drained cavity with no residual compartments prior to catheter removal
- Evaluate for vascular communication in case of transcatheter bleeding
- Confirm patency of the urinary or biliary system after stent insertion before removal of the safety catheter
- Assess patency of indwelling drainage catheters
- Assess position of indwelling drainage catheters

COMMON CONTRAINDICATIONS

- No absolute contraindications
- Pregnancy
- Care should be taken during injection of contrast media in a potentially infected system to avoid bacterial seeding

POSSIBLE COMPLICATIONS

- Catheter dislodgment and loss of access
- Pain
- Contrast extravasation
- Septic shock *(fever, chills with hypotension)*

PREPROCEDURAL ASSESSMENT AND PLANNING [2, 3]

- History, indications, and physical examination *(Appendix 1* in Chap. 149*)*
- Evaluation of diagnostic imaging studies to determine the position of the indwelling catheter, the size of the remaining cavity, and relevant anatomy

B. Taslakian (✉)
Department of Radiology, New York University Langone Medical Center, 660 First Ave, New York, NY 10016, USA
e-mail: btaslakian@gmail.com

B. Taslakian et al. (eds.), *Procedural Dictations in Image-Guided Intervention*,
DOI 10.1007/978-3-319-40845-3_74

- Periprocedural management of coagulation status *(Appendices 2* in Chap. 150 *and 3* in Chap. 151*)*
- Antibiotic prophylaxis: Not routinely recommended unless persistent infection is suspected
- Imaging modality for guidance: Fluoroscopy
- Positioning: Supine, prone, oblique, lateral decubitus

PROCEDURE NOTE

Procedure: Fluoroscopy- guided tubography (sinography)
Staff: [_]
Fellow: [_]
Resident: [_]
Clinical Information: Describe history and list indications
Allergies: None known/Allergic to [specify/type of allergy]
Anesthesia: Not required
Medications: List any relevant medications used
Contrast Material: (_) mL of [type] contrast material was used for injection
Field: Sterile
Procedure classification: Clean-contaminated/Contaminated
Position: Supine/Prone/Oblique/Left/Right lateral decubitus
Monitoring: Intravenous access line was secured and vital signs were continuously monitored by nursing staff throughout the procedure
Total fluoroscopy time: (_) minutes
Cumulative radiation dose: (_) mGy

Description of Procedure:

The risks, benefits, alternatives, and the procedure itself were explained to the patient/patient's Power of Attorney/legal guardian, and informed written/verbal consent was obtained. The site of the procedure was identified and marked. Time out was performed to confirm the correct patient, procedure, and site.

The skin and previously inserted indwelling catheter were prepped and draped in the usual sterile fashion. (_) mL of contrast media was injected slowly through the catheter under fluoroscopy visualization to delineate the catheter, the cavity/gallbladder/biliary tree/urinary system, showing [specify the findings].

The catheter was left in place, and attached to a drainage system.

The catheter was removed over a ( )-French [type] guidewire under direct fluoroscopy visualization and sterile dressing was applied.

The patient was transferred to the floor/discharged home following the procedure in a stable condition. Staff was present and scrubbed for the entire procedure.

Intra-Procedure Findings: List all relevant findings.
Immediate Complications: None encountered during or directly after the procedure. List complications if any.
Post-Procedure Plan: Specify the plan according to the findings.

Impression:

- Tubography, as described above.
- The indwelling catheter was removed without complications.
- The patient tolerated the procedure well and left the interventional unit in stable condition.
- List any other relevant or important information/findings.

Reference

1. Maher MM, Kealey S, McNamara A, O'Laoide R, Gibney RG, Malone DE. Management of visceral interventional radiology catheters: a troubleshooting guide for interventional radiologists. Radiographics. 2002;22(2):305–22.
2. Taslakian B, Sebaaly MG, Al-Kutoubi A. Patient evaluation and preparation in vascular and interventional radiology: what every interventional radiologist should know (part 1: patient assessment and laboratory tests). Cardiovasc Intervent Radiol. 2016;39(3): 325–33.
3. Taslakian B, Sebaaly MG, Al-Kutoubi A. Patient evaluation and preparation in vascular and interventional radiology: what every interventional radiologist should know (part 2: patient preparation and medications). Cardiovasc Intervent Radiol. 2016;39(4):489–99. doi: 10.1007/s00270-015-1239-4. [Epub 2015 Nov 25].

Part XII
Vascular Interventional Procedures: Aorta

Introduction by Jamal J. Hoballah, Section Reviewer

The endovascular technology has transformed the management of aortic aneurysmal disease during the past two decades. Formidable thoracic and abdominal incisions have been replaced with small groin incisions and percutaneous approaches.

Endovascular treatment is currently being offered for the majority of abdominal aortic aneurysms. The percentage of patients with aortic aneurysmal disease who are candidates or amenable to endovascular treatment continues to grow. This is paralleled by the continuous development of technology addressing anatomical challenges that test its efficacy and durability. Devices dealing with short and angulated infrarenal necks are becoming available and supplemented by chimney and snorkel techniques. Fenestrated and branched grafts are being used to address renal and visceral involvement. The endovascular treatment had also given rise to complications specific to this technology such as endoleaks and graft migration. The framework for endovascular treatment relies on angiography, insertion and accurate deployment of the device and management of endoleaks. Attempts to cover all the various devices and approaches in the management of aortic aneurysm disease are beyond the scope of this book. In this section, selected representative procedures for endovascular treatment of thoracic and abdominal aortic aneurysms. and their complications will be covered. We provide a comprehensive list of procedural reports that covers these interventions, with up-to-date explanatory notes, synopsis of the indications and contraindications, and potential complications in an organized and practical format.

Section Chapters

Aortography and Selective Angiography

75

Bedros Taslakian, Karim Rebeiz and Peter Sawan

INTRODUCTION

Diagnostic catheter arteriography continues to be the gold standard for the evaluation of many vascular abnormalities, including hypervascular tumors, arteriovenous malformations, arteriovenous fistulae, and sources of bleeding.

COMMON INDICATIONS [1–3]

Aortography:

- Acute traumatic aortic injury
- Aortic dissection and aneurysm
- Aortitis
- Congenital anomalies
- Evaluation of aorta and its branches prior to, during, and following percutaneous endovascular aortic procedures
- Preoperative mapping of vascular anatomy

Arteriography:

- Evaluation of vascular disorders
- Evaluation of vascular complications of diseases, surgery, and trauma
- Evaluation prior to, during, and following selective percutaneous endovascular procedures
- Diagnosis and localization of hypervascular tumors

COMMON CONTRAINDICATIONS [1–3]

- Hemodynamic instability with multisystem dysfunction
- Uncontrolled severe hypertension and congestive heart failure
- Uncorrectable bleeding disorders
- Recent myocardial infarction
- Significant cardiac arrhythmias and electrolyte imbalance
- Past history of allergic reaction to iodinated contrast media or renal dysfunction *(consider alternative contrast agents such as carbon dioxide or gadolinium)*
- Pregnancy
- Recent imaging of the gastrointestinal tract using positive intraluminal contrast *(in case of abdominal arteriography)*
- Uncooperative patient
- Active bacteremia and sepsis
- Pheochromocytoma
- Active large vessel vasculitis and connective tissue disorders *(increased risk of puncture*

B. Taslakian
Department of Radiology, New York University Langone Medical Center, 660 First Ave, New York, NY 10016, USA
e-mail: btaslakian@gmail.com

K. Rebeiz · P. Sawan (✉)
Department of Radiology, Memorial Sloan Kettering Cancer Center, 1275 York Avenue, New York 10065, NY, USA
e-mail: sawanp@mskcc.org

K. Rebeiz
e-mail: krebeiz00@gmail.com

B. Taslakian et al. (eds.), *Procedural Dictations in Image-Guided Intervention*,
DOI 10.1007/978-3-319-40845-3_75

site complications, vascular injury, and thrombosis)
- Local conditions at the vascular access sites such as infection, preexisting pseudoaneurysm, hematoma, inguinal hernia, fresh incision, and recent injuries *(an alternative access site should be selected)*

POSSIBLE COMPLICATIONS [1–4]

- Access site complications *(e.g., hematoma, retroperitoneal hemorrhage, pseudoaneurysm, arteriovenous fistula, thrombosis)*
- Nausea, vomiting, and vasovagal syncope
- Fever and chills
- Contrast-induced allergic reaction
- Contrast-induced nephropathy
- Arterial perforation or dissection
- Catheter or guidewire breakage
- Limb amputation *(rare)*
- Risks related to any minimally invasive procedure performed under conscious sedation *(e.g., allergy to medications)*
- Mortality

PREPROCEDURAL ASSESSMENT AND PLANNING [2, 3, 5–7]

- History, indications, and physical examination *(Appendix 1* in Chap. 149*)*. Document indications of the procedure, lower or upper extremity pulses and vital signs
- Evaluation of diagnostic imaging studies to determine the relevant vascular anatomy and assess the access site
- Periprocedural management of coagulation status *(Appendices 2* in Chap. 150 *and 3* in Chap. 151*)*
- Antibiotic prophylaxis: Not routinely recommended [2, 3, 5] *(Appendices 4* in Chap. 152 *and 5* in Chap. 153*)*
- Imaging modality for guidance: Fluoroscopy; combined with ultrasound for arterial puncture
- Positioning: Supine
- Arterial access: Common femoral artery, left brachial artery [1, 4]
- Patient preparation:
  - Start intravenous fluids the night before angiography in order to ensure adequate hydration, combined with effective monitoring of fluid status
  - Insert a urinary catheter or ask the patient to void before the procedure depending on the estimated time of the procedure
  - Considerations for patients with specific diseases or conditions, patients on specific medications or patients with history of multiple comorbidities: consult with the referring clinician, and obtain subspecialty consultation as needed

PROCEDURE NOTE

Procedure: Catheter-directed diagnostic aortography/selective angiography/superselective angiography
Staff: [_]
Fellow: [_]
Resident: [_]
Clinical History and Indications: Describe history and list indications
Allergies: None known/Allergic to [specify/type of allergy]
Anesthesia: Local anesthesia/Conscious sedation
Medications: List any relevant medications used
Contrast Material: (_) mL of [type] contrast material was used for intra-arterial injection
Field: Sterile
Procedure classification: Clean
Position: Supine
Monitoring: Intravenous access line was secured and vital signs were continuously monitored by nursing staff/anesthesia team throughout the procedure
Total fluoroscopy time: (_) minutes
Cumulative radiation dose: (_) mGy

Description of Procedure *(retrograde femoral catheterization, Seldinger technique, aortography):*

The risks, benefits, alternatives, and procedure itself were explained to the patient/patient's Power of Attorney/patient's legal guardian, and informed written/verbal consent was obtained. Time out was performed to confirm the correct patient, procedure, and site. The site of the procedure was identified and marked.

The skin of both groins were shaved, prepped, and draped in the usual sterile fashion. The right/left common femoral artery as well as the inguinal ligament were located by palpation/ultrasound and marked. The site of arterial puncture was determined using combined information from palpation, ultrasound, and fluoroscopy over the middle of the medial third of the femoral head. Local anesthesia was administered. Common femoral artery access was obtained using a (_)-gauge [type] needle and the Seldinger technique under direct ultrasound visualization/by palpation. Once good pulsatile arterial flow was detected, a (_)-inch [type] guidewire was advanced through the needle, up through the common femoral artery, into the aorta under direct fluoroscopic visualization and a (_)-French vascular sheath was placed.

Heparinized saline infusion was started into the femoral arterial sheath. Subsequently, a (_)-French, (_)-cm-long [pigtail/type] catheter was advanced into the abdominal/thoracic aorta over a (_)-inch [hydrophilic/type] guidewire under direct fluoroscopic visualization and placed at the level of [specify anatomic location]. The vascular catheter was used to perform a digital subtraction aortogram, by injecting (_) mL of contrast at a flow rate of (_) mL/sec using an automated injector. Digital subtraction angiography images were obtained at (_) frames per second during suspended respiration in an anterior–posterior projection/and [specify other projections if obtained].

Following the procedure the right/left femoral artery sheath was removed and adequate hemostasis was achieved by compression for (_) minutes/using [type] vascular closure device. The lower extremity pulses were checked following the procedure and were [comparable to the pre-procedure pulses/specify if otherwise needed]. The patient was transferred to the floor/recovery room for close monitoring following the procedure in a stable condition. Staff was present for the entire procedure.

Description of Procedure *(left brachial or axillary artery catheterization, Seldinger technique, aortography):*

The risks, benefits, alternatives, and procedure itself were explained to the patient/patient's Power of Attorney/patient's legal guardian, and informed written/verbal consent was obtained. Time out was performed to confirm the correct patient, procedure, and site. The site of the procedure was identified and marked.

The left arm was abducted adequately. Baseline axillary, brachial, radial, and ulnar pulses were obtained and documented in the chart. The skin of left arm was prepped and draped in the usual sterile fashion. The site of the left axillary/brachial arterial puncture was determined using combined information from palpation, ultrasound, and fluoroscopy along the lateral axillary fold over the proximal humeral neck/distal humerus. Local anesthesia was administered. Left axillary/brachial artery access was obtained using a (_)-gauge [type] needle and the Seldinger technique under direct ultrasound visualization/by palpation. Once good pulsatile arterial flow was detected, a (_)-inch [type] guidewire was advanced through the needle, up the axillary/brachial artery, into the thoracic aorta under direct fluoroscopic visualization. A (_) French, (_)-cm-long, [vascular/type] sheath was placed. Heparinized saline infusion was started into the arterial sheath. Subsequently, a (_)-French, (_)-cm-long [pigtail/type] catheter was advanced into the abdominal/ascending/descending thoracic aorta over a (_)-inch [hydrophilic/type] guidewire under direct fluoroscopic visualization and the tip was placed at the level of [specify anatomic location]. The vascular catheter was used to perform a digital subtraction aortogram, by injecting (_) mL of contrast at a flow rate of (_) mL/sec using an automated injector. Digital subtraction angiography images were obtained at (_) frames per second during suspended respiration in an anterior–posterior projection/and [specify other projections if obtained].

Following the procedure the arterial sheath was removed and adequate hemostasis was achieved by compression for (_) minutes. The upper extremity pulses were checked following the procedure and were [comparable to the pre-procedure pulses/specify if otherwise needed]. The patient was transferred to the floor/recovery room for close monitoring following the procedure in a stable condition. Staff was present for the entire procedure.

Description of Procedure *(retrograde femoral catheterization, Seldinger technique, selective/superselective arteriography):*
The risks, benefits, alternatives, and procedure itself were explained to the patient/patient's Power of Attorney/patient's legal guardian, and informed written/verbal consent was obtained. Time out was performed to confirm the correct patient, procedure, and site. The site of the procedure was identified and marked.

The skin of both groins were shaved, prepped, and draped in the usual sterile fashion. The right/left femoral artery as well as the inguinal ligament were located by palpation/ultrasound and marked. The site of arterial puncture was determined using combined information from palpation, ultrasound, and fluoroscopy over the middle of the medial third of the femoral head. Local anesthesia was administered. Femoral artery access was obtained using (_)-gauge [type] needle and the Seldinger technique under direct ultrasound visualization/by palpation. Once good pulsatile arterial flow was detected, a (_)-inch [type] guidewire was advanced through the needle into the aorta under direct fluoroscopic visualization and a (_)-French vascular sheath was placed.

Heparinized saline infusion was started into the femoral arterial sheath. Subsequently, a (_)-French, (_)-cm-long [type] catheter was advanced into the abdominal/thoracic aorta over a (_)-inch [hydrophilic/type] guidewire under direct fluoroscopic visualization and the [name] artery was selectively catheterized. After confirming the catheter location by manual contrast injection, digital subtraction angiography of the [specify anatomic location/organ/vessel] was performed by injecting (_) mL of contrast media manually/using an automated injector at a rate of (_) mL/sec. Following this, a (_)-French [type] coaxial microcatheter was advanced into the previously inserted catheter and superselective catheterization of the [name] artery was performed. Digital subtraction angiography was performed by manual injection of (_) mL contrast material using (_) mL syringe.

Following the procedure the right/left femoral artery sheath was removed and adequate hemostasis was achieved by compression for (_) minutes/using [type] vascular closure device. The femoral pulses were checked following the procedure and were [comparable to the pre-procedure pulses/specify if otherwise needed]. The patient was transferred to the floor/recovery room for close monitoring following the procedure in a stable condition. Staff was present for the entire procedure.

Intra-Procedure Findings: List all relevant findings.

Immediate Complications: None encountered during or directly after the procedure. List complications if any.

Post-Procedure Plan [1, 3]**:**

- Keep patient complete bed rest with the right/left leg extended for (6) hours *[adjust depending on the puncture site]*.
- Check the right/left groin/[specify the puncture site if different] for any bleeding or hematoma formation every 15 min for 1 h, then every 30 min for 1 h, then every hour for 4 h; inform interventional radiology team if any signs of bleeding are observed *[adjust depending on the puncture site]*.
- Check and document lower extremity pulses every 30 min for 2 h then every 1 h for 4 h *[adjust depending on the puncture site]*.
- Monitor vital signs every 15 min for 1 h, then every 30 min for 4 h; notify interventional radiology team if systolic blood pressure <95 mmHg, or heart rate >110 beats/min.
- Resume diet and previous orders as needed and if otherwise not contraindicated.
- Continue adequate intravenous hydration and monitor fluid (intake–output) status.

- Check complete blood count and creatinine on the day following the procedure or as clinically indicated.
- Perform regular neurological examination when the procedure includes manipulation in the ascending thoracic aorta, aortic arch or brachiocephalic arteries.

Impression:

- Aortography/selective/superselective angiography of the [name the artery] as described above.
- The patient tolerated the procedure well and left the interventional unit in stable condition.
- The patient was unstable and the procedure was canceled/terminated prematurely.
- List any other relevant or important information/finding.

References

1. Kandarpa K, Gardiner GA Jr, Keller FS. Diagnostic arteriography. In: Kandarpa K, Machan L, editors. Handbook of interventional radiologic procedures. 4th ed. Philadelphia: Lippincott Williams & Wilkins; 2011. p. 61–84.
2. Heran MK, Marshalleck F, Temple M, Grassi CJ, Connolly B, Towbin RB, et al. Joint quality improvement guidelines for pediatric arterial access and arteriography: from the Societies of Interventional Radiology and Pediatric Radiology. J Vasc Interv Radiol. 2010;21(1):32–43.
3. American College of Radiology. ACR–SIR–SPR practice parameter for performance of arteriography. Reston, VA: American College of Radiology; 2014.
4. Kaufman JA. Invasive vascular diagnosis. In: Mauro MA, Murphy KPJ, Thomson KR, Venbrux AC, Morgan RA, editors. Image-guided interventions. 2nd ed. Philadelphia: Saunders Elsevier; 2014. p. 11–32.
5. Venkatesan AM, Kundu S, Sacks D, Wallace MJ, Wojak JC, Rose SC, et al. Practice guidelines for adult antibiotic prophylaxis during vascular and interventional radiology procedures. J Vasc Interv Radiol. 2010;21(11):1611–30.
6. Taslakian B, Sebaaly MG, Al-Kutoubi A. Patient evaluation and preparation in vascular and interventional radiology: what every interventional radiologist should know (part 1: patient assessment and laboratory tests). Cardiovasc Intervent Radiol. 2016;39(3):325–33.
7. Taslakian B, Sebaaly MG, Al-Kutoubi A. Patient evaluation and preparation in vascular and interventional radiology: what every interventional radiologist should know (part 2: patient preparation and medications). Cardiovasc Intervent Radiol. 2016;39(4):489–99. doi: 10.1007/s00270-015-1239-4. [Epub 2015 Nov 25].

Endovascular Abdominal Aortic Aneurysm Repair (EVAR)

76

Bedros Taslakian

Abbreviations

AAA	Abdominal aortic aneurysm
EVAR	Endovascular abdominal aortic aneurysm repair
IMA	Inferior mesenteric artery
SMA	Superior mesenteric artery
ACT	Activated clotting time

INTRODUCTION

Abdominal aortic aneurysm (AAA) is an abnormal dilatation of the abdominal aorta greater than 50 % of the normal proximal segment, or dilatation greater than 3 cm. Factors associated with development of AAA include smoking, increasing age, coronary artery disease, hypercholesterolemia, peripheral vascular disease, hypertension, connective tissue disorders, and family history. Continuous expansion of AAAs results in an increased risk of rupture and distal embolization. Risk factors for AAA rupture include aneurysm size, rate of expansion, poorly controlled hypertension, chronic obstructive pulmonary disease, and smoking. Surgical repair of AAA has traditionally been the standard of care. Endovascular abdominal aortic aneurysm repair (EVAR) is now an established safe alternative therapy. Fenestrated and branching endovascular grafts have increased the indications for EVAR when the anatomical arrangements are suboptimal for a straight EVAR such as neck length <10 mm.

COMMON INDICATIONS [1–4]

Indications for EVAR are the same as those for an open surgical approach

- Known or suspected rupture in the presence of appropriate anatomy
- Symptomatic AAA regardless of diameter, a potential sign of impending rupture *(e.g., tender or painful aneurysm)*
- Rapidly expending AAA *(>1 cm increase in diameter in 12 months)*
- Asymptomatic fusiform aneurysm with a diameter of >5.5 cm for men; >5.0 cm for women

B. Taslakian (✉)
Department of Radiology, New York University Langone Medical Center, 660 First Ave, New York, NY 10016, USA
e-mail: btaslakian@gmail.com

B. Taslakian et al. (eds.), *Procedural Dictations in Image-Guided Intervention*,
DOI 10.1007/978-3-319-40845-3_76

- AAA with penetrating atherosclerotic ulcer or saccular aneurysm (pseudoaneurysm) twice the diameter of normal infrarenal aorta
- Inflammatory AAAs
- Smaller AAAs with concomitant iliac aneurysms requiring repair
- Smaller AAAs with associated thrombotic/embolic complications
- Ideal anatomic inclusion criteria are:
  - Proximal neck length *(segment of aorta between the origin of the lowest renal artery and superior aspect of the aneurysm)*: 15 mm or greater
  - Proximal neck diameter: 33 mm or under depending on the endograft device
  - Proximal neck angulation: <60°
  - Neck thrombus: minimal; thrombus greater than 2 mm in depth involving more than 25 % of the proximal neck circumference is considered unfavorable
  - Diameter of the distal aorta of at least 18 mm if a bifurcated device is to be deployed to accommodate the bifurcated endograft

COMMON CONTRAINDICATIONS [1–4]

- Predominant bowel supply by a hypertrophied inferior mesenteric artery (IMA) in the setting of significant superior mesenteric artery (SMA) stenosis; revascularization of the SMA may be required
- Anatomic or clinical factors that render the patient unsuitable for EVAR *(i.e., absence of appropriate proximal and distal landing zones, absence of suitable access vessels, severe hemodynamic instability)*
- Concomitant disease with short life expectancy *(relative contraindication)*
- Renal insufficiency *(relative contraindication; use reduced amounts of diluted contrast, alternative contrast such as carbon dioxide or gadolinium)*
- Severe contrast reactions *(relative contraindication; can use alternative contrast such as carbon dioxide or gadolinium)*

POSSIBLE COMPLICATIONS [1–4]

- Vascular access site-related complications; 1–10 %: hematoma, infection, lymphocele, access artery injuries *(thrombosis, dissection, pseudoaneurysm, arteriovenous fistula formation, vessel perforation, vascular avulsion)*
- Ischemic complications due to dislodgment of thrombotic and atheromatous deposits, with microembolization into supplying arteries, interruption of collateral or supplying arteries and/or due to thrombosis of endograft components
  - EVAR-induced colonic ischemia; 1–3 %
  - Spinal cord ischemia; 0.21 %
  - Renal ischemia/infarction
- Conversion to open surgical repair; 0.9 %
- Renal dysfunction due to endograft coverage of the renal artery, thrombotic renal artery occlusion, or distal embolization of the renal artery branches, contrast-induced nephropathy; 2 %
- Graft migration; 1.8–3.6 %
- Graft stenosis or thrombosis
- Limb occlusion due to kinking of the endograft limb; 0–5 %
- Graft infection; 0.2–1 %
- Reintervention; 19.2 %
- Rupture of AAA
- Endoleak *(leakage of blood into the aneurysmal sac outside the endograft but not leakage outside the vascular compartment)*; 25–44 %
- Perioperative mortality; 0–6 %
- Abdominal compartment syndrome after EVAR for ruptured AAA *(in patients in whom a large retroperitoneal hematoma and diffuse visceral edema cause elevated intraabdominal pressure and multiorgan dysfunction)*

PREPROCEDURAL ASSESSMENT AND PLANNING [1, 4]

- History, indications, and physical examination *(Appendix 1* in Chap. 149*)*. Document indications of the procedure, lower or upper extremity pulses, and vital signs
- Evaluation of diagnostic imaging studies to determine the relevant vascular anatomy, assess the access vessels, and obtain accurate diameter and length measurements
- Periprocedural management of coagulation status *(Appendices 2* in Chap. 150 *and 3* in Chap. 151*)*
- Antibiotic prophylaxis: Routinely recommended *(first choice agent: 1 g cefazolin intravenously)* [3, 5] *(Appendices 4* in Chap. 152 *and 5* in Chap. 153*)*
- Imaging modality for guidance: Fluoroscopy; combined with ultrasound for arterial puncture
- Positioning: Supine
- Vascular access: carefully assess the quality of common femoral and iliac arteries. The site through which the main endograft body is inserted will be selected based on the preoperative planning and measurements. Usually right femoral artery is used to insert the main endograft body; if severely diseased, operators may decide to use the left side. The contralateral femoral artery is then used to deploy the contralateral endograft limb. Left brachial/axillary artery can be used for angiography.
- Preprocedural embolization of the internal iliac artery if the common iliac aneurysm extends to the iliac bifurcation, as the external iliac artery is the target site for distal endograft attachment. Prior to embolization, it should be confirmed that the contralateral internal iliac artery is patent and the bowel perfusion is not reliable on the internal iliac arteries. Bilateral internal iliac artery embolization might be performed in patients with bilateral common iliac artery aneurysms extending to the level of iliac bifurcation, if the patient is high risk of surgical aortic repair. Bilateral embolization is preferably staged 1 to 2 weeks apart. The use of branched iliac endograft when available is another option to avoid internal iliac embolization and preserve hypogastric flow.
- Patient preparation:
  - Start intravenous fluids the night before angiography in order to ensure adequate hydration, combined with effective monitoring of fluid status
  - Insert a urinary catheter before the procedure
  - Considerations for patients with specific diseases or conditions, patients on specific medications, or patients with history of multiple comorbidities: consult with the referring clinician, and obtain subspecialty consultation as needed

PROCEDURE NOTE

Procedure: Endovascular repair of abdominal aortic aneurysm
Staff: [_]
Fellow: [_]
Resident: [_]
Clinical History and Indications: Describe history and list indications
Allergies: None known/Allergic to [specify/type of allergy]
Anesthesia: Regional anesthesia with monitored conscious sedation/General anesthesia
Medications: List any relevant medications used
Contrast Material: (_) mL of [type] contrast material was used for intra-arterial injection
Field: Sterile
Procedure classification: Clean
Position: Supine
Monitoring: Intravenous access line was secured and vital signs were continuously monitored by nursing staff/anesthesia team throughout the procedure
Total fluoroscopy time: (_) minutes
Cumulative radiation dose: (_) mGy

Description of Procedure:

The risks, benefits, alternatives, and procedure itself were explained to the patient/patient's

Power of Attorney/patient's legal guardian, and informed written consent was obtained. Time out was performed to confirm the correct patient, procedure, and site. The site of the vascular access was identified and marked.

The skin of both groins were shaved, prepped, and draped in the usual sterile fashion. Right *(side used for deploying the main body)* common femoral artery access was obtained via surgical cutdown/arteriotomy and a (_)-French vascular sheath was introduced.

Percutaneous access of the right common femoral artery was obtained under ultrasound guidance. Two vascular closure devices were applied without tying for performing the procedure percutaneously.

The left *(side used for deploying the contralateral limb)* common femoral artery as well as the inguinal ligament were located by palpation/ultrasound and marked. The site of arterial puncture was determined using combined information from palpation, ultrasound, and fluoroscopy over the middle of the medial third of the femoral head. Common femoral artery access was obtained using a (_)-gauge [type] needle and the Seldinger technique under direct ultrasound visualization/by palpation/surgical arteriotomy. Once good pulsatile arterial flow was detected, a (_)-inch [type] guidewire was advanced through the needle, up through the common femoral artery, into the aorta under direct fluoroscopic visualization and a (_)-French vascular sheath was placed.

Heparinized saline infusion was started into the femoral arterial sheaths. A baseline activated clotting time (ACT) was obtained and systemic heparinazation was started by injecting (_) international units of heparin intravenously to achieve an ACT of 250–300 s. The ACT was measured regularly throughout the procedure.

Subsequently, a (_)-French, (_)-cm-long [pigtail/type] graduated marker catheter was advanced via the left (contralateral) access into the abdominal aorta over a (_)-inch [hydrophilic/type] guidewire under direct fluoroscopic visualization and placed at the level of [specify anatomic location]. The vascular catheter was used to perform a digital subtraction aortogram, by injecting (_) mL of contrast at a flow rate of (_) mL/sec using an automated injector. Digital subtraction angiography images were obtained at (_) frames per second during suspended respiration in an anterior–posterior projection/and [specify other projections if obtained]. The level of the lowest renal artery was marked (pay special attention to the presence of accessory renal arteries).

The right (main body) arterial access was used to advance a (_)-French diagnostic catheter over a (_)-inch hydrophilic wire to the level of the descending aorta, which was then exchanged for a (_)-inch superstiff [type] guidewire.

Then, the (_)-French introducer sheath was advanced over the superstiff guidewire into the aorta. The main body of the endograft device [specify type, length and diameter] was advanced over the superstiff guidewire so that the superior end of the endograft was positioned at the level of the lowest renal artery under magnified fluoroscopy control. Intermittent angiography was performed using the contralateral access site/upper extremity access to confirm the position of the endograft immediately distal to the lowest renal artery. After confirming appropriate position, the trunk and contralateral limb were deployed under fluoroscopy control exposing the contralateral gate. Repeat aortography was performed confirming the correct location of the endograft and continued patency of the renal arteries.

The pigtail catheter introduced through the left (contralateral) femoral artery (outside the graft) was then withdrawn over a guidewire and a (_)-French angled tip diagnostic [type] catheter was introduced over a (_)-inch hydrophilic wire to cannulate the gate of the contralateral limb of the endograft.

Due to difficulty in cannulation of the contralateral limb gate, the ipsilateral limb was fully deployed and the delivery system was removed under fluoroscopic guidance. A (_)-French angled tip catheter was introduced over a (_)-inch guidewire from the right femoral artery access into the endograft and the wire was snared through the left femoral artery access using a [type] snare.

Due to difficulty in cannulation of the contralateral limb opening, a left brachial arterial access was obtained and a (_)-French vascular sheath was inserted. The contralateral limb was then antegradely catheterized using a (_)-French angled tip catheter introduced over a (_)-inch guidewire from the left brachial access.

Once the contralateral gate is cannulated, the hydrophilic catheter was advanced into the descending aorta. The catheter was exchanged to a pigtail marker catheter. The wire was removed and the pig tail was pulled back into the body of the endograft and rotated to confirm intragraft position. After confirming appropriate position, the pigtail was readvanced into the suprarenal aorta and a (_)-inch superstiff [type] guidewire was advanced and positioned in the descending aorta through the contralateral access. An angiogram was then performed through the left sheath to identify the origin of the hypogastric artery allowing to measure the distance to the gate and select the length of the contralateral limb. Then, the left femoral sheath was exchanged to a 12 French sheath. The contralateral limb [specify type of graft, length, diameter] was introduced over the superstiff guidewire and after confirming position, it was deployed in place to land just proximal to the common iliac bifurcation (unless there is aneurysmal extension beyond the bifurcation and internal iliac artery embolization was performed before the procedure).

The endograft, ipsilateral limb, contralateral limb and extension were balloon dilated using a (_) x (_) mm [type] compliant balloon to achieve maximum profile.

All stiff guidewires were removed after introducing a pigtail catheter from one limb and leaving the balloon catheter through the other limb to maintain access in case of any complications were observed during angiography. Then completion angiography was performed by injecting (_) mL of contrast at a rate of (_) mL/second showing patent renal and hypogastric arteries and absence of endoleak [specify if otherwise noted].

The right and left femoral sheaths were removed and arteriotomies were surgically repaired. The femoral sheaths vascular closure devices were then fully deployed and tied. The patient was transferred to the intensive care unit/recovery room after the procedure in a stable/critical condition for further close monitoring. Staff was present during the entire procedure.

Intra-Procedure Findings: List all relevant findings.

Immediate Complications: None encountered during or directly after the procedure. List complications if any.

Post-Procedure Plan [1, 2, 4, 6]**:**

- Keep patient complete bed rest with the right/left leg extended for 6 h *[adjust depending on the puncture site]*.
- Check the right/left groin/[specify the puncture site if different] for any bleeding or hematoma formation every 15 min for 1 h, then every 30 min for 1 h, then every hour for 4 h; inform interventional radiology team if signs of bleeding are observed *[adjust depending on the puncture site]*.
- Check and document lower extremity pulses every 30 min for 2 h then every 1 h for 4 h *[adjust depending on the puncture site]*.
- Monitor vital signs every 15 min for 1 h, then every 30 min for 4 h; notify interventional radiology team if systolic blood pressure <95 mmHg, or heart rate >110 beats/min.
- Continue adequate intravenous hydration and monitor fluid (intake–output) status.
- Check complete blood count and creatinine on the day following the procedure or as clinically indicated.
- Perform regular neurological examination when the procedure includes manipulation in the ascending thoracic aorta, aortic arch or brachiocephalic arteries.
- Start patients on antiplatelet therapy and statins.
- Perform post-procedural physical examination and imaging surveillance at 1–3 month, 6 months, and then yearly if no endoleak is detected.

- If endoleak is detected, perform post-procedural physical examination and imaging surveillance every 6 months for the first 2 years and yearly thereafter unless treatment is indicated.

Impression:

- Endovascular repair of abdominal aortic aneurysm, as described above.
- The patient tolerated the procedure well and left the interventional unit in stable condition.
- The patient was unstable and the procedure was canceled/terminated prematurely.
- List any other relevant or important information/finding.

References

1. Patel PJ. Stent-Grafts for abdominal aortic aneurysms. In: Kandarpa K, Machan L, editors. Handbook of interventional radiologic procedures. 4th ed. Philadelphia: Lippincott Williams & Wilkins; 2011. p. 188–98.
2. Bryce Y, Rogoff P, Romanelli D, Reichle R. Endovascular repair of abdominal aortic aneurysms: vascular anatomy, device selection, procedure, and procedure-specific complications. Radiographics. 2015;35(2):593–615.
3. Walker TG, Kalva SP, Yeddula K, Wicky S, Kundu S, Drescher P, et al. Clinical practice guidelines for endovascular abdominal aortic aneurysm repair: written by the Standards of Practice Committee for the Society of Interventional Radiology and endorsed by the Cardiovascular and Interventional Radiological Society of Europe and the Canadian Interventional Radiology Association. J Vasc Interv Radiol. 2010;21(11):1632–55.
4. Chun J, Thompson MM, Morgan RA. Aortic endografting. In: Mauro MA, Murphy KPJ, Thomson KR, Venbrux AC, Morgan RA, editors. Image-guided interventions. 2nd ed. Philadelphia: Saunders Elsevier; 2014. p. 311–20.
5. Venkatesan AM, Kundu S, Sacks D, Wallace MJ, Wojak JC, Rose SC, et al. Practice guidelines for adult antibiotic prophylaxis during vascular and interventional radiology procedures. J Vasc Interv Radiol. 2010;21(11):1611–30.
6. Uthoff H, Peña C, Katzen BT, et al. Current clinical practice in postoperative endovascular aneurysm repair imaging surveillance. J Vasc Interv Radiol. 2012;23(9):1152–9, e6.

Percutaneous Transluminal Embolization of Type II Endoleak

77

Eric T. Aaltonen

Abbreviations

EVAR	Endovascular aneurysm repair
IMA	Inferior mesenteric artery
CT	Computed tomography
US	Ultrasound

INTRODUCTION

Endovascular aneurysm repair (EVAR) of abdominal aortic aneurysms has become a widely accepted alternative to open repair with similar survival and rupture outcomes. There are five subtypes of endoleak following EVAR; type II endoleak is the most common (40 %) and involves perigraft blood flow via an artery arising from the aneurysm sac [1]. There are two subtypes of type II endoleaks, single vessel inflow and outflow is characterized as IIA and multiple inflow/outflow vessels are characterized as IIB. The annual incidence of type II endoleaks following endovascular aneurysm repair is approximately 5–8 % [2, 3]. The presence of a type II endoleak on imaging is associated with a very low risk of rupture if there is no accompanying increase in aneurysm sac diameter and these endoleaks often resolve spontaneously. However, growth of the aneurysm sac associated with a type II endoleak is concerning for impending rupture. A 5 mm interval increase in maximum diameter of the sac over a 6-month period is a widely accepted treatment threshold [4]. Treatment of a type II endoleak requires cessation of the inflow/outflow of perigraft blood by embolization either via a percutaneous transluminal or transarterial approach. These two techniques have been shown to have similar success and complication outcomes [5]. Regardless of technique, the sac must be embolized centrally much like the nidus of an arteriovenous malformation to achieve success. Percutaneous puncture of the aneurysm sac can be achieved by a translumbar or transabdominal approach and is typically performed with computed tomography (CT), ultrasound (US), or fluoroscopic guidance.

E.T. Aaltonen (✉)
Department of Radiology, New York University Langone Medical Center, 660 1st Avenue, New York, NY 10016, USA
e-mail: eric.aaltonen@nyumc.org

B. Taslakian et al. (eds.), *Procedural Dictations in Image-Guided Intervention*,
DOI 10.1007/978-3-319-40845-3_77

COMMON INDICATIONS [4, 6]

Absolute Indications:

- 5 mm or greater increase in maximum aneurysm sac diameter over a 6-month period during EVAR surveillance

Relative Indications:

- Less than 5 mm increase in maximum aneurysm sac diameter over a 6-month surveillance period
- 5 mm or greater increase in maximum aneurysm sac diameter over a surveillance period longer than 6 months

COMMON CONTRAINDICATIONS

- Unsafe window for percutaneous access to aneurysm sac
- Severe coagulopathy that cannot be corrected *(relative contraindication)*

POSSIBLE COMPLICATIONS [4, 7]

- Endograft perforation
- Endograft infection
- Hemorrhage/hematoma
- Nontarget embolization *(ischemia secondary to embolic material in distal IMA branches)*
- Injury to adjacent structures *(overlying bowel, kidneys, inferior vena cava, other vasculature)*

PREPROCEDURAL ASSESSMENT AND PLANNING [8–10]

- History, indications, and physical examination *(Appendix 1* in Chap. 149*)*
- Evaluation of diagnostic imaging studies to determine the relevant anatomy and a safe approach for percutaneous access to aneurysm sac
- Periprocedural management of coagulation status *(Appendices 2* in Chap. 150 *and 3* in Chap. 151*)*
- Antibiotic prophylaxis: Not routinely recommended [8] *(Appendices 4* in Chap. 152 *and 5* in Chap. 153*)*
- Imaging modality for guidance: CT or US
- Positioning: Supine for transabdominal approach, prone for translumbar approach

PROCEDURE NOTE

Procedure: Percutaneous transluminal embolization of type II endoleak
Staff: [_]
Fellow: [_]
Resident: [_]
Clinical History and Indications: Describe history and indication *(include date of endograft placement and specify interval increase in aneurysm sac diameter and length of surveillance period)*
Allergies: None known/Allergic to [specify/type of allergy]
Anesthesia: Local anesthesia/Conscious sedation/General anesthesia
Medications: List any relevant medications used
Contrast Material: (_) mL of [type] contrast material was used for intravenous injection *(CT)*/None (US)
Field: Sterile
Procedure classification: Clean
Position: Supine/Prone
Monitoring: Intravenous access line was secured and vital signs were continuously monitored by nursing staff/anesthesia team throughout the procedure
Total fluoroscopy time: (_) min
Cumulative radiation dose: (_) mGy

Description of Procedure:

The risks, benefits, alternatives, and procedure itself were explained to the patient/patient's Power of Attorney/patient's legal guardian, and informed written consent was obtained. Time out was performed to confirm the correct patient, procedure, and site. The site of the procedure was identified and marked.

The patient was positioned supine/prone, with the arms placed above the head. The patient's abdomen/back was prepped and draped in usual sterile fashion. Limited CT/US examination was performed to visualize the aneurysm sac and determine a safe approach for percutaneous access. Local anesthesia was administered. The chosen access site was punctured under CT/US guidance using a (…)-gauge [type] needle. The needle was advanced into the aneurysm sac using CT/CT fluoroscopy/real-time US guidance. Once the needle tip was properly placed in perfused portion of the aneurysm demonstrating contrast enhancement *(CT)*/color Doppler flow *(US)* and confirmed with free return of blood, embolization was performed using [embolic material of choice —coils, N-isobutyl cyanoacrylate (glue), ethylene vinyl alcohol polymer (Onyx), gelfoam, thrombin]. Embolization was performed to stasis and confirmed with repeat CT/lack of Doppler signal on US.

The needle was removed and adequate hemostasis was achieved at the percutaneous access site. Sterile dressing was applied and the patient was transferred to the floor/recovery room following the procedure in a stable condition. Staff was present for the entire procedure.

Intra-Procedure Findings: List all relevant findings.

Immediate Complications: None encountered during or directly after the procedure. List complications if any.

Post-Procedure Plan [5, 6]**:**

- Bed rest for 2 h with patient positioned to keep percutaneous access site down *[positioning depends on access site location].*
- Check the access site for any bleeding or hematoma formation every 15 min for 1 h, then every 30 min for 1 h; inform interventional radiology team if any complications are observed.
- Monitor vital signs every 15 min for 1 h, then every 30 min for 1 h; notify interventional radiology team if systolic blood pressure <90 mmHg, or heart rate >110 beats/min.
- Resume diet and previous orders as needed and if not otherwise contraindicated.
- Continue adequate intravenous hydration and monitor fluid (intake–output) status.
- Follow up imaging, typically with CT angiography, recommended at 1 month, 6 months, 12 months, and annually thereafter to monitor aneurysm sac for continued/new expansion. Continued growth of aneurysm sac may require additional embolization or open surgical repair.

Impression:

- Percutaneous transluminal embolization of abdominal aortic aneurysm type II endoleak using [embolic material above].
- The patient tolerated the procedure well and left the interventional unit in stable condition.
- The patient was unstable and the procedure was canceled/terminated prematurely.
- List any other relevant or important information/finding.

References

1. Bashir MR, Ferral H, Jacobs C, McCarthy W, Goldin M. Endoleaks after endovascular abdominal aortic aneurysm repair: management strategies according to CT findings. AJR Am J Roentgenol. 2009;192(4):W178–86.
2. van Marrewijk C, Buth J, Harris PL, Norgren L, Nevelsteen A, Wyatt MG. Significance of endoleaks after endovascular repair of abdominal aortic aneurysms: the EUROSTAR experience. J Vasc Surg. 2002;35(3):461–73.
3. Mehta M, Sternbach Y, Taggert JB, Kreienberg PB, Roddy SP, Paty PS, et al. Long-term outcomes of secondary procedures after endovascular aneurysm repair. J Vasc Surg. 2010;52(6):1442–9.
4. Hausegger KA. Endoleaks: Classification, Diagnosis, and Treatment. In: Mauro MA, Murphy KPJ, Thomson KR, Venbrux AC, Morgan RA, editors. Image-guided interventions. 2nd ed. Philadelphia: Saunders Elsevier; 2014. p. 334–47.
5. Stavropoulos SW, Park J, Fairman R, Carpenter J. Type 2 endoleak embolization comparison: translumbar versus modified transarterial embolization. J Vasc Interv Radiol. 2009;20(10):1299–302.
6. Lookstein RA, Giordano CF. Diagnosis and Management of Endoleaks. In: Kandarpa K, Machan L, editors. Handbook of interventional radiologic procedures. 4th ed. Philadelphia: Lippincott Williams & Wilkins; 2011. p. 198–205.
7. Sarac TP, Gibbons C, Vargas L, Liu J, Srivastava S, Bena J, et al. Long-term follow-up of type II endoleak

embolization reveals the need for close surveillance. J Vasc Surg. 2012;55(1):33–40.
8. Venkatesan AM, Kundu S, Sacks D, Wallace MJ, Wojak JC, Rose SC, et al. Practice guidelines for adult antibiotic prophylaxis during vascular and interventional radiology procedures. J Vasc Interv Radiol. 2010;21:1611–30.
9. Taslakian B, Sebaaly MG, Al-Kutoubi A. Patient evaluation and preparation in vascular and interventional radiology: what every interventional radiologist should know (part 1: patient assessment and laboratory tests). Cardiovasc Intervent Radiol. 2016;39 (3):325–33.
10. Taslakian B, Sebaaly MG, Al-Kutoubi A. Patient evaluation and preparation in vascular and interventional radiology: what every interventional radiologist should know (part 2: patient preparation and medications). Cardiovasc Intervent Radiol. 2016;39 (4):489–99. doi: 10.1007/s00270-015-1239-4. [Epub 2015 Nov 25].

Thoracic Endovascular Aortic Repair (TEVAR) and Aortic Fenestration

78

Bedros Taslakian

INTRODUCTION

Open surgical repair is the conventional method for the treatment of abnormalities of the ascending thoracic aorta, requiring cardiopulmonary bypass and median sternotomy. With the recent advances in minimally invasive surgical techniques, endovascular stent graft placement has become an accepted and more widely used alternative to traditional surgical repair of descending thoracic aortic disease. In cases of aortic aneurysm, the aim of stenting is to provide a durable conduit for aortic blood flow across the extent of the aneurysm and subsequent depressurization and thrombosis of aneurysm sac and eventual stabilization or regression in size. In type B dissection, treatment consists of covering the primary entry tear and reexpanding the true lumen by redirecting the blood flow into the true lumen, and facilitating thrombosis of at least the proximal false lumen; this decompresses the false lumen and restores patency of the true lumen. Flap fenestration with or without stent placement can be performed to create an artificial tear in the distal dissection septum thereby allowing outflow from the false lumen to decompress the false lumen which is usually at a higher pressure than the true lumen. This enhanced communication of flow between the true and false lumens reduces the risk of further dissection, and relieves the obstruction of branch vessels due to compression of the true lumen by the false lumen.

B. Taslakian (✉)
Department of Radiology, New York University Langone Medical Center, 660 First Ave, New York, NY 10016, USA
e-mail: btaslakian@gmail.com

COMMON INDICATIONS [1–5]

Indications for thoracic aortic stent graft repair:

- Symptomatic descending thoracic aortic aneurysm regardless of size
- Asymptomatic descending thoracic aortic aneurysm >5.5 cm or >2× diameter of adjacent normal aorta
- Asymptomatic descending thoracic aortic aneurysm growing >1 cm per year or >5 mm over a 6-month period
- Penetrating atherosclerotic aortic ulcers with depth greater than 10 mm or diameter wider than 20 mm
- Acute complicated Stanford type B dissection; associated with rupture, malperfusion, uncontrolled hypertension, persistent pain, and retrograde extension of dissection proximal to the left subclavian artery
- Chronic Stanford type B dissection with dilatation of the false lumen >1 cm per year, *(INSTEAD trial showed that stent graft treatment of patients with subacute or chronic aortic dissection offers no benefit in terms of reducing the risk of aortic rupture or enhancing life expectancy)*

B. Taslakian et al. (eds.), *Procedural Dictations in Image-Guided Intervention*,
DOI 10.1007/978-3-319-40845-3_78

- Acute traumatic aortic injury; with intramural hematoma (grade 2), pseudoaneurysm (grade 3), or transection or rupture (grade 4)
- Intramural hematoma
- Aortic fistula
- Mycotic aneurysm
- Acute aortic rupture
- Thoracoabdominal aneurysms with initial aortic debranching followed by stent graft placement

Indications for percutaneous aortic fenestration in patients with aortic dissection:
- Mesenteric ischemia due to obstruction of mesenteric arteries
- Renal failure, pain, or severe uncontrollable renovascular hypertension due to renal artery obstruction
- Paraplegia or paraparesis due to spinal artery involvement
- Severe peripheral ischemia with rest pain or severe claudication
- Severe compression/obliteration of the true lumen

COMMON CONTRAINDICATIONS [1, 4]

Absolute contraindications:
- Suspected infection
- Allergies to device materials

Relative contraindications:
- Contrast allergy
- Renal insufficiency
- Short life expectancy
- Unfavorable anatomy: inadequate proximal or distal seal zones, tortuosity, lack of vascular access options, or extremes of aortic diameter *(may be possible to overcome with advanced endovascular procedures such as branching grafts or "chimney" procedures)*

POSSIBLE COMPLICATIONS [1–4]

- Vascular access site-related complications; hematoma, infection, lymphocele, access artery injuries *(thrombosis, dissection, pseudoaneurysm, arteriovenous fistula formation, vessel perforation, vascular avulsion)*
- Postimplantation syndrome *(back pain, mild elevation of white count, low-grade fever, elevation of C-reactive protein)*
- Ischemic complications due to dislodgment of thrombotic and atheromatous deposits, with microembolization into supplying arteries, interruption of collateral or supplying arteries and/or due to thrombosis of endograft components
  - Spinal cord ischemia
  - Cerebrovascular accident
  - Visceral ischemia
- Intra-procedural aortic perforation and conversion to open surgical repair
- Iliac artery rupture
- New dissection or extension of an existing dissection
- Contrast-induced nephropathy
- Graft migration; *1–2.8 %*
- Graft collapse, stenosis, or thrombosis
- Graft malposition or incomplete expansion
- Graft infection
- Endoleak; *3.9–15.3 %*
- Late aortic perforation and subsequent fistula formation
- Aortotracheal/esophageal fistula
- Mortality

PREPROCEDURAL ASSESSMENT AND PLANNING [1–4, 6]

- History, indications, and physical examination *(Appendix 1* in Chap. 149*)*. Document indications of the procedure, lower and upper extremity pulses, and vital signs.
- Evaluation of recent (within 3 month) diagnostic imaging studies to determine the relevant vascular anatomy, assess the access vessels and obtain accurate diameter and length measurements. Reformatting in multiple planes is essential for accurate measurements. In cases of dissection, the precise relationship of each major branch vessel to the dissection flap, and relative position and

size of the true and false lumens should be assessed.

- Anatomic selection criteria: Lending zones; normal aortic segments >20 mm in length are required distal to the left subclavian artery and proximal to the celiac trunk. Aortic angulation of <60° is preferred.
- Periprocedural management of coagulation status *(Appendices 2* in Chap. 150 *and 3* in Chap. 151*)*
- Antibiotic prophylaxis: Routinely recommended *(first choice agent: 1 g cefazolin intravenously)* [6] *(Appendices 4* in Chap. 152 *and 5* in Chap. 153*)*
- Imaging modality for guidance: Fluoroscopy
- Positioning: Supine
- Vascular access: Carefully assess the quality of common femoral and iliac arteries. Adequate caliber to accommodate delivery systems or requirement for a surgical conduit. Usually right femoral artery is used. For aortic dissections, select an access site that allows entrance into the true lumen. Typically, the false lumen does not extend as far as the common femoral artery, and puncture at this level usually provides access to the true lumen (correlate with diagnostic imaging findings). The contralateral femoral artery and/or left brachial/axillary artery can be used for angiography or introduction of intravascular ultrasound device which can be of great value in cases of dissection to differentiate the true from the false lumen.
- In cases when the left subclavian artery coverage is required to obtain an adequate proximal seal *(particularly in dissection or traumatic aortic transection cases):*
  - Preoperative duplex ultrasound of the carotid and vertebral arteries should be performed.
  - Consideration given to performing preemptive left carotid-subclavian bypass or subclavian transposition, specifically in patients with prior internal mammary coronary bypass or a dominant left vertebral artery. TEVAR can then be completed as a second-stage procedure with embolization of the native subclavian artery to prevent type II endoleak.
- Patient preparation:
  - Start intravenous fluids the night before angiography in order to ensure adequate hydration, combined with effective monitoring of fluid status.
  - Insert a urinary catheter before the procedure depending on the estimated time of the procedure.
  - Considerations for patients with specific diseases or conditions, patients on specific medications, or patients with history of multiple comorbidities; obtain subspecialty consultation as needed.
  - Prophylactic cerebrospinal fluid drainage: Patient with perioperative hypotension *(mean arterial pressure < 70 mm Hg)*, aortic treatment length > 20 cm, endograft coverage between the levels of T8 and L2, and prior history of abdominal aortic aneurysm repair.

PROCEDURE NOTE

Procedure: Thoracic endovascular aortic repair/aortic fenestration with/without endovascular stent graft repair
Staff: [_]
Fellow: [_]
Resident: [_]
Clinical History and Indications: Describe history and list indications
Allergies: None known/Allergic to [specify/type of allergy]
Anesthesia: Local anesthesia (rarely)/Regional anesthesia with monitored conscious sedation/General anesthesia
Medications: List any relevant medications used
Contrast Material: (_) mL of [type] contrast material was used for intra-arterial injection
Field: Sterile
Procedure classification: Clean
Position: Supine

Monitoring: Intravenous access line was secured and vital signs were continuously monitored by nursing staff/anesthesia team throughout the procedure
Total fluoroscopy time: (_) min
Cumulative radiation dose: (_) mGy

Description of Procedure *(endovascular graft repair of thoracic aorta):*

The risks, benefits, alternatives, and procedure itself were explained to the patient/patient's Power of Attorney/patient's legal guardian, and informed written consent was obtained. Time out was performed to confirm the correct patient, procedure, and site. The site of the vascular access was identified and marked.

The patient was positioned supine on the fluoroscopy table. General/regional anesthesia with monitored sedation was performed. The left arm was positioned at 90 degrees to allow for angiography. The skin of both groins and left arm were shaved, prepped, and draped in the usual sterile fashion. A right radial arterial line was obtained for continuous arterial pressure monitoring. Right femoral artery access was obtained via surgical cutdown/arteriotomy/surgical conduit and a (_)-French sheath was introduced.

Left common femoral artery access was obtained using a (_)-gauge [type] needle and the Seldinger technique under direct ultrasound visualization/by palpation. Once arterial flow was detected, a (_)-inch [type] guidewire was advanced through the needle into the aorta under direct fluoroscopic visualization and a (_)-French vascular sheath was placed.

Left brachial artery access was also obtained for lateral angiography, using a (_)-gauge [type] needle and the Seldinger technique under direct ultrasound visualization/by palpation. Once arterial flow was detected, a (_)-inch [type] guidewire was advanced through the needle, into the aortic arch under direct fluoroscopic visualization and a (_)-French vascular sheath was placed.

Heparinized saline infusion was started into the arterial sheaths. Systemic heparinization was also achieved by injecting (_) international units of heparin intravenously and a baseline activated clotting time (ACT) was obtained (typically 250–300 s preferred).

Subsequently, a (_)-French, [pigtail/type] marker catheter was advanced via the left femoral/brachial access into the ascending aorta/proximal aortic arch over a (_)-inch [hydrophilic/type] guidewire under direct fluoroscopic visualization. The vascular catheter was used to perform a digital subtraction aortogram, by injecting (_) mL of contrast at a flow rate of (_) mL/s using an automated injector. Digital subtraction angiography images were obtained at (_) frames per second during suspended respiration in a left anterior oblique projection, perpendicular to the aortic arch and [specify other projections if obtained].

The right femoral arterial access was used to advance a (_)-French diagnostic catheter over a (_)-inch hydrophilic wire to the level of the proximal aortic arch, which was then exchanged for a (_)-inch superstiff [type] guidewire.

Then, the introducer sheath was advanced over the superstiff guidewire with continuous fluoroscopic guidance. The endograft device [specify type, length and diameter] was then advanced over the superstiff guidewire with continuous fluoroscopic guidance angled perpendicular to the proximal landing zone, so that the superior end of the endograft was positioned at an appropriate level [specify location of proximal lending zone]. Intermittent angiography was performed using the contralateral access site/upper extremity access to confirm the position of the endograft. After reconfirming appropriate positioning, the respiration was suspended and the endograft was deployed under continuous fluoroscopy control as per manufacturer instructions. Repeat aortography was performed confirming the correct location of the endograft. Then the delivery catheter was carefully withdrawn under continuous fluoroscopy. The endograft was balloon dilated using a (_) × (_) mm [type] compliant balloon to achieve maximum profile (balloon dilation should be avoided in cases of aortic dissection).

All stiff guidewires were removed and completion aortography was performed confirming the correct location of the endograft, continued patency of the arch branch vessels and absence of endoleaks [specify if otherwise].

The left femoral and brachial vascular sheaths were removed and hemostasis was achieved by compression/using [type] occlusion device. The right femoral sheath was also removed and arteriotomy was surgically repaired. The patient was transferred to the intensive care unit/ recovery room after the procedure in a stable/critical condition for further close monitoring. Staff was present during the entire procedure. There was excellent flow into both feet at the completion of the procedure.

Description of Procedure *(endovascular aortic fenestration with/without stent graft placement):*

The risks, benefits, alternatives, and procedure itself were explained to the patient/patient's Power of Attorney/patient's legal guardian, and informed written consent was obtained. Time out was performed to confirm the correct patient, procedure, and site. The site of the vascular access was identified and marked.

The patient was positioned supine on the fluoroscopy table. General/regional anesthesia with monitored sedation was performed. The left arm was positioned at 90° to allow for angiography. The skin of both groins and left arm were shaved, prepped, and draped in the usual sterile fashion. A right radial arterial line was obtained for continuous arterial pressure monitoring. Right femoral artery access was obtained via surgical arteriotomy/surgical conduit and a (_)-French sheath was introduced.

Left common femoral artery access was obtained using a (_)-gauge [type] needle and the Seldinger technique under direct ultrasound visualization/by palpation. Once arterial flow was detected, a (_)-inch [type] guidewire was advanced through the needle into the aorta under direct fluoroscopic visualization and a (_)-French vascular sheath was placed.

Left brachial artery access was also obtained, using a (_)-gauge [type] needle and the Seldinger technique under direct ultrasound visualization/ by palpation. Once arterial flow was detected, a (_)-inch [type] guidewire was advanced through the needle, into the aortic arch under direct fluoroscopic visualization and a (_)-French vascular sheath was placed. Heparinized saline infusion was started into the arterial sheaths.

Subsequently, a (_)-French [pigtail/type] catheter was advanced via the left femoral access into the ascending aorta/proximal aortic arch over a (_)-inch J-tip [hydrophilic/type] guidewire under direct fluoroscopic visualization. Then the catheter was exchanged for an endovascular ultrasound device and location within the true lumen was confirmed.

A marker catheter was advanced through the left arm access over a (_)-inch hydrophilic wire into the true lumen and location was confirmed using the endovascular ultrasound. The vascular catheter was used to perform a limited digital subtraction aortogram, by injecting (_) mL of contrast at a flow rate of (_) mL/s using an automated injector. Digital subtraction angiography images were obtained at (_) frames per second during suspended respiration in a left anterior oblique projection, perpendicular to the aortic arch and [specify other projections if obtained]. The location of the intimal tear was identified and the catheter was carefully directed into the false lumen over the hydrophilic guidewire. Pressure measurements of the true and false lumens were obtained showing significant gradient/no significant pressure gradients (fenestration will not be beneficial in this case).

The true lumen was then cannulated through the right femoral access using a (_) French [type] catheter advanced over a (_)-inch J-tip hydrophilic wire. The catheter was then exchanged for a (_)-French guiding sheath. Location was confirmed within the true lumen using the intravascular ultrasound. The hydrophilic wire was then exchanged for a (_)-inch [stiff] wire and a curved, hollow metal [type] needle was introduced through the sheath over the wire into the aorta and placed above the level to be punctured. The intravascular ultrasound transducer was then positioned at the intended level of the puncture [usually in the infrarenal aorta, although fenestrations at several levels may be required to achieve equalization of pressures/The level chosen for puncture should allow enough space for the stylet to pass through the flap without puncturing the far wall of the aorta and directed away from major branch vessels]. The metal stylet, with a coaxially mounted (_)-French catheter, was inserted to just inside the needle tip. Under fluoroscopic and intravascular ultrasound control, the needle assembly was pulled back and rotated until it was seen at intravascular ultrasound indenting the flap at the point required for puncture. The stylet was then advanced 1–2 cm through the flap. The stylet was removed and the catheter was advanced in position across the flap. A stiff J-tip guidewire was then advanced into the false lumen through the catheter. A (_)-French vascular [type] catheter was introduced over the stiff wire into the false lumen to confirm satisfactory entry and measure false lumen pressure. With an over-the-wire exchange technique, an appropriately sized (15–20 mm), low-profile [type] balloon catheter was inserted through the sheath and, under intravascular ultrasound guidance, the balloon was positioned across the flap and inflated to dilate the fenestrated flap. Luminal pressures were again measured [document pressure in the true and false lumen/If there is a residual gradient, consider whether to enlarge the fenestration with a larger balloon (no larger than 20 mm) or to create a second fenestration].

Following the fenestration, the stiff guidewire was removed. A (_)-French, (_)-cm-long [pigtail/type] marker catheter was advanced via the left femoral/brachial access into the ascending aorta/proximal aortic arch over a (_)-inch [hydrophilic/type] guidewire under direct fluoroscopic visualization. The vascular catheter was used to perform a digital subtraction aortogram, by injecting (_) mL of contrast at a flow rate of (_) mL/s using an automated injector. Digital subtraction angiography images were obtained at (_) frames per second during suspended respiration in a left anterior oblique projection, perpendicular to the aortic arch and [specify other projections if obtained].

The right femoral arterial access was used to advance a (_)-French diagnostic catheter over a (_)-inch hydrophilic wire to the level of the proximal aortic arch, which was then exchanged for a (_)-inch superstiff [type] guidewire.

Then, the introducer sheath was advanced over the superstiff guidewire with continuous fluoroscopic guidance. The endograft device [specify type, length and diameter] was advanced over the superstiff guidewire with continuous fluoroscopic guidance angled perpendicular to the proximal landing zone, so that the superior end of the endograft was positioned at an appropriate level to cover the proximal intimal tear [specify location of proximal lending zone]. Intermittent angiography was performed using the contralateral access site/upper extremity access to confirm the position of the endograft. After reconfirming appropriate position, the respiration was suspended and the endograft was deployed under continuous fluoroscopy control as per manufacturer instructions. Repeat aortography was performed confirming the correct location of the endograft. Then the delivery catheter was carefully withdrawn under continuous fluoroscopy. No balloon dilatation should be performed in case of dissection.

All stiff guidewires were removed and completion aortography was performed confirming the correct location of the endograft, continued patency of the arch branch vessels and absence of endoleaks [specify if otherwise].

The left femoral and brachial vascular sheaths were removed and hemostasis was achieved by compression/using [type] occlusion device. The right femoral sheath was also removed and arteriotomy was surgically repaired. The patient was transferred to the intensive care unit/recovery room after the procedure in a stable/critical condition for further close monitoring. Staff was present during the entire procedure.

Intra-Procedure Findings: List all relevant findings.

Immediate Complications: None encountered during or directly after the procedure. List complications if any.

Post-Procedure Plan [1]:

- Keep patient complete bed rest with the right/left leg extended for 6 h [adjust depending on the puncture site].
- Check the right/left groin/[specify the puncture site if different] for any bleeding or hematoma formation every 15 min for 1 h, then every 30 min for 1 h, then every hour for 4 h; inform interventional radiology team if any signs of bleeding are observed [adjust depending on the puncture site].
- Check and document lower extremity pulses every 30 min for 2 h then every 1 h for 4 h [adjust depending on the puncture site].
- Monitor vital signs every 15 min for 1 h, then every 30 min for 4 h; notify interventional radiology team if systolic blood pressure <100 mm Hg, or heart rate >110 beats/min. Maintain mean arterial pressure over 100 mm Hg.
- Drain CSF catheter as needed to keep CSF pressure below mmHg
- Continue adequate intravenous hydration and monitor fluid (intake–output) status.
- Check complete blood count and creatinine on the day following the procedure or as clinically indicated.
- Perform regular neurological examination and monitor for signs and symptoms of paraplegia or paraparesis, or stroke.
- Perform post-procedural physical examination and imaging surveillance at 1, 6, and 12 months, and then yearly if no endoleak is detected.
- If endoleak is detected, perform post-procedural physical examination and imaging surveillance every 6 months for the first 2 years and yearly thereafter unless treatment is indicated.

Impression:

- Thoracic endovascular aortic repair/aortic fenestration with/without stent graft placement, as described above.
- The patient tolerated the procedure well and left the interventional unit in stable condition.
- The patient was unstable and the procedure was canceled/terminated prematurely.
- List any other relevant or important information/finding.

References

1. Wang DS, Dake MD. Stent-Grafts for Thoracic Aortic Aneurysms and Dissections. In: Kandarpa K, Machan L, editors. Handbook of interventional radiologic procedures. 4th ed. Philadelphia: Lippincott Williams & Wilkins; 2011. p. 171–80.
2. Wang GJ, Fairman RM. Endovascular repair of the thoracic aorta. Semin Intervent Radiol. 2009;26(1):17–24.
3. Bean MJ, Johnson PT, Roseborough GS, Black JH, Fishman EK. Thoracic aortic stent-grafts: utility of multidetector CT for pre- and postprocedure evaluation. Radiographics. 2008 Nov-Dec;28(7):1835-51.
4. Nation DA, Wang GJ. TEVAR: Endovascular Repair of the Thoracic Aorta. Semin Intervent Radiol. 2015;32 (3):265–71.
5. Hartnell GG, Gates J. Aortic fenestration: a why, when, and how-to guide. Radiographics. 2005;25(1):175–89.
6. Venkatesan AM, Kundu S, Sacks D, Wallace MJ, Wojak JC, Rose SC, et al. Practice guidelines for adult antibiotic prophylaxis during vascular and interventional radiology procedures. J Vasc Interv Radiol. 2010;21(11):1611–30.

79 Transarterial Embolization of Type II Endoleak

Eric T. Aaltonen

Abbreviation

EVAR Endovascular aneurysm repair

INTRODUCTION

Endovascular aneurysm repair (EVAR) of abdominal aortic aneurysms has become a widely accepted alternative to open repair with similar survival and rupture outcomes. There are five subtypes of endoleak following EVAR; type II endoleak is the most common (40 %) and involves perigraft blood flow via an artery arising from the aneurysm sac [1]. There are two subtypes of type II endoleaks; single vessel inflow and outflow is characterized as IIA and multiple inflow/outflow vessels are characterized as IIB. The annual incidence of type II endoleaks following endovascular aneurysm repair is approximately 5–8 % [2, 3]. The presence of a type II endoleak on imaging is associated with a very low risk of rupture if there is no accompanying increase in aneurysm sac diameter and these endoleaks often resolve spontaneously. However, growth of the aneurysm sac associated with a type II endoleak is concerning for impending rupture. A 5 mm interval increase in maximum diameter of the sac over a 6-month period is a widely accepted treatment threshold [4]. Treatment of a type II endoleak requires cessation of the inflow/outflow of perigraft blood by embolization either via a transarterial or percutaneous transluminal approach. These two techniques have been shown to have similar success and complication outcomes [5]. Regardless of technique, the sac must be embolized centrally much like the nidus of an arteriovenous malformation to achieve success. Transarterial embolization of the inflow vessel only without embolization of the sac may lead to recruitment of other side branches and continued endoleak [4].

COMMON INDICATIONS [4, 6]

Absolute Indications:

- 5 mm or greater increase in maximum aneurysm sac diameter over a 6-month period during EVAR surveillance

Relative Indications:

- Less than 5 mm increase in maximum aneurysm sac diameter over a 6-month surveillance period

E.T. Aaltonen (✉)
Department of Radiology, New York University Langone Medical Center, 660 1st Avenue, New York, NY 10016, USA
e-mail: eric.aaltonen@nyumc.org

B. Taslakian et al. (eds.), *Procedural Dictations in Image-Guided Intervention*,
DOI 10.1007/978-3-319-40845-3_79

- 5 mm or greater increase in maximum aneurysm sac diameter over a surveillance period longer than 6 months

COMMON CONTRAINDICATIONS

- Severe allergy to intravenous contrast or impaired renal function *(consider CO_2 angiography or percutaneous approach)*
- Severe coagulopathy that cannot be corrected *(relative contraindication)*

POSSIBLE COMPLICATIONS [4, 7]

General (angiography-related) complications:
- Hemorrhage *(puncture-site hematoma, retroperitoneal hematoma if "high" puncture above inguinal ligament)*
- Pseudoaneurysm *(superficial femoral artery "low" puncture)*
- Arteriovenous fistula *(puncture-site artery)*
- Thrombosis of the femoral artery
- Distal embolization
- Contrast-induced allergic reaction
- Contrast-induced nephropathy
- Arterial perforation or dissection
- Catheter or guidewire breakage
- Limb amputation *(rare)*
- Risks related to any minimally invasive procedure performed under conscious sedation *(e.g., allergy to medications)*

Procedure-specific complications:
- Nontarget embolization *(ischemia secondary to embolic material in distal inferior mesenteric artery branches)*

PREPROCEDURAL ASSESSMENT AND PLANNING [8–10]

- History, indications, and physical examination *(Appendix 1* in Chap. 148*)* including distal pulses
- Evaluation of diagnostic imaging studies to determine probable source and approach to vessel causing retrograde filling of aneurysm sac *(often the source is the inferior mesenteric artery and a microcatheter is used to directly catheterize the artery and sac* via *the arc of Riolan from the superior mesenteric artery)*
- Periprocedural management of coagulation status *(Appendices 2* in Chap. 149 *and 3* in Chap. 150*)*
- Antibiotic prophylaxis: Not routinely recommended [8] *(Appendices* in Chap. 151 *and* in Chap. 152*)*
- Imaging modality for guidance: Fluoroscopy
- Positioning: Supine
- Arterial access: Common femoral artery, left radial/brachial artery

PROCEDURE NOTE

Procedure: Transarterial embolization of type II endoleak
Staff: [_]
Fellow: [_]
Resident: [_]
Clinical History and Indications: Describe history and indication; *(include date of endograft placement and specify interval increase in aneurysm sac diameter and length of surveillance period)*
Allergies: None known/Allergic to [specify/type of allergy]
Anesthesia: Local anesthesia/Conscious sedation/General anesthesia
Medications: List any relevant medications used
Contrast Material: (_) mL of [type] contrast material was used for intra-arterial injection
Field: Sterile
Procedure classification: Clean
Position: Supine
Monitoring: Intravenous access line was secured and vital signs were continuously monitored by nursing staff/anesthesia team throughout the procedure
Total fluoroscopy time: (_) min
Cumulative radiation dose: (_) mGy
Description of Procedure *(inferior mesenteric artery is source of endoleak):*

The risks, benefits, alternatives, and procedure itself were explained to the patient/patient's

Power of Attorney/patient's legal guardian, and informed written consent was obtained. Time out was performed to confirm the correct patient, procedure, and site. The site of the arterial access was identified and marked.

The patient was positioned supine and the right/left groin was prepped and draped in usual sterile fashion. The right/left common femoral artery as well as the inguinal ligament were located by palpation/ultrasound and marked. The site of arterial puncture was determined using combined information from palpation, ultrasound, and fluoroscopy over the middle of the medial third of the femoral head. Local anesthesia was administered. Common femoral artery access was obtained using a (_)-gauge [type] needle and the Seldinger technique under direct ultrasound visualization/by palpation. Once pulsatile arterial flow was detected, a (_)-inch [type] guidewire was advanced through the needle, up through the common femoral artery, into the aorta under direct fluoroscopic visualization and a (_)-French vascular sheath was placed.

Heparinized saline infusion was initiated through the sidearm of the femoral arterial sheath. Subsequently, a (_)-French, (_) cm-long [type] catheter was advanced into the abdominal aorta over a (0.035)-inch [hydrophilic/type] guidewire under direct fluoroscopic visualization, the superior mesenteric artery was selectively catheterized and angiography was performed using (_) mL of contrast and demonstrated [specify findings]. Following this, superselective catheterization of the arc of Riolan was performed using a (_)-French [type] coaxial microcatheter. Angiography was performed using (_) mL of contrast demonstrating a type II endoleak within the aneurysm sac arising from the inferior mesenteric artery and being supplied by the arc of Riolan. The microcatheter was advanced retrogradely through the inferior mesenteric artery via the arc of Riolan and directly into the aneurysm sac. Embolization of the sac was performed using [embolic material of choice—coils, *N*-isobutyl cyanoacrylate (glue), ethylene vinyl alcohol polymer (Onyx), gelfoam, thrombin; specify type, amount of embolizing material, size/number of coils]. Embolization was performed to stasis with additional embolic material placed within the inferior mesenteric artery as the microcatheter was partially withdrawn. Repeat angiography performed using (_) mL of contrast with the microcatheter in the arc of Riolan demonstrated no residual enhancement of the aneurysm sac.

Following the procedure, the right/left femoral artery sheath was removed and adequate hemostasis was achieved with manual compression for (_) min/using the [type] vascular closure device. The femoral and distal pulses were checked following the procedure and were [comparable to the pre-procedure pulses/specify if otherwise needed]. Sterile dressing was applied and the patient was transferred to the floor/recovery room following the procedure in stable condition. Staff was present for the entire procedure.

Description of Procedure (*lumbar artery is source of endoleak*):
The risks, benefits, alternatives, and procedure itself were explained to the patient/patient's Power of Attorney/patient's legal guardian, and informed written consent was obtained. Time out was performed to confirm the correct patient, procedure, and site. The site of the arterial access was identified and marked.

The patient was positioned supine and the right/left groin was prepped and draped in usual sterile fashion. The right/left common femoral artery as well as the inguinal ligament were located by palpation/ultrasound and marked. The site of arterial puncture was determined using combined information from palpation, ultrasound, and fluoroscopy over the middle of the medial third of the femoral head. Local anesthesia was administered. Common femoral artery access was obtained using a (_)-gauge [type] needle and the Seldinger technique under direct ultrasound visualization/by palpation. Once pulsatile arterial flow was detected, a (_)-inch [type] guidewire was advanced through the needle, up through the common femoral artery, into the aorta under direct fluoroscopic visualization and a (_)-French vascular sheath was placed.

Heparinized saline infusion was initiated through the sidearm of the femoral arterial sheath. Subsequently, a (_)-French, (_) cm-long [type] catheter was advanced into the abdominal aorta over a (0.035)-inch [hydrophilic/type] guidewire under direct fluoroscopic visualization and the right/left internal iliac artery was selectively catheterized and angiography was performed using (_) mL of contrast demonstrating [specify findings]. Following this, superselective catheterization of the iliolumbar artery was performed using a (_)-French [type] coaxial microcatheter. Angiography performed using (_) mL of contrast demonstrated a type II endoleak within the aneurysm sac from a lumbar artery arising from the iliolumbar artery. The microcatheter was advanced retrogradely through the lumbar artery via the iliolumbar artery and directly into the aneurysm sac. Embolization of the sac was performed using [embolic material of choice—coils, *N*-isobutyl cyanoacrylate (glue), ethylene vinyl alcohol polymer (Onyx), gelfoam, thrombin; specify type, amount of embolizing material, size/number of coils]. Embolization was performed to stasis with additional embolic material placed within the lumbar artery as the microcatheter was partially withdrawn. Repeat angiography performed using (_) mL of contrast with the microcatheter in the iliolumbar/internal iliac artery demonstrated no residual enhancement of the aneurysm sac.

Following the procedure the right/left femoral artery sheath was removed and adequate hemostasis was achieved with manual compression for ( ) min/using the [type] vascular closure device. The femoral and distal pulses were checked following the procedure and were [comparable to the pre-procedure pulses/specify if otherwise needed].Sterile dressing was applied and the patient was transferred to the floor/recovery room following the procedure in stable condition. Staff was present for the entire procedure.

Intra-Procedure Findings: List all relevant findings.

Immediate Complications: None encountered during or directly after the procedure. List complications if any.

Post-Procedure Plan [5, 6]:

- Bed rest for (2–6) h with right/left leg straight.
- Check the arterial access site at the right/left groin for any bleeding or hematoma formation every 15 min for 1 h, then every 30 min for 1 h; inform interventional radiology team if any complications are observed.
- Monitor vital signs every 15 min for 1 h, then every 30 min for 1 h; notify interventional radiology team if systolic blood pressure <90 mm Hg, or heart rate >110 beats/min.
- Resume diet and previous orders as needed and if not otherwise contraindicated.
- Continue adequate intravenous hydration and monitor fluid (intake–output) status.
- Follow up imaging, typically with CT angiography, recommended at 1 month, 6 months, 12 months, and annually thereafter to monitor aneurysm sac for continued/new expansion. Continued growth of aneurysm sac may require additional embolization or open surgical repair.

Impression:

- Transarterial embolization of abdominal aortic aneurysm type II endoleak using [embolic material above].
- The patient tolerated the procedure well and left the interventional unit in stable condition.
- The patient was unstable and the procedure was canceled/terminated prematurely.
- List any other relevant or important information/finding.

References

1. Bashir MR, Ferral H, Jacobs C, McCarthy W, Goldin M. Endoleaks after endovascular abdominal aortic aneurysm repair: management strategies according to CT findings. AJR Am J Roentgenol. 2009;192(4):W178–86.

2. van Marrewijk C, Buth J, Harris PL, Norgren L, Nevelsteen A, Wyatt MG. Significance of endoleaks after endovascular repair of abdominal aortic aneurysms: the EUROSTAR experience. J Vasc Surg. 2002;35(3):461–73.
3. Mehta M, Sternbach Y, Taggert JB, Kreienberg PB, Roddy SP, Paty PS, et al. Long-term outcomes of secondary procedures after endovascular aneurysm repair. J Vasc Surg. 2010;52(6):1442–9.
4. Hausegger KA. Endoleaks: classification, diagnosis, and treatment. In: Mauro MA, Murphy KPJ, Thomson KR, Venbrux AC, Morgan RA, editors. Image-guided interventions. 2nd ed. Philadelphia: Saunders Elsevier; 2014. p. 334–47.
5. Stavropoulos SW, Park J, Fairman R, Carpenter J. Type 2 endoleak embolization comparison: translumbar versus modified transarterial embolization. J Vasc Interv Radiol. 2009;20(10):1299–302.
6. Lookstein RA, Giordano CF. Diagnosis and Management of Endoleaks. In: Kandarpa K, Machan L, editors. Handbook of interventional radiologic procedures. 4th ed. Philadelphia: Lippincott Williams & Wilkins; 2011. p. 198–205.
7. Sarac TP, Gibbons C, Vargas L, Liu J, Srivastava S, Bena J, et al. Long-term follow-up of type II endoleak embolization reveals the need for close surveillance. J Vasc Surg. 2012;55(1):33–40.
8. Venkatesan AM, Kundu S, Sacks D, Wallace MJ, Wojak JC, Rose SC, et al. Practice guidelines for adult antibiotic prophylaxis during vascular and interventional radiology procedures. J Vasc Interv Radiol. 2010;21:1611–30.
9. Taslakian B, Sebaaly MG, Al-Kutoubi A. Patient evaluation and preparation in vascular and interventional radiology: what every interventional radiologist should know (part 1: patient assessment and laboratory tests). Cardiovasc Intervent Radiol. 2016;39 (3):325–33.
10. Taslakian B, Sebaaly MG, Al-Kutoubi A. Patient evaluation and preparation in vascular and interventional radiology: what every interventional radiologist should know (part 2: patient preparation and medications). Cardiovasc Intervent Radiol. 2016;39 (4):489–99. doi: 10.1007/s00270-015-1239-4. [Epub 2015 Nov 25].

Part XIII
Vascular Interventional Procedures: Systemic Veins

Introduction by John A. Kaufman, Section Reviewer

Interventions in the central systemic veins have a very important role in Interventional Radiology (IR). The impact of a well-placed, reliably functioning central venous access on a patient's quality of life is huge. Vena cava filters can be life-saving devices for patients with venous thromboembolism who cannot be anticoagulated. Recanalization and stent placement in the central veins is becoming both more prevalent and easier as better tools and devices become available. Overall, central venous interventions are a big part of many IR practices, and are often essential for optimal patient care.

One of the hallmarks of patients needing central venous interventions is their varied pathologies. These patients can originate on almost any service in the hospital, or any physician's office. This provides a unique opportunity for interventionalists to contribute to the care of the patients by providing consultation and assisting in the management of the venous component of their health. For example, the interventionalist who places a retrievable or convertible IVC filter should take responsibility for following that patient and helping the referring physician decide when filtration is no longer necessary. The interventionalist may place and remove dozens of filters each year, but most physicians manage just a handful of these patients. In summary, these are important procedures, and ideal for a consultative IR practice.

This section provides a comprehensive list of procedural reports that covers a vast majority of procedures performed in the systemic veins, with up-to-date explanatory notes, synopsis of the indications and contraindications, and potential complications in an organized and practical format.

Section Chapters

Brachiocephalic/Subclavian Venoplasty and Stenting

80

Howayda Al Mrad and Joelle Wazen

INTRODUCTION

Central venous stenosis is commonly associated with intravenous device placement such as dialysis catheters. Patients on hemodialysis are more affected as they usually require device placement and have a turbulent blood flow at the level of their arteriovenous fistula. A rarer cause of central vein occlusion is primary upper extremity deep venous thrombosis such as Paget-Schroetter syndrome/effort-induced thrombosis and thoracic outlet syndrome, in which the vein is subject to extrinsic anatomic compression by the mediastinal structures. Endovascular techniques have largely replaced the direct surgical approach in the treatment of brachiocephalic and subclavian venous stenosis due to their relative safety and efficacy. Stent placement shows excellent technical results and helps preserve vascular access for a substantial period of time; however, repeated intervention is required to maintain patency. Self expanding stents are preferred in these locations.

H. Al Mrad (✉)
Department of Radiology, American University of Beirut Medical Center, Beirut 1107 2020, Lebanon
e-mail: mourad.howayda@gmail.com

J. Wazen
Department of Diagnostic Radiology, UMass Memorial Medical Center, Worcester, MA, USA
e-mail: joelle.wazen@gmail.com

INDICATIONS [1–7]

- Venous stenosis due to previous history of central venous device placement
- Late stenosis after surgical decompression
- Symptomatic hemodialysis shunt dysfunction and arm swelling due to central venous obstruction
- Stenting after unsuccessful venoplasty *(i.e., residual stenosis or restenosis)*
- Primary upper extremity deep venous thrombosis if residual stenosis develops following surgical decompression, thrombectomy, or thrombolysis

COMMON CONTRAINDICATION [2, 3, 5, 8]

- Benign subclavian vein obstruction secondary to compression syndromes *(Paget-Schroetter syndrome, thoracic outlet syndrome)*, requiring surgical decompression first

POSSIBLE COMPLICATIONS [1, 2, 5, 8]

- Bleeding from puncture site
- Venous thrombosis and rupture
- Restenosis
- Pneumothorax
- Air embolism
- Migration of the stent

B. Taslakian et al. (eds.), *Procedural Dictations in Image-Guided Intervention*,
DOI 10.1007/978-3-319-40845-3_80

- Infection
- Stent compression or fracture *(due to external compression by normal adjacent anatomic structures)*
- Cardiac perforation *(very rare)*
- Hemothorax or hemomediastium

PREPROCEDURAL ASSESSMENT AND PLANNING [9–11]

- History, indications, and physical examination *(Appendix 1* in Chap. 149*)*
- Evaluation of diagnostic imaging studies to determine the relevant vascular anatomy, and presence of normal variants and venous thrombosis/occlusion. This will assure preprocedural selection of an appropriate access site and effective planning to avoid complications and limit procedure time.
- Periprocedural management of coagulation status *(Appendices 2* in Chap. 150 *and 3* in Chap. 151*)*
- Antibiotic prophylaxis: Not routinely recommended [9] *(Appendices 4* in Chap. 152 *and 5* in Chap. 153*)*
- Imaging modality for guidance: Fluoroscopy, combined with ultrasound for access venotomy
- Positioning: Supine
- Venous access: Brachial, basilic vein, cephalic vein (less desirable)

PROCEDURE NOTE

Procedure: Left/Right subclavian/brachiocephalic angioplasty/and stenting
Staff: [_]
Fellow: [_]
Resident: [_]
Clinical History and Indications: Describe history and list indications
Allergies: None known/Allergic to [specify/type of allergy]
Anesthesia: Local anesthesia/conscious sedation
Medications: List any relevant medications used
Contrast Material: (_) mL of [type] contrast material was used for venography
Field: Sterile
Procedure classification: Clean
Position: Supine
Monitoring: Intravenous access line was secured and vital signs were continuously monitored by nursing staff/anesthesia team throughout the procedure
Total fluoroscopy time: (_) min
Cumulative radiation dose: (_) mGy

Description of the procedure:
The risks, benefits, alternatives, and the procedure itself were explained to the patient/patient's Power of Attorney/legal guardian, and informed written/verbal consent was obtained. The site of the procedure was identified and marked. Time out was performed to confirm the correct patient, procedure and site. The site of the venous access was identified and marked.

The right/left arm was cleaned and draped in the usual sterile fashion. Ultrasound examination was performed to determine the site of venous puncture. Local anesthesia was administered. The left/right basilic/brachial/cephalic vein was punctured under ultrasound guidance using a (_)-gauge [type] needle. Once good venous flow was detected, a (_)-inch [type] guidewire was advanced through the needle under direct fluoroscopic visualization. A small skin incision was made and a (_)-French vascular sheath was advanced over the guidewire. Peripheral venogram was performed by injecting (_) mL of [-type] contrast through the sheath and digital subtraction angiography images were obtained showing [specify findings]. Digital road-mapping was also performed to identify the site and length of stenosis as well as the diameter of the normal vein. Through the sheath, a (_) French [angiographic/type] catheter was inserted over a (0.035)-inch [hydrophilic/type] guidewire to navigate through the point of stricture/obstruction, which was successfully crossed. The hydrophilic guidewire was exchanged for a (_)-inch [type] guidewire which was advanced into the inferior vena cava to provide adequate support. Following this, a (_) mm [type] balloon catheter was inserted over the guidewire and venoplasty was performed by inflating the balloon manually with iodinated contrast material using a (_)-mL syringe/inflation device, under fluoroscopy visualization until the "waist" at the stricture site disappeared. The balloon was left inflated for (_) min and the inflation was repeated on (_) consecutive occasions. Then, a (_)-cm-ong, (_)-mm [type] stent was deployed at the site of the stenosis/obstruction. The stent was dilated to the required size using balloon dilatation. Completion venography was performed for documentation and future reference.

The sheath was removed and adequate hemostasis was achieved at the venotomy site by compression for (_) minutes. Sterile dressing was applied and the patient was transferred to the floor/recovery room following the procedure in a stable condition. Staff was present for the entire procedure.

Intra-procedure Findings: List all relevant findings.

Immediate Complications: None encountered during or directly after the procedure. List complications if any.

Post-procedure Plan [1, 2, 8]**:**

- Keep patient complete bed rest with the right/left arm extended for (2–3) h.
- Check the puncture site for any bleeding or hematoma formation every 15 min for 1 h, then every 30 min for 2 h; inform interventional radiology team if any complications are observed.
- Monitor vital signs every 15 min for 1 h, then every 30 min for 2 h; notify interventional radiology team if systolic blood pressure <95 mmHg, or heart rate >110 beats/min.
- Resume diet and previous orders as needed and if not otherwise contraindicated.
- Continue adequate intravenous hydration and monitor fluid (intake–output) status.
- Check complete blood count, creatinine, and blood urea nitrogen on the day following the procedure or as clinically indicated.
- Lifelong 325 mg daily aspirin, if not otherwise contraindicated.
- Warfarin for patients with underlying venous thrombosis for 3–6 months following the procedure.
- Follow-up venography at one month to assess for restenosis and stent patency.

Impression:

- Left/Right brachiocephalic/subclavian venoplasty/and stenting as described above.
- The patient tolerated the procedure well and left the interventional unit in stable condition.
- The patient was unable to tolerate the procedure which was canceled/terminated prematurely.
- List any other relevant or important information/finding.

References

1. Kaufman JA. Upper extremity, neck, and central thoracic veins. In: Kaufman JA, Lee MJ, editors. Vascular and interventional radiology: the requisites. 2nd ed. Philadelphia: Elsevier; 2014. p. 136–58.
2. Kurli V, Singh CK, Ingraham Clark TW. Acute upper extremity deep venous thrombosis. In: Mauro MA, Murphy KPJ, Thomson KR, Venbrux AC, Zollikofer CL, editors. Image-guided interventions. Philadelphia: Saunders Elsevier; 2008. P. 1088–94.
3. Gottmann U, Sadick M, Kleinhuber K, Benck U, Huck K, Krämer BK, et al. Central vein stenosis in a dialysis patient: a case report. J Med Case Rep. 2012;6(1):189.
4. Kundu S. Central venous obstruction management. Semin Intervent Radiol. 2009;26(2):115–21.
5. Hammer F, Becker D, Goffette P, Mathurin P. Crushed stents in benign left brachiocephalic vein stenoses. J Vasc Surg. 2000;32(2):392–6.
6. Haage P, Vorwerk D, Piroth W, Schuermann K, Guenther RW. Treatment of hemodialysis-related central venous stenosis or occlusion: results of primary wallstent placement and follow-up in 50 patients 1. Radiology. 1999;212(1):175–80.
7. Vesely TM, Hovsepian DM, Pilgram TK, Coyne DW, Shenoy S. Upper extremity central venous obstruction in hemodialysis patients: treatment with wallstents. Radiology. 1997;204(2):343–8.
8. Mather MN, Hallisey MJ. Venous Angioplasty and Stents. In: Kandarpa K, Machan L, editors. Handbook of interventional radiologic procedures. 4th ed. Philadelphia: Lippincott Williams & Wilkins; 2011. p. 432–8.

9. Venkatesan AM, Kundu S, Sacks D, Wallace MJ, Wojak JC, Rose SC, et al. Practice guidelines for adult antibiotic prophylaxis during vascular and interventional radiology procedures. J Vasc Interv Radiol. 2010;21(11):1611–30.
10. Taslakian B, Sebaaly MG, Al-Kutoubi A. Patient evaluation and preparation in vascular and interventional radiology: what every interventional radiologist should know (part 1: patient assessment and laboratory tests). Cardiovasc Intervent Radiol. 2016;39(3):325–33.
11. Taslakian B, Sebaaly MG, Al-Kutoubi A. Patient evaluation and preparation in vascular and interventional radiology: what every interventional radiologist should know (part 2: patient preparation and medications). Cardiovasc Intervent Radiol. 2016;39(4):489–99. doi: 10.1007/s00270-015-1239-4. [Epub 2015 Nov 25].

Inferior Vena Cava Filter Insertion

81

Bedros Taslakian

Abbreviations

VTE	Venous thromboembolism
IVC	Inferior vena cava

INTRODUCTION

Venous thromboembolism (VTE) is a common cause of morbidity and mortality in hospitalized and surgical patients. Inferior vena cava (IVC) filter placement is essential in patients with recurrent pulmonary thromboembolisms despite adequate anticoagulation or when anticoagulation is contraindicated. The ideal location for filter placement for preventing lower-extremity and pelvic venous thromboembolism is the infrarenal IVC, whereas other locations can be selected in specific cases. Several factors should be taken into consideration when selecting the IVC filter; such as the clinical settings in which the filter is used, magnetic resonance imaging compatibility of the device, and the ease of placement and removal. Retrievable IVC filters are available; can be left in place as a permanent implant or removed when the indication for filter placement resolves.

B. Taslakian (✉)
Department of Radiology, New York University Langone Medical Center, 660 First Ave, New York, NY 10016, USA
e-mail: btaslakian@gmail.com

COMMON INDICATIONS [1–3]

Absolute Indications: *Documented VTE with one or more of the following:*

- Contraindication to anticoagulation
- Anticoagulation-induced bleeding
- Progression or recurrence of VTE despite adequate anticoagulation
- Inability to achieve or maintain therapeutic anticoagulation
- Massive, life-threatening pulmonary embolism with residual deep venous thrombosis

Relative Indications: *Documented VTE with one or more of the following:*

- Documented progression of iliofemoral thrombosis despite adequate anticoagulation
- Iliocaval thrombus
- Massive, free-floating inferior vena cava thrombus
- Before initiation of thrombolytic therapy for iliocaval thrombosis
- Non-compliant patients or inability to monitor patient during treatment
- Increased risk of anticoagulation-induced bleeding, such as patients with frequent falls
- Limited cardiac or pulmonary reserve

B. Taslakian et al. (eds.), *Procedural Dictations in Image-Guided Intervention*,
DOI 10.1007/978-3-319-40845-3_81

Indications for prophylactic filter placement: *Patients with no documented VTE and one of the following:*

- Trauma patient with increased risk of VTE
- Closed head and spinal cord injury
- Multiple fractures involving the long and pelvic bones
- Perioperative prophylaxis in patients with a history or increased risk of VTE
- Critically ill patients with a history or increased risk of VTE and a contraindication to anticoagulation

COMMON CONTRAINDICATIONS [1–3]

- Complete IVC occlusion/thrombosis
- Absent IVC
- Filter cannot be safely accommodated within a very small or large IVC
- Documented allergy to filter material
- Inability to image during filter placement *(e.g., pregnancy)*
- Lack of access to the inferior vena cava *(i.e., all access veins are occluded)*
- Severe coagulopathy that cannot be corrected *(relative contraindication)*
- Past history of allergic contrast material reaction and impaired renal function *(procedure can be performed using alternative contrast agents such as CO_2 or gadolinium)*

POSSIBLE COMPLICATIONS [1–3]

- Access site complications *(e.g., hematoma, thrombosis of access vein, arterial injury)*
- Contrast-induced nephropathy and allergic reaction
- Malposition of the filter
- Malfunctions of the filter leading to recurrent pulmonary thromboembolism
- Malfunction of the deployment system during insertion
- Venous and IVC thrombosis
- Filter fracture and migration
- Filter infection
- IVC perforation during the procedure or due to penetration of filter parts through the wall
- Mortality

PREPROCEDURAL ASSESSMENT AND PLANNING [4–6]

- History, indications, and physical examination *(Appendix 1* in Chap. 149*)*
- Evaluation of diagnostic imaging studies to determine the relevant vascular anatomy and presence of normal variants and venous thrombosis/occlusion. This will assure preprocedural selection of an appropriate access vein and effective planning to avoid complications and limit procedure time.
- Periprocedural management of coagulation status *(Appendices 2* in Chap. 150 *and 3* in Chap. 151*)*
- Antibiotic prophylaxis: Not routinely recommended [4] *(Appendices 4* in Chap. 152 *and 5* in Chap. 153*)*
- Imaging modality for guidance: Fluoroscopy, combined with ultrasound for access venotomy
- Positioning: Supine
- Venous access: Internal jugular vein, femoral vein

PROCEDURE NOTE

Procedure: Placement of inferior vena cava filter
Staff: [_]
Fellow: [_]
Resident: [_]
Clinical History and Indications: Describe history and list indications
Allergies: None known/Allergic to [specify/type of allergy]
Anesthesia: Local anesthesia/conscious sedation
Medications: List any relevant medications used
Contrast Material: (_) mL of [type] contrast material was used for venography
Field: Sterile
Procedure classification: Clean
Position: Supine

Monitoring: Intravenous access line was secured and vital signs were continuously monitored by nursing staff/anesthesia team throughout the procedure
Total fluoroscopy time: (_) min
Cumulative radiation dose: (_) mGy

Description of Procedure *(Jugular Approach):*
The risks, benefits, alternatives, and procedure itself were explained to the patient/patient's Power of Attorney/patient's legal guardian, and informed written/verbal consent was obtained. Time out was performed to confirm the correct patient and procedure. The site of the venous access was identified and marked.

The patient was positioned supine, with the neck turned to the contralateral side. The patient's left/right cervical and upper thoracic regions were prepped and draped in the usual sterile fashion. Ultrasound examination was performed to determine the site of venous puncture. Local anesthesia was administered. The left/right internal jugular vein was punctured under ultrasound guidance using a (_)-gauge [type] needle. Once good venous flow was detected, a (0.018)-inch [type] guidewire was advanced through the needle under direct fluoroscopic visualization and placed in the superior vena cava. A small skin incision was made and a (_)-French vascular sheath was advanced over the guidewire. Then, a (_)-French pigtail catheter was advanced into the Inferior vena cava over a (0.035)-inch [hydrophilic/type] guidewire, and its tip was positioned at the confluence of the iliac veins. Cavogram was performed by injecting (_) mL of [type] contrast, at a rate of (15–20 mL/s) and digital subtraction angiography imaging was performed at (_) frames per second during suspended respiration in an anterior–posterior projection/[specify other projections if obtained]. The contralateral iliac vein and renal veins were identified as inflow of unopacified blood/by reflux of contrast into the venous orifices/by selective catheterization. The size of the inferior vena cava was estimated at (_) cm in diameter.

Following this, the pigtail catheter and the short vascular sheath were exchanged over a (0.035)-inch [type] guidewire for a (_)-French, (_)-cm-long [specify type] filter delivery sheath, under fluoroscopy guidance. The filter delivery system was advanced through the sheath and positioned in the desired location below the lowest renal vein/[specify location]. The sheath was withdrawn to expose the filter which was deployed under continuous fluoroscopy guidance in the infrarenal vena cava/[specify filter apex location relative to vertebral body anatomy]. Completion cavogram was performed using the delivery sheath to document the filter position and exclude complications.

The sheath was removed and adequate hemostasis was achieved at the venotomy site by compression for (_) minutes. Sterile dressing was applied and the patient was transferred to the floor/recovery room following the procedure in a stable condition. Staff was present for the entire procedure.

Description of Procedure *(Femoral Approach):*
The risks, benefits, alternatives, and procedure itself were explained to the patient/patient's Power of Attorney/patient's legal guardian, and informed written/verbal consent was obtained. Time out was performed to confirm the correct patient and procedure. The site of the venous access was identified and marked.

The skin of both groins were shaved, prepped and draped in the usual sterile fashion. The right/left common femoral vein was located by palpation/ultrasound and marked. Local anesthesia was administered and a small skin incision was made. Femoral venous access was obtained using a (_)-gauge [type] needle under direct ultrasound visualization/by palpation. Once good venous flow was detected, a (_)-inch [type] guidewire was advanced through the needle, up through the femoral vein into the inferior vena cava under direct fluoroscopic visualization and a (_)-French, (_)-cm-long vascular sheath was placed.

Then, a (_)-French pigtail catheter was advanced into the inferior vena cava over a (0.035)-inch [hydrophilic/type] guidewire, and its tip was positioned at the confluence of the iliac veins. Cavogram was performed by injecting (_) mL of [type] contrast, at a rate of (15–20 mL/s) and digital subtraction angiography imaging was performed at (_) frames per second during suspended respiration in an anterior–posterior projection/[specify other projections if obtained]. The contralateral iliac vein and renal veins were identified as inflow of unopacified blood/by reflux of contrast into orifices of veins/by selective catheterization. The size of the inferior vena cava was estimated at (_) cm in diameter.

Following this, the pigtail catheter and the short vascular sheath were exchanged over a (0.035)-inch [type] guidewire for a (_)-French, (_)-cm-long [specify type] filter delivery sheath, under fluoroscopy guidance. The filter delivery system was advanced through the sheath and positioned in the desired location below the lowest renal vein/[specify other location]. The sheath was withdrawn to expose the filter, which was deployed under continuous fluoroscopy guidance in the infrarenal vena cava/[specify filter apex location relative to vertebral body anatomy]. Completion cavogram was performed using the delivery sheath to document position and exclude complications.

The sheath was removed and adequate hemostasis was achieved at the venotomy site by compression for (_) min. Sterile dressing was applied and the patient was transferred to the floor/recovery room following the procedure in a stable condition. Staff was present for the entire procedure.

Intra-Procedure Findings: List all relevant findings.

Immediate Complications: None encountered during or directly after the procedure. List complications if any.

Post-Procedure Plan [1–3]:

- Keep patient complete bed rest with the right/left leg extended/head elevated for (2–3) hours *[adjust depending on the venotomy site]*.
- Check the puncture site for any bleeding or hematoma formation every 15 min for 1 h, then every 30 min for 2 h; inform interventional radiology team if any complications are observed.
- Monitor vital signs every 15 min for 1 h, then every 30 min for 2 h; notify interventional radiology team if systolic blood pressure <95 mmHg, or heart rate >110 beats/minute.
- Resume diet and previous orders as needed and if not otherwise contraindicated.
- Continue adequate intravenous hydration and monitor fluid (intake–output) status.
- Check complete blood count, creatinine, and blood urea nitrogen on the day following the procedure or as clinically indicated.
- Observe for developing limb edema, which may indicate caval thrombosis or new deep venous thrombosis.
- For permanent filters, perform regular abdominal imaging studies, every 3 to 5 years, to check filter position and integrity.
- For temporary filters, schedule regular follow-up visits during the temporal window of retrievability to assess anticoagulation status and determine the timing for safe filter removal.

Impression:

- Insertion of inferior vena cava filter as described above.
- The patient tolerated the procedure well and left the interventional unit in stable condition.
- The patient was unstable and the procedure was canceled/terminated prematurely.
- List any other relevant or important information/finding.

References

1. Binkert CA. Caval Filtration. In: Mauro MA, Murphy KPJ, Thomson KR, Venbrux AC, Morgan RA, editors. Image-guided interventions. 2nd ed. Philadelphia: Saunders Elsevier; 2014. p. 781–9.
2. Williamson JA, Kaufman JA. Vena Caval Filters. In: Kandarpa K, Machan L, editors. Handbook of interventional radiologic procedures. 4th ed. Philadelphia: Lippincott Williams & Wilkins; 2011. p. 376–90.

3. Caplin DM, Nikolic B, Kalva SP, Ganguli S, Saad WE, Zuckerman DA. Quality improvement guidelines for the performance of inferior vena cava filter placement for the prevention of pulmonary embolism. J Vasc Interv Radiol. 2011;22(11):1499–506.
4. Venkatesan AM, Kundu S, Sacks D, Wallace MJ, Wojak JC, Rose SC, et al. Practice guidelines for adult antibiotic prophylaxis during vascular and interventional radiology procedures. J Vasc Interv Radiol. 2010;21(11):1611–30.
5. Taslakian B, Sebaaly MG, Al-Kutoubi A. Patient evaluation and preparation in vascular and interventional radiology: what every interventional radiologist should know (part 1: patient assessment and laboratory tests). Cardiovasc Intervent Radiol. 2016;39(3):325–33.
6. Taslakian B, Sebaaly MG, Al-Kutoubi A. Patient evaluation and preparation in vascular and interventional radiology: what every interventional radiologist should know (part 2: patient preparation and medications). Cardiovasc Intervent Radiol. 2016;39(4):489–99. doi: 10.1007/s00270-015-1239-4. [Epub 2015 Nov 25].

Inferior Vena Cava Filter Retrieval

82

Bedros Taslakian

Abbreviations

VTE Venous thromboembolism

INTRODUCTION

Retrievable filters may be placed with the intent of either temporary or permanent filtration. These filters are designed to allow percutaneous filter removal or repositioning during a device-specific window of retrievability. Placement of a retrievable filter with the intent to discontinue filtration follows the same indications used for permanent vena cava filters. The decision to use these filters therefore is based on the anticipated required duration of protection against clinically significant venous thromboembolism (VTE) and/or risk of pharmacologic VTE therapy or prophylaxis. Discontinuation of caval filtration is generally recommended when the indication for the caval interruption is no longer present and is not anticipated to recur or when the risk of recurrent VTE is estimated to be less than the risk of leaving the filter in place.

B. Taslakian (✉)
Department of Radiology, New York University Langone Medical Center, New York, NY, USA
e-mail: btaslakian@gmail.com

COMMON INDICATIONS [1–3]

Absolute Indications: *the filter is a source of major complication:*

- Filter migration
- Malpositioned filter
- Intracardiac migration of the filter
- Symptomatic penetration of the wall of vena cava by filter limbs
- Filter dysfunction due to change in position or structural damage

Relative Indications:

- Effective pharmacological VTE therapy or prophylaxis is achieved
- Resolution of risk factors for VTE
- Discontinuation of filtration to avoid lifelong anticoagulation after resolution of VTE and its risk factors

COMMON CONTRAINDICATIONS [2, 3]

- Delayed removal exceeding the specified temporal window of retrievability
- Persistent indication for vena caval filtration
- Large retained thrombus within the filter

B. Taslakian et al. (eds.), *Procedural Dictations in Image-Guided Intervention*,
DOI 10.1007/978-3-319-40845-3_82

- Failure to achieve adequate pharmacological VTE therapy or prophylaxis
- Noncompliant patients with the pharmacological therapy or follow-up appointments
- High-risk state for recurrent VTE
- Short *(i.e., <6 months)* life expectancy
- Lack of vascular access for filter retrieval
- Retrieval may be postponed in patients with severe coagulopathy; however, interruption of therapeutic or prophylactic anticoagulation is discouraged before filter removal

POSSIBLE COMPLICATIONS [1–3]

- Access site complications *(e.g., hematoma, thrombosis of access vein, arterial injury)*
- Contrast-induced nephropathy and allergic reaction
- Filter fracture and migration
- Embolization of a retained thrombus within the filter
- Inferior vena cava perforation/laceration/stenosis
- Failure of retrieval
- Cardiac arrhythmias

PREPROCEDURAL ASSESSMENT AND PLANNING [4, 5]

- History, indications, and physical examination *(Appendix 1* in Chap. 149*)*; assess for the absence of signs and symptoms of new, recurrent, or progressive VTE
- Evaluation of diagnostic imaging studies to determine the relevant vascular anatomy and assess filter type, location, and integrity, as well as the presence of a large trapped thrombus, caval penetration, and filter migration. This will assure absence of contraindications for filter removal and selection of an appropriate venous access. Duplex examination of the lower extremities is also indicated to exclude the presence of deep venous thrombosis.
- Periprocedural management of coagulation status *(Appendices 2* in Chap. 150 *and 3* in Chap. 151*)*
- Antibiotic prophylaxis: Not routinely recommended *(Appendices 4* in Chap. 152 *and 5* in Chap. 153*)*
- Imaging modality for guidance: Fluoroscopy; combined with ultrasound for access venotomy
- Positioning: Supine
- Venous access: Jugular vein, femoral vein *(depending on the type of the filter)* [2]

PROCEDURE NOTE

Procedure: Removal of inferior vena cava filter
Staff: [_]
Fellow: [_]
Resident: [_]
Clinical History and Indications: Describe history and list indications
Allergies: None known/Allergic to [specify/type of allergy]
Anesthesia: Local anesthesia/conscious sedation
Medications: List any relevant medications used
Contrast Material: (_) mL of [type] contrast material was used for venography
Field: Sterile
Procedure classification: Clean
Position: Supine
Monitoring: Intravenous access line was secured and vital signs were continuously monitored by nursing staff/anesthesia team throughout the procedure
Total fluoroscopy time: (_) min
Cumulative radiation dose: (_) mGy

Description of Procedure *(Jugular Approach):* The risks, benefits, alternatives and procedure itself were explained to the patient/patient's Power of Attorney/patient's legal guardian, and informed written/verbal consent was obtained. Time out was performed to confirm the correct patient and procedure. The site of the venous puncture was determined and marked.

The patient was positioned supine, with the neck turned to the contralateral side. The patient's left/right cervical and upper thoracic regions were prepped and draped in sterile fashion. Ultrasound examination was performed to determine the site of venous puncture. Local anesthesia was administered. The left/right internal jugular vein was punctured under ultrasound guidance using a (_)-gauge [type] needle. Once good venous flow was detected, a (0.018)-inch [type] guidewire was advanced through the needle under direct fluoroscopic visualization and placed in the superior vena cava. A small skin incision was made and a (_)-French vascular sheath was advanced over the guidewire. Then, a (_)-French pigtail catheter was advanced into the inferior vena cava over a (0.035)-inch [hydrophilic/type] guidewire, and its tip was positioned below the filter. Cavogram was performed by injecting (_) mL of [type] contrast, at a rate of (15–20 mL/s) and digital subtraction angiography imaging was performed at (_) frames per second during suspended respiration in an anterior–posterior projection/[specify other projections if obtained].

Following this, the pigtail catheter and short vascular sheath were exchanged over a (0.035)-inch [type] guidewire for a (_)-French, (_)-cm-long [specify type] sheath, under fluoroscopy guidance. The sheath was advanced into the inferior vena cava and placed above the apex of the filter. Through the sheath, a vascular retrieval snare/[type] filter retrieval device was advanced, the filter was grasped and removed by maintaining the filter in stable position and pushing the guiding retrieval catheter over the filter/maintaining the guiding retrieval catheter in stable position and pulling the filter into the catheter (these techniques are based on the manufacturer's instructions). Once the filter was entirely within the retrieval device, it was pulled out the vascular sheath and inspected for integrity. Completion cavogram was performed using the vascular sheath to exclude complications.

The vascular sheath was removed and adequate hemostasis was achieved at the venotomy site by compression for (_) min. Sterile dressing was applied and the patient was transferred to the floor/recovery room following the procedure in a stable condition. Staff was present for the entire procedure.

Description of Procedure *(Femoral Approach):*
The risks, benefits, alternatives and procedure itself were explained to the patient/patient's Power of Attorney/patient's legal guardian, and informed written/verbal consent was obtained. Time out was performed to confirm the correct patient and procedure.

The skin of both groins were shaved, prepped and draped in the usual sterile fashion. The right/left common femoral vein was located by palpation/ultrasound and marked. Local anesthesia was administered and a small skin incision was made. Femoral venous access was obtained using an (_)-gauge [type] needle under direct ultrasound visualization/by palpation. Once good venous flow was detected, a (_)-inch [type] guidewire was advanced through the needle into the inferior vena cava under direct fluoroscopic visualization and a (_)-French, (_)-cm-long vascular sheath was placed.

Then, a (_)-French pigtail catheter was advanced into the inferior vena cava over a (0.035)-inch [hydrophilic/type] guidewire and its tip was positioned at the confluence of the iliac veins. Cavogram was performed by injecting (_) mL of [type] contrast, at a rate of (15–20 mL/s) and digital subtraction angiography imaging was performed at (_) frames per second during suspended respiration in an anterior–posterior projection/[specify other projections if obtained].

Following this, the pigtail catheter and short vascular sheath were exchanged over a (0.035)-inch [type] guidewire for a (_)-French, (_)-cm -long [specify type] sheath, under fluoroscopy guidance. The sheath was advanced into the inferior vena cava and placed below the filter. Through the sheath, a vascular retrieval snare/[type] filter retrieval device was advanced, the filter was grasped and removed by maintaining the filter in stable position and pushing the guiding retrieval catheter over the filter/maintaining the guiding retrieval catheter in stable position and pulling the filter into the catheter (these techniques are based on the manufacturer's instructions). Once the filter was entirely within the retrieval device, it was pulled out the vascular sheath and inspected for integrity. Completion cavogram was performed using the vascular sheath to exclude complications.

The vascular sheath was removed and adequate hemostasis was achieved at the venotomy site by compression for (_) minutes. Sterile dressing was applied and the patient was transferred to the floor/recovery room following the procedure in a stable condition. Staff was present for the entire procedure.

Intra-Procedure Findings: List all relevant findings.

Immediate Complications: None encountered during or directly after the procedure. List complications if any.

Post-Procedure Plan [2, 3]:

- Keep patient complete bed rest with the right/left leg extended/head elevated for (2–3) h *[adjust depending on the venotomy site]*.
- Check the puncture site for any bleeding or hematoma formation every 15 min for 1 h, then every 30 min for 2 h; inform interventional radiology team if any complications are observed.
- Monitor vital signs every 15 min for 1 h, then every 30 min for 4 h; notify interventional radiology team if systolic blood pressure <95 mm Hg, or heart rate >110 beats/minute.
- Resume diet and previous orders as needed and if not otherwise contraindicated.
- Continue adequate intravenous hydration and monitor fluid (intake–output) status.
- Check complete blood count, creatinine and blood urea nitrogen on the day following the procedure or as clinically indicated.
- Continue primary VTE treatment or prophylaxis as indicated.
- Regular follow-up to monitor for new, recurrent, or progressive deep venous thrombosis or VTE.

Impression:

- Removal of inferior vena cava filter as described above.
- The patient tolerated the procedure well and left the interventional unit in stable condition.
- The patient was unstable and the procedure was canceled/terminated prematurely.
- List any other relevant or important information/finding.

References

1. Binkert CA. Caval filtration. In: Mauro MA, Murphy KPJ, Thomson KR, Venbrux AC, Morgan RA, editors. Image-guided interventions. 2nd ed. Philadelphia: Saunders Elsevier; 2014. p. 781–9.
2. Williamson JA, Kaufman JA. Vena Caval Filters. In: Kandarpa K, Machan L, editors. Handbook of interventional radiologic procedures. 4th ed. Philadelphia: Lippincott Williams & Wilkins; 2011. p. 376–90.
3. Kaufman JA, Kinney TB, Streiff MB, Sing RF, Proctor MC, Becker D, et al. Guidelines for the use of retrievable and convertible vena cava filters: report from the Society of Interventional Radiology multidisciplinary consensus conference. J Vasc Interv Radiol. 2006;17(3):449–59.
4. Taslakian B, Sebaaly MG, Al-Kutoubi A. Patient evaluation and preparation in vascular and interventional radiology: what every interventional radiologist should know (part 1: patient assessment and laboratory tests). Cardiovasc Intervent Radiol. 2016;39(3):325–33.
5. Taslakian B, Sebaaly MG, Al-Kutoubi A. Patient evaluation and preparation in vascular and interventional radiology: what every interventional radiologist should know (part 2: patient preparation and medications). Cardiovasc Intervent Radiol. 2016;39(4):489–99. doi: 10.1007/s00270-015-1239-4. [Epub 2015 Nov 25].

Inferior Vena Cavogram

83

Howayda Al Mrad and Joelle Wazen

Abbreviations

IVC Inferior vena cava

INTRODUCTION

While magnetic resonance imaging and computed tomography may be the modalities of choice to assess the inferior vena cava (IVC), cavography is the only method that exactly delineates the luminal anatomy and hemodynamics of the inferior vena cava. Furthermore, cavography is well used prior to, during, and following endovascular interventional procedures, such as IVC filter placement and IVC stenting. Cavography naturally involves contrast use; iodinated contrast material may be generally used; but for patients with renal insufficiency and previous history of allergic reaction, gadolinium, and CO_2 are preferable.

H. Al Mrad (✉)
Department of Diagnostic Radiology, American University of Beirut Medical Center, Riad El-Solh, Beirut 10017 2020, Lebanon
e-mail: mourad.howayda@gmail.com

J. Wazen
Department of Diagnostic Radiology, UMass Memorial Medical Center, Worcester, MA, USA
e-mail: joelle.wazen@gmail.com

COMMON INDICATIONS [1–4]

- Evaluation prior to, during, and following IVC filter placement or removal
- Evaluation prior to, during, and following IVC stenting or reconstruction
- Suspected anatomical variants and congenital malformations
- Suspected IVC occlusive diseases
- Suspected extrinsic compression
- Suspected mural/intra-luminal lesion

COMMON CONTRAINDICATIONS [3]

No absolute contraindications since the availability of gadolinium and CO_2 contrast media.

Relative contraindications:
- Pregnancy
- Previous severe contrast reaction
- Severely compromised cardiopulmonary status

B. Taslakian et al. (eds.), *Procedural Dictations in Image-Guided Intervention*,
DOI 10.1007/978-3-319-40845-3_83

COMMON COMPLICATIONS [5]

- Access site complications (e.g., *hematoma, thrombosis of access vein, arterial injury)*
- Access vein phlebitis
- IVC perforation
- Contrast allergy to iodinated contrast
- Contrast-induced nephropathy

PREPROCEDURAL ASSESSMENT AND PLANNING [6, 7]

- History, indications and physical examination *(Appendix 1 in* Chap. 149*)*
- Evaluation of diagnostic imaging studies to determine the relevant vascular anatomy
- Periprocedural management of coagulation status *(Appendices 2 in* Chap. 150 *and 3* in Chap. 151*)*
- Antibiotic prophylaxis: Not routinely recommended *(Appendices 4* in Chap. 152 *and 5* in Chap. 153*)*
- Imaging modality for guidance: Fluoroscopy; combined with ultrasound for access venotomy
- Positioning: Supine
- Venous access: Internal jugular vein, femoral vein

PROCEDURE NOTE

Procedure: Inferior vena cavogram
Staff: [_]
Fellow: [_]
Resident: [_]
Clinical History and Indications: Describe history and list indications
Allergies: None known/Allergic to [specify/type of allergy]
Anesthesia: Local anesthesia/conscious sedation
Medications: List any relevant medications used
Contrast Material: (_) mL of [type] contrast material was used for venography
Field: Sterile
Procedure classification: Clean
Position: Supine
Monitoring: Intravenous access line was secured and vital signs were continuously monitored by nursing staff/anesthesia team throughout the procedure
Total fluoroscopy time: (_) minutes
Cumulative radiation dose: (_) mGy

Description of the procedure *(Femoral Approach):*
The risks, benefits, alternatives and the procedure itself were explained to the patient/patient's Power of Attorney/legal guardian, and informed written/verbal consent was obtained. Time out was performed to confirm the correct patient and procedure.

The right/left inguinal area was cleaned and draped in the usual sterile fashion. Local anesthesia was infused at the skin entry site. The common femoral vein was located and punctured with a (_)-gauge [type] needle. Using the Seldinger technique, a (_)-inch [type] guidewire was advanced through the needle, up the common femoral vein into to the inferior vena cava under direct fluoroscopic visualization. A (_)-inch [type] pigtail catheter was then advanced over the guidewire and placed at the confluence of the common iliac veins.

Cavogram was performed by injecting (_) mL of [type] contrast, at a rate of (15–20 mL/s) and digital subtraction angiography imaging was performed at (_) frames per second during suspended respiration in an anterior–posterior projection/[specify other projections if obtained].

The venous sheath was removed and adequate hemostasis was achieved at the venotomy site by compression for (_) minutes. Sterile dressing was applied and the patient was transferred to the floor/recovery room following the procedure in a stable condition. Staff was present for the entire procedure.

Description of the procedure *(Jugular Approach)*:
The risks, benefits, alternatives and the procedure itself were explained to the patient/patient's Power of Attorney/legal guardian, and informed written/verbal consent was obtained. Time out

was performed to confirm the correct patient and procedure.

The patient was positioned supine, with the neck turned to the contralateral side. The patient's left/right cervical and upper thoracic regions were prepped and draped in the usual sterile fashion. Ultrasound examination was performed to determine the site of venous puncture. Local anesthesia was administered. The left/right internal jugular vein was punctured under ultrasound guidance using a (_)-gauge [type] needle. Once good venous flow was detected, a (0.018)-in. [type] guidewire was advanced through the needle under direct fluoroscopic visualization and placed in the superior vena cava. A small skin incision was made and a (_)-French vascular sheath was advanced over the guidewire. Then, a (_)-French pigtail catheter was advanced into the inferior vena cava over a (0.035)-in. [hydrophilic/type] guidewire, and its tip was positioned at the confluence of the iliac veins.

Cavogram was performed by injecting (_) mL of [type] contrast, at a rate of (15–20 mL/s) and digital subtraction angiography imaging was performed at (_) frames per second during suspended respiration in an anterior–posterior projection/[specify other projections if obtained].

The venous sheath was removed and adequate hemostasis was achieved at the venotomy site by compression for (_) minutes. Sterile dressing was applied and the patient was transferred to the floor/recovery room following the procedure in a stable condition. Staff was present for the entire procedure.

Intra-Procedure Findings: List all relevant findings.

Immediate Complications: None encountered during or directly after the procedure. List complications if any.

Post-Procedure Plan:

- Keep patient complete bed rest with the right/ left leg extended/head elevated for (2–3) h *[adjust depending on the venotomy site].*
- Check the puncture site for any bleeding or hematoma formation every 15 min for 1 h, then every 30 min for 2 h; inform interventional radiology team if any complications are observed.
- Monitor vital signs every 15 min for 1 h, then every 30 min for 2 h; notify interventional radiology team if systolic blood pressure <95 mmHg, or heart rate >110 beats/minute.
- Resume diet and previous orders as needed and if otherwise not contraindicated.
- Check complete blood count, creatinine and blood urea nitrogen on the day following the procedure or as clinically indicated.

Impression:

- Inferior vena cavogram.
- The patient tolerated the procedure well and left the interventional unit in a stable condition.
- The patient was unstable and the procedure was canceled/terminated prematurely.
- List any other relevant or important information/finding.

References

1. Kaufman JA. Inferior vena cava and tributaries. In: Kaufman JA, Lee MJ, editors. Vascular and interventional radiology: the requisites. 2nd ed. Philadelphia: Elsevier; 2014. p. 287–308.
2. Saad WE. IR for liver transplant. In: Kandarpa K, Machan L, editors. Handbook of interventional radiologic procedures. 4th ed. Philadelphia: Lippincott Williams & Wilkins; 2011. p. 398–407.
3. Aruny JE. Venography. In: Kandarpa K, Machan L, editors. Handbook of interventional radiologic procedures. 4th ed. Philadelphia: Lippincott Williams & Wilkins; 2011. p. 96–108.
4. Dewald CL, Jensen CC, Park YH, Hanks SE, Harrell DS, Peters GL, et al. Vena cavography with CO2 versus with iodinated contrast material for inferior vena cava filter placement: a prospective evaluation. Radiol. 2000;216(3):752–7.
5. Techniques of angiographic investigations of the inferior vena cava. In: Chermet J, Bigot JM editors. Venography of the inferior vena cava and its branches. Berlin: Springer-Verlag; 1980. p. 1–5.

6. Taslakian B, Sebaaly MG, Al-Kutoubi A. Patient evaluation and preparation in vascular and interventional radiology: what every interventional radiologist should know (part 1: patient assessment and laboratory tests). Cardiovasc Intervent Radiol. 2016;39(3):325–33.
7. Taslakian B, Sebaaly MG, Al-Kutoubi A. Patient evaluation and preparation in vascular and interventional radiology: what every interventional radiologist should know (part 2: patient preparation and medications). Cardiovasc Intervent Radiol. 2016;39(4):489–99. doi: 10.1007/s00270-015-1239-4. [Epub 2015 Nov 25].

Peripherally Inserted Central Catheter (PICC)

84

Bedros Taslakian

Abbreviations

PICC	Peripherally inserted central catheter
TPN	Total parental nutrition

INTRODUCTION

Image-guided peripherally inserted central catheters (PICC), which are inserted through a peripheral vein, are well tolerated by patients and have relatively low rate of complications. The access vein can be selected based on the operator's preference and presence of sufficiently distended patent vein. Some operators will choose the largest vein in the upper nondependent arm above the elbow as their access vein, whereas others will routinely select the basilic vein located away from brachial artery to avoid the risk of inadvertent arterial puncture. The cephalic vein which is prone to spasm and thrombosis, and the brachial vein which is located in close proximity to the artery, can also be catheterized. PICC lines can be used from 1 to 12 weeks for continuous or intermittent infusions, as well as frequent blood sampling. Multi-lumen catheters facilitate the infusion of incompatible agents, whereas catheters with a large internal lumen are optimal for infusion of viscous liquids or when rapid infusion of blood products is indicated.

COMMON INDICATIONS [1–4]

- Continuous or frequent administration of intravenous medications or fluids
- Rapid infusion of viscous liquids or blood products
- Administration of cytotoxic medications or chemotherapy that cause venous inflammation in the peripheral veins
- Total parental nutrition (TPN)
- Contraindications for the placement of a permanent venous access (e.g., *coagulopathy, active infection)*
- Infusion of hypertonic agents
- Frequent blood sampling *(rarely a separate indication)*

B. Taslakian (✉)
Department of Radiology, New York University Langone Medical Center, 660 First Ave, New York, NY 10016, USA
e-mail: btaslakian@gmail.com

B. Taslakian
NYU Langone Medical Center, New York, NY 10016, USA

B. Taslakian et al. (eds.), *Procedural Dictations in Image-Guided Intervention*,
DOI 10.1007/978-3-319-40845-3_84

COMMON CONTRAINDICATIONS [1, 2, 4, 5]

- Past history of allergic contrast material reaction and impaired renal function *(the procedure can be performed without contrast media injection)*
- Central venous thrombosis or occlusion
- Difficulty identifying suitable patent peripheral vein
- Focal cellulitis, radiation-induced injury, or burn *(different site can be selected for insertion)*
- Previous mastectomy or axillary lymph node dissection *(different side can be selected for insertion)*
- Patients on hemodialysis *(significant rate of peripheral venous thrombosis)*
- Patients in whom hemodialysis is anticipated (e.g., *renal transplant, chronic renal disease)*

POSSIBLE COMPLICATIONS [1–4]

- Access-site related (e.g., *hematoma, inadvertent arterial injury*).
- Cardiac arrhythmias
- Venous thrombosis
- Catheter site infection and bacteremia
- Malposition when inserted without fluoroscopy guidance
- Catheter dislodgment
- Catheter malfunction due to thrombosis or fibrin sheath formation
- Catheter fracture and embolization of fragments

PREPROCEDURAL ASSESSMENT AND PLANNING [2, 6–8]

- History, indications, and physical examination *(Appendix 1* in Chap. 149*)*
- Evaluation of diagnostic imaging studies to determine the relevant vascular anatomy, and presence of normal variants and venous thrombosis. This will assure adequate planning of the procedure and proper access vein selection.
- Periprocedural management of coagulation status *(Appendices 2* in Chap. 150 *and 3* in Chap. 151*)*
- Antibiotic prophylaxis: Not routinely recommended [2, 6] *(Appendices 4* in Chap. 152 *and 5* in Chap. 153*)*
- Imaging modality for guidance: Ultrasound, fluoroscopy, combined ultrasound/fluoroscopy
- Positioning: Supine
- Venous access: Peripheral vein, preferably in the upper extremity

PROCEDURE NOTE

Procedure: Single-/double-lumen peripherally inserted central catheter placement
Staff: [_]
Fellow: [_]
Resident: [_]
Clinical History and Indications: Describe history and list indications
Allergies: None known/Allergic to [specify/type of allergy]
Anesthesia: Local anesthesia/conscious sedation
Medications: List any relevant medications used
Contrast Material: None/(_) mL of [type] contrast material was used for venography
Field: Sterile
Procedure classification: Clean
Position: Supine
Monitoring: Intravenous access line was secured and vital signs were continuously monitored by nursing staff/anesthesia team throughout the procedure
Total fluoroscopy time: (_) minutes
Cumulative radiation dose: (_) mGy

Description of Procedure:
The risks, benefits, alternatives and procedure itself were explained to the patient/patient's Power of Attorney/patient's legal guardian, and

informed written/verbal consent was obtained. Time out was performed to confirm the correct patient and procedure.

The right/left upper extremity was prepped and draped in the usual sterile fashion. A tourniquet was placed to distend the veins. Ultrasound examination was performed to locate an adequately distended patent peripheral vein and determine the site of venous puncture. The [name the vein] vein was selected for puncture. Local anesthesia was administered. Venous access was obtained using a (_)-gauge [type] needle, under direct ultrasound visualization/by palpation. Once good venous flow was detected, a (_)-inch [type] guidewire was advanced through the needle under direct fluoroscopic visualization and its tip was placed at the cavoatrial junction/ [specify location if the wire could not be advanced centrally]. The required catheter length was measured using the guidewire/estimated *(bedside procedure)* and the catheter was cut to the required length. A small skin incision was made and a (_)-French [peel away/type] sheath was placed into the access vein over the guidewire.

The stiffener of the sheath was removed and the catheter was advanced through the sheath using a stiffening stylet/guidewire to the desired position. After confirming adequate position of the catheter tip at the cavoatrial junction [specify location if otherwise] by imaging, the sheath was removed, the catheter was anchored to the skin and sterile dressing was applied. The catheter was flushed with normal saline and loaded with (_) mL of (10–100) IU/mL heparin solution. Spot fluoroscopy image/chest radiograph was obtained to document catheter tip position for future reference.

The patient was transferred to the floor/recovery room/discharged home following the procedure in a stable condition. Staff was present for the entire procedure.

Intra-Procedure Findings: List all relevant findings.

Immediate Complications: None encountered during or directly after the procedure. List complications if any.

Post-Procedure Plan [1, 2]:

- Always aspirate and discard contents of lumen prior to each use to avoid flushing the intraluminal heparin into the systemic circulation.
- After each use and before capping the lumen, flush the lumen with 10 mL of normal saline followed by instillation of heparin solution (10–100 IU/mL) based on the specific luminal volume of the catheter to maintain patency.
- When not in use, flush the lumen with normal saline followed by instillation of heparin solution 2–3 times per week.
- Apply sterile dressing after disinfecting the skin with chlorhexidine-based preparation twice weekly.
- Check for signs of catheter-related infection regularly and take the appropriate measures when observed.

Impression:

- (_)-French single-/double- lumen peripherally inserted central catheter placement through [specify peripheral vein] as described above.
- The patient tolerated the procedure well and left the interventional unit in stable condition.
- Document the maximum injection rate of power injectable catheters.
- The patient was unstable/unable to tolerate the procedure and the procedure was canceled/terminated prematurely.
- List any other relevant or important information/finding.

References

1. Hughes JA, Cantwell CP, Waybill PN. Peripherally inserted central catheters and nontunneled central venous catheters. In: Mauro MA, Murphy KPJ, Thomson KR, Venbrux AC, Morgan RA, editors. Image-guided interventions. 2nd ed. Philadelphia: Saunders Elsevier; 2014. p. 861–8.
2. Regalado S, Funaki B. Central venous access. In: Kandarpa K, Machan L, editors. Handbook of interventional radiologic procedures. 4th ed. Philadelphia: Lippincott Williams & Wilkins; 2011. p. 354–70.

3. Marcy PY. Central venous access: techniques and indications in oncology. Eur Radiol. 2008;18 (10):2333–44.
4. Dariushnia SR, Wallace MJ, Siddiqi NH, Towbin RB, Wojak JC, Kundu S, et al. Quality improvement guidelines for central venous access. J Vasc Interv Radiol. 2010;21(7):976–81.
5. Hoggard J, Saad T, Schon D, Vesely TM, Royer T. Guidelines for venous access in patients with chronic kidney disease. A position statement from the american society of diagnostic and interventional nephrology, clinical practice committee and the association for vascular access. Semin Dial. 2008;21(2):186–91.
6. Venkatesan AM, Kundu S, Sacks D, Wallace MJ, Wojak JC, Rose SC, et al. Practice guidelines for adult antibiotic prophylaxis during vascular and interventional radiology procedures. J Vasc Interv Radiol. 2010;21(11):1611–30.
7. Taslakian B, Sebaaly MG, Al-Kutoubi A. Patient evaluation and preparation in vascular and interventional radiology: what every interventional radiologist should know (part 1: patient assessment and laboratory tests). Cardiovasc Intervent Radiol. 2016;39(3):325–33.
8. Taslakian B, Sebaaly MG, Al-Kutoubi A. Patient evaluation and preparation in vascular and interventional radiology: what every interventional radiologist should know (part 2: patient preparation and medications). Cardiovasc Intervent Radiol. 2016;39(4):489–99. doi: 10.1007/s00270-015-1239-4. [Epub 2015 Nov 25].

Placement of Non-tunneled Central Venous Catheter

85

Bedros Taslakian and Jad Chokr

INTRODUCTION

Central venous catheters, which are used for infusion therapy, exchange therapy, phlebotomy, and hemodynamic monitoring, are invaluable in modern medical practice. Non-tunneled central venous catheters can be inserted for short-term continuous or intermittent use. The right internal jugular vein is the preferred access vein, has a straight course toward the right atrium simplifying catheter placement and carries a lower risk of complications. On the other hand, the femoral veins are the least optimal site of venous access because of higher rate of catheter-related infection and occlusion.

COMMON INDICATIONS [1–4]

- Rapid infusion of viscous liquids or blood products
- Administration of cytotoxic medications or chemotherapy that cause venous inflammation in the peripheral veins
- Total parental nutrition (TPN)
- Contraindications for the placement of a permanent venous access *(e.g., coagulopathy, active infection)*
- Infusion of hypertonic agents
- Exchange therapy *(e.g., short-term hemodialysis and plasmapheresis)*
- Hemodynamic monitoring *(i.e., central venous pressure measurement)*
- Lack of peripheral venous access *(e.g., emergency venous access)*

COMMON CONTRAINDICATIONS [1, 2, 4, 5]

- Past history of allergic contrast material reaction and impaired renal function *(procedure can be performed without contrast media injection)*
- Venous thrombosis or occlusion
- Focal cellulitis, radiation-induced injury, or burn
- Coagulopathy that cannot be corrected

Specific contraindications to subclavian central line insertion *(higher rate of stenosis/occlusion)*

- Patients on hemodialysis
- Patients in whom hemodialysis is anticipated *(e.g., renal transplant, chronic kidney disease)*

B. Taslakian (✉)
Department of Radiology, New York University Langone Medical Center, 660 First Ave, New York, NY 10016, USA
e-mail: btaslakian@gmail.com

J. Chokr
Department of Diagnostic Radiology, Neuroradiology Division, Banner University Medical Center, Tucson, AZ, USA
e-mail: Jad_1986@hotmail.com

B. Taslakian et al. (eds.), *Procedural Dictations in Image-Guided Intervention*,
DOI 10.1007/978-3-319-40845-3_85

POSSIBLE COMPLICATIONS [1–5]

- Pleural transgression causing pneumothorax, hemothorax, or intrapleural infusion
- Arterial puncture with subsequent cannulation or injury
- Venous perforation
- Focal hemorrhage and hematoma at the venotomy site
- Subclavian vein stenosis
- Thrombophlebitis
- Cardiac arrhythmia
- Catheter site infection and bacteremia
- Catheter malposition when inserted without fluoroscopy guidance
- Catheter dislodgment
- Catheter malfunction due to occlusion or fibrin sheath formation
- Catheter fracture and embolization of fragments
- Cardiac injury and tamponade

PREPROCEDURAL ASSESSMENT AND PLANNING [6–8]

- History, indications, and physical examination *(Appendix 1* in Chap. 149*)*
- Evaluation of diagnostic imaging studies to determine the relevant vascular anatomy, and presence of normal variants and venous thrombosis/occlusion. This will assure adequate planning of the procedure and proper access selection.
- Periprocedural management of coagulation status *(Appendices 2* in Chap. 150 *and 3* in Chap. 151*)*
- Antibiotic prophylaxis: No consensus, although not routinely recommended [6] *(Appendices 4* in Chap. 152 *and 5* in Chap. 153*)*
- Imaging modality for guidance: Ultrasound, fluoroscopy, combined ultrasound/fluoroscopy
- Positioning: Supine, in Trendelenburg position
- Venous access: Subclavian vein, internal jugular vein *(note: femoral vein can be used as an emergency access)*

PROCEDURE NOTE

Procedure: Percutaneous left/right internal jugular/subclavian central line insertion [(_) French [type] single-/double-/triple- lumen]
Staff: [_]
Fellow: [_]
Resident: [_]
Clinical History and Indications: Describe history and list indications
Allergies: None known/Allergic to [specify/type of allergy]
Anesthesia: Local anesthesia/conscious sedation
Medications: List any relevant medications used
Contrast Material: None/(_) mL of [type] contrast material was used
Field: Sterile
Procedure classification: Clean
Position: Supine
Monitoring: Intravenous access line was secured and vital signs were continuously monitored by nursing staff/anesthesia team throughout the procedure
Total fluoroscopy time: (_) minutes
Cumulative radiation dose: (_) mGy

Description of Procedure:
The risks, benefits, alternatives and procedure itself were explained to the patient/patient's Power of Attorney/patient's legal guardian, and informed written/verbal consent was obtained. Time out was performed to confirm the correct patient and procedure.

The patient was positioned supine, in slight trendelenburg, with the neck turned to the contralateral side. The patient's left/right cervical and upper thoracic regions were prepped and draped in sterile fashion. Ultrasound examination was performed to determine the site of venous puncture. Local anesthesia was administered. The left/right internal jugular/subclavian vein was punctured under ultrasound guidance using a (_)-gauge [type] needle. Once good venous flow was detected, a (_)-inch [type] guidewire was advanced through the needle under direct fluoroscopic visualization and its tip was placed centrally. A small skin incision was made and a (_)-French dilator was advanced over the guidewire to dilate the subcutaneous tissue. The dilator was removed and a (_) French [type] single-/double-/triple-lumen central venous catheter was advanced over the guidewire, with the tip placed at the [specify location]. The catheter was then anchored to the skin, using nonabsorbable sutures. At time of procedure completion, all ports were aspirated and flushed properly with normal saline. The ports were loaded with (_) mL of (10–100) IU/mL heparin solution and capped. Spot fluoroscopy image/chest radiograph was obtained to document catheter tip position for future reference.

The patient was transferred to the floor/recovery room following the procedure in a stable condition. Staff was present for the entire procedure.

Intra-Procedure Findings: List all relevant findings.

Immediate Complications: None encountered during or directly after the procedure. List complications if any.

Post-Procedure Plan [1, 2]:

- Always aspirate and discard contents of lumen prior to each use to avoid flushing the intraluminal heparin into the systemic circulation.
- After each use and before capping the ports, flush the lumens with 10 mL of normal saline followed by instillation of heparin solution (10–100 IU/mL) based on the specific luminal volume of the catheter to maintain patency and function.
- When not in use, flush the ports with normal saline followed by instillation of heparin solution 2–3 times per week.
- Apply sterile dressing after disinfecting the skin with chlorhexidine-based preparation as needed.
- Check for signs of catheter-related skin infection regularly and take the appropriate measures if any detected.

Impression:

- Insertion of right/left internal jugular/subclavian nontunneled central line [(_) French [type] single-/double-/triple- lumen].
- The patient tolerated the procedure well and left the interventional unit in stable condition.
- The patient was unstable and the procedure was canceled/terminated prematurely.
- List any other relevant or important information/finding.

References

1. Hughes JA, Cantwell CP, Waybill PN. Peripherally inserted central catheters and nontunneled central venous catheters. In: Mauro MA, Murphy KPJ, Thomson KR, Venbrux AC, Morgan RA, editors. Image-guided interventions. 2nd ed. Philadelphia: Saunders Elsevier; 2014. p. 861–8.
2. Regalado S, Funaki B. Central venous access. In: Kandarpa K, Machan L, editors. Handbook of interventional radiologic procedures. 4th ed. Philadelphia: Lippincott Williams & Wilkins; 2011. p. 354–70.
3. Marcy PY. Central venous access: techniques and indications in oncology. Eur Radiol. 2008;18(10):2333–44.
4. Dariushnia SR, Wallace MJ, Siddiqi NH, Towbin RB, Wojak JC, Kundu S, et al. Quality improvement guidelines for central venous access. J Vasc Interv Radiol. 2010;21(7):976–81.
5. Hoggard J, Saad T, Schon D, Vesely TM, Royer T. Guidelines for venous access in patients with chronic kidney disease. A position statement from the American society of diagnostic and interventional nephrology, clinical practice committee and the association for vascular access. Semin Dial. 2008;21(2):186–91.
6. Venkatesan AM, Kundu S, Sacks D, Wallace MJ, Wojak JC, Rose SC, et al. Practice guidelines for adult antibiotic prophylaxis during vascular and interventional radiology procedures. J Vasc Interv Radiol. 2010;21(11):1611–30.
7. Taslakian B, Sebaaly MG, Al-Kutoubi A. Patient evaluation and preparation in vascular and interventional radiology: what every interventional radiologist should know (part 1: patient assessment and laboratory tests). Cardiovasc Intervent Radiol. 2016;39(3):325–33.
8. Taslakian B, Sebaaly MG, Al-Kutoubi A. Patient evaluation and preparation in vascular and interventional radiology: what every interventional radiologist should know (part 2: patient preparation and medications). Cardiovasc Intervent Radiol. 2016;39(4):489–99. doi: 10.1007/s00270-015-1239-4. [Epub 2015 Nov 25].

86 Placement of Subcutaneous Central Venous Port

Bedros Taslakian

INTRODUCTION

Subcutaneous ports provide a safe and effective method of venous infusion when intermittent central venous access is required over a long time frame ranging from months to years. They have the lowest rate of infectious complications among central venous catheters because of their nonexposed location. The right internal jugular vein is the preferred access vein; it has a straight course toward the right atrium simplifying catheter placement and therefore the lowest risk of complications. Ports are accessed through the skin with a noncoring needle that penetrates the self-sealing silicone septum. The device may have one or two lumens, each with a dedicated access port.

COMMON INDICATIONS [1–4]

- Intermittent long-term administration of cytotoxic medication, antibiotics, or chemotherapy
- Intermittent long-term administration of total parental nutrition
- Intermittent long-term infusion of blood products
- Erythrocytapheresis
- Therapeutic plasma exchange

COMMON CONTRAINDICATIONS [1, 2, 4, 5]

- Past history of allergic contrast material reaction and impaired renal function *(procedure can be performed without contrast media injection)*
- Lack of a suitable vein for access due to venous thrombosis or occlusion
- Focal cellulitis or radiation-induced injury
- Severe skin involvement due to scleroderma, graft-versus-host disease, or Stevens-Johnson syndrome
- Allergy to catheter material *(procedure can be performed without contrast media injection)*
- Coagulopathy that cannot be corrected
- Active infection or bacteremia
- Severely neutropenic patients

Specific contraindications to subclavian access: *(higher rate of stenosis/occlusion)*

- Patients on hemodialysis
- Patients in whom hemodialysis is anticipated (e.g., *renal transplant, chronic kidney disease)*

B. Taslakian (✉)
Department of Radiology, New York University Langone Medical Center, 40 Waterside Plaza, Apt 17E, New York, NY 10010, USA
e-mail: btaslakian@gmail.com

B. Taslakian et al. (eds.), *Procedural Dictations in Image-Guided Intervention*,
DOI 10.1007/978-3-319-40845-3_86

POSSIBLE COMPLICATIONS [1–6]

- Pleural transgression causing pneumothorax, hemothorax, or intrapleural infusion
- Arterial puncture with subsequent cannulation or injury
- Venous perforation
- Focal hemorrhage and hematoma at the venotomy site
- Air embolism
- Thrombophlebitis and pulmonary thromboembolism
- Venous stenosis or occlusion
- Cardiac arrhythmia
- Subcutaneous pocket infection
- Catheter-related bloodstream infection
- Catheter migration and dislodgment
- Catheter malfunction due to thrombosis, fibrin sheath formation, or kinking
- Catheter fracture *(pinch-off syndrome)* and embolization of fragments
- Cardiac injury and tamponade
- Thoracic duct injury

PREPROCEDURAL ASSESSMENT AND PLANNING [1–3, 7–9]

- History, indications, and physical examination *(Appendix 1* in Chap. 149*)*
- Evaluation of diagnostic imaging studies to determine the relevant vascular anatomy, and presence of normal variants and venous thrombosis/occlusion. This will assure adequate planning of the procedure and proper access selection.
- Periprocedural management of coagulation status *(Appendices 2* in Chap. 150 *and 3 in* Chap. 151*)*
- Antibiotic prophylaxis: No consensus, although some prefer routine prophylaxis given the severity of complications and difficulty in treating infected ports in immunocompromised patients [1–3, 7] *(Appendices 4* in Chap. 152 *and 5* in Chap. 153*)*
- Imaging modality for guidance: Ultrasound, fluoroscopy, combined ultrasound/fluoroscopy
- Positioning: Supine, in Trendelenburg position
- Venous access: Internal jugular vein *(preferred, right > left)*, external jugular vein, subclavian vein *(should be avoided)* [1, 2, 5]

PROCEDURE NOTE

Procedure: Left/right internal jugular/subclavian subcutaneous port implantation [(_) French (#) lumen].
Staff: [_]
Fellow: [_]
Resident: [_]
Clinical History and Indications: Describe history and list indications
Allergies: None known/Allergic to [specify/type of allergy]
Anesthesia: Local anesthesia/conscious sedation
Medications: List any relevant medications used
Contrast Material: None/(_) mL of [type] contrast material was used for venography
Field: Sterile
Procedure classification: Clean
Position: Supine in slight Trendelenburg
Monitoring: Intravenous access line was secured and vital signs were continuously monitored by nursing staff/anesthesia team throughout the procedure
Total fluoroscopy time: (_) minutes
Cumulative radiation dose: (_) mGy

Description of Procedure:
The risks, benefits, alternatives and procedure itself were explained to the patient/patient's Power of Attorney/patient's legal guardian, and informed written/verbal consent was obtained. Time out was performed to confirm the correct patient and procedure.

The patient was positioned supine, in slight trendelenburg, with the neck turned to the contralateral side. The patient's left/right cervical and upper thoracic regions were prepped and draped in sterile fashion. Ultrasound examination was performed to determine the site of venous puncture. Local anesthesia was administered. The left/right internal jugular/subclavian vein was punctured under ultrasound guidance using a (_)-gauge [type] needle. Once good venous flow was detected, a (0.018)-in. [type] guidewire was advanced through the needle under direct fluoroscopic visualization and placed centrally. A small skin incision was made and a (5)-French dilator was advanced over the guidewire, through which the wire was exchanged for a (0.035)-in. [stiff/type] guidewire that was advanced into the superior vena cava. The dilator was removed. The intended port placement site and the tunnel tract were anesthetized using a long needle. A single skin incision was made in the chest wall parallel to the dermatomes and an adequately sized subcutaneous pocket was created using blunt dissection. Following this, a tunneling device was advanced from the pocket to the neck venotomy site, making a gentle curve in the subcutaneous tract. The required catheter length was measured with the guidewire and the catheter was cut to appropriate length. Following this, an appropriately sized peel-away sheath was placed through the jugular access over the existing guidewire. A (_)-French catheter, attached to the port, was pulled through the tunnel, advanced through the peel-away sheath and its tip was positioned at the cavoatrial junction.

The neck venotomy site was closed with skin glue/subcutaneous suture. The port was placed into the pocket and fixed in place with absorbable sutures. The pocket was closed with a two-layer closure. The deep layer was closed with (3–0) absorbable sutures and the cutaneous layer was closed with skin glue/a running subcuticular (4–0) absorbable suture. At time of procedure completion, the port was accessed with a non-coring needle, aspirated, flushed with saline to check for leaks, and loaded with (_) mL of (10–100) IU/mL heparin solution. The skin was cleaned with normal saline and chlorhexidine solution and sterile occlusive dressing was applied. Spot fluoroscopy image was obtained to document catheter tip position for future reference.

The patient was transferred to the floor/recovery room/discharged home following the procedure in a stable condition. Staff was present for the entire procedure.

Intra-Procedure Findings: List all relevant findings.

Immediate Complications: None encountered during or directly after the procedure. List complications if any.

Post-Procedure Plan [1, 2]:

- Apply sterile dressing after disinfecting the skin with chlorhexidine-based preparation daily until the site is healed.
- Always aspirate and discard contents of lumen prior to each use to avoid flushing the intraluminal heparin into the systemic circulation.
- After each use, flush the port with 10 mL of normal saline followed by instillation of heparin solution (10–100 IU/mL) based on the specific luminal volume of the catheter to maintain patency and function.
- When not in use, flush the port with normal saline followed by instillation of heparin solution 2–3 times per week.
- Check for signs of port-related skin infection regularly and take the appropriate measures if any detected.

Impression:

- Placement of right/left internal jugular/subclavian subcutaneous port [(_) French (#) lumen].
- The patient tolerated the procedure well and left the interventional unit in stable condition.
- The patient was unstable and the procedure was canceled/terminated prematurely.
- List any other relevant or important information/finding.

References

1. Dixon RG. Subcutaneous ports. In: Mauro MA, Murphy KPJ, Thomson KR, Venbrux AC, Morgan RA, editors. Image-guided interventions. 2nd ed. Philadelphia: Saunders Elsevier; 2014. p. 876–90.
2. Regalado S, Funaki B. Central venous access. In: Kandarpa K, Machan L, editors. Handbook of interventional radiologic procedures. 4th ed. Philadelphia: Lippincott Williams & Wilkins; 2011. p. 354–70.
3. Funaki B. Chest port insertion. Semin Intervent Radiol. 2005;22(3):242–4.

4. Dariushnia SR, Wallace MJ, Siddiqi NH, Towbin RB, Wojak JC, Kundu S, et al. Quality improvement guidelines for central venous access. J Vasc Interv Radiol. 2010;21(7):976–81.
5. Hoggard J, Saad T, Schon D, Vesely TM, Royer T. Guidelines for venous access in patients with chronic kidney disease. A position statement from the American society of diagnostic and interventional nephrology, clinical practice committee and the association for vascular access. Semin Dial. 2008;21(2):186–91.
6. Funaki B. Subcutaneous chest port infection. Semin Intervent Radiol. 2005;22(3):245–7.
7. Venkatesan AM, Kundu S, Sacks D, Wallace MJ, Wojak JC, Rose SC, et al. Practice guidelines for adult antibiotic prophylaxis during vascular and interventional radiology procedures. J Vasc Interv Radiol. 2010;21(11):1611–30.
8. Taslakian B, Sebaaly MG, Al-Kutoubi A. Patient evaluation and preparation in vascular and interventional radiology: what every interventional radiologist should know (part 1: patient assessment and laboratory tests). Cardiovasc Intervent Radiol. 2016;39(3):325–33.
9. Taslakian B, Sebaaly MG, Al-Kutoubi A. Patient evaluation and preparation in vascular and interventional radiology: what every interventional radiologist should know (part 2: patient preparation and medications). Cardiovasc Intervent Radiol. 2016;39(4):489–99. doi: 10.1007/s00270-015-1239-4. [Epub 2015 Nov 25].

Placement of Tunneled Central Venous Catheter

87

Bedros Taslakian

INTRODUCTION

Peripherally inserted or tunneled central venous catheters are suitable in cases when frequent access is needed over a relatively short or intermediate period of time. Tunneled central venous catheters are durable devices and show significantly lower rate of catheter-related infection when compared to the non-tunneled catheters allowing a safe, long-term venous access for chronic patients. The right internal jugular vein is the preferred access vein, allowing a straight course toward the right atrium which simplifies catheter placement, and therefore carries a lower risk of complications.

COMMON INDICATIONS [1–4]

- Intermediate to long-term administration of cytotoxic medication or chemotherapy
- Intermediate to long-term total parental nutrition
- Chronic exchange therapy (e.g., *hemodialysis and plasmapheresis)*

B. Taslakian (✉)
Department of Radiology, New York University Langone Medical Center, 660 First Ave, New York, NY 10016, USA
e-mail: btaslakian@gmail.com

COMMON CONTRAINDICATIONS [1–5]

- Past history of allergic contrast material reaction and impaired renal function *(procedure can be performed without contrast media injection)*
- Lack of a suitable vein for access due to venous thrombosis or occlusion
- Focal cellulitis or radiation-induced injury
- Severe skin involvement due to scleroderma, graft-versus-host disease, or Stevens-Johnson syndrome
- Allergy to catheter material
- Coagulopathy that cannot be corrected
- Active infection or bacteremia

Specific contraindications to subclavian access: *(higher rate of stenosis/occlusion)*

- Patients on hemodialysis
- Patients in whom hemodialysis is anticipated (e.g., *renal transplant, chronic kidney disease)*

POSSIBLE COMPLICATIONS [1–6]

- Pleural transgression causing pneumothorax, hemothorax, or intrapleural infusion
- Arterial puncture with subsequent cannulation or injury
- Venous perforation
- Focal hemorrhage and hematoma at the venotomy site

B. Taslakian et al. (eds.), *Procedural Dictations in Image-Guided Intervention*,
DOI 10.1007/978-3-319-40845-3_87

- Thrombophlebitis and pulmonary thromboembolism
- Venous stenosis or occlusion
- Cardiac arrhythmia
- Tunnel-site and catheter-related bloodstream infection
- Tip malposition when inserted without fluoroscopy guidance
- Subclavian vein stenosis
- Catheter dislodgment
- Catheter malfunction due to thrombosis, fibrin sheath formation, or kinking
- Catheter fracture and embolization of fragments
- Cardiac injury and tamponade

PREPROCEDURAL ASSESSMENT AND PLANNING [2, 7–9]

- History, indications, and physical examination *(Appendix 1* in Chap. 149*)*
- Evaluation of diagnostic imaging studies to determine the relevant vascular anatomy, and presence of normal variants and venous thrombosis/occlusion. This will assure adequate planning of the procedure and proper access vein selection.
- Periprocedural management of coagulation status *(Appendices 2* in Chap. 150 *and 3* in Chap. 151*)*
- Antibiotic prophylaxis: No consensus, although not routinely recommended [2, 7] *(Appendices 4* in Chap. 152 *and 5* in Chap. 153*)*
- Imaging modality for guidance: Ultrasound, fluoroscopy, combined ultrasound/fluoroscopy
- Positioning: Supine, in Trendelenburg position
- Venous access: Internal jugular vein (preferred, right > left), external jugular vein, subclavian vein *(should be avoided in dialysis patients)* [1, 2, 5]

PROCEDURE NOTE

Procedure: Tunneled left/right internal jugular/external jugular/subclavian central line insertion [(_) French [type] single-/double-lumen]
Staff: [_]
Fellow: [_]
Resident: [_]
Clinical History and Indications: Describe history and list indications
Allergies: None known/Allergic to [specify/type of allergy]
Anesthesia: Local anesthesia/conscious sedation
Medications: List any relevant medications used
Contrast Material: None/(_) mL of [type] contrast material was used for venography
Field: Sterile
Procedure classification: Clean
Position: Supine, in slight Trendelenburg
Monitoring: Intravenous access line was secured and vital signs were continuously monitored by nursing staff/anesthesia team throughout the procedure
Total fluoroscopy time: (_) minutes
Cumulative radiation dose: (_) mGy

Description of Procedure:
The risks, benefits, alternatives, and procedure itself were explained to the patient/patient's Power of Attorney/patient's legal guardian, and informed written/verbal consent was obtained. Time out was performed to confirm the correct patient and procedure.

The patient was positioned supine, in slight trendelenburg, with the neck turned to the contralateral side. The patient's left/right cervical and upper thoracic regions were prepped and draped in sterile fashion. Ultrasound examination was performed to determine the site of venous puncture. Local anesthesia was administered. The left/right internal jugular/external jugular/subclavian vein was punctured under ultrasound guidance using a (_)-gauge [type] needle. Once good venous flow was detected, a (0.018)-in.

[type] guidewire was advanced through the needle under direct fluoroscopic visualization and placed centrally. A small skin incision was made and a (5)-French dilator was advanced over the guidewire to dilate the subcutaneous tissue. The guidewire was exchanged for a (0.035)-in. [stiff/type] guidewire, its tip was advanced into the superior vena cava and the dilator was removed. The intended subcutaneous path of the tunnel was anesthetized using a long needle. A small skin incision was made in the chest wall at the desired catheter entry site and the tunneling device was advanced through the skin incision toward the neck venotomy site, making a gentle curve in the tract.

Following this, a (_)-French peel-away sheath was placed through the jugular access over the existing stiff guidewire. A (_)-French tunneled catheter was pulled through the tunnel to a point that the retention cuffs were placed appropriately within the tunnel. The catheter was cut to suitable length and advanced through the peel-away sheath and its tip was positioned at the cavoatrial junction. The neck venotomy site was closed with skin glue/subcutaneous suture. The catheter was then anchored to the skin, using nonabsorbable sutures. At time of procedure completion, all ports were aspirated, flushed properly with normal saline, loaded with (_) mL of (10–100) IU/mL heparin solution and capped. Spot fluoroscopy image was obtained to document catheter tip position for future reference.

The patient was transferred to the floor/recovery room/discharged home following the procedure in a stable condition. Staff was present for the entire procedure.

Intra-Procedure Findings: List all relevant findings.

Immediate Complications: None encountered during or directly after the procedure. List complications if any.

Post-Procedure Plan [1, 2]:

- Remove the anchoring sutures within 10–14 days after catheter placement.
- Always aspirate and discard contents of lumen prior to each use to avoid flushing the intraluminal heparin into the circulation.
- After each use and before capping the lumen, flush the lumens with 10 mL of normal saline followed by instillation of heparin solution (10–100 IU/mL) based on the specific luminal volume of the catheter to maintain patency and function.
- When not in use, flush the lumen with normal saline followed by instillation of heparin solution 2–3 times per week.
- Apply sterile dressing after disinfecting the skin with chlorhexidine-based preparation, as needed.
- Check for signs of catheter-related skin infection regularly and take the appropriate measures if any detected.

Impression:

- Insertion of right/left internal jugular/subclavian tunneled central line [(_) French [type] single-/double- lumen].
- The patient tolerated the procedure well and left the interventional unit in stable condition.
- The patient was unable to tolerate the procedure which was canceled/terminated prematurely.
- List any other relevant or important information/finding.

References

1. Bream PR Jr. Tunneled central venous catheters. In: Mauro MA, Murphy KPJ, Thomson KR, Venbrux AC, Morgan RA, editors. Image-guided interventions. 2nd ed. Philadelphia: Saunders Elsevier; 2014. p. 869–75.
2. Regalado S, Funaki B. Central venous access. In: Kandarpa K, Machan L, editors. Handbook of interventional radiologic procedures. 4th ed. Philadelphia: Lippincott Williams & Wilkins; 2011. p. 354–70.
3. Marcy PY. Central venous access: techniques and indications in oncology. Eur Radiol. 2008;18(10):2333–44.
4. Dariushnia SR, Wallace MJ, Siddiqi NH, Towbin RB, Wojak JC, Kundu S, et al. Quality improvement guidelines for central venous access. J Vasc Interv Radiol. 2010;21(7):976–81.
5. Hoggard J, Saad T, Schon D, Vesely TM, Royer T. Guidelines for venous access in patients with chronic kidney disease. A position statement from the American society of diagnostic and interventional nephrology, clinical practice committee and the association for vascular access. Semin Dial. 2008;21(2):186–91.

6. Wilcox TA. Catheter-related bloodstream infections. Semin Intervent Radiol. 2009;26(2):139–43.
7. Venkatesan AM, Kundu S, Sacks D, Wallace MJ, Wojak JC, Rose SC, et al. Practice guidelines for adult antibiotic prophylaxis during vascular and interventional radiology procedures. J Vasc Interv Radiol. 2010;21(11):1611–30.
8. Taslakian B, Sebaaly MG, Al-Kutoubi A. Patient evaluation and preparation in vascular and interventional radiology: what every interventional radiologist should know (part 1: patient assessment and laboratory tests). Cardiovasc Intervent Radiol. 2016;39(3):325–33.
9. Taslakian B, Sebaaly MG, Al-Kutoubi A. Patient evaluation and preparation in vascular and interventional radiology: what every interventional radiologist should know (part 2: patient preparation and medications). Cardiovasc Intervent Radiol. 2016;39(4):489–99. doi: 10.1007/s00270-015-1239-4. [Epub 2015 Nov 25].

88 Superior Vena Cava Stent Insertion

Joelle Wazen and Howayda Al Mrad

INTRODUCTION

Superior vena cava (SVC) syndrome often requires immediate evaluation and intervention. It is most commonly caused by neoplastic involvement by external compression, intravascular thrombosis, or both, with lung cancer being responsible in the majority of cases. Other less common causes are radiation induced mediastinal fibrosis, indwelling devices, such as catheters or pacemakers, and to a lesser extent infections such as syphilis and tuberculosis. Percutaneous stent insertion, a minimally invasive option, yields immediate resolution of symptoms with a low complication rate making it an acceptable first-line treatment.

COMMON INDICATIONS [1–5]

- Malignant SVC syndrome
- Covered stents for transmural malignant invasion of the SVC
- Benign SVC syndrome, less frequently, but typically cases requiring immediate relief of symptoms

COMMON CONTRAINDICATION [1, 2, 4]

- Contraindication to anticoagulation or thrombolytic therapy
- Advanced disease in cancer patients with short-life expectancy *(relative contraindication)*
- Anatomic variations presenting technical difficulties *(relative contraindication)*

POSSIBLE COMPLICATIONS [1, 2, 4]

- Bleeding from puncture site
- Stent thrombosis
- Mediastinal hematoma
- Hemothorax
- Stent migration
- Infection
- Pulmonary embolism
- Venous perforation
- Cardiac puncture and tamponade *(rare)*
- Cardiac arrhythmia

J. Wazen
Department of Diagnostic Radiology, UMass Memorial Medical Center, Worcester, MA, USA
e-mail: joelle.wazen@gmail.com

H. Al Mrad (✉)
Department of Radiology, American University of Beirut Medical Center, Riad Elsolh, 1107 2020, Beirut, Lebanon
e-mail: mourad.howayda@gmail.com

B. Taslakian et al. (eds.), *Procedural Dictations in Image-Guided Intervention*,
DOI 10.1007/978-3-319-40845-3_88

PREPROCEDURAL ASSESSMENT AND PLANNING [6–8]

- History, indications, and physical examination *(Appendix 1* in Chap. 149*)*
- Evaluation of diagnostic imaging studies to determine the relevant vascular anatomy, and presence of normal variants and venous thrombosis/occlusion. This will assure preprocedural selection of an appropriate access site and effective planning to avoid complications and limit procedure time.
- Periprocedural management of coagulation status *(Appendices 2* in Chap. 150 *and 3* in Chap. 151*)*
- Antibiotic prophylaxis: Not routinely recommended [6] *(Appendices 4* in Chap. 152 *and 5* in Chap. 153*)*
- Imaging modality for guidance: Fluoroscopy; combined with ultrasound for access venotomy
- Positioning: Supine
- Venous access: femoral, brachial, or basilic vein

PROCEDURE NOTE

Procedure: Superior vena cava stenting
Staff: [_]
Fellow: [_]
Resident: [_]
Clinical History and Indications: Describe history and list indications
Allergies: None known/Allergic to [specify/type of allergy]
Anesthesia: Local anesthesia/conscious sedation
Medications: List any relevant medications used
Contrast Material: (_) mL of [type] contrast material was used
Field: Sterile
Procedure classification: Clean
Position: Supine
Monitoring: Intravenous access line was secured and vital signs were continuously monitored by nursing staff/anesthesia team throughout the procedure
Total fluoroscopy time: (_) minutes
Cumulative radiation dose: (_) mGy

Description of the procedure *(Femoral approach):*
The risks, benefits, alternatives, and the procedure itself were explained to the patient/patient's Power of Attorney/legal guardian, and informed written/verbal consent was obtained. The site of the procedure was identified and marked. Time out was performed to confirm the correct patient and procedure.

The skin of both groins were shaved, prepped, and draped in the usual sterile fashion. The right/left common femoral vein was located by palpation/ultrasound and marked. Local anesthesia was administered and a small skin incision was made. Femoral venous access was obtained using a (_)-gauge [type] needle under direct ultrasound visualization/by palpation. Once good venous flow was detected, a (_)-inch [type] guidewire was advanced through the needle into the cava under direct fluoroscopic visualization and a (_)-French, (_)-cm-long vascular sheath was placed, with the tip of the sheath placed at the level of [name the anatomic location].

Then, a (_)-French pigtail catheter was advanced into the superior vena cava over a (0.035)-in [hydrophilic/type] guidewire. Cavogram was performed by injecting (_) mL of [type] contrast, at a rate of (15–20 mL/s) and digital subtraction angiography was performed at (_) frames per second during suspended respiration in an anterior–posterior projection/[specify other projections if obtained]. Through the sheath, a (_) French [angiographic/type] catheter was inserted over a (0.035)-in [hydrophilic/type] guidewire to navigate through the point of stricture/obstruction, which was successfully crossed. The hydrophilic guidewire was exchanged for a (_)-inch [stiff/type] guidewire which was advanced into a stable location to provide adequate support. Following this, a (_) mm [type] balloon catheter was inserted over the guidewire and venoplasty was performed by inflating the balloon manually with iodinated contrast material using a (_)-mL syringe/inflation device, under fluoroscopy visualization until the "waist" at the stricture site disappeared. Then, a (_)-cm-long, (_)-mm [type] stent was deployed at the site of the stenosis/obstruction. The stent was dilated to the required size using balloon dilatation. Completion venography was performed for documentation and future reference.

The sheath was removed and adequate hemostasis was achieved at the venotomy site by compression for (_) minutes. Sterile dressing was applied and the patient was transferred to the floor/recovery room following the procedure in a stable condition. Staff was present for the entire procedure.

Description of the procedure *(Brachial or basilic vein approach):*
The risks, benefits, alternatives and the procedure itself were explained to the patient/patient's Power of Attorney/legal guardian, and informed written/verbal consent was obtained. The site of the procedure was identified and marked. Time out was performed to confirm the correct patient and procedure.

The right/left arm was cleaned and draped in the usual sterile fashion. Ultrasound examination was performed to determine the site of venous puncture. Local anesthesia was administered. The left/right basilic/brachial vein was punctured under ultrasound guidance using a (_)-gauge [type] needle. Once good venous flow was detected, a (_)-inch [type] guidewire was advanced through the needle under direct fluoroscopic visualization. A small skin incision was made and a (_)-French vascular sheath was advanced over the guidewire. Then, a (_)-French [pigtail/type] catheter was advanced into the [right/left brachiocephalic vein/superior vena cava] over a (0.035)-in [hydrophilic/type] guidewire. Venography was performed by injecting (_) mL of [type] contrast, at a rate of (_) mL/s and digital subtraction angiography was performed at (_) frames per second during suspended respiration in an anterior–posterior projection/[specify other projections if obtained]. Digital road-mapping was also performed to identify the site and length of stenosis as well as the diameter of the normal vein. Through the sheath, a (_) French [angiographic/type] catheter was inserted over a (0.035)-in [hydrophilic/type] guidewire to navigate through the point of stricture/obstruction, which was successfully crossed. The hydrophilic guidewire was exchanged for a (_)-inch [stiff/type] guidewire which was advanced into the inferior vena cava to provide adequate support. Following this, a (_) mm [type] balloon catheter was inserted over the guidewire and venoplasty was performed by inflating the balloon manually with iodinated contrast material using a (_)-mL syringe/inflation device, under fluoroscopy visualization until the "waist" at the stricture site disappeared. The balloon was left inflated for (_) minutes and the inflation was repeated on (_) consecutive occasions. Then, a (_)-cm-long, (_)-mm [type] stent was deployed at the site of the stenosis/obstruction. The stent was dilated to the required size using balloon dilatation. Completion venography was performed for documentation and future reference.

Intra-Procedure Findings: List all relevant findings.

Immediate Complications: None encountered during or directly after the procedure. List complications if any.

Post-Procedure Plan [1–5]:

- Keep patient complete bed rest with the right/left leg/arm extended for (2–3) h.
- Check the puncture site for any bleeding or hematoma formation every 15 min for 1 h, then every 30 min for 2 h; inform interventional radiology team if any complications are observed.
- Monitor vital signs every 15 min for 1 h, then every 30 min for 2 h; notify interventional radiology team if systolic blood pressure <95 mmHg, or heart rate >110 beats/min.

- Resume diet and previous orders as needed and if not otherwise contraindicated.
- Continue adequate intravenous hydration and monitor fluid (intake-output) status.
- Check complete blood count, creatinine, and blood urea nitrogen on the day following the procedure or as clinically indicated.
- Daily aspirin [4] for 1 or more months [2, 5], or lifelong [3], with or without additional antiplatelets or anticoagulation [4, 5].
- Follow-up venography at 1 month to assess for restenosis and stent patency.

Impression:

- Superior vena cava stenting, as described above.
- The patient tolerated the procedure well and left the interventional unit in stable condition.
- The patient was unstable during/unable to tolerate the procedure which was canceled/ terminated prematurely.
- List any other relevant or important information/finding.

References

1. Bechara CF, Lin PH. Superior vena cava occlusion. In: Cronenwett JL, Johnston KW, editors. Rutherford's vascular surgery. 8th ed. Philadelphia: Saunders Elsevier; 2014. p. 982–88e2.
2. Dodelinger R. Chronic upper extremity/superior vena cava occlusive disease. In: Mauro MA, Murphy KPJ, Thomson KR, Venbrux AC, Zollikofer CL, editors. Image-guided interventions. Philadelphia: Saunders Elsevier; 2008. p. 1055–65.
3. Mather MN, Hallisey MJ. Venous angioplasty and stents. In: Kandarpa K, Machan L, editors. Handbook of interventional radiologic procedures. 4th ed. Philadelphia: Lippincott Williams & Wilkins; 2011. p. 432–8.
4. Lanciego C, Pangua C, Chacón JI, Velasco J, Boy RC, Viana A, et al. Endovascular stenting as the first step in the overall management of malignant superior vena cava syndrome. Am J Roentgenol. 2009;193(2): 549–58.
5. Gross CM, Krämer J, Waigand J, Uhlich F, Schröder G, Thalhammer C, et al. Stent implantation in patients with superior vena cava syndrome. Am J Roentgenol. 1997;169(2):429–32.
6. Venkatesan AM, Kundu S, Sacks D, Wallace MJ, Wojak JC, Rose SC, et al. Practice guidelines for adult antibiotic prophylaxis during vascular and interventional radiology procedures. J Vasc Interv Radiol. 2010;21(11):1611–30.
7. Taslakian B, Sebaaly MG, Al-Kutoubi A. Patient evaluation and preparation in vascular and interventional radiology: what every interventional radiologist should know (part 1: patient assessment and laboratory tests). Cardiovasc Intervent Radiol. 2016;39(3):325–33.
8. Taslakian B, Sebaaly MG, Al-Kutoubi A. Patient evaluation and preparation in vascular and interventional radiology: what every interventional radiologist should know (part 2: patient preparation and medications). Cardiovasc Intervent Radiol. 2016;39(4):489–99. doi: 10.1007/s00270-015-1239-4. [Epub 2015 Nov 25].

Superior Vena Cavogram

89

Joelle Wazen and Howayda Al Mrad

Abbreviations

SVC Superior vena cava

INTRODUCTION

Cavography is considered the gold standard for evaluating the superior vena cava (SVC) in general and superior vena cava syndrome specifically. It helps delineate accurate anatomy while providing information on the venous hemodynamics. Other less common SVC interventions not necessarily related to SVC pathology may also require cavography. For instance, SVC filter insertion in recurrent upper extremity deep vein thrombosis.

COMMON INDICATIONS [1–5]

- Suspected SVC obstruction or stenosis
- Evaluation prior to and following SVC stenting
- Evaluation prior to and following SVC filter insertion

COMMON CONTRAINDICATION [1]

No absolute contraindications since the availability of Gadolinium and CO_2 contrast media.

Relative contraindications:

- Pregnancy
- Previous severe contrast reaction
- Severely compromised cardiopulmonary status

POSSIBLE COMPLICATIONS [1]

- Access site complications *(e.g., hematoma, thrombosis of access vein, arterial injury)*
- Contrast extravasation in case venous perforation
- Contrast allergy to iodinated contrast
- Contrast-induced nephropathy
- Access vein phlebitis

J. Wazen
Department of Diagnostic Radiology, UMass Memorial Medical Center, Worcester, MA, USA
e-mail: joelle.wazen@gmail.com

H. Al Mrad (✉)
Department of Radiology, American University of Beirut Medical Center, Riad Elsolh, 1107 2020, Beirut, Lebanon
e-mail: mourad.howayda@gmail.com

B. Taslakian et al. (eds.), *Procedural Dictations in Image-Guided Intervention*,
DOI 10.1007/978-3-319-40845-3_89

PREPROCEDURAL ASSESSMENT AND PLANNING [6, 7]

- History, indications, and physical examination *(Appendix 1* in Chap. 149*)*
- Periprocedural management of coagulation status *(Appendices 2* in Chap. 150 *and 3* in Chap. 151*)*
- Antibiotic prophylaxis: Not routinely recommended *(Appendices 4* in Chap. 152 *and 5* in Chap. 153*)*
- Imaging modality for guidance: Fluoroscopy, combined with ultrasound for access venotomy
- Positioning: Supine
- Venous access: Brachial/basilic vein, femoral vein

PROCEDURE NOTE

Procedure: Superior vena cavogram
Staff: [_]
Fellow: [_]
Resident: [_]
Clinical History and Indications: Describe history and list indications
Allergies: None known/Allergic to [specify/type of allergy]
Anesthesia: Local anesthesia/conscious sedation
Medications: List any relevant medications used
Contrast Material: (_) mL of [type] contrast material was used for venography
Field: Sterile
Procedure classification: Clean
Position: Supine
Monitoring: Intravenous access line was secured and vital signs were continuously monitored by nursing staff/anesthesia team throughout the procedure
Total fluoroscopy time: (_) minutes
Cumulative radiation dose: (_) mGy

Description of the procedure *(Femoral approach):*
The risks, benefits, alternatives, and the procedure itself were explained to the patient/patient's Power of Attorney/legal guardian, and informed written/verbal consent was obtained. The site of the procedure was identified and marked. Time out was performed to confirm the correct patient and procedure.

The skin of both groins were shaved, prepped, and draped in the usual sterile fashion. The right/left common femoral vein was located by palpation/ultrasound and marked. Local anesthesia was administered and a small skin incision was made. Femoral venous access was obtained using a (_)-gauge [type] needle under direct ultrasound visualization/by palpation. Once good venous flow was detected, a (_)-inch [type] guidewire was advanced through the needle into the inferior vena cava under direct fluoroscopic visualization and a (_)-French, (_)-cm-long vascular sheath was placed, with the tip of the sheath placed at the level of [name the anatomic location].

Then, a (_)-French pigtail catheter was advanced into the upper superior vena cava/right/left brachiocephalic vein over a (0.035)-inch [hydrophilic/type] guidewire. Cavogram was performed by injecting (_) mL of [type] contrast, at a rate of (15 to 20) mL/s and digital subtraction angiography was performed at (_) frames per second during suspended respiration in an anterior–posterior projection/[specify other projections if obtained].

The sheath was removed and adequate hemostasis was achieved at the venotomy site by compression for (_) minutes. Sterile dressing was applied and the patient was transferred to the floor/recovery room following the procedure in a stable condition. Staff was present for the entire procedure.

Description of the procedure *(Bilateral brachial or basilic vein approach):*
The risks, benefits, alternatives, and the procedure itself were explained to the patient/patient's Power of Attorney/legal guardian, and informed written/verbal consent was obtained. The site of the procedure was identified and marked. Time out was performed to confirm the correct patient and procedure.

Both arms were cleaned and draped in the usual sterile fashion. Ultrasound examination was performed to determine the site of venous puncture.

Local anesthesia was administered. The left basilic/brachial vein was punctured under ultrasound guidance using a (_)-gauge [type] needle. Once good venous flow was detected, a (_)-inch [type] guidewire was advanced through the needle under direct fluoroscopic visualization. A small skin incision was made and a (_)-French vascular sheath was advanced over the guidewire. Vascular access was secured in the same fashion on the right side and a (_)-French vascular sheath was placed in the right basilic/brachial vein. Then, a (_)-French [pigtail/type] catheter was advanced into the [right and left brachiocephalic veins/upper superior vena cava] over a (0.035)-in. [hydrophilic/type] guidewire. Venography was performed by injecting (_) mL of [type] contrast, at a rate of (15–20) mL/s and digital subtraction angiography was performed at (_) frames per second during suspended respiration in an anterior–posterior projection/ [specify other projections if obtained].

The vascular sheath was removed and adequate hemostasis was achieved at the venotomy sites by compression for (_) minutes. Sterile dressings were applied and the patient was transferred to the floor/recovery room following the procedure in a stable condition. Staff was present for the entire procedure.

Intra-Procedure Findings: List all relevant findings.

Immediate Complications: None encountered during or directly after the procedure. List complications if any.

Post-Procedure Plan [1]:

- For femoral puncture, keep patient in complete bed rest with the right/left leg extended for (2–3) h.
- Check the puncture site for any bleeding or hematoma formation every 15 min for 1 h, then every 30 min for 2 h; inform interventional radiology team if any complications are observed.
- Monitor vital signs every 15 min for 1 h, then every 30 min for 2 h; notify interventional radiology team if systolic blood pressure <95 mmHg, or heart rate >110 beats/minute.
- Resume diet and previous orders as needed and if not otherwise contraindicated.
- Continue adequate intravenous hydration and monitor fluid (intake-output) status.
- Check complete blood count, creatinine and blood urea nitrogen on the day following the procedure or as clinically indicated.
- Follow-up venography at one month to assess for restenosis and stent patency.

Impression:

- Superior vena cavogram.
- The patient tolerated the procedure well and left the interventional unit in stable condition.
- The patient was unstable during/unable to tolerate the procedure which was canceled/ terminated prematurely.
- List any other relevant or important information/finding.

References

1. Aruny JE. Venography. In: Kandarpa K, Machan L, editors. Handbook of interventional radiologic procedures. 4th ed. Philadelphia: Lippincott Williams & Wilkins; 2011. p. 96–108.
2. Gillespie DL, Caliste XA. Venography. In: Cronenwett JL, Johnston KW, editors. Rutherford's vascular surgery. 8th ed. Philadelphia: Saunders Elsevier; 2014. p. 307–24.e2.
3. Dodelinger RF, Kaufman JA. Superior vena cava occlusive disease. In: Mauro MA, Murphy KPJ, Thomson KR, Venbrux AC, Zollikofer CL, editors. Image-guided interventions. 2nd ed. Philadelphia: Saunders Elsevier; 2014. p. 743–49.e1.
4. Usoh F, Hingorani A, Ascher E, Shiferson A, Tran V, Marks N, et al. Long-term follow-up for superior vena cava filter placement. Ann Vasc Surg. 2009;23 (3):350–4.
5. Shimm DS, Logue GL, Rigsby LC. Evaluating the superior vena cava syndrome. JAMA. 1981;245 (9):951–3.
6. Taslakian B, Sebaaly MG, Al-Kutoubi A. Patient evaluation and preparation in vascular and interventional radiology: what every interventional radiologist should know (part 1: patient assessment and laboratory tests). Cardiovasc Intervent Radiol. 2016;39 (3):325–33.
7. Taslakian B, Sebaaly MG, Al-Kutoubi A. Patient evaluation and preparation in vascular and interventional radiology: what every interventional radiologist should know (part 2: patient preparation and medications). Cardiovasc Intervent Radiol. 2016;39(4):489–99. doi: 10.1007/s00270-015-1239-4. [Epub 2015 Nov 25].

Part XIV

Vascular Interventional Procedures: Visceral Arteries

Introduction by Aghiad Al-Kutoubi, Section Reviewer

Disease of the visceral artery is perhaps less commonly seen in practice than the remainder of the vascular tree but can have serious clinical consequences. Advances in cross-sectional imaging have shifted the balance towards noninvasive imaging in the first instance particularly with CT angiography. Pre-planning with the benefit of 3D angiographic information allows appropriate selection of the access route, type of catheter and also type of device when necessary. Traumatic injury to the abdominal organs particularly the spleen is now frequently handled by endovascular means leaving surgery for the cases of complex nature.

This section provides a comprehensive list of procedural reports that covers the vast majority of the currently performed vascular procedures in the visceral arteries with up-to-date explanatory notes, synopsis of the indications and contraindications, and potential complications in an organized and practical format.

Section Chapters

Abdominal Visceral Arteriography 90

Bedros Taslakian and Sela Batouzian

INTRODUCTION

Diagnostic visceral catheter arteriography continues to be the gold standard for the evaluation of many vascular abnormalities, including hypervascular tumors, arteriovenous malformations, arteriovenous fistulae, and sources of bleeding.

COMMON INDICATIONS [1–3]

- Evaluation and treatment planning in acute or chronic intestinal ischemia
- Evaluation and treatment planning in acute or chronic gastrointestinal bleeding
- Evaluation of primary vascular disorders *(e.g., aneurysms, pseudoaneurysms, vascular malformations, vasculitis, arteriovenous fistulae, occlusive vascular disorders)*
- Evaluation of vascular complications of diseases, surgery, and traumatic abdominal injuries
- Evaluation prior to, during, and following selective percutaneous endovascular procedures
- Diagnosis and localization of intra-abdominal hypervascular tumors
- Evaluation of mesenteric, splenic, and portal vein patency and hemodynamics
- Preoperative mapping of vascular anatomy
- Preoperative and postoperative evaluation of transplanted organs

COMMON CONTRAINDICATIONS [1–3]

- Hemodynamic instability with multisystem dysfunction
- Uncontrolled severe hypertension or congestive heart failure
- Recent myocardial infarction
- Significant cardiac arrhythmias and electrolyte imbalance
- Uncorrectable bleeding disorders
- Pregnancy
- Uncooperative patient
- Past history of allergic reaction to iodinated contrast media or severe renal dysfunction
- Recent imaging of the gastrointestinal tract using positive intraluminal contrast
- Active bacteremia and sepsis
- Pheochromocytoma
- Active large vessel vasculitis and connective tissue disorders *(increased risk of puncture site complications, vascular injury, and thrombosis)*
- Local conditions at the vascular access site such as infection, preexisting pseudoa-

B. Taslakian (✉)
Department of Radiology, New York University Langone Medical Center, 660 First Ave, New York, NY 10016, USA
e-mail: btaslakian@gmail.com

S. Batouzian
Coronary Care Unit (CCU), Clemenceau Medical Center (CMC), Beirut, Lebanon
e-mail: sela.batouzian1@gmail.com

B. Taslakian et al. (eds.), *Procedural Dictations in Image-Guided Intervention*,
DOI 10.1007/978-3-319-40845-3_90

neurysm, hematoma, inguinal hernia, fresh incision, and recent injuries *(an alternative access site should be selected)*

POSSIBLE COMPLICATIONS [1–4]

- Access site complications *(e.g., hematoma, retroperitoneal hemorrhage, pseudoaneurysm, arteriovenous fistula, thrombosis)*
- Nausea, vomiting, and vasovagal syncope
- Fever and chills
- Contrast-induced allergic reaction
- Contrast-induced nephropathy
- Arterial perforation or dissection
- Catheter or guidewire breakage
- Limb amputation *(rare)*
- Risks related to any minimally invasive procedure performed under conscious sedation *(e.g., allergy to medications)*

PREPROCEDURAL ASSESSMENT AND PLANNING [2, 3, 5–7]

- History, indications, and physical examination *(Appendix 1* in Chap. 149*)*. Document indications of the procedure, lower or upper extremity pulses, and vital signs
- Evaluation of diagnostic imaging studies to determine the relevant vascular anatomy and assess the access vessels
- Periprocedural management of coagulation status *(Appendices 2* in Chap. 150 *and 3* in Chap. 151*)*
- Antibiotic prophylaxis: Not routinely recommended [2, 3, 5] *(Appendices 4* in Chap. 152 *and 5* in Chap. 153*)*
- Imaging modality for guidance: Fluoroscopy; combined with ultrasound for arterial puncture
- Positioning: Supine
- Arterial access: Common femoral artery *(preferred)*, left brachial artery, left axillary artery [1, 4]
- Patient preparation:
  – Start intravenous fluids the night before angiography in order to ensure adequate hydration, combined with effective monitoring of fluid status
  – Insert a urinary catheter or ask the patient to void before the procedure depending on the estimated time of the procedure
  – Considerations for patients with specific diseases or conditions, patients on specific medications, or patients with history of multiple comorbidities: consult with the referring clinician, and obtain subspecialty consultation as needed

PROCEDURE NOTE

Procedure: Catheter-directed diagnostic angiography of [name the organ/artery]
Staff: [_]
Fellow: [_]
Resident: [_]
Clinical History and Indications: Describe history and list indications
Allergies: None known/Allergic to [specify/type of allergy]
Anesthesia: Local anesthesia/Conscious sedation
Medications: List any relevant medications used
Contrast Material: (_) mL of [type] contrast material was used for intra-arterial injection
Field: Sterile
Procedure classification: Clean
Position: Supine
Monitoring: Intravenous access line was secured and vital signs were continuously monitored by nursing staff/anesthesia team throughout the procedure
Total fluoroscopy time: (_) minutes
Cumulative radiation dose: (_) mGy

Description of Procedure *(Femoral artery approach)*:
The risks, benefits, alternatives, and procedure itself were explained to the patient/patient's Power of Attorney/patient's legal guardian, and informed written/verbal consent was obtained. Time out was performed to confirm the correct patient, procedure, and site. The site of the procedure was identified and marked.

The skin of both groins were shaved, prepped, and draped in the usual sterile fashion. The right/left common femoral artery as well as the inguinal ligament were located by palpation/ultrasound and marked. The site of arterial puncture was determined using combined information from palpation, ultrasound and fluoroscopy over the middle of the medial third of the femoral head. Local anesthesia was administered. Common femoral artery access was obtained using a (_)-gauge [type] needle and the Seldinger technique under direct ultrasound visualization/by palpation. Once good pulsatile arterial flow was detected, a (_)-inch [type] guidewire was advanced through the needle, up through the common femoral artery, into the aorta under direct fluoroscopic visualization and a (_)-French vascular sheath was placed.

Heparinized saline infusion was started into the femoral arterial sheath. Subsequently, a (_)-French, (_)-cm-long [type] catheter was advanced into the abdominal/thoracic aorta over a (0.035)-in. [hydrophilic/type] guidewire under direct fluoroscopic visualization, the catheter was formed and the [name] artery was selectively catheterized. After confirming the catheter location by contrast injection, digital subtraction angiography of the [specify anatomic location/vessel] was performed by injecting (_) mL of contrast manually/using automated injector at a rate of (_) mL/sec. Delayed images were obtained to delineate the venous/portovenous circulation. Following this, a (_)-French [type] coaxial microcatheter was advanced into the previously inserted catheter and superselective catheterization of the [name arterial branch] artery was performed. Digital subtraction angiography was performed by manual injection of (_) mL contrast material using (_) mL syringe.

Following the procedure the right/left femoral artery sheath was removed and adequate hemostasis was achieved by compression for (_) minutes/using [type] vascular closure device. The lower extremity pulses were checked following the procedure and were [comparable to the preprocedure pulses/specify if otherwise needed]. The patient was transferred to the floor/recovery room for close monitoring following the procedure in a stable condition. Staff was present for the entire procedure.

Intra-Procedure Findings: List all relevant findings.

Immediate Complications: None encountered during or directly after the procedure. List complications if any.

Post-Procedure Plan [1–3]:

- Keep patient in complete bed rest with the right/left leg extended for (6) h *[adjust depending on the puncture site]*.
- Check the right/left groin/[specify the puncture site if different] for any bleeding or hematoma formation every 15 min for 1 h, then every 30 min for 1 h, then every hour for 4 h; inform interventional radiology team if any signs of bleeding are observed *[adjust depending on the puncture site]*.
- Check and document lower extremity pulses every 30 min for 2 h then every 1 h for 4 h *[adjust depending on the puncture site]*.
- Monitor vital signs every 15 min for 1 h, then every 30 min for 4 h; notify interventional radiology team if systolic blood pressure <95 mmHg, or heart rate >110 beats/minute.
- Resume diet and previous orders as needed and if otherwise not contraindicated.
- Continue adequate intravenous hydration and monitor fluid (intake-output) status.
- Check complete blood count and creatinine on the day following the procedure or as clinically indicated.
- Perform regular neurological examination when the procedure includes manipulation in the ascending thoracic aorta, aortic arch, or brachiocephalic arteries.

Impression:

- Selective/superselective angiography of the [name the artery] as described above.
- The patient tolerated the procedure well and left the interventional unit in stable condition.
- The patient was unstable and the procedure was canceled/terminated prematurely.
- List any other relevant or important information/finding.

References

1. Kandarpa K, Gardiner GA Jr, Keller FS. Diagnostic arteriography. In: Kandarpa K, Machan L, editors. Handbook of interventional radiologic procedures. 4th ed. Philadelphia: Lippincott Williams & Wilkins; 2011. p. 61–84.
2. Heran MK, Marshalleck F, Temple M, Grassi CJ, Connolly B, Towbin RB, et al. Joint quality improvement guidelines for pediatric arterial access and arteriography: from the Societies of Interventional Radiology and Pediatric Radiology. J Vasc Interv Radiol. 2010;21(1):32–43.
3. American College of Radiology. ACR–SIR–SPR practice parameter for performance of arteriography. Reston, VA: American College of Radiology; 2014.
4. Kaufman JA. Invasive vascular diagnosis. In: Mauro MA, Murphy KPJ, Thomson KR, Venbrux AC, Morgan RA, editors. Image-guided interventions. 2nd ed. Philadelphia: Saunders Elsevier; 2014. p. 11–32.
5. Venkatesan AM, Kundu S, Sacks D, Wallace MJ, Wojak JC, Rose SC, et al. Practice guidelines for adult antibiotic prophylaxis during vascular and interventional radiology procedures. J Vasc Interv Radiol. 2010;21(11):1611–30.
6. Taslakian B, Sebaaly MG, Al-Kutoubi A. Patient evaluation and preparation in vascular and interventional radiology: what every interventional radiologist should know (part 1: patient assessment and laboratory tests). Cardiovasc Intervent Radiol. 2016;39 (3):325–33.
7. Taslakian B, Sebaaly MG, Al-Kutoubi A. Patient evaluation and preparation in vascular and interventional radiology: what every interventional radiologist should know (part 2: patient preparation and medications). Cardiovasc Intervent Radiol. 2016;39(4):489–99. doi: 10.1007/s00270-015-1239-4. [Epub 2015 Nov 25].

Celiac and Superior Mesenteric Artery Angioplasty and Stenting

91

Maen Aboul Hosn

INTRODUCTION

Chronic mesenteric ischemia is caused by long-standing atherosclerotic disease in more than 90 % of cases and it usually involves two or more mesenteric vessels. It typically presents as intermittent transient episodes of inadequate intestinal blood supply and manifests as "food fear," postprandial pain, nausea, diarrhea, and weight loss. Although both open and endovascular revascularization have similar technical success and survival rates, the endovascular approach is associated with lower patency and higher recurrence rates, with increased need for repeat intervention. As such it is reserved for patients with poor nutritional status as a bridge to surgery or in those with short life expectancy or hostile abdomen.

COMMON INDICATIONS [1–4]

- Chronic mesenteric ischemia without peritonitis
- Bridge to open revascularization

M. Aboul Hosn (✉)
Department of Vascular Surgery, University of Iowa Hospitals and Clinics, 200 Hawkins Dr, Iowa City, IA 52242, USA
e-mail: maen-aboulhosn@uiowa.edu

COMMON CONTRAINDICATIONS [1–3]

- Peritonitis
- Bowel necrosis
- Extrinsic compression as the cause of stenosis
- Coagulopathy

POSSIBLE COMPLICATIONS [2]

General (angiography-related) complications:
- Hemorrhage *(puncture-site hematoma, retroperitoneal hematoma if "high" puncture above inguinal ligament)*
- Pseudoaneurysm *(superficial femoral artery "low" puncture)*
- Arteriovenous fistula *(puncture-site artery)*
- Thrombosis of the femoral artery
- Distal embolization
- Contrast-induced allergic reaction
- Contrast-induced nephropathy
- Arterial perforation or dissection
- Catheter or guide-wire breakage
- Limb amputation *(rare)*
- Risks related to any minimally invasive procedure performed under conscious sedation *(e.g., allergy to medications)*

Procedure-specific complications:
- Mesenteric arterial occlusion/dissection
- Worsening bowel ischemia

B. Taslakian et al. (eds.), *Procedural Dictations in Image-Guided Intervention*,
DOI 10.1007/978-3-319-40845-3_91

PREPROCEDURAL ASSESSMENT AND PLANNING

- History, indications, and physical examination *(Appendix 1* in Chap. 149*)*. Document indications of the procedure and vital signs.
- Evaluation of diagnostic imaging studies to determine the relevant vascular anatomy and assess the access site
- Periprocedural management of coagulation status *(Appendices 2* in Chap. 150 *and 3* in Chap. 151*)*
- Antibiotic prophylaxis: Not routinely recommended, unless the patient is at high risk of developing stent infection [5] *(Appendices 4* in Chap. 152 *and 5* in Chap. 153*)*
- Imaging modality for guidance: Fluoroscopy; combined with ultrasound for arterial puncture
- Positioning: Supine

PROCEDURE NOTE

Procedure: Celiac/superior mesenteric artery angioplasty and stenting
Staff: [_]
Fellow: [_]
Resident: [_]
Clinical Information: Describe history and list indications
Allergies: No known drug allergy/Allergic to (specify)
Anesthesia: Local anesthesia/Monitored conscious sedation
Medications: List any relevant medications used (sedation, antibiotics, intravenous heparin)
Contrast Material: (_) mL of [type] contrast material was used for intra-arterial injection
Field: Sterile
Procedure Classification: Clean
Position: Supine
Monitoring: Intravenous access was secured and vitals were continuously monitored by nursing staff/anesthesia team throughout the procedure
Total fluoroscopy time: (_) minutes
Cumulative radiation dose: (_) mGy

Description of Procedure:
The risks, benefits, alternatives, and procedure itself were explained to the patient/patient's Power of Attorney/patient's legal guardian, and informed written consent was obtained. Time out was performed to confirm the correct patient, procedure, and site. The site of the procedure was identified and marked.

The skin of both groins/left antecubital fossa were shaved, prepped, and draped in the usual sterile fashion. The right/left common femoral/left brachial artery was located by palpation/ultrasound and marked. The site of arterial puncture was determined using combined information from palpation, ultrasound, and fluoroscopy over the middle of the medial third of the femoral head. Local anesthesia was administered. Common femoral/brachial artery access was obtained using a (_)-gauge [type] needle and the Seldinger technique under direct ultrasound visualization/by palpation. Once good pulsatile arterial flow was detected, a (_)-inch [type] guidewire was advanced through the needle, into the aorta under direct fluoroscopic visualization and a (_)-French vascular sheath was placed.

A (_)-French pigtail catheter/Omni flush catheter was advanced over a (_)-inch [type] wire to the abdominal aorta and angiographic runs were performed delineating the flow to the celiac artery, superior mesenteric artery, and both renal arteries. The patient was fully anticoagulated using intravenous heparin (80–100 U/kg). Then, the short sheath was exchanged with a long (_)-French Flexor/Ansel/Arrow Flex sheath and its tip was placed in proximity to the celiac artery/superior mesenteric artery takeoff. A (_)-French Cobra/SOS/Berenstein catheter was used to maneuver the glide wire into the celiac artery/superior mesenteric artery distally and the catheter was advanced over it. Selective mesenteric angiography was performed confirming the presence of the catheter tip within the vessel lumen and absence of any dissection. Then, the wire was re-advanced beyond the level of the stenosis into a distal branch and a (_) × (_) mm low profile angioplasty balloon was advanced over the guidewire and placed across the stenotic segment. After the balloon was insufflated to achieve predilatation, a (_) × (_) mm balloon-expandable stent was advanced and deployed to cover the entire lesion, with 1–2 mm of the stent flaring into the aorta. A completion angiogram was performed through the sheath showing a patent stent with no evidence of residual stenosis. The procedure was concluded at this point. An ACT level was measured and then the femoral artery sheath was removed and adequate hemostasis was achieved by compression for (_) minutes/using [type] vascular closure device. The lower extremity pulses were checked following the procedure and were [comparable to the preprocedure pulses/specify if otherwise needed]. The patient was transferred to the floor/recovery room for close monitoring following the procedure in a stable condition. Staff was present for the entire procedure.

Intra-Procedure Findings: List all relevant radiologic findings.

Immediate Complications: None encountered during or directly after the procedure. List the complications if any.

Post-Procedure Plan [1–3, 6]:

Standard post-angiogram management plan

- Keep patient complete in bed rest with the right/left leg extended for 6 h *[adjust depending on the puncture site]*.
- Check the right/left groin/[specify the puncture site if different] for any bleeding or hematoma formation every 15 min for 1 h, then every 30 min for 1 h, then every hour for 4 h; inform interventional radiology team if any signs of bleeding are observed *[adjust depending on the puncture site]*.
- Check and document lower extremity pulses every 30 min for 2 h then every 1 h for 4 h *[adjust depending on the puncture site]*.
- Monitor vital signs every 15 min for 1 h, then every 30 min for 4 h; notify interventional radiology team if systolic blood pressure <95 mmHg, or heart rate >110 beats/minute.
- Resume diet and previous orders as needed and if otherwise not contraindicated.
- Continue adequate intravenous hydration and monitor fluid (intake-output) status.
- Check complete blood count and creatinine on the day following the procedure or as clinically indicated.
- Perform regular neurological examination when the procedure includes manipulation in the ascending thoracic aorta, aortic arch, or brachiocephalic arteries.

Procedure-specific management plan:

- Perform regular abdominal exam for signs of peritonitis.
- Start patient on 300 mg of clopidogrel (if not administered before the procedure) and maintain on 75 mg/day for 6 to 8 weeks.
- Start patient on 325 mg of aspirin on the day of the procedure and then 75 mg per day, indefinitely.

Impression:

- Celiac/superior mesenteric artery angioplasty and stenting as described above.
- The patient tolerated the procedure well and left the interventional unit in a stable condition.
- The procedure was cancelled/terminated prematurely.
- List any other relevant of important information/finding.

References

1. Pecoraro F, Rancic Z, Lachat M, Mayer D, Amann-Vesti B, Pfammatter T, et al. Chronic mesenteric ischemia: critical review and guidelines for management. Ann Vasc Surg. 2013;27(1):113–22.
2. Oderich GS, Tallarita T, Gloviczki P, Duncan AA, Kalra M, Misra S, et al. Mesenteric artery complications during angioplasty and stent placement for atherosclerotic chronic mesenteric ischemia. J Vasc Surg. 2012;55(4):1063–71.
3. Oderich GS, Bower TC, Sullivan TM, Bjarnason H, Cha S, Gloviczki P. Open versus endovascular revascularization for chronic mesenteric ischemia: risk-stratified outcomes. J Vasc Surg. 2009;49(6):1472–79.e3.
4. Chang JB, Stein TA. Mesenteric ischemia: acute and chronic. Ann Vasc Surg. 2003;17(3):323–8.

5. Venkatesan AM, Kundu S, Sacks D, Wallace MJ, Wojak JC, Rose SC, et al. Practice guidelines for adult antibiotic prophylaxis during vascular and interventional radiology procedures. J Vasc Interv Radiol. 2010;21(11):1611–30.
6. Atkins MD, Kwolek CJ, LaMuraglia GM, Brewster DC, Chung TK, Cambria RP. Surgical revascularization versus endovascular therapy for chronic mesenteric ischemia: a comparative experience. J Vasc Surg. 2007;45(6):1162–71.

Embolization for Management of Acute Non-variceal Gastrointestinal Hemorrhage

92

Anne M. Covey

Abbreviations

GI Gastrointestinal

INTRODUCTION

Angiography and transarterial intervention has become a mainstay in the treatment of acute non-variceal gastrointestinal (GI) hemorrhage. GI hemorrhage can be divided into "upper" involving the esophagus, stomach, and duodenum that are predominantly supplied by branches of the gastroduodenal artery and "lower" involving the jejunum to the anus supplied by branches of the superior and inferior mesenteric arteries and branches of the internal iliac artery. Rich collateral supply of the upper, and to a lesser degree lower GI tract allow for safe selective embolization with minimal risk of ischemia.

Common causes of upper GI arterial bleeding include gastric or duodenal ulcers, Mallory Weiss tear, gastritis, and visceral pseudoaneurysm (e.g., post pancreatitis). Lower GI hemorrhage is often caused by diverticular disease, tumors, and angiodysplasia. It is important to remember, that even severe GI bleeding is intermittent and if the patient is not actively bleeding at the time of contrast injection, the site may not be identified. If the site of bleeding is known to be the stomach or duodenum based on CT angiography or endoscopy, empiric embolization of the left gastric or gastroduodenal artery may be considered.

In some cases, maintaining patency of the parent vessel is important; for example hemorrhage from a gastroduodenal artery stump after pancreaticoduodenectomy or internal iliac blow-out after pelvic surgery, and in such cases covered stent placement is a good option to keep in mind.

Safe and effective treatment of a patient with acute GI hemorrhage requires multidisciplinary input from surgeons, radiologists, and gastroenterologists to determine the best strategy for diagnosis and treatment. Many patients can be treated definitively at endoscopy using sclerosis, banding, or clipping. It is important for the operator to have a detailed understanding of the relevant vascular anatomy and the tools at their disposal.

A.M. Covey (✉)
Department of Radiology, Division of Interventional Radiology, Memorial Sloan Kettering Cancer Center, 1275 York Ave, New York, NY 10065, USA
e-mail: coveya@mskcc.org

B. Taslakian et al. (eds.), *Procedural Dictations in Image-Guided Intervention*,
DOI 10.1007/978-3-319-40845-3_92

COMMON INDICATIONS [1–3]

- Acute hemorrhage involving the stomach, duodenum, or colon not amenable to endoscopic treatment
- Acute hemorrhage involving the small bowel

COMMON CONTRAINDICATIONS [1, 2]

- Anaphylactic contrast reaction
- Uncontrolled coagulopathy

POSSIBLE COMPLICATIONS [4]

General (angiography-related) complications:
- Hemorrhage *(puncture-site hematoma, retroperitoneal hematoma if "high" puncture above inguinal ligament)*
- Pseudoaneurysm *(superficial femoral artery "low" puncture)*
- Arteriovenous fistula *(puncture-site artery)*
- Thrombosis of the femoral artery
- Distal embolization
- Contrast-induced allergic reaction
- Contrast-induced nephropathy
- Arterial perforation or dissection
- Catheter or guide-wire breakage
- Risks related to any minimally invasive procedure performed under conscious sedation *(e.g., allergy to medications)*

Embolization (procedure-specific) complications:
- Non-target embolization
- Ischemic bowel necrosis

PREPROCEDURAL ASSESSMENT AND PLANNING

- History, indications, and physical examination *(Appendix 1* in Chap. 149*)*
- Evaluation of diagnostic imaging studies including nuclear medicine bleeding scan, arterial phase CT to determine the location of the hemorrhage, or vascular abnormality and the relevant vascular anatomy
- Periprocedural management of coagulation status *(Appendices 2* in Chap. 150 *and 3* in Chap. 151*)*
- Antibiotic prophylaxis: Not routinely recommended *(Appendices 4* in Chap. 152 *and 5* in Chap. 153*)*
- Imaging modality for guidance: Fluoroscopy; combined with ultrasound for access vessel puncture.
- Positioning: Supine

PROCEDURE NOTE

Procedure: Fluoroscopic guided visceral angiogram and embolization of [specify arterial branch/es]
Staff: [_]
Fellow: [_]
Resident: [_]
Clinical Information: Describe history and list indications
Allergies: None known/Allergic to [specify/type of allergy]
Anesthesia: Local anesthesia/conscious sedation/general anesthesia
Medications: List any relevant medications used (sedation)
Contrast Used: (_) mL of [type] contrast media was used for angiography
Field: Sterile
Procedure classification: Clean
Position: Supine
Monitoring: Intravenous access line was secured and vital signs were continuously monitored by nursing staff/anesthesia team throughout the procedure
Total fluoroscopy time: (_) minutes
Cumulative radiation dose: (_) mGy

Description of Procedure:
The risks, benefits, alternatives, and the procedure itself were explained to the patient/patient's Power of Attorney/patient's legal guardian, and informed written/verbal consent was obtained. The site of the procedure was identified and

marked. Time out was performed to confirm the correct patient, procedure, and site.

The skin of both groins were shaved, prepped, and draped in the usual sterile fashion. The right/left femoral artery as well as the inguinal ligament were located by palpation/ultrasound and marked. The site of arterial puncture was determined using combined information from palpation, ultrasound and fluoroscopy over the middle of the medial third of the femoral head. Local anesthesia was administered. Femoral artery access was obtained using a (_)-gauge [type] needle and the Seldinger technique, double-/single- wall entry under direct ultrasound visualization/by palpation. Once good pulsatile arterial flow was detected, a (_)-inch [type] guidewire was advanced through the needle, into the aorta under direct fluoroscopic visualization and a (_)-French vascular sheath was placed.

A (_) French [Cobra/Sos/other] angiographic catheter was advanced over a (_)-inch [type] guidewire into the aorta and used to select the celiac/superior mesenteric/inferior mesenteric/ other artery. Digital subtraction angiography was performed. After identification of active extravasation/vascular abnormality [specify], the target vessel [specify vessel] was subselectively catheterized with a (_)-French [type] microcatheter. Embolization of the [specify vessel] was performed with (0.018 micro/0.025/0.035 macro coils) extending across the abnormality/ proximal to the abnormality. At the end of the procedure, completion angiography with the catheter positioned in the [name of vessel] demonstrated no further extravasation/vascular abnormality.

The catheter and sheath were removed and hemostasis of the puncture site was achieved by manual compression for (_) minutes/using a [type] vascular closure device.

The patient was transferred to the floor/ recovery room/ICU following the procedure in a guarded/stable condition. Staff was present for the entire procedure.

Intra-Procedure Findings: List all relevant findings.

Immediate Complications: None encountered during or directly after the procedure. List complications if any.

Post-Procedure Plan: [5]:

- If a closure device is used successfully, keep right/left leg straight for (1–4) h and abstain from strenuous activities.
- If manual compression is used for hemostasis, keep right/left leg straight for (4–6) h and abstain from strenuous activities.
- If arterial sheath is left in place, keep right/left leg straight and abstain from activities.
- Check pedal pulses every 30 min for (2–4) h
- Observe right/left puncture site for bleeding every 15 min for 1 h, then every 30 min for 1 h, then every 1 h for 2 h.
- Inform interventional radiology team if systolic blood pressure < 95 mm Hg, heart rate > 100 beats per minute, or if any abdominal pain develops.
- Follow serial hemoglobin and hematocrit every 4–6 h for 24 h to assess response to embolization

Impression:

- Visceral angiography demonstrating active extravasation/vascular abnormality/neither from the [name vessel]. Embolization of the [name vessel] was performed with [name embolic agent].
- The patient tolerated the procedure well and left the interventional unit in guarded/stable condition.
- The patient was unstable and the procedure was canceled/terminated prematurely.
- List any other relevant or important information/finding.

References

1. McPherson SJ, Patel R. Management of upper GI hemorrhage. In: Mauro MA, Murphy KP, Thompson KR, Venbrux AC, Morgan RA, editors. Image-guided interventions. Philadelphia PA: Elsevier Saunders; 2014. p. 362–73.

2. Darcy M. Management of lower GI hemorrhage. In: Mauro MA, Murphy KP, Thompson KR, Venbrux AC, Morgan RA, editors. Image-guided interventions. Philadelphia, PA: Elsevier Saunders; 2014. p. 374–9.
3. Millward SF. ACR appropriateness criteria on treatment of acute nonvariceal GI tract bleeding. J Am Coll Radiol. 2008;5(4):550–4.
4. Loffroy R, Rao P, Ota S, De Lin M, Kwak BK, Geschwind JF. Embolization of acute nonvariceal upper GI hemorrhage resistant to endoscopic treatment: results and predictors of recurrent bleeding. Cardiovasc Intervent Radiol. 2010;33(6):1088–100.
5. Darcy M. Acute gastrointestinal arterial bleeding. In: Kandarpa Machan, editor. Handbook of interventional radiologic procedures. 4th ed. Philadelphia, PA: Lippincott Williams & Wilkins; 2011. p. 233–9.

Embolization of the Splenic Artery in Nontraumatized Patients

93

Bedros Taslakian and Sela Batouzian

INTRODUCTION

Catheter-directed splenic embolization can be used to induce global or segmental infarction of the splenic tissue and has been advocated for the intentional infarction of splenic tissue to reduce its consumptive activity. Efficient infarction of splenic tissue is achieved by embolization of the intrasplenic branches due to the presence of collateral circulation principally via the short gastric arteries and because intrasplenic arterial vascularization is represented by terminal vessels. Partial catheter-mediated infarction of the splenic tissues allows maintenance of the spleen's immunologic function while reducing sequestration and destruction of the blood elements and preoperative reduction of splenic volume in massive splenomegaly. It has shown better results and significantly lower complication rate when compared to complete splenic embolization.

COMMON INDICATIONS [1–4]

- Hypersplenism and pancytopenia secondary to hematologic disorders *(e.g., idiopathic thrombocytopenic purpura, thalassemia, hereditary spherocytosis, autoimmune hemolytic anemia)*
- Liver cirrhosis associated with portal hypertension *(hypersplenism and pancytopenia, recurrent gastroesophageal visceral hemorrhage, hepatic encephalopathy)*
- Pancytopenia secondary to lymphoma and leukemia
- Hypersplenism and pancytopenia secondary to congenital diseases *(e.g., Gaucher disease, biliary atresia)*
- Hypersplenism and pancytopenia secondary to portal vein thrombosis
- Chemotherapy-induced bone marrow suppression or hypersplenism leading to pancytopenia
- Intolerance to immunosuppressive agents *(i.e., pancytopenia)*
- Hypersplenism and pancytopenia secondary to idiopathic hypersplenism
- Before laparoscopic splenectomy in selected group of patients *(e.g., high operative risk, refusal of blood transfusion)*

B. Taslakian (✉)
Department of Radiology, New York University Langone Medical Center, 660 First Ave, New York, NY 10016, USA
e-mail: btaslakian@gmail.com

S. Batouzian
Coronary Care Unit (CCU), Clemenceau Medical Center (CMC), Beirut, Lebanon
e-mail: sela.batouzian1@gmail.com

B. Taslakian et al. (eds.), *Procedural Dictations in Image-Guided Intervention*,
DOI 10.1007/978-3-319-40845-3_93

COMMON CONTRAINDICATIONS [1–4]

- Past history of allergy to intravenous contrast media or impaired renal function *(consider CO_2 for angiography)*
- Pregnancy
- Uncorrected coagulopathy
- Acute or chronic infection of spleen
- Systemic infection
- Massive splenomegaly *(consider staged partial embolization)*

POSSIBLE COMPLICATIONS [1–4]

General (angiography-related) complications:
- Hemorrhage *(puncture-site hematoma, retroperitoneal hematoma if "high" puncture above inguinal ligament)*
- Pseudoaneurysm *(superficial femoral artery "low" puncture)*
- Arteriovenous fistula *(puncture-site artery)*
- Thrombosis of the femoral artery
- Distal embolization
- Contrast-induced allergic reaction
- Contrast-induced nephropathy
- Arterial perforation or dissection
- Catheter or guidewire breakage
- Limb amputation *(rare)*
- Risks related to any minimally invasive procedure performed under conscious sedation *(e.g., allergy to medications)*

Embolization (procedure-specific) related complications:
- Postembolization syndrome *(fever, nausea, pain)*, as side effect of the embolization
- Pleural effusion, ascites, left lower lobe atelectasis
- Nontarget embolization causing organ infarction *(pancreatitis and necrosis of gastric wall)*
- Splenic perforation
- Splenic abscess formation
- Pneumococcal pneumonia and sepsis
- Splenic vein thrombosis
- Splenic regeneration requiring repeat embolization
- Mortality

PREPROCEDURAL ASSESSMENT AND PLANNING [1–7]

- History, indications, and physical examination *(Appendix 1* in Chap. 149*)*. Document indications of the procedure, lower or upper extremity pulses, and vital signs
- Evaluation of diagnostic imaging studies to determine the relevant vascular anatomy and identify all potential sites of injury and occult sources of bleeding
- Periprocedural management of coagulation status *(Appendices 2* in Chap. 150 *and 3* in Chap. 151*)*
- Antibiotic prophylaxis: Routinely recommended [1–5] *(Appendices 4* in Chap. 152 *and 5* in Chap. 153*)*
- Pneumococcal vaccine (14-valent vaccine) should be administered a few days before the procedure [1–4]
- Imaging modality for guidance: Fluoroscopy; combined with ultrasound for arterial puncture
- Positioning: Supine
- Arterial access: Common femoral artery *(preferred)*, left brachial artery, left axillary artery

PROCEDURE NOTE

Procedure: Catheter-directed partial/complete embolization of the splenic artery
Staff: [_]
Fellow: [_]
Resident: [_]
Clinical History and Indications: Describe history and list indications
Allergies: None known/Allergic to [specify/type of allergy]

Anesthesia: Local anesthesia/Conscious sedation/ General anesthesia
Medications: List any relevant medications used
Contrast Material: (_) mL of [type] contrast material was used for intra-arterial injection
Field: Sterile
Procedure classification: Clean
Position: Supine
Monitoring: Intravenous access line was secured and vital signs were continuously monitored by nursing staff/anesthesia team throughout the procedure
Total fluoroscopy time: (_) minutes
Cumulative radiation dose: (_) mGy

Description of Procedure *(coil embolization of the intrasplenic branches of the splenic artery):* The risks, benefits, alternatives, and procedure itself were explained to the patient/ patient's Power of Attorney/patient's legal guardian, and informed written/verbal consent was obtained. Time out was performed to confirm the correct patient, procedure, and site. The site of the procedure was identified and marked.

The skin of both groins were shaved, prepped and draped in the usual sterile fashion. The right/left common femoral artery as well as the inguinal ligament were located by palpation/ ultrasound and marked. The site of arterial puncture was determined using combined information from palpation, ultrasound, and fluoroscopy over the middle of the medial third of the femoral head. Local anesthesia was administered. Common femoral artery access was obtained using (_)-gauge [type] needle and the Seldinger technique under direct ultrasound visualization/ by palpation. Once good pulsatile arterial flow was detected, a (_)-inch [type] guidewire was advanced through the needle, into the aorta under direct fluoroscopic visualization and a (_)-French vascular sheath was placed.

Heparinized saline infusion was started into the femoral arterial sheath. Subsequently, a (_)-French, (_) cm-long [type] catheter was advanced into the abdominal aorta over a (_)-inch [hydrophilic/type] guidewire under direct fluoroscopic visualization and the celiac artery was selectively catheterized. The catheter was then advanced into the splenic artery under fluoroscopy and selective splenic artery angiography was performed by manual injection of (_) mL of contrast demonstrating [specify findings]. Following this, superselective catheterization of intrasplenic segmental arterial branches supplying the [specify anatomic location] was performed using a (_)-French [type] coaxial microcatheter. Superselective embolization was performed using (number) detachable microcoils {(_) cm length/(_) mm diameter}/PVA particles [type/size] until complete stasis was achieved. Parenchymal angiography was performed by manual injection of (_) mL contrast media in the splenic artery proximal to the coils and the volume of the remaining viable splenic tissue was estimated at around (_) %.

Following the procedure the right/left femoral artery sheath was removed and adequate hemostasis was achieved by compression for (_) minutes/using [type] vascular closure device. The lower extremity pulses were checked following the procedure and were [comparable to the pre-procedure pulses/specify if otherwise needed]. The patient was transferred to the floor/ recovery room for close monitoring following the procedure in a stable condition. Staff was present for the entire procedure.

Intra-Procedure Findings: List all relevant findings.

Immediate Complications: None encountered during or directly after the procedure. List complications if any.

Post-Procedure Plan [1, 2]:

Standard post-angiogram management plan

- Keep patient complete bed rest with the right/left leg extended for 6 h *[adjust depending on the puncture site]*.
- Check the right/left groin/[specify the puncture site if different] for any bleeding or hematoma formation every 15 min for 1 h, then every 30 min for 1 h, then every hour for 4 h; inform interventional radiology team if any signs of bleeding are observed *[adjust depending on the puncture site]*.
- Check and document lower extremity pulses every 30 min for 2 h then every 1 h for 4 h *[adjust depending on the puncture site]*.
- Monitor vital signs every 15 min for 1 h, then every 30 min for 4 h; notify interventional radiology team if systolic blood pressure <95 mmHg, or heart rate >110 beats/minute.
- Resume diet and previous orders as needed and if otherwise not contraindicated.
- Continue adequate intravenous hydration and monitor fluid (intake–output) status.
- Check complete blood count and creatinine on the day following the procedure or as clinically indicated.
- Perform regular neurological examination when the procedure includes manipulation in the ascending thoracic aorta, aortic arch or brachiocephalic arteries.

Procedure-specific management plan:

- Follow-up physical examination and laboratory studies, and hematological assessment at 2 and 4 weeks.
- Start adequate intravenous antibiotic coverage to reduce the risk of abscess formation.
- Perform cross-sectional imaging prior to discharge or after 1 month to evaluate the extent of splenic infarction.
- Manage postembolization syndrome conservatively using appropriate antiemetic and analgesic medication and adequately hydrate the patient.
- Provide specific instructions to minimize the risk of splenic rupture *(e.g., avoid contact sports)*.

Impression:

- Catheter-directed partial/complete splenic embolization, as described above.
- The patient tolerated the procedure well and left the interventional unit in stable condition.
- The patient was unstable and the procedure was canceled/terminated prematurely.
- List any other relevant or important information/finding.

References

1. Kos S, Liu DM, Ho SGF. Solid organ embolization. In: Kandarpa K, Machan L, editors. Handbook of interventional radiologic procedures. 4th ed. Philadelphia: Lippincott Williams & Wilkins; 2011. p. 274–80.
2. Dondelinger RF. Splenic embolization in nontraumatized patients. In: Mauro MA, Murphy KPJ, Thomson KR, Venbrux AC, Morgan RA, editors. Image-guided interventions. 2nd ed. Philadelphia: Saunders Elsevier; 2014. p. 503–7.
3. Madoff DC, Denys A, Wallace MJ, Murthy R, Gupta S, Pillsbury EP, et al. Splenic arterial interventions: anatomy, indications, technical considerations, and potential complications. Radiographics. 2005;25 (Suppl 1):S191–211.
4. Smith M, Ray CE. Splenic artery embolization as an adjunctive procedure for portal hypertension. Semin Intervent Radiol. 2012;29(2):135–9.
5. Venkatesan AM, Kundu S, Sacks D, Wallace MJ, Wojak JC, Rose SC, et al. Practice guidelines for adult antibiotic prophylaxis during vascular and interventional radiology procedures. J Vasc Interv Radiol. 2010;21(11):1611–30.
6. Taslakian B, Sebaaly MG, Al-Kutoubi A. Patient evaluation and preparation in vascular and interventional radiology: what every interventional radiologist should know (part 1: patient assessment and laboratory tests). Cardiovasc Intervent Radiol. 2016;39(3):325–33.
7. Taslakian B, Sebaaly MG, Al-Kutoubi A. Patient evaluation and preparation in vascular and interventional radiology: what every interventional radiologist should know (part 2: patient preparation and medications). Cardiovasc Intervent Radiol. 2016;39(4):489–99. doi: 10.1007/s00270-015-1239-4. [Epub 2015 Nov 25].

Embolization of the Splenic Artery in Traumatic Splenic Injury

94

Bedros Taslakian and Sela Batouzian

INTRODUCTION

The treatment of traumatic splenic injuries has changed dramatically over the past years, from surgical to nonsurgical management, thus decreasing the occurrence of fatal post-splenectomy sepsis or impaired resistance to certain encapsulated organisms. Splenic artery embolization has been proposed to reduce the failure rate of conservative management. In the settings of distal focal pseudoaneurysm, arteriovenous fistulas or contrast extravasation supplied by a discrete vessel, superselective embolization is performed using microcoils deployed as distally as possible, in the affected small arterial branches. Superselective distal embolization tends to preserve perfusion to the remaining splenic parenchyma. On the other hand, proximal embolization with coils is preferred in patients with a high risk for splenic rupture, patients who become hemodynamically unstable during angiography or in whom extensive vascular injury involving multiple arterial branches is detected. Proximal embolization decreases the volume of splenic arterial blood flow and thus allows the spleen to heal without infarction.

COMMON INDICATIONS [1–5]

Still controversial and may vary depending on the local management protocols

- Grade III or IV splenic laceration with borderline hemodynamic lability or transfusion requirements greater than 4 units of packed red blood cells over 24 h
- Contrast extravasation on CT angiography
- Segmental splenic infarction, which indicates splenic arterial branch injury
- Intrasplenic pseudoaneurysm, because of relatively high risk of delayed bleeding
- Intrasplenic arteriovenous fistula, because of relatively high risk of delayed bleeding
- Recurrent hemodynamic lability and transfusion requirement, suggestive of delayed splenic rupture
- Evidence of rebleeding after initial splenic artery embolization

COMMON CONTRAINDICATIONS [1, 2, 5]

Absolute contraindications:

- Hemodynamic instability despite adequate resuscitation, requiring emergent surgical exploration

B. Taslakian (✉)
Department of Radiology, New York University Langone Medical Center, 660 First Ave, New York, NY 10016, USA
e-mail: btaslakian@gmail.com

S. Batouzian
Coronary Care Unit (CCU), Clemenceau Medical Center (CMC), Beirut, Lebanon
e-mail: sela.batouzian1@gmail.com

B. Taslakian et al. (eds.), *Procedural Dictations in Image-Guided Intervention*,
DOI 10.1007/978-3-319-40845-3_94

- Associated injuries such as bowel perforation, requiring emergent surgical exploration

Relative contraindications (benefits should be weighed against risks):

- Past history of allergy to intravenous contrast media
- Pregnancy
- Impaired renal function
- Penetrating splenic trauma

POSSIBLE COMPLICATIONS [1–3, 5, 6]

General (angiography-related) complications:

- Hemorrhage *(puncture-site hematoma, retroperitoneal hematoma if "high" puncture above inguinal ligament)*
- Pseudoaneurysm *(superficial femoral artery "low" puncture)*
- Arteriovenous fistula *(puncture-site artery)*
- Thrombosis of the femoral artery
- Distal embolization
- Contrast-induced allergic reaction
- Contrast-induced nephropathy
- Arterial perforation or dissection
- Catheter or guidewire breakage
- Limb amputation *(rare)*
- Risks related to any minimally invasive procedure performed under conscious sedation *(e.g., allergy to medications)*

Embolization (procedure-specific) related complications:

- Nontarget embolization causing organ infarction *(pancreatitis and necrosis of gastric wall)*
- Postembolization syndrome *(fever, nausea, pain)*
- Splenic infarction, mainly with distal embolization or proximal embolization with undersized coils
- Septicemia
- Splenic abscess and pseudocyst formation
- Failure to control bleeding and delayed hemorrhage
- Splenic vein thrombosis

PREPROCEDURAL ASSESSMENT AND PLANNING [7–9]

- History, indications, and physical examination *(Appendix 1* in Chap. 149*)*. Document indications of the procedure, lower or upper extremity pulses and vital signs
- Evaluation of diagnostic imaging studies to determine the relevant vascular anatomy and identify all potential sites of injury and occult sources of bleeding
- Periprocedural management of coagulation status *(Appendices 2* in Chap. 150 *and 3* in Chap. 151*)*
- Antibiotic prophylaxis: Routinely recommended [7] *(Appendices 4* in Chap. 152 *and 5* in Chap. 153*)*
- Imaging modality for guidance: Fluoroscopy; combined with ultrasound for arterial puncture
- Positioning: Supine
- Arterial access: Common femoral artery *(preferred)*, left brachial artery, left axillary artery

PROCEDURE NOTE

Procedure: Catheter-directed proximal/distal superselective embolization of the splenic artery
Staff: [_]
Fellow: [_]
Resident: [_]
Clinical History and Indications: Describe history and list indications
Allergies: None known/Allergic to [specify/type of allergy]
Anesthesia: Local anesthesia/Conscious sedation/General anesthesia
Medications: List any relevant medications used
Contrast Material: (_) mL of [type] contrast material was used for intra-arterial injection
Field: Sterile
Procedure classification: Clean
Position: Supine
Monitoring: Intravenous access line was secured and vital signs were continuously monitored by

nursing staff/anesthesia team throughout the procedure
Total fluoroscopy time: (_) minutes
Cumulative radiation dose: (_) mGy

Description of Procedure *(superselective coil embolization of the intrasplenic arterial branches):* The risks, benefits, alternatives, and procedure itself were explained to the patient/patient's Power of Attorney/patient's legal guardian, and informed written/verbal consent was obtained. Time out was performed to confirm the correct patient, procedure, and site. The site of the procedure was identified and marked.

The skin of both groins were shaved, prepped, and draped in the usual sterile fashion. The right/left common femoral artery as well as the inguinal ligament were located by palpation/ultrasound and marked. The site of arterial puncture was determined using combined information from palpation, ultrasound, and fluoroscopy over the middle of the medial third of the femoral head. Local anesthesia was administered. Common femoral artery access was obtained using a (_)-gauge [type] needle and the Seldinger technique under direct ultrasound visualization/by palpation. Once good pulsatile arterial flow was detected, a (_)-inch [type] guidewire was advanced through the needle, into the aorta under direct fluoroscopic visualization and a (_)-French vascular sheath was placed.

Heparinized saline infusion was started into the femoral arterial sheath. Subsequently, a (_)-French, (_) cm-long [type] catheter was advanced into the abdominal aorta over a (_)-inch [hydrophilic/type] guidewire under direct fluoroscopic visualization and the celiac artery was selectively catheterized. The catheter was then advanced into the splenic artery under fluoroscopy and selective splenic artery angiography was performed by manual injection of (_) mL of contrast demonstrating [specify findings]. Following this, superselective catheterization of intrasplenic segmental arterial branches supplying the [specify anatomic location] was performed using a (_)-French [type] coaxial microcatheter. Superselective embolization was performed using (number) detachable coils [(_) cm length/(_) mm diameter] until complete stasis was achieved. Digital subtraction splenic angiography was then performed and adequate occlusion of the branch artery, and absence of contrast extravasation was confirmed.

Following the procedure the right/left femoral artery sheath was removed and adequate hemostasis was achieved by compression for (_) minutes/using [type] vascular closure device. The lower extremity pulses were checked following the procedure and were comparable to the preprocedure pulses/specify if otherwise needed. The patient was transferred to the floor/recovery room/ICU for close monitoring following the procedure in a stable condition. Staff was present for the entire procedure.

Description of Procedure *(Proximal coil embolization of the splenic artery):*

The risks, benefits, alternatives, and procedure itself were explained to the patient/patient's Power of Attorney/patient's legal guardian, and informed written/verbal consent was obtained. Time out was performed to confirm the correct patient, procedure, and site. The site of the procedure was identified and marked.

The skin of both groins were shaved, prepped, and draped in the usual sterile fashion. The right/left common femoral artery as well as the inguinal ligament were located by palpation/ultrasound and marked. The site of arterial puncture was determined using combined information from palpation, ultrasound, and fluoroscopy over the middle of the medial third of the femoral head. Local anesthesia was administered. Common femoral artery access was obtained using a (_)-gauge [type] needle and the Seldinger technique under direct ultrasound visualization/by palpation. Once good pulsatile arterial flow was detected, a (_)-inch [type] guidewire was advanced through the needle, into the aorta under direct fluoroscopic visualization and a (_)-French vascular sheath was placed.

Heparinized saline infusion was started into the femoral arterial sheath. Subsequently, a (_)-French, (_) cm-long [type] catheter was advanced into the abdominal aorta over a (_)-inch [hydrophilic/type] guidewire under direct fluoroscopic visualization and the celiac artery was selectively catheterized. The catheter was then advanced into the splenic artery under fluoroscopy and selective splenic artery angiography was performed by manual injection of (_) mL of contrast demonstrating [specify findings]. The catheter was then positioned just distal to the origin of the dorsal pancreatic artery and embolization was performed using (number) detachable coils [(_) cm length/(_) mm diameter] until stasis was achieved. Digital subtraction splenic angiography was then performed confirming adequate occlusion of the splenic artery, and absence of contrast extravasation.

Following the procedure the right/left femoral artery sheath was removed and adequate hemostasis was achieved by compression for (_) minutes/using [type] vascular closure device. The lower extremity pulses were checked following the procedure and were comparable to the preprocedure pulses/specify if otherwise needed. The patient was transferred to the floor/recovery room/ICU for close monitoring following the procedure in a stable condition. Staff was present for the entire procedure.

Intra-Procedure Findings: List all relevant findings.

Immediate Complications: None encountered during or directly after the procedure. List complications if any.

Post-Procedure Plan [1, 2]:

Standard post-angiogram management plan

- Keep patient complete bed rest with the right/left leg extended for 6 h *[adjust depending on the puncture site]*.
- Check the right/left groin/[specify the puncture site if different] for any bleeding or hematoma formation every 15 min for 1 h, then every 30 min for 1 h, then every hour for 4 h; inform interventional radiology team if any signs of bleeding are observed *[adjust depending on the puncture site]*.
- Check and document lower extremity pulses every 30 min for 2 h then every 1 h for 4 h *[adjust depending on the puncture site]*.
- Monitor vital signs every 15 min for 1 h, then every 30 min for 4 h; notify interventional radiology team if systolic blood pressure <95 mmHg, or heart rate >110 beats/min.
- Resume diet and previous orders as needed and if otherwise not contraindicated.
- Continue adequate intravenous hydration and monitor fluid (intake–output) status.
- Check complete blood count and creatinine on the day following the procedure or as clinically indicated.
- Perform regular neurological examination when the procedure includes manipulation in the ascending thoracic aorta, aortic arch or brachiocephalic arteries.

Procedure-specific management plan:

- Follow-up physical examination and laboratory studies closely for signs of persistent or delayed hemorrhage.
- Start adequate antibiotic and deep venous thrombosis prophylaxis as needed.
- Perform cross-sectional imaging within a minimum of 3 weeks if not otherwise indicated to evaluate the presence of pseudoaneurysm formation and recurrent bleeding caused by delayed rupture.
- Manage postembolization syndrome conservatively using appropriate antiemetic and analgesic medication and with adequate hydration.

Impression:

- Catheter-directed superselective distal/proximal splenic artery embolization, as described above.
- The patient tolerated the procedure well and left the interventional unit in stable condition.
- The patient was unstable and the procedure was canceled/terminated prematurely.
- List any other relevant or important information/finding.

References

1. Mathur VV, Sclafani SJA. Trauma management. In: Kandarpa K, Machan L, editors. Handbook of interventional radiologic procedures. 4th ed. Philadelphia: Lippincott Williams & Wilkins; 2011. p. 245–57.

2. Dondelinger RF. Management of trauma to the liver and spleen. In: Mauro MA, Murphy KPJ, Thomson KR, Venbrux AC, Morgan RA, editors. Image-guided interventions. 2nd ed. Philadelphia: Saunders Elsevier; 2014. p. 491–502.
3. Madoff DC, Denys A, Wallace MJ, Murthy R, Gupta S, Pillsbury EP, et al. Splenic arterial interventions: anatomy, indications, technical considerations, and potential complications. Radiographics. 2005;25 (Suppl 1):S191–211.
4. Stassen NA, Bhullar I, Cheng JD, Crandall ML, Friese RS, Guillamondegui OD, et al. Selective nonoperative management of blunt splenic injury: an Eastern Association for the Surgery of Trauma practice management guideline. J Trauma Acute Care Surg. 2012;73(5 Suppl 4):S294–300.
5. Imbrogno BF, Ray CE. Splenic artery embolization in blunt trauma. Semin Interv Radiol. 2012;29(2):147–9.
6. Angle JF, Siddiqi NH, Wallace MJ, Kundu S, Stokes L, Wojak JC, et al. Quality improvement guidelines for percutaneous transcatheter embolization: Society of Interventional Radiology Standards of Practice Committee. J Vasc Interv Radiol. 2010;21 (10):1479–86.
7. Venkatesan AM, Kundu S, Sacks D, Wallace MJ, Wojak JC, Rose SC, et al. Practice guidelines for adult antibiotic prophylaxis during vascular and interventional radiology procedures. J Vasc Interv Radiol. 2010;21(11):1611–30.
8. Taslakian B, Sebaaly MG, Al-Kutoubi A. Patient evaluation and preparation in vascular and interventional radiology: what every interventional radiologist should know (part 1: patient assessment and laboratory tests). Cardiovasc Intervent Radiol. 2016;39(3):325–33.
9. Taslakian B, Sebaaly MG, Al-Kutoubi A. Patient evaluation and preparation in vascular and interventional radiology: what every interventional radiologist should know (part 2: patient preparation and medications). Cardiovasc Intervent Radiol. 2016;39(4):489–99. doi: 10.1007/s00270-015-1239-4. [Epub 2015 Nov 25].

Embolization of Visceral Aneurysms and Pseudoaneurysms

95

Bedros Taslakian and Sela Batouzian

INTRODUCTION

False aneurysms, also known as pseudoaneurysms, of the visceral arteries are vascular abnormalities that represent focus of contained hemorrhage due to a disruption in arterial wall continuity. False aneurysms can be iatrogenic or posttraumatic in origin or secondary to arterial wall damage from periarterial infectious or inflammatory processes such as pancreatitis, in addition to other causes. Pseudoaneurysms always require treatment regardless of their size, because of the high likelihood of rupture with subsequent acute gastrointestinal, peritoneal, or retroperitoneal hemorrhage. The risk of rupture of true aneurysms, however, is lower and management is based on the size, symptoms, rate of growth, and vascular territory.

COMMON INDICATIONS [1–4]

- Pseudoaneurysms, regardless of the size or associated symptoms
- True aneurysms in pregnant women, or liver transplant recipients regardless of the size or associated symptoms
- True aneurysms measuring 2.0–2.5 cm in diameter or larger in nonpregnant women of childbearing age
- Symptomatic visceral true aneurysms, causing ischemic complications, hemorrhage, or renovascular hypertension
- Visceral true aneurysms increasing in size on follow-up imaging studies
- Splenic artery aneurysm in patients with portal hypertension
- Splenic artery aneurysm measuring 2.5 cm or larger

COMMON CONTRAINDICATIONS

Contraindications of angiography and arterial access (see Chap. 75).

Specific procedure-related contraindications:
- Infection within the target vascular structure or bacteremia
- Solitary kidney *(renal artery aneurysms)*
- Ruptured aneurysm or pseudoaneurysm in hemodynamically unstable patients not responding to fluid resuscitation

B. Taslakian (✉)
Department of Radiology, New York University Langone Medical Center, 660 First Ave, New York, NY 10016, USA
e-mail: btaslakian@gmail.com

S. Batouzian
Coronary Care Unit (CCU), Clemenceau Medical Center (CMC), Beirut, Lebanon
e-mail: sela.batouzian1@gmail.com

B. Taslakian et al. (eds.), *Procedural Dictations in Image-Guided Intervention*,
DOI 10.1007/978-3-319-40845-3_95

POSSIBLE COMPLICATIONS [1–4]

General (angiography-related) complications:

- Hemorrhage *(puncture-site hematoma, retroperitoneal hematoma if "high" puncture above inguinal ligament)*
- Pseudoaneurysm *(superficial femoral artery "low" puncture)*
- Arteriovenous fistula *(puncture-site artery)*
- Thrombosis of the femoral artery
- Distal embolization
- Contrast-induced allergic reaction
- Contrast-induced nephropathy
- Arterial perforation or dissection
- Catheter or guidewire breakage
- Limb amputation *(rare)*
- Risks related to any minimally invasive procedure performed under conscious sedation *(e.g., allergy to medications)*

Embolization (procedure-specific) related complications:

- Aneurysm perforation
- Nonselective embolization causing target organ infarction
- Nontarget organ embolization *(e.g., pancreatitis, cholecystitis, gastric wall necrosis)*
- Postembolization syndrome *(fever, nausea, pain)*
- Abscess formation
- Rupture after successful embolization
- Reperfusion after embolization

PREPROCEDURAL ASSESSMENT AND PLANNING [5–7]

- History, indications, and physical examination *(Appendix 1* in Chap. 149*)*. Document indications of the procedure, lower or upper extremity pulses, and vital signs.
- Evaluation of diagnostic imaging studies to determine the relevant vascular anatomy
- Periprocedural management of coagulation status *(Appendices 2* in Chap. 150 *and 3* in Chap. 151*)*
- Antibiotic prophylaxis: Recommended if there is high likelihood of causing organ infarction [5] *(Appendices 4* in Chap. 152 *and 5* in Chap. 153*)*
- Imaging modality for guidance: Fluoroscopy; combined with ultrasound for arterial puncture
- Positioning: Supine
- Arterial access: Common femoral artery *(preferred)*, left brachial artery, left axillary artery

PROCEDURE NOTE

Procedure: Catheter-directed embolization of [name the artery] aneurysm/pseudoaneurysm
Staff: [_]
Fellow: [_]
Resident: [_]
Clinical History and Indications: Describe history and list indications
Allergies: None known/Allergic to [specify/type of allergy]
Anesthesia: Local anesthesia/Conscious sedation/General anesthesia
Medications: List any relevant medications used
Contrast Material: (_) mL of [type] contrast material was used for intra-arterial injection
Field: Sterile
Procedure classification: Clean
Position: Supine
Monitoring: Intravenous access line was secured and vital signs were continuously monitored by nursing staff/anesthesia team throughout the procedure
Total fluoroscopy time: (_) minutes
Cumulative radiation dose: (_) mGy

Description of Procedure: *(front- door and back- door "sandwich" embolization):*
The risks, benefits, alternatives, and procedure itself were explained to the patient/patient's Power of Attorney/patient's legal guardian, and informed written/verbal consent was obtained. Time out was performed to confirm the correct patient, procedure, and site. The site of the procedure was identified and marked.

The skin of both groins were shaved, prepped, and draped in the usual sterile fashion. The right/left common femoral artery as well as the inguinal ligament were located by palpation/ ultrasound and marked. The site of arterial puncture was determined using combined information from palpation, ultrasound, and fluoroscopy over the middle of the medial third of the femoral head. Local anesthesia was administered. Common femoral artery access was obtained using (_)-gauge [type] needle and the Seldinger technique under direct ultrasound visualization/ by palpation. Once good pulsatile arterial flow was detected, a (_)-inch [type] guidewire was advanced through the needle into the aorta under direct fluoroscopic visualization and a (_)-French vascular sheath was placed.

Heparinized saline infusion was started into the femoral arterial sheath. Subsequently, a (_)-French, (_) cm-long [type] catheter was advanced into the abdominal aorta over a (_)-inch [hydrophilic/type] guidewire under direct fluoroscopic visualization and the [name the artery] artery was selectively catheterized. Digital subtraction angiography was performed by injecting (_) mL of contrast. Following this, the catheter was advanced into the [name artery/arterial branch] and angiography was performed. Embolization of the pseudoaneurysm/aneurysm was performed by occluding the distal outflow first and then the proximal inflow/feeding arteries. The distal outflow [name the artery/arterial branch] artery was canalized beyond the pseudoaneurysm/aneurysm neck using a (_)-French [type] catheter which was advanced over a (_)-inch [type] guidewire and was embolized by deploying (number) [type] detachable coils [(_) cm length/(_) mm diameter]/(_) mm/Amplatzer plug. Complete occlusion of the outflow vessel was documented by performing angiography and the catheter was withdrawn and placed proximal to the pseudoaneurysm/aneurysm neck. The inflow artery was embolized by deploying (number) [type] detachable coils [(_) cm length/(_) mm diameter]/(_) mm/Amplatzer plug. Completion angiography was performed confirming adequate occlusion of the aneurysm and feeding arteries, and absence of contrast extravasation.

Following the procedure the right/left femoral artery sheath was removed and adequate hemostasis was achieved by compression for (_) minutes/using [type] vascular closure device. The femoral pulses were checked following the procedure and were [comparable to the pre-procedure pulses/specify if otherwise needed]. The patient was transferred to the floor/recovery room/ICU for close monitoring following the procedure in a stable condition. Staff was present for the entire procedure.

Description of Procedure: *(placement of covered stent graft across the neck of the aneurysm):* The risks, benefits, alternatives, and procedure itself were explained to the patient/patient's Power of Attorney/patient's legal guardian, and informed written/verbal consent was obtained. Time out was performed to confirm the correct patient, procedure, and site. The site of the procedure was identified and marked.

The skin of both groins were shaved, prepped, and draped in the usual sterile fashion. The right/left common femoral artery as well as the inguinal ligament were located by palpation/ ultrasound and marked. The site of arterial puncture was determined using combined information from palpation, ultrasound, and fluoroscopy over the middle of the medial third of the femoral head. Local anesthesia was administered. Common femoral artery access was obtained using a (_)-gauge [type] needle and the Seldinger technique under direct ultrasound visualization/ by palpation. Once good pulsatile arterial flow was detected, a (_)-inch [type] guidewire was advanced through the needle into the aorta under direct fluoroscopic visualization and a (_)-French vascular sheath was placed.

Heparinized saline infusion was started into the femoral arterial sheath. Subsequently, a (_)-French, (_) cm-long [type] catheter was advanced into the abdominal aorta over a (_)-inch [hydrophilic/type] guidewire under direct fluoroscopic visualization and the [name the artery] artery was selectively catheterized. Digital subtraction angiography was performed by injecting (_) mL of contrast. Following this, the catheter was advanced into the [name artery/ arterial branch] over the guidewire and angiography was performed. After identifying the pseudoaneurysm neck and side branch arteries, the catheter was exchanged over the guidewire for a stent delivery device and a (_) mm long, (_) mm diameter [type] covered stent was deployed across the neck of the pseudoaneurysm/aneurysm, excluding it while maintaining distal perfusion. Completion angiography was performed confirming complete exclusion of the aneurysm/pseudoaneurysm, patency of the artery, and absence of contrast extravasation.

Following the procedure the right/left femoral artery sheath was removed and adequate hemostasis was achieved by compression for (_) minutes/using [type] vascular closure device. The lower extremity pulses were checked following the procedure and were [comparable to the pre-procedure pulses/specify if otherwise needed]. The patient was transferred to the floor/recovery room for close monitoring following the procedure in a stable condition. Staff was present for the entire procedure.

Description of Procedure: *(stent-assisted coil placement- using uncovered stent across aneurysmal neck):*
The risks, benefits, alternatives, and procedure itself were explained to the patient/patient's Power of Attorney/patient's legal guardian, and informed written/verbal consent was obtained. Time out was performed to confirm the correct patient, procedure, and site. The site of the procedure was identified and marked.

The skin of both groins were shaved, prepped, and draped in the usual sterile fashion. The right/left common femoral artery as well as the inguinal ligament were located by palpation/ultrasound and marked. The site of arterial puncture was determined using combined information from palpation, ultrasound, and fluoroscopy over the middle of the medial third of the femoral head. Local anesthesia was administered. Common femoral artery access was obtained using a (_)-gauge [type] needle and the Seldinger technique under direct ultrasound visualization/by palpation. Once good pulsatile arterial flow was detected, a (_)-inch [type] guidewire was advanced through the needle into the aorta under direct fluoroscopic visualization and a (_)-French vascular sheath was placed.

Heparinized saline infusion was started into the femoral arterial sheath. Subsequently, a (_)-French, (_) cm-long [type] catheter was advanced into the abdominal aorta over a (_)-inch [hydrophilic/type] guidewire under direct fluoroscopic visualization and the [name the artery] artery was selectively catheterized. Digital subtraction angiography was performed by injecting (_) mL of contrast. Following this, the catheter was advanced into the [name artery/arterial branch] over the guidewire and angiography was performed. After identifying the pseudoaneurysm neck and side branch arteries, the catheter was exchanged for a stent delivery device and a (_) mm long, (_) mm diameter [type] uncovered stent was deployed across the neck of the pseudoaneurysm/aneurysm. Then, a (_)-French [type] coaxial microcatheter was advanced into the previously inserted catheter and its tip was positioned inside the pseudoaneurysm/aneurysm sac which was packed through the stent struts with (number) [type] detachable coils [(_) cm length/(_) mm diameter]. Completion angiography was performed confirming complete exclusion of the aneurysm/pseudoaneurysm, patency of the artery, and absence of contrast extravasation.

Following the procedure the right/left femoral artery sheath was removed and adequate hemostasis was achieved by compression for (_) minutes/using [type] vascular closure device. The lower extremity pulses were checked following the procedure and were [comparable to the pre-procedure pulses/specify if otherwise needed]. The patient was transferred to the floor/recovery room/ICU for close monitoring following the procedure in a stable condition. Staff was present for the entire procedure.

Intra-Procedure Findings: List all relevant findings.

Immediate Complications: None encountered during or directly after the procedure. List complications if any.

Post-Procedure Plan [1–3]: *Standard post-angiogram management plan:*

- Keep patient complete bed rest with the right/left leg extended for 6 h *[adjust depending on the puncture site]*.
- Check the right/left groin/[specify the puncture site if different] for any bleeding or hematoma formation every 15 min for 1 h, then every 30 min for 1 h, then every hour for 4 h; inform interventional radiology team if any signs of bleeding are observed *[adjust depending on the puncture site]*.
- Check and document lower extremity pulses every 30 min for 2 h then every 1 h for 4 h *[adjust depending on the puncture site]*.
- Monitor vital signs every 15 min for 1 h, then every 30 min for 4 h; notify interventional radiology team if systolic blood pressure <95 mmHg, or heart rate >110 beats/min.
- Resume diet and previous orders as needed and if otherwise not contraindicated.
- Continue adequate intravenous hydration and monitor fluid (intake–output) status.
- Check complete blood count and creatinine on the day following the procedure or as clinically indicated.
- Perform regular neurological examination when the procedure includes manipulation in the ascending thoracic aorta, aortic arch or brachiocephalic arteries.

Procedure-specific management plan:

- Perform cross-sectional imaging to assess aneurysmal sac perfusion and its size as well as the organ perfusion prior to discharge and at 1, 3, and 6 months after the procedure.
- Manage postembolization syndrome conservatively using appropriate antiemetic and analgesic medication and adequately hydrate the patient.
- Follow-up physical examination and laboratory studies, and hematological assessment at 2 and 4 weeks.

Impression:

- Catheter-directed embolization of [name] artery aneurysm/pseudoaneurysm/stent grafting of [name] artery, as described above.
- The patient tolerated the procedure well and left the interventional unit in stable condition.
- The patient was unstable and the procedure was canceled/terminated prematurely.
- List any other relevant or important information/finding.

References

1. Kos S, Martin ML, Machan L. Visceral aneurysms. In: Kandarpa K, Machan L, editors. Handbook of interventional radiologic procedures. 4th ed. Philadelphia: Lippincott Williams & Wilkins; 2011. p. 239–45.
2. Jackson JE. Management of visceral aneurysms. In: Mauro MA, Murphy KPJ, Thomson KR, Venbrux AC, Morgan RA, editors. Image-guided interventions. 2nd ed. Philadelphia: Saunders Elsevier; 2014. p. 508–15.
3. Chadha M1, Ahuja C. Visceral artery aneurysms: diagnosis and percutaneous management. Semin Intervent Radiol. 2009;26(3):196–206.
4. Madoff DC, Denys A, Wallace MJ, Murthy R, Gupta S, Pillsbury EP, et al. Splenic arterial interventions: anatomy, indications, technical considerations, and potential complications. Radiographics. 2005;25 (Suppl 1):S191–211.
5. Venkatesan AM, Kundu S, Sacks D, Wallace MJ, Wojak JC, Rose SC, et al. Practice guidelines for adult antibiotic prophylaxis during vascular and interventional radiology procedures. J Vasc Interv Radiol. 2010;21(11):1611–30.
6. Taslakian B, Sebaaly MG, Al-Kutoubi A. Patient evaluation and preparation in vascular and interventional radiology: what every interventional radiologist should know (part 1: patient assessment and laboratory tests). Cardiovasc Intervent Radiol. 2016;39 (3):325–33.
7. Taslakian B, Sebaaly MG, Al-Kutoubi A. Patient evaluation and preparation in vascular and interventional radiology: what every interventional radiologist should know (part 2: patient preparation and medications). Cardiovasc Intervent Radiol. 2016;39(4):489–99. doi: 10.1007/s00270-015-1239-4. [Epub 2015 Nov 25].

Thrombolysis for Management of Acute Mesenteric Ischemia

96

Maen Aboul Hosn

INTRODUCTION

Acute mesenteric ischemia is a life-threatening condition characterized by acute interruption of the major blood vessels supplying the bowel. The superior mesenteric artery is the mesenteric vessel most commonly involved. Early diagnosis and intervention is key before bowel necrosis ensues. The treatment approach depends on the underlying etiology *(mesenteric arterial embolism/thrombosis, mesenteric vein thrombosis)* and it usually involves open exploration and revascularization especially when bowel compromise is suspected. Catheter-directed thrombolysis is utilized in cases of distal mesenteric embolization without clinical evidence of bowel necrosis or peritonitis.

COMMON INDICATIONS [1–4]

- Acute embolic mesenteric ischemia without peritonitis
- Onset of symptoms <8 h

M. Aboul Hosn (✉)
Department of Vascular Surgery, University of Iowa Hospitals and Clinics, 200 Hawkins Dr, Iowa City, IA 52242, USA
e-mail: maen-aboulhosn@uiowa.edu

COMMON CONTRAINDICATIONS [1–3]

- Peritonitis
- Bowel necrosis
- Active internal bleeding
- Coagulopathy
- Recent cerebrovascular event
- Neurosurgical intervention within 3 months
- Major trauma
- Organ biopsy

POSSIBLE COMPLICATIONS [1, 2]

General (angiography-related) complications:
- Hemorrhage *(puncture-site hematoma, retroperitoneal hematoma if "high" puncture above inguinal ligament)*
- Pseudoaneurysm *(superficial femoral artery "low" puncture)*
- Arteriovenous fistula *(puncture-site artery)*
- Thrombosis of the femoral artery
- Distal embolization
- Contrast-induced allergic reaction
- Contrast-induced nephropathy
- Arterial perforation or dissection
- Catheter or guidewire breakage
- Limb amputation *(rare)*
- Risks related to any minimally invasive procedure performed under conscious sedation *(e.g., allergy to medications)*

B. Taslakian et al. (eds.), *Procedural Dictations in Image-Guided Intervention*,
DOI 10.1007/978-3-319-40845-3_96

Thrombolysis (procedure-specific) related complications:

- Worsening bowel ischemia
- Intracranial hemorrhage
- Internal hemorrhage

PREPROCEDURAL ASSESSMENT AND PLANNING [5, 6]

- History, indications, and physical examination *(Appendix 1* in Chap. 149*)*. Document indications of the procedure and vital signs. Rule out any contraindications to lytic therapy
- Evaluation of diagnostic imaging studies to determine the relevant vascular anatomy and assess the access site
- Periprocedural management of coagulation status *(Appendices 2* in Chap. 150 *and 3* in Chap. 151*)*
- Antibiotic prophylaxis: Not routinely recommended *(Appendices 4* in Chap. 152 *and 5* in Chap. 153*)*
- Imaging modality for guidance: Fluoroscopy; combined with ultrasound for arterial puncture
- Positioning: Supine

PROCEDURE NOTE

Procedure: Catheter-directed thrombolysis for acute occlusion of superior mesenteric artery.
Staff: [_]
Fellow: [_]
Resident: [_]
Clinical Information: Describe history and list indications
Allergies: No known drug allergy/Allergic to (specify)
Anesthesia: Local anesthesia/Monitored conscious sedation
Medications: List any relevant medications used (sedation, heparin, thrombolytic agent)
Contrast Material: (_) mL of [type] contrast material was used for angiography
Field: Sterile
Procedure Classification: Clean
Position: Supine
Monitoring: Intravenous access was secured and vitals were continuously monitored by nursing staff/anesthesia team throughout the procedure
Total fluoroscopy time: (_) minutes
Cumulative radiation dose: (_) mGy

Description of Procedure:
The risks, benefits, alternatives, and the procedure itself were explained to the patient/patient's Power of Attorney/legal guardian, and informed written consent was obtained. The site of the procedure was identified and marked. Time out was performed to confirm the correct patient, procedure, and site.

Intravenous unfractionated heparin was started and continued throughout the procedure. The groin area was prepped and draped in the usual sterile manner. After infiltrating the skin with 1 % Lidocaine, and using ultrasound guidance, the right/left common femoral artery was accessed retrogradely with a micropuncture kit and the position of the microwire was confirmed by fluoroscopy. A small nick in the skin was done using a 11 blade and the microsheath was exchanged with a (_)-French sheath over an exchange wire. A (_)-inch glidewire was advanced into the abdominal aorta. A (_)-French pigtail catheter/Omni flush catheter was advanced over the wire to the abdominal aorta and angiographic runs were performed delineating the flow to the celiac artery, superior mesenteric artery, and both renal arteries. Next, the short sheath was exchanged with a long (_)-French Flexor/Ansel/Arrow Flex sheath and its tip was placed in proximity to the superior mesenteric artery takeoff. Using lateral projections, a (_)-French Cobra/SOS/Berenstein catheter was used to maneuver the glidewire into the superior mesenteric artery distally and the catheter was advanced over it. Selective mesenteric angiography was performed confirming the presence and location of the mesenteric occlusion/clot. The glidewire was passed beyond the level of the occlusion and was then exchanged with a (_)-inch Bentson wire/stiff glidewire/Amplatz wire. The long sheath was then engaged at the orifice of the superior mesenteric artery. Next, a (_)-French multi-sidehole catheter was advanced proximal to/across the area of occlusion for delivery of the lytic solution. An initial bolus of (5–10) mg of rtPA was administered into the clot and then an infusion of (0.5–1.5) mg/hour was started. The sheath was secured to the skin with a 3-0 Nylon suture for a planned repeat angiogram in 24 h and a dry dressing was applied over the catheter exit site. Staff was present for the entire procedure.

Intra-Procedure Findings: List all relevant radiologic findings.

Immediate Complications: None encountered during or directly after the procedure. List the complications if any.

Post-Procedure Plan [1–3]**:**

- Patient observation for 24 h in a monitored unit.
- Keep patient complete bed rest with the right/left leg extended.
- Check the right/left groin for any bleeding or hematoma formation every 15 min for 1 h, then every 30 min.
- Check and document lower extremity pulses every 30 min for 2 h then every 1 h.
- Continuous vital signs monitoring; notify interventional radiology team if systolic blood pressure <95 mmHg, or heart rate >110 beats/min.
- Continue adequate intravenous hydration and monitor fluid (intake–output) status.
- Perform regular neurological examination every hour and inform interventional radiology team if any signs of neurological deficit develop.
- Check for increasing abdominal pain and signs of bleeding.
- Serial fibrinogen, D-dimer, and lactic acid levels.
- Repeat angiogram in 24 h.

Impression:

- Catheter-directed thrombolysis for acute occlusion of superior mesenteric artery as described above.
- The patient tolerated the procedure well and left the interventional unit in a stable condition.
- The patient was unstable and the procedure was canceled/terminated prematurely.
- List any other relevant or important information/finding.

References

1. Jia Z, Jiang G, Tian F, Zhao J, Li S, Wang K, et al. Early endovascular treatment of superior mesenteric occlusion secondary to thromboemboli. Eur J Vasc Endovasc Surg. 2014;47(2):196–203.
2. Acosta S, Björck M. Modern treatment of acute mesenteric ischaemia. Br J Surg. 2014;101(1):e100–8.
3. Heiss P, Loewenhardt B, Manke C, Hellinger A, Dietl KH, Schlitt HJ, et al. Primary percutaneous aspiration and thrombolysis for the treatment of acute embolic superior mesenteric artery occlusion. Eur Radiol. 2010;20(12):2948–58.
4. Schoots IG, Levi MM, Reekers JA, Lameris JS, van Gulik TM. Thrombolytic therapy for acute superior mesenteric artery occlusion. J Vasc Interv Radiol. 2005;16(3):317–29.
5. Taslakian B, Sebaaly MG, Al-Kutoubi A. Patient evaluation and preparation in vascular and interventional radiology: what every interventional radiologist should know (part 1: patient assessment and laboratory tests). Cardiovasc Intervent Radiol. 2016;39(3): 325–33.
6. Taslakian B, Sebaaly MG, Al-Kutoubi A. Patient evaluation and preparation in vascular and interventional radiology: what every interventional radiologist should know (part 2: patient preparation and medications). Cardiovasc Intervent Radiol. 2016;39(4): 489–99. doi: 10.1007/s00270-015-1239-4. [Epub 2015 Nov 25].

Part XV

Vascular Interventional Procedures: Renal Vascular System

Introduction by Aghiad Al-Kutoubi, Section Reviewer

Interventional radiologists play a pivotal role in the prompt diagnosis and percutaneous treatment of many renal vascular abnormalities in native or transplanted kidneys. These minimally invasive procedures can either obviate open surgery or stabilize the patient's condition prior to open surgical reintervention.

Recent data have suggested that renal artery angioplasty and stenting are not as effective in the management of hypertension and preservation of renal function; however, the procedure is still required in cases of severe atherosclerotic stenosis as well as in other cases of renal vascular hypertension in the younger age group and in the context of renal transplantation. As an adjunct to treatment of complex thoraco-abdominal aneurysms with branching devices, renal artery stenting requires advanced skills and experience.

Intervention on the renal arteries in the context of aneurysms and trauma also requires pre-planning preferably with cross-sectional angiography to overcome the complex anatomical branching patterns and minimize contrast load.

Renal denervation was initially promising in the treatment of essential hypertension but more careful evaluation is probably required before this technique becomes established in clinical practice.

This section provides a comprehensive list of procedural reports that covers the vast majority of the currently performed procedures in the renal vascular system with up-to-date explanatory notes, synopsis of the indications and contraindications, and potential complications in an organized and practical format.

Section Chapters

Catheter-Directed Embolization of Renal Artery in Nontraumatized Patients

97

Mikhael Georges Sebaaly

INTRODUCTION

Renal artery embolization was introduced more than 30 years ago. The use of renal artery embolization in nontraumatized patients has decreased. But, there remain certain conditions where selective or total renal artery embolization is the mainstay of care.

COMMON INDICATIONS [1–6]

- Arteriocalyceal fistula
- Arteriovenous fistulas in patients with persistent gross hematuria, hemodynamic instability or deterioration of renal function and in patients with high-flow fistulas
- Inoperable renal cell carcinoma with hematuria or paraneoplastic symptoms *(paraneoplastic hypocalcemia)*
- Inoperable renal cell carcinoma with no symptoms to reduce tumor burden, used with immune-stimulating therapy
- Tumor with extensive venous involvement
- In Jehovah's witnesses to decrease the amount of blood loss intraoperatively
- Patient with single kidney containing tumor
- Renal angiomyolipoma ≥ 4 cm in diameter
- Prior to radiofrequency ablation of well-defined peripheral malignant tumor
- Ruptured bleeding benign tumors in cases of pregnancy
- Massive protein loss secondary to end-stage renal disease
- Intractable hypertension in end-stage renal disease
- Transplanted kidney with graft intolerance syndrome as an alternative to surgical removal
- Persistent urinary leakage in failing kidneys
- Peripheral renal artery aneurysm *(size > 20 mm in men and postmenopausal women, any size in women of child-bearing age and patients with severe hypertension)*
- Central renal artery aneurysm not amenable to stent graft placement

COMMON CONTRAINDICATIONS

Absolute contraindications:

- Acute infection

Relative contraindications:

- Past history of allergy to intravenous contrast media *(consider CO_2)*
- Uncorrected coagulopathy
- Single kidney

M.G. Sebaaly (✉)
Department of Diagnostic Radiology, American University of Beirut Medical Center (AUBMC), Riad El-Solh, 1107 2020, Beirut, Lebanon
e-mail: ms246@aub.edu.lb

B. Taslakian et al. (eds.), *Procedural Dictations in Image-Guided Intervention*,
DOI 10.1007/978-3-319-40845-3_97

POSSIBLE COMPLICATIONS [6, 7]

General (angiography-related) complications:

- Hemorrhage *(puncture-site hematoma, retroperitoneal hematoma if "high" puncture above inguinal ligament)*
- Pseudoaneurysm *(superficial femoral artery "low" puncture)*
- Arteriovenous fistula *(puncture-site artery)*
- Thrombosis of the femoral artery
- Distal embolization
- Contrast-induced allergic reaction
- Contrast-induced nephropathy
- Arterial perforation or dissection
- Catheter or guidewire breakage
- Limb amputation *(rare)*
- Risks related to any minimally invasive procedure performed under conscious sedation *(e.g., allergy to medications)*

Procedure-specific complications:

- Severe hypertension after selective renal artery embolization
- Postembolization syndrome due to necrosis of large masses
- Thromboembolism
- Inadvertent embolization of nontarget tissues
- Hemolysis, acute bronchospasm, pulmonary hypertension, disseminated intravascular coagulation, and fatal cardiovascular collapse in cases of ethanol embolization

PREPROCEDURAL ASSESSMENT AND PLANNING [8–10]

- History, indications, and physical examination *(Appendix 1* in Chap. 149*)*
- Evaluation of diagnostic imaging studies and physiologic tests to determine the relevant vascular anatomy, anatomic relations, physiologic and pathologic conditions
- Periprocedural management of coagulation status *(Appendices 2* in Chap. 150 *and 3* in Chap. 151*)*
- Antibiotic prophylaxis: Recommended, if intent to create infarction or high likelihood of tissue infarction [8] *(Appendices 4* in Chap. 152 *and 5* in Chap. 153*)*
- Imaging modality for guidance: Fluoroscopy; combined with ultrasound for access artery puncture
- Positioning: Supine
- Arterial access: Common femoral artery

PROCEDURE NOTE

Procedure: Catheter-directed embolization of the left/right renal artery
Staff: [_]
Fellow: [_]
Resident: [_]
Clinical Information: Describe history and list indications
Allergies: None known/Allergic to [specify/type of allergy]
Anesthesia: Local anesthesia/Conscious sedation/General anesthesia
Medications: List any relevant medications used (sedation, antibiotics)
Contrast Used: (_) mL of [type] contrast media was used for intra-arterial injection
Field: Sterile
Procedure classification: Clean
Position: Supine
Monitoring: Intravenous access line was secured and vital signs were continuously monitored by nursing staff/anesthesia team throughout the procedure
Total fluoroscopy time: (_) minutes
Cumulative radiation dose: (_) mGy

Description of Procedure:

The risks, benefits, alternatives, and the procedure itself were explained to the patient/patient's Power of Attorney/patient's legal guardian, and informed written consent was obtained. The site of the puncture was identified and marked. Time out was performed to confirm the correct patient, procedure, and site.

The skin of both groins were shaved, prepped, and draped in the usual sterile fashion. The right/left femoral artery as well as the inguinal ligament were located by palpation/ultrasound and marked. The site of arterial puncture was determined using combined information from palpation, ultrasound, and fluoroscopy over the middle of the medial third of the femoral head. Local anesthesia was administered. Femoral artery access was obtained using (_)-gauge [type] needle and the Seldinger technique, double-/single- wall entry under direct ultrasound visualization/by palpation. Once good pulsatile arterial flow was detected, a (_)-inch [type] guidewire was advanced through the needle, up the femoral artery, into the aorta under direct fluoroscopic visualization and a (_)-French vascular sheath was placed.

Subsequently, a (_)-French, (_) cm-long [type] catheter was advanced into the abdominal aorta over a (_)-inch [hydrophilic/type] guidewire under direct fluoroscopic visualization and the right/left renal artery was selectively catheterized. The catheter was then advanced into the right/left renal artery and selective renal angiography was performed by manual injection of (_) mL of contrast demonstrating [specify findings]. A (2.9)-French microcatheter was advanced into the branch supplying the tumor/pseudoaneurysm. Following this, the selected branch was embolized using [specify size and number] coils/small fractions of alcohol was injected over a period of (_) minutes/[specify size and amount in mL] nanometer particles followed by glue./A balloon catheter was advanced and inflated in the main renal artery leading to its obstruction. Then, (_) mL of ethanol/(_) mL Ethibloc mixed with Lipiodol/(_) mL bucrylate mixed with Lipiodol was injected into the renal artery distal to the balloon.

Then, under fluoroscopy renal artery angiography was performed by manual injection of (_) mL of contrast demonstrating [total cessation of flow].

Following the procedure the right/left femoral artery sheath was removed and adequate homeostasis was achieved by (_) minute compression/using [type] vascular closure device. The femoral pulses were checked following the procedure and were [comparable to the pre-procedure pulses/specify if otherwise needed]. The patient was transferred to the floor/recovery room for close monitoring following the procedure in a stable condition. Staff was present and scrubbed for the entire procedure.

Intra-Procedure Findings: List all relevant findings.

Immediate Complications: None encountered during or directly after the procedure. List complications if any.

Post-Procedure Plan:

Standard post-angiogram management plan

- Keep patient complete bed rest with the right/left leg extended for 6 h *[adjust depending on the puncture site]*.
- Check the right/left groin/[specify the puncture site if different] for any bleeding or hematoma formation every 15 min for 1 h, then every 30 min for 1 h, then every hour for 4 h; inform interventional radiology team if any signs of bleeding are observed *[adjust depending on the puncture site]*.
- Check and document lower extremity pulses every 30 min for 2 h then every 1 h for 4 h *[adjust depending on the puncture site]*.
- Monitor vital signs every 15 min for 1 h, then every 30 min for 4 h; notify interventional radiology team if systolic blood pressure <95 mmHg, or heart rate >110 beats/minute.
- Resume diet and previous orders as needed and if otherwise not contraindicated.
- Continue adequate intravenous hydration and monitor fluid (intake–output) status.
- Check complete blood count and creatinine on the day following the procedure or as clinically indicated.
- Perform regular neurological examination when the procedure includes manipulation in the ascending thoracic aorta, aortic arch or brachiocephalic arteries.

Embolization-specific management plan:

- Anti-inflammatory and antiemetic medications.
- Analgesia by for 1 to 2 days using patient controlled analgesia via automated pump system.

Impression:

- Catheter-directed embolization of left/right renal artery/branch, as described above.

- The patient tolerated the procedure well and left the interventional unit in a stable condition.
- The patient was unstable and the procedure was canceled/terminated prematurely.
- List any other relevant or important information/finding.

References

1. Kehagias D, Mourikis D, Kousaris M, Chatziioannou A, Vlahos L. Management of renal angiomyolipoma by selective arterial embolization. Urol Int. 1998;60:113–7.
2. Ishijima H, Ishizaka H, Sakurai M, Ito K, Endo K. Partial renal embolization for pediatric renovascular hypertension secondary to fibromuscular dysplasia. Cardiovasc Intervent Radiol. 1997;20:383–6.
3. Tacke J, Mahnken A, Bücker A, Rohde D, Günther RW. Nephron-sparing percutaneous ablation of a 5 cm renal cell carcinoma by superselective emboliza- tion and percutaneous RF-ablation. Rofo. 2001;173(11):980–3.
4. De Baere T, Lagrange C, Kuoch V, Morice P, Court B, Roche A. Transcatheter ethanol renal ablation in 20 patients with persistent urine leaks: an alternative to surgical nephrectomy. J Urol. 2000;164:1148–52.
5. Frey GT, Sella DM, Atwell TD. Image-Guided Renal Intervention. Radiol Clin North Am. 2015;53(5):1005–19.
6. Muller A, Rouvière O. Renal artery embolization-indications, technical approaches and outcomes. Nat Rev Nephrol. 2015;11(5):288–301.
7. Varma PP, Malik N, Khullar D, Ahmed S, Sakhuja V, Chugh KS. Fatal intracerebral hemorrhage associated with severe hypertension following renal artery embolization. Int J Artif Organs. 1993;16:720–1.
8. Venkatesan AM, Kundu S, Sacks D, Wallace MJ, Wojak JC, Rose SC, et al. Practice guidelines for adult antibiotic prophylaxis during vascular and interventional radiology procedures. J Vasc Interv Radiol. 2010;21(11):1611–30.
9. Taslakian B, Sebaaly MG, Al-Kutoubi A. Patient evaluation and preparation in vascular and interventional radiology: what every interventional radiologist should know (part 1: patient assessment and laboratory tests). Cardiovasc Intervent Radiol. 2016;39(3):325–33.
10. Taslakian B, Sebaaly MG, Al-Kutoubi A. Patient evaluation and preparation in vascular and interventional radiology: what every interventional radiologist should know (part 2: patient preparation and medications). Cardiovasc Intervent Radiol. 2016;39(4):489–99. doi: 10.1007/s00270-015-1239-4. [Epub 2015 Nov 25].

Embolization of Renal Angiomyolipoma

98

Hearns W. Charles

Abbreviations

PEComas	Perivascular epithelioid cell tumors
AML	Angiomyolipoma
TSC	Tuberous sclerosis complex
RCC	Renal cell carcinoma

INTRODUCTION

Renal angiomyolipomas are highly vascular tumors that contain various quantities of disorganized triphasic differentiated cells composed of adipose, smooth muscle, and vascular endothelial cells [1, 2]. They belong to a family of neoplasms called perivascular epithelioid cell tumors (PEComas), which include pulmonary lymphangioleiomyomatosis. PEComas are characterized by the proliferation of unique epithelioid cells distributed around blood vessels [3]. The estimated overall prevalence of angiomyolipoma worldwide is 0.3–3 % [1, 2]. In most cases (80–90 %), angiomyolipoma presents clinically as an isolated condition (i.e., sporadic angiomyolipoma); in the remaining 10–20 % of cases, angiomyolipoma (AML) presents in association with tuberous sclerosis complex (TSC) [2]. TSC is an autosomal dominant disease that leads to the formation of tumors in multiple organs, including brain, lungs, skin, liver, and kidneys [4]. 70–90 % of individuals with TSC have renal AML by adulthood [5–7]. Most cases of sporadic AML are asymptomatic and are discovered incidentally during radiographic procedures [2, 8]. This may be prompted by radiographic investigation of clinical evidence of internal hemorrhage of unknown origin. Surveillance imaging and embolization have led to a significant reduction in morbidity and mortality in patients with TSC [9]. In some TSC cases, large number of infiltrative AMLs can compromise normal kidney parenchyma, leading to loss of renal function. However, the long-term effects of such tumors on renal function can be quite variable, with some patients having progression to end-stage renal disease. Others, with low to moderate AML tumor burden, have normal or variably impaired estimated glomerular filtration rate.

Although AMLs are typically benign, epithelioid AMLs can display varying degrees of

H.W. Charles (✉)
Department of Radiology, Division of Interventional Radiology, New York University Langone Medical Center, 660 First Avenue, 7th Floor, New York, NY 10016, USA
e-mail: hearns.charles@nyumc.org

B. Taslakian et al. (eds.), *Procedural Dictations in Image-Guided Intervention*,
DOI 10.1007/978-3-319-40845-3_98

epithelial atypia and can behave aggressively, recurring and metastasizing to distant sites in patients with TSC, leading to their possible misclassification as renal cell carcinoma (RCC) [10–12].

When an AML reaches a certain size, it has an increased risk of spontaneous bleeding [13]. This is also affected by intralesional presence of microaneurysms [14]. For this reason, medical, interventional, and surgical treatment modalities represent the different methods of management.

COMMON INDICATIONS [15]

Absolute Indications:
- AML size ≥ 4 cm
- Clinical evidence of bleeding and any size AML

Relative Indications:
- AML size >3 cm with documented growth

COMMON CONTRAINDICATIONS

Absolute contraindications:
- Active infection

Relative contraindications:
- Coagulopathy
- History of allergic reaction to iodinated contrast
- Significant renal insufficiency

POSSIBLE COMPLICATIONS

General (angiography-related) complications:
- Hemorrhage *(puncture-site hematoma, retroperitoneal hematoma if "high" puncture above inguinal ligament)*
- Pseudoaneurysm *(superficial femoral artery "low" puncture)*
- Arteriovenous fistula *(puncture-site artery)*
- Thrombosis of the femoral artery
- Distal embolization
- Contrast-induced allergic reaction
- Contrast-induced nephropathy
- Arterial perforation, dissection, and pseudoaneurysm formation
- Catheter or guidewire breakage
- Limb amputation *(rare)*
- Risks related to any minimally invasive procedure performed under conscious sedation *(e.g., allergy to medications)*

Procedure-specific complications:
- Nontarget embolization; renal parenchymal infarction
- Postembolization renal infection/abscess formation

PREPROCEDURAL ASSESSMENT AND PLANNING

- History and physical examination *(assess need for anesthesia)*
- Evaluation of diagnostic imaging studies (CT or MRI) to determine: number and size of AML(s); unilateral or bilateral renal tumoral disease; relevant vascular anatomy and presence of normal variants. This is for procedure and embolization planning and to avoid complications and limit procedure time.
- Periprocedural management of coagulation status *(Appendices 2* in Chap. 150 *and 3* in Chap. 151*)*
- Antibiotic prophylaxis: Recommended because of likelihood of infarction [16] *(Appendices 4* in Chap. 152 *and 5* in Chap. 153*)*
- Imaging modality for guidance: Fluoroscopy
- Positioning: Supine
- Arterial access: Common femoral artery

PROCEDURE NOTE

Procedure: Left/right renal arteriogram and transarterial embolization of left/right renal Angiomyolipoma (AML)
Staff: [_]
Fellow: [_]
Resident: [_]

Clinical Information: Describe history and list indications
Allergies: None known/Allergic to [specify/type of allergy]
Anesthesia: Conscious sedation was administered and physiologic monitoring was carried out throughout the procedure by the radiology nursing staff
Medications: List any relevant medications used
Contrast Material: (_) mL of [type] nonionic contrast material
Field: Sterile
Procedure classification: Clean
Position: Supine
Total fluoroscopy time: (_) minutes
Cumulative radiation dose: (_) mGy

Description of Procedure:
Informed consent was obtained from the patient, following a discussion on the risks, benefits, and alternatives to the procedure.

Sterile technique and fluoroscopic guidance were used to catheterize the right common femoral artery using a (_)-French introducer sheath. Through this, over a (0.035)-in. [type] wire, a (_)-French [type] catheter was advanced and used to catheterize the left/right renal artery with subsequent branch superselection using a (3)-French [type] microcatheter. Angiography was performed showing [specify findings].

Following superselective microcatheterization of the arterial branch supply to the angiomyolipoma, embolization was performed using a (7:5) ratio of (95 %) ethanol: lipiodol solution (total, 1.5 mL). The quaternary arterial branch supply to the aforementioned pseudoaneurysm was embolized using a small amount (0.3 mL) of 1:3 n-BCA: lipiodol suspension.

Postembolization completion angiography was performed.

The catheters were then removed and, contrast injection via the introducer sheath showed a normal appearance of the right external iliac and common femoral arteries. The sheath was removed, with simultaneous deployment of [type] arterial closure device, and ancillary manual compression applied to effect hemostasis. The patient was then transferred to the floor/recovery room in a stable condition. Staff was present during the entire procedure.

Intra-Procedure Findings: List all relevant findings.

Preembolization contrast examination shows:

- Normal caliber and course of the proximal left/right renal artery.
- Large, approximately (_)-cm hypervascular mass extending from left/right renal upper/lower pole with a dominant upper/lower polar tertiary single arterial branch supply consistent with known AML. There is associated arterial steal from the remainder of the kidney. Within this mass, centrally, there is delayed enhancement of a (_) × (_) cm tubular structure consistent with an intralesional aneurysm. On the venous phase, there is opacification of a secondary tubular structure superior to the aforementioned aneurysm measuring (_) × (_) cm, having flow characteristics of a venous varix or malformation. There are additional curvilinear areas of contrast appearing in venous phase medial to pseudoaneurysm with similar flow pattern.
- Left renal vein appears normal.

Postembolization angiogram shows:

- Devascularization of a vast majority of the AML with no flow seen to the pseudoaneurysm or the aforementioned venous structures, and excellent deposition of the embolic agent within the mass and these vascular structures.
- Minimal residual fine vascularity to a small portion of the [specify] aspect of the large mass via otherwise normal small peripheral branches of the [specify]. Normal parenchyma would be sacrificed with embolization at this level at this time. Further embolization was not performed.
- Improved opacification of the normal left/right kidney, including a rim of parenchyma along the [specify] aspect of the AML.
- Wide patency of the renal vein.

Immediate complications: None encountered during or directly after the procedure. List complications if any.

Post-Procedure Plan:

- Keep patient in complete bed rest with the right leg extended for (_) hours.
- Check the (right groin) access site for any bleeding or hematoma formation every 15 min × 4, then every 30 min × 2, then every 1 h × 2.
- Check neurovascular exam: (right groin) access and popliteal, and ankle arterial pulses; every 15 min × 4, then every 30 min × 2, then every 1 h × 2
- Inform interventional radiology team for any access site bleeding or hematoma formation.
- Monitor vital signs every 15 min × 4, then every 30 min × 2, then every 1 h × 2.
- Notify Interventional Radiology team if systolic blood pressure ≥ 130 mmHg or ≤ 90 mmHg; or diastolic BP > 100 mmHg.
- Notify Interventional Radiology team if heart rate ≥ 100 BPM or ≤ 60 BPM, at extension [_]. If not during regular work hours, page beeper number [_].
- Notify physician if patient unable to void 6 h following the procedure.
- Resume diet and previous orders as needed and if not otherwise contraindicated.
- Encourage fluid intake and continue routine monitoring (intake/output) status.
- Pain control as clinically indicated.

Impression:

- Large left/right renal angiomyolipoma, with associated vascular steal from the normal kidney and associated intralesional aneurysm and varices.
- AML embolization using liquid embolic agents, as described above.
- Improved visualization of the normal renal parenchyma following AML embolization.

References

1. Bissler JJ, Kingswood JC. Renal angiomyolipomata. Kidney Int. 2004;66:924–34.
2. Wagner BJ, Wong-You-Cheong JJ, Davis CJ Jr. Adult renal hamartomas. RadioGraphics. 1997;17:155–69.
3. Prasad SR, Sahani DV, Mino-Kenudson M, Narra VR, Humphrey PA, Menias CO, et al. Neoplasms of the perivascular epithelioid cell involving the abdomen and the pelvis: cross-sectional imaging findings. J Comput Assist Tomogr. 2007;31:688–96.
4. Astrinidis A, Henske EP. Tuberous sclerosis complex: linking growth and energy signaling pathways with human disease. Oncogene. 2005;24:7475–81.
5. Ewalt DH, Sheffield E, Sparagana SP, Delgado MR, Roach ES. Renal lesion growth in children with tuberous sclerosis complex. J Urol. 1998;160:141–5.
6. Stillwell TJ, Gomez MR, Kelalis PP. Renal lesions in tuberous sclerosis. J Urol 1987;138:477–481.
7. O'Callaghan FJ, Noakes MJ, Martyn CN, Osborne JP. An epidemiological study of renal pathology in tuberous sclerosis complex. BJU Int. 2004;94:853–7.
8. Koo KC, Kim WT, Ham WS, Lee JS, Ju HJ, Choi YD. Trends of presentation and clinical outcome of treated renal angiomyolipoma. Yonsei Med J. 2010;51:728–34.
9. Shepherd CW, Gomez MR, Lie JT, Crowson CS. Causes of death in patients with tuberous sclerosis. Mayo Clin Proc. 1991;66:792–6.
10. Park HK, Zhang S, Wong MK, Kim HL. Clinical presentation of epithelioid angiomyolipoma. Int J Urol. 2007;14:21–5.
11. Eble JN. Angiomyolipoma of kidney. Semin Diagn Pathol. 1998;15:21–40.
12. Bjornsson J, Short MP, Kwiatkowski DJ, Henske EP. Tuberous sclerosis-associated renal cell carcinoma: clinical, pathological, and genetic features. Am J Pathol. 1996;149:1201–8.
13. Oesterling JE, Fishman EK, Goldman SM, Marshall FF. The management of renal angiomyolipoma. J Urol. 1986;135:1121–4.
14. Yamakado K, Tanaka N, Nakagawa T, Kobayashi S, Yanagawa M, Takeda K. Renal angiomyolipoma: relationships between tumor size, aneurysm formation, and rupture. Radiology. 2002;225:78–82.
15. Rabenou RA, Charles HW. Differentiation of sporadic versus tuberous sclerosis complex-associated angiomyolipoma. AJR. 2015;205:292–301.
16. Venkatesan AM, Kundu S, Sacks D, Wallace MJ, Wojak JC, Rose SC, et al. Practice guidelines for adult antibiotic prophylaxis during vascular and interventional radiology procedures. J Vasc Interv Radiol. 2010;21(11):1611–30.

Management of Acute Renal Ischemia

99

Mikhael Georges Sebaaly

Abbreviations

US	Ultrasound
ACEI	Angiotensin converting enzyme inhibitor
ARB	Angiotensin receptor blocker

INTRODUCTION

Acute renal ischemia is impaired renal perfusion leading to diminished renal excretory function. If the ischemia affects both kidneys or a solitary functioning kidney, the patient may present with acute renal failure. Several factors affect the degree of ischemia, such as gradual occlusion of the renal artery, which leads to formation of collateral perfusion to the kidney, and hence these patients may benefit from delayed revascularization. Endovascular techniques are not used commonly in all acute renal ischemia, but they are beneficial in some cases.

COMMON INDICATIONS [1–4]

- Trauma with renal artery dissection
- Trauma with renal artery avulsion
- Thromboembolic events in the renal artery
- Renal artery atherosclerosis with acute stenosis due to plaque ulceration
- Aortic dissection leading to renal hypoperfusion
- Renal artery occlusion post endovascular intervention
- Critical renal artery stenosis in patients starting on ACEI/ARB

COMMON CONTRAINDICATIONS [5, 6]

Absolute contraindications:

- Hemodynamic instability despite adequate resuscitation, requiring emergent surgical exploration in cases of trauma
- Associated injuries such as bowel perforation, requiring emergent surgical exploration

Relative contraindications (benefits of intervention should be weighed against risks of management):

- Past history of allergy to intravenous contrast media
- Pregnancy

M.G. Sebaaly (✉)
Department of Diagnostic Radiology, American University of Beirut Medical Center (AUBMC), Riad El-Solh, 1107 2020, Beirut, Lebanon
e-mail: ms246@aub.edu.lb

B. Taslakian et al. (eds.), *Procedural Dictations in Image-Guided Intervention*,
DOI 10.1007/978-3-319-40845-3_99

- Significant irreversible ischemic parenchymal damage *(more than 24 h of ischemia)*

POSSIBLE COMPLICATIONS [7]

General (angiography-related) complications:

- Hemorrhage *(puncture-site hematoma, retroperitoneal hematoma if "high" puncture above inguinal ligament)*
- Pseudoaneurysm *(superficial femoral artery "low" puncture)*
- Arteriovenous fistula *(puncture-site artery)*
- Thrombosis of the femoral artery
- Distal embolization
- Contrast-induced allergic reaction
- Contrast-induced nephropathy
- Arterial perforation or dissection
- Catheter or guidewire breakage
- Limb amputation *(rare)*
- Risks related to any minimally invasive procedure performed under conscious sedation *(e.g., allergy to medications)*

Angioplasty (Procedure-specific) complications:

- Residual stenosis
- Dissection related to guidewire manipulation
- Arterial rupture
- Distal atheroembolization
- Emergent nephrectomy or surgical bypass
- Perinephric hematoma

PREPROCEDURAL ASSESSMENT AND PLANNING [8–10]

- History, indications, and physical examination *(Appendix 1* in Chap. 149*)*
- Evaluation of diagnostic imaging studies and physiologic test to determine the relevant vascular anatomy, anatomic relations, physiologic and pathologic conditions
- Periprocedural management of coagulation status *(Appendices 2* in Chap. 150 *and 3* in Chap. 151*)*
- Antibiotic prophylaxis: Not routinely recommended [8] *(Appendices 4* in Chap. 152 *and 5* in Chap. 153*)*
- Imaging modality for guidance: Fluoroscopy
- Positioning: Supine
- Arterial access: Transfemoral/transbrachial route

PROCEDURE NOTE

Procedure: Right/Left renal Artery Angioplasty/stenting and thrombolysis
Staff: [_]
Fellow: [_]
Resident: [_]
Clinical Information: Describe history and list indications
Allergies: None known/Allergic to [specify/type of allergy]
Anesthesia: Local anesthesia/conscious sedation/general anesthesia
Medications: List any relevant medications used
Contrast Used: (_) mL of [type] contrast media was used for angiography
Field: Sterile
Procedure classification: Clean
Position: Supine
Monitoring: Intravenous access line was secured and vital signs were continuously monitored by nursing staff/anesthesia team throughout the procedure.
Total fluoroscopy time: (_) minutes
Cumulative radiation dose: (_) mGy

Description of Procedure:
The risks, benefits, alternatives, and the procedure itself were explained to the patient/patient's Power of Attorney/patient's legal guardian, and informed written/verbal consent was obtained. The site of the puncture was identified and marked. Time out was performed to confirm the correct patient, procedure, and site.

The skin of both groins/left antecubital fossa were shaved, prepped and draped in the usual sterile fashion. The right/left femoral/left brachial artery was located by palpation/ultrasound and marked. The site of arterial puncture was determined using combined information from palpation, ultrasound, and fluoroscopy. Local anesthesia was administered. Femoral/brachial artery access was obtained using a (_)-gauge [type] needle and the Seldinger technique, double-/single-wall entry under direct ultrasound visualization/by palpation. Once good pulsatile arterial flow was detected, a (_)-inch [type] guidewire was advanced through the needle, up the femoral/brachial artery, into the aorta under direct fluoroscopic visualization and a (_)-French vascular sheath was placed.

Subsequently, a (_)-French, (_) cm-long [type] catheter was advanced into the abdominal aorta over a (_)-inch [hydrophilic/type] guidewire under direct fluoroscopic visualization and the right/left renal artery was selectively catheterized. The catheter was then advanced into the renal artery under fluoroscopy and selective renal artery angiography was performed by manual injection of (_) mL of contrast demonstrating [specify findings]. Following this, the catheter was advanced to the level of the obstruction with wire projecting beyond its tip, local thrombolytic agent [specify agent] was injected intra-arterially for [_] hours/transcatheter aspiration thrombectomy using [specify type of device]/the lesion was crossed so that the catheter is aligned along the long axis of the lesion. Then, a [_] mm balloon expandable stent was inflated slowly until it assumed a dumbbell configuration and a [type/size] stent was deployed. Then angiography was repeated by manual injection of (_) mL of contrast demonstrating [specify findings].

Following the procedure the right/left femoral/brachial artery sheath was removed and adequate hemostasis was achieved by (_) minute compression/using [type] vascular closure device.

The lower extremity/radial pulses were checked following the procedure and were [comparable to the pre-procedure pulses/specify if otherwise needed]. The patient was transferred to the floor/recovery room for close monitoring following the procedure in a stable condition. Staff was present and scrubbed for the entire procedure.

Intra-Procedure Findings: List all relevant findings.

Immediate Complications: None encountered during or directly after the procedure. List complications if any.

Post-Procedure Plan:

Standard post-angiogram management plan

- Keep patient complete bed rest with the right/left leg extended for 6 h *[adjust depending on the puncture site]*.
- Check the right/left groin/[specify the puncture site if different] for any bleeding or hematoma formation every 15 min for 1 h, then every 30 min for 1 h, then every hour for 4 h; inform interventional radiology team if any signs of bleeding are observed *[adjust depending on the puncture site]*.
- Check and document lower extremity pulses every 30 min for 2 h then every 1 h for 4 h *[adjust depending on the puncture site]*.
- Monitor vital signs every 15 min for 1 h, then every 30 min for 4 h; notify interventional radiology team if systolic blood pressure <95 mmHg, or heart rate >110 beats/minute.
- Resume diet and previous orders as needed and if otherwise not contraindicated.
- Continue adequate intravenous hydration and monitor fluid (intake–output) status.
- Check complete blood count and creatinine on the day following the procedure or as clinically indicated.
- Perform regular neurological examination when the procedure includes manipulation in the ascending thoracic aorta, aortic arch or brachiocephalic arteries.

Procedure-specific management plan:

- Renal duplex study after 1–2 weeks, then after 6 months, then annually for 3 years.
- Clopidogrel for 3 months, then lifetime 81 mg/325 mg of aspirin per day.
- Perform renal duplex study if there is evidence of decline in renal function or worsening hypertension.
- Resume antihypertensive therapy, ACEI/ARB as first-line.

- Adequate control of diabetes and dyslipidemia.
- Resume lifetime anticoagulation in case of embolic causes *(atrial fibrillation).*

Impression:

- Right/Left renal artery angioplasty/stenting and thrombolysis, as described above.
- The patient tolerated the procedure well and left the interventional unit in a stable condition.
- The procedure was canceled/terminated prematurely.
- List any other relevant or important information/finding.

References

1. Bruce LM, Croce MA, Santaniello JM, Miller PR, Lyden SP, Fabian TC. Blunt renal artery injury: incidence, diagnosis and management. Am Surg. 2001;67:550–4.
2. Gluck G, Croitoru M, Deleanu D, Platon P. Local thrombolytic treatment for renal arterial embolism. Eur Urol. 2000;38:339–43.
3. van de Ven PJ, Kaatee R, Beutler JJ, Beek FJ, Woittiez AJ, Buskens E, et al. Arterial stenting and balloon angioplasty in ostial atherosclerotic renovascular disease: a randomised trial. Lancet. 1999;353:282–6.
4. Rysavá R, Zabka J, Peregrin JH, Tesar V, Merta M, Rychlik I. Acute renal failure due to bilateral renal artery thrombosis associated with primary antiphospholipid syndrome. Nephrol Dial Transplant. 1998;13:2645–7.
5. Cognet F, Garcier JM, Dranssart M, Defraissinette B, Cercueil JP, Ravel A, et al. Percutaneous transluminal renal angioplasty in atheroma with renal failure: long term outcomes in 99 patients. Eur Radiol. 2001;11:2524–30.
6. Muray S, Martín M, Amoedo ML, García C, Jornet AR, Vera M, et al. Rapid decline in renal function reflects reversibility and predicts outcome after angioplasty in renal artery stenosis. Am J Kidney Dis. 2002;39:60–6.
7. Nakayama T, Okaneya T, Kinebuchi Y, Murata Y, Iizuka K. Thrombolytic therapy for traumatic unilateral renal artery thrombosis. Int J Urol. 2006;13:168–70.
8. Venkatesan AM, Kundu S, Sacks D, Wallace MJ, Wojak JC, Rose SC, et al. Practice guidelines for adult antibiotic prophylaxis during vascular and interventional radiology procedures. J Vasc Interv Radiol. 2010;21(11):1611–30.
9. Taslakian B, Sebaaly MG, Al-Kutoubi A. Patient evaluation and preparation in vascular and interventional radiology: what every interventional radiologist should know (part 1: patient assessment and laboratory tests). Cardiovasc Intervent Radiol. 2016;39 (3):325–33.
10. Taslakian B, Sebaaly MG, Al-Kutoubi A. Patient evaluation and preparation in vascular and interventional radiology: what every interventional radiologist should know (part 2: patient preparation and medications). Cardiovasc Intervent Radiol. 2016;39 (4):489–99. doi: 10.1007/s00270-015-1239-4. [Epub 2015 Nov 25].

Renal Arteriography

100

Bedros Taslakian

INTRODUCTION

Diagnostic renal catheter arteriography continues to be the gold standard for the evaluation of many vascular abnormalities, including fibromuscular hyperplasia, hypervascular tumors, arteriovenous malformations, aneurysms, arteriovenous fistulae, and sources of bleeding.

COMMON INDICATIONS [1–3]

- Renovascular hypertension
- Progressive renal insufficiency to evaluate for renovascular occlusive disease
- Penetrating or blunt traumatic renal injury
- Evaluation of primary vascular disorders *(e.g., aneurysms, pseudoaneurysms, vascular malformations, vasculitis, arteriovenous fistulae)*
- Diagnosis and localization of hypervascular tumors in the kidney
- Hematuria of unknown cause
- Postoperative evaluation of transplanted kidney
- Evaluation prior to, during and following selective percutaneous endovascular procedures

COMMON CONTRAINDICATIONS [1–3]

- Hemodynamic instability with multisystem dysfunction
- Uncontrolled severe hypertension and congestive heart failure
- Recent myocardial infarction
- Significant cardiac arrhythmias and electrolyte imbalance
- Uncorrectable bleeding disorders
- Pregnancy
- Past history of allergic reaction to iodinated contrast media or renal dysfunction *(consider alternative contrast agents such as carbon dioxide or gadolinium)*
- Recent imaging of the gastrointestinal tract using positive intraluminal contrast
- Uncooperative patient
- Active bacteremia and sepsis
- Pheochromocytoma
- Active large vessel vasculitis and connective tissue disorders *(increased risk of puncture site complications, vascular injury, and thrombosis)*
- Local conditions at the vascular access site such as infection, preexisting pseudoaneurysm, hematoma, inguinal hernia, fresh incision, and recent injuries *(an alternative access site should be selected)*

B. Taslakian (✉)
Department of Radiology, New York University Langone Medical Center, 660 First Ave, New York, NY 10016, USA
e-mail: btaslakian@gmail.com

B. Taslakian et al. (eds.), *Procedural Dictations in Image-Guided Intervention*,
DOI 10.1007/978-3-319-40845-3_100

POSSIBLE COMPLICATIONS [1–4]

- Access site complications *(e.g., hematoma, retroperitoneal hemorrhage, pseudoaneurysm, arteriovenous fistula, thrombosis)*
- Nausea, vomiting, and vasovagal syncope
- Fever and chills
- Contrast-induced allergic reaction
- Contrast-induced nephropathy
- Arterial perforation or dissection
- Catheter or guidewire breakage
- Limb amputation *(rare)*
- Mortality

PREPROCEDURAL ASSESSMENT AND PLANNING [2, 3, 5–7]

- History, indications, and physical examination *(Appendix 1* in Chap. 149*)*. Document indications of the procedure, lower or upper extremity pulses, and vital signs
- Evaluation of diagnostic imaging studies to determine the relevant vascular anatomy and assess the access vessels
- Periprocedural management of coagulation status *(Appendices 2* in Chap. 150 *and 3* in Chap. 151*)*
- Antibiotic prophylaxis: Not routinely recommended [2, 3, 5] *(Appendices 4* in Chap. 152 *and 5* in Chap. 153*)*
- Imaging modality for guidance: Fluoroscopy; combined with ultrasound for arterial puncture
- Positioning: Supine
- Arterial access: Common femoral artery *(preferred)*, left brachial artery, left axillary artery [1, 4]
- Patient preparation:
  - Start intravenous fluids the night before angiography in order to ensure adequate hydration, combined with effective monitoring of fluid status
  - Insert a urinary catheter or ask the patient to void before the procedure depending on the estimated time of the procedure
  - Considerations for patients with specific diseases or conditions, patients on specific medications, or patients with history of multiple comorbidities: consult with the referring clinician, and obtain subspecialty consultation as needed

PROCEDURE NOTE

Procedure: Catheter-directed diagnostic left/right/bilateral renal angiography
Staff: [_]
Fellow: [_]
Resident: [_]
Clinical History and Indications: Describe history and list indications
Allergies: None known/Allergic to [specify/type of allergy]
Anesthesia: Local anesthesia/Conscious sedation
Medications: List any relevant medications used
Contrast Material: (_) mL of [type] contrast material was used for intra-arterial injection
Field: Sterile
Procedure classification: Clean
Position: Supine
Monitoring: Intravenous access line was secured and vital signs were continuously monitored by nursing staff/anesthesia team throughout the procedure
Total fluoroscopy time: (_) minutes
Cumulative radiation dose: (_) mGy

Description of Procedure: *(Femoral artery approach)*
The risks, benefits, alternatives, and procedure itself were explained to the patient/patient's Power of Attorney/patient's legal guardian, and informed written/verbal consent was obtained. Time out was performed to confirm the correct patient, procedure, and site. The site of the procedure was identified and marked.

The skin of both groins were shaved, prepped, and draped in the usual sterile fashion. The right/left common femoral artery as well as the inguinal ligament were located by palpation/ultrasound and marked. The site of arterial puncture was determined using combined information from palpation, ultrasound, and fluoroscopy over the middle of the medial third of the femoral head. Local anesthesia was administered. Common femoral artery access was obtained using a (_)-gauge [type] needle and the Seldinger technique under direct ultrasound visualization/by palpation. Once good pulsatile arterial flow was detected, a (_)-inch [type] guidewire was advanced through the needle, up through the common femoral artery, into the aorta under direct fluoroscopic visualization and a (_)-French vascular sheath was placed.

Heparinized saline infusion was started into the femoral arterial sheath. Subsequently, a (_)-French, (_)-cm-long [type] catheter was advanced into the abdominal/thoracic aorta over a (_)-inch [hydrophilic/type] guidewire under direct fluoroscopic visualization and the left/right renal artery was selectively catheterized. After confirming the catheter location by contrast injection, digital subtraction angiography was performed by injecting (_) mL of contrast media manually/using automated injector at a rate of (_) mL/sec. Delayed images were obtained to delineate the renal venous circulation.

Following the procedure the right/left femoral artery sheath was removed and adequate hemostasis was achieved by compression for (_) minutes/using [type] vascular closure device. The femoral pulses were checked following the procedure and were [comparable to the pre-procedure pulses/specify if otherwise needed]. The patient was transferred to the floor/recovery room for close monitoring following the procedure in a stable condition. Staff was present for the entire procedure.

Intra-Procedure Findings: List all relevant findings.

Immediate Complications: None encountered during or directly after the procedure. List complications if any.

Post-Procedure Plan [1–3]:

- Keep patient complete bed rest with the right/left leg extended for 6 h *[adjust depending on the puncture site]*.
- Check the right/left groin/[specify the puncture site if different] for any bleeding or hematoma formation every 15 min for 1 h, then every 30 min for 1 h, then every hour for 4 h; inform interventional radiology team if any signs of bleeding are observed *[adjust depending on the puncture site]*.
- Check and document lower extremity pulses every 30 min for 2 h then every 1 h for 4 h *[adjust depending on the puncture site]*.
- Monitor vital signs every 15 min for 1 h, then every 30 min for 4 h; notify interventional radiology team if systolic blood pressure < 95 mmHg, or heart rate > 110 beats/min.
- Resume diet and previous orders as needed and if otherwise not contraindicated.
- Continue adequate intravenous hydration and monitor fluid (intake–output) status.
- Check complete blood count and creatinine on the day following the procedure or as clinically indicated.
- Perform regular neurological examination when the procedure includes manipulation in the ascending thoracic aorta, aortic arch or brachiocephalic arteries.

Impression:

- Selective/superselective right/left/bilateral renal arteriography, as described above.
- The patient tolerated the procedure well and left the interventional unit in stable condition.
- The procedure was canceled/terminated prematurely.
- The patient refused to undergo/complete the procedure.
- List any other relevant or important information/finding.

References

1. Kandarpa K, Gardiner GA Jr, Keller FS. Diagnostic arteriography. In: Kandarpa K, Machan L, editors. Handbook of interventional radiologic procedures. 4th ed. Philadelphia: Lippincott Williams & Wilkins; 2011. p. 61–84.
2. Heran MK, Marshalleck F, Temple M, Grassi CJ, Connolly B, Towbin RB, et al. Joint quality improvement guidelines for pediatric arterial access and arteriography: from the societies of interventional radiology and pediatric radiology. J Vasc Interv Radiol. 2010;21(1):32–43.

3. American College of Radiology. ACR–SIR–SPR practice parameter for performance of arteriography. Reston, VA: American College of Radiology; 2014.
4. Kaufman JA. Invasive vascular diagnosis. In: Mauro MA, Murphy KPJ, Thomson KR, Venbrux AC, Morgan RA, editors. Image-guided interventions. 2nd ed. Philadelphia: Saunders Elsevier; 2014. p. 11–32.
5. Venkatesan AM, Kundu S, Sacks D, Wallace MJ, Wojak JC, Rose SC, et al. Practice guidelines for adult antibiotic prophylaxis during vascular and interventional radiology procedures. J Vasc Interv Radiol. 2010;21(11):1611–30.
6. Taslakian B, Sebaaly MG, Al-Kutoubi A. Patient evaluation and preparation in vascular and interventional radiology: what every interventional radiologist should know (part 1: patient assessment and laboratory tests). Cardiovasc Intervent Radiol. 2016;39(3):325–33.
7. Taslakian B, Sebaaly MG, Al-Kutoubi A. Patient evaluation and preparation in vascular and interventional radiology: what every interventional radiologist should know (part 2: patient preparation and medications). Cardiovasc Intervent Radiol. 2016;39(4):489–99. doi: 10.1007/s00270-015-1239-4. [Epub 2015 Nov 25].

101 Renal Artery Angioplasty and Stent Placement

Mikhael Georges Sebaaly

Abbreviations

PTRA Percutaneous transluminal renal artery angioplasty

INTRODUCTION

Percutaneous transluminal renal artery angioplasty (PTRA) is indicated in the treatment of renovascular hypertension and in an effort to restore or prevent further decline of renal function in cases of renal insufficiency. Renovascular hypertension is the most common cause of secondary hypertension. It accounts for 5 % of all hypertension causes. Renovascular hypertension can be caused either by atherosclerosis of the renal artery or due to fibromuscular dysplasia. Renal artery stenosis or occlusion may also lead to progressive renal insufficiency due to nephrosclerosis.

COMMON INDICATIONS [1–5]

- Angiographically documented renal artery stenosis causing 10 % systolic pressure gradient across the stenotic lesion with one of the following:
  - Poor blood pressure control in patients receiving optimal therapy
  - Multiple antihypertensive medications are needed to achieve adequate control of the blood pressure
  - Lateralization of renal vein renin secretion to the affected side with suppression of the unaffected side
  - Positive radionuclide renogram with angiotensin converting enzyme inhibitor challenge
  - Renal insufficiency with asymmetrical loss of renal mass documented by serial imaging examinations
  - Renal insufficiency associated with renal artery stenosis of >50 %
- Renal artery stenosis in a transplanted kidney associated with hypertension, renal insufficiency, or both
- Renal bypass saphenous graft stenosis associated with hypertension, renal insufficiency or both
- Unexplained pulmonary edema *(e.g., pulmonary edema with normal left ventricular function)*
- Unstable angina *(patients with renal artery stenosis and unstable angina may show improvement of symptoms post PTRA)*

M.G. Sebaaly (✉)
Department of Diagnostic Radiology, American University of Beirut Medical Center (AUBMC), Riad El-Solh, 1107 2020, Beirut, Lebanon
e-mail: ms246@aub.edu.lb

B. Taslakian et al. (eds.), *Procedural Dictations in Image-Guided Intervention*,
DOI 10.1007/978-3-319-40845-3_101

COMMON CONTRAINDICATIONS [5]

Absolute contraindications:

- Hemodynamically unstable patient
- Insignificant stenosis by pressure gradient measurement across the lesion
- Marked renal atrophy *(kidneys measuring less than 7 cm pole-to-pole)*

Relative contraindications:

- Past history of allergy to intravenous contrast media *(consider CO_2)*
- Pregnancy
- Impaired renal function
- Uncorrected coagulopathy
- Long segment disease with total occlusion
- Atherosclerosis plaque extending into the renal artery *(ostial lesion)*
- Severe atherosclerotic aortic disease *(increased risk of atheroma embolization)*
- Contemplated surgical replacement of the aorta

POSSIBLE COMPLICATIONS [5, 6]

General (angiography-related) complications:

- Hemorrhage *(puncture-site hematoma, retroperitoneal hematoma if "high" puncture above inguinal ligament)*
- Pseudoaneurysm *(superficial femoral artery "low" puncture)*
- Arteriovenous fistula *(puncture-site artery)*
- Thrombosis of the femoral artery
- Distal embolization
- Contrast-induced allergic reaction
- Contrast-induced nephropathy
- Arterial perforation or dissection
- Catheter or guide-wire breakage
- Limb amputation *(rare)*
- Risks related to any minimally invasive procedure performed under conscious sedation *(e.g., allergy to medications)*

Angioplasty (procedure-specific) complications:

- Local thrombus at site of angioplasty
- Renal artery dissection
- Renal artery branch perforation
- Peripheral renal embolus
- Perinephric hematoma
- Segmental infarction of the kidney
- Nephrectomy or surgical bypass
- Worsening renal function due to microcholesterol embolization or contrast-induced nephropathy

PREPROCEDURAL ASSESSMENT AND PLANNING [7–9]

- History, indications, and physical examination *(Appendix 1* in Chap. 149*)*
- Evaluation of diagnostic imaging studies and physiologic test to determine the relevant vascular anatomy (e.g., the number and orientation of the renal arteries and lesion characteristics), physiologic, and pathologic conditions
- Periprocedural management of coagulation status *(Appendices 2* in Chap. 150 *and 3* in Chap. 151*)*
- Antibiotic prophylaxis: Not routinely recommended unless the procedure is high risk *(cases of repeat intervention within 7 days, prolonged indwelling arterial sheath, or prolonged duration of procedure)* [7]. Some authors suggest routine use of prophylactic antibiotics [6] *(Appendices 4* in Chap. 152 *and 5* in Chap. 153*)*.
- Medications: Continue all regular medications, with the exception of diuretics to avoid dehydration *(consult with the primary clinician)*. Unless otherwise contraindicated, place the patient on acetylsalicylic acid (aspirin) before the procedure (325-mg) and loading dose of clopidogrel (300- to 600-mg).
- Imaging modality for guidance: Fluoroscopy; combined with ultrasound for arterial puncture
- Positioning: Supine
- Arterial access: Transfemoral route is preferred; transbrachial or transradial route as an alternative [6]

PROCEDURE NOTE

Procedure: Right/Left renal artery angioplasty and stent placement
Staff: [_]

Fellow: [_]
Resident: [_]
Clinical Information: Describe history and list indications
Allergies: None known/Allergic to [specify/type of allergy]
Anesthesia: Local anesthesia/Conscious sedation
Medications: List any relevant medications used (sedation, antibiotics)
Contrast Used: (_) mL of [type] contrast media was used for angiography
Field: Sterile
Procedure classification: Clean
Position: Supine
Monitoring: Intravenous access line was secured and vital signs were continuously monitored by nursing staff/anesthesia team throughout the procedure
Total fluoroscopy time: (_) minutes
Cumulative radiation dose: (_) mGy

Description of Procedure:

The risks, benefits, alternatives, and the procedure itself were explained to the patient/patient's Power of Attorney/patient's legal guardian, and informed written consent was obtained. The site of the puncture was identified and marked. Time out was performed to confirm the correct patient, procedure, and site.

The skin of both groins were shaved, prepped, and draped in the usual sterile fashion. The right/left femoral artery as well as the inguinal ligament were located by palpation/ultrasound and marked. The site of arterial puncture was determined using combined information from palpation, ultrasound, and fluoroscopy over the middle of the medial third of the femoral head. Local anesthesia was administered. Femoral artery access was obtained using (_)-gauge [type] needle and the Seldinger technique, double- / single-wall entry under direct ultrasound visualization/by palpation. Once good pulsatile arterial flow was detected, a (_)-inch [type] guidewire was advanced through the needle, up the femoral artery, into the aorta under direct fluoroscopic visualization and a (_)-French vascular sheath was placed. (_) units of unfractionated heparin were administered intravenously *(dose of 50–70 U/kg is administered to increase the activated clotting time (ACT) to longer than 220 s).*

Subsequently, a (_)-French, (_) cm-long [type] catheter was advanced into the abdominal aorta over a (_)-inch [hydrophilic/type] guidewire under direct fluoroscopic visualization and the right/left renal artery was selectively catheterized. Then, selective renal artery angiography was performed by manual injection of (_) mL of contrast demonstrating [specify findings]. Following this, a (_)-French, (_) cm-long Flexor/Ansel vascular sheath was advanced over the guidewire and positioned at [specify location]. A (_) × (_) mm [type] balloon expandable stent deploying catheter was advanced over the guidewire and the catheter was aligned along the long axis of the lesion with its markers across the lesion. Then, the balloon expandable stent was deployed by inflating the balloon. The balloon was deflated and the deploying device was removed. Then selective renal angiography was repeated by manual injection of (_) mL of contrast demonstrating good flow/residual stenosis.

Following the procedure the right/left femoral artery sheath was removed and adequate hemostasis was achieved by (_) minute-compression/using [type] vascular closure device.

The femoral pulses were checked following the procedure and were [comparable to the pre-procedure pulses/specify if otherwise needed]. The patient was transferred to the floor/recovery room for close monitoring following the procedure in a stable condition. Staff was present and scrubbed for the entire procedure.

Intra-Procedure Findings: List all relevant findings.

Immediate Complications: None encountered during or directly after the procedure. List complications if any.

Post-Procedure Plan:

Standard post-angiogram management plan

- Keep patient complete bed rest with the right/left leg extended for 6 h *[adjust depending on the puncture site]*.

- Check the right/left groin/[specify the puncture site if different] for any bleeding or hematoma formation every 15 min for 1 h, then every 30 min for 1 h, then every hour for 4 h; inform interventional radiology team if any signs of bleeding are observed *[adjust depending on the puncture site]*.
- Check and document lower extremity pulses every 30 min for 2 h then every 1 h for 4 h *[adjust depending on the puncture site]*.
- Monitor vital signs every 15 min for 1 h, then every 30 min for 4 h; notify interventional radiology team if systolic blood pressure <95 mmHg, or heart rate > 110 beats/min.
- Resume diet and previous orders as needed and if otherwise not contraindicated.
- Continue adequate intravenous hydration and monitor fluid (intake-output) status.
- Check complete blood count and creatinine on the day following the procedure or as clinically indicated.
- Perform regular neurological examination when the procedure includes manipulation in the ascending thoracic aorta, aortic arch, or brachiocephalic arteries.

Procedure-specific management plan:

- Consider post-procedure heparin in patients demonstrating slow blood flow in the stent on immediate post-procedure angiography.
- Renal duplex study after 1 or 2 weeks, then at 6 months, then annually for 3 years.
- Clopidogrel for 3 months, then lifetime 81–325 mg of aspirin per day.
- Perform renal duplex study if decline in renal function or worsening hypertension.
- Resume antihypertensive therapy, ACEI/ARB as first-line.
- Adequate control of diabetes and dyslipidemia.
- Follow blood pressure and renal function periodically.

Impression:

- Left/Right renal artery angioplasty and stent placement, as described above.
- The patient tolerated the procedure well and left the interventional unit in a stable condition.
- The patient was unstable and the procedure was canceled/terminated prematurely.
- List any other relevant or important information/finding.

References

1. Maxwell MH, Bleifer KH, Franklin SS, Varady PD. Cooperative study of renovascular hypertension. Demographic analysis of the study. JAMA. 1972;220:1195–204.
2. Zhang Y, Ge JB, Qian JY, Ye ZB. Prevalence and risk factors of atherosclerotic renal artery stenosis in 1,200 Chinese patients undergoing coronary angiography. Nephron Clin Pract. 2006;104:c185–92.
3. Rundback JH, Sacks D, Kent KC, Cooper C, Jones D, Murphy T, et al. Guidelines for the use of renal artery stents in clinical trials. Circulation. 2002;106:1572–85.
4. De Bruyne B, Manoharan G, Pijls NH, Verhamme K, Madaric J, Bartunek J, et al. Assessment of renal artery stenosis severity by pressure gradient measurements. J Am Coll Cardiol. 2006;48:1851–5.
5. Trost DR, Sos TA. Renal Artery Angioplasty and Stents. In: Kandarpa K, Machan L, editors. Handbook of interventional radiologic procedures. 4th ed. Philadelphia: Lippincott Williams & Wilkins; 2011. p. 205–18.
6. Carr TM 3rd, Sabri SS, Turba UC, Park AW, Saad WE, Angle JF, et al. Stenting for atherosclerotic renal artery stenosis. Tech Vasc Interv Radiol. 2010;13(2):134–45.
7. Venkatesan AM, Kundu S, Sacks D, Wallace MJ, Wojak JC, Rose SC, et al. Practice guidelines for adult antibiotic prophylaxis during vascular and interventional radiology procedures. J Vasc Interv Radiol. 2010;21(11):1611–30.
8. Taslakian B, Sebaaly MG, Al-Kutoubi A. Patient evaluation and preparation in vascular and interventional radiology: what every interventional radiologist should know (part 1: patient assessment and laboratory tests). Cardiovasc Intervent Radiol. 2016;39(3):325–33.
9. Taslakian B, Sebaaly MG, Al-Kutoubi A. Patient evaluation and preparation in vascular and interventional radiology: what every interventional radiologist should know (part 2: patient preparation and medications). Cardiovasc Intervent Radiol. 2016;39(4):489–99. doi: 10.1007/s00270-015-1239-4. [Epub 2015 Nov 25].

Renal Sympathetic Denervation 102

Mikhael Georges Sebaaly

INTRODUCTION

Hypertension is one of the most common diseases in the world. Controlling the blood pressure is the only proven measure that can decrease the complications of hypertension. Renal sympathetic denervation is a promising technique in the control of the blood pressure in uncontrolled hypertension and severe intolerable side effects of antihypertensive therapy. This procedure has no major morbidities according to conducted studies.

COMMON INDICATIONS [1]

- Resistant hypertension despite multiple antihypertensive drugs
- Intolerable side effects of antihypertensive medications
- Patient post renal transplant with hypertension due to the native kidneys

M.G. Sebaaly (✉)
Department of Diagnostic Radiology, American University of Beirut Medical Center (AUBMC), Riad El-Solh, Beirut 1107 2020, Lebanon
e-mail: ms246@aub.edu.lb

COMMON CONTRAINDICATIONS [2]

Absolute contraindications:
- Renal artery stenosis
- Unsuitable renal artery anatomy *(less than 4 mm in diameter, less than 20 mm in length, multiple renal arteries)*
- Stenotic valvular heart disease
- Unstable angina within 6 months
- Cerebrovascular accident within 6 months
- Myocardial infarction within 6 months
- Previous renal artery intervention

Relative contraindications:
- Past history of allergy to intravenous contrast media *(consider CO2)*
- Pregnancy
- Impaired renal function

POSSIBLE COMPLICATIONS [1, 3, 4]

General (angiography-related) complications:
- Hemorrhage *(puncture-site hematoma, retroperitoneal hematoma if "high" puncture above inguinal ligament)*
- Pseudoaneurysm *(superficial femoral artery "low" puncture)*
- Arteriovenous fistula *(puncture-site artery)*
- Thrombosis of the femoral artery
- Distal embolization
- Contrast-induced allergic reaction
- Contrast-induced nephropathy
- Arterial perforation or dissection

B. Taslakian et al. (eds.), *Procedural Dictations in Image-Guided Intervention*,
DOI 10.1007/978-3-319-40845-3_102

- Catheter or guidewire breakage
- Limb amputation *(rare)*
- Risks related to any minimally invasive procedure performed under conscious sedation *(e.g., allergy to medications)*

Renal sympathetic denervation (procedure-specific) complications:

- Severe drop in blood pressure after the procedure
- Urinary tract infection
- Paraesthesias
- Transient back pain
- Transient intra-procedural bradycardia
- Progression of atherosclerotic lesion in renal arteries if present
- Renal artery dissection
- Minor renal artery spasm or edema

PREPROCEDURAL ASSESSMENT AND PLANNING [5, 6]

- History, indications, and physical examination *(Appendix 1* in Chap. 149*)*
- Evaluation of diagnostic imaging studies and physiologic tests to determine the relevant vascular anatomy, anatomic relations, physiologic, and pathologic conditions
- Periprocedural management of coagulation status *(Appendices 2* in Chap. 150 *and 3* in Chap. 151*)*
- Imaging modality for guidance: Fluoroscopy; combined with ultrasound for arterial puncture
- Positioning: Supine
- Arterial access: Transfemoral route for the majority of cases

PROCEDURE NOTE

Procedure: Renal sympathetic denervation
Staff: [_]
Fellow: [_]
Resident: [_]
Clinical Information: Describe history and list indications
Allergies: None known/Allergic to [specify/type of allergy]
Anesthesia: Local anesthesia with conscious sedation/general anesthesia
Medications: List any relevant medications used
Contrast Used: (_) mL of [type] contrast media was used for angiography
Field: Sterile
Procedure classification: Clean
Position: Supine
Monitoring: Intravenous access line was secured and vital signs were continuously monitored by nursing staff/anesthesia team throughout the procedure
Total fluoroscopy time: (_) minutes
Cumulative radiation dose: (_) mGy

Description of Procedure:

The risks, benefits, alternatives, and the procedure itself were explained to the patient/patient's Power of Attorney/patient's legal guardian, and informed written consent was obtained. The site of the puncture was identified and marked. Time out was performed to confirm the correct patient, procedure and site.

The skin of both groins was shaved, prepped, and draped in the usual sterile fashion. The right/left femoral artery as well as the inguinal ligament were located by palpation/ultrasound and marked. The site of arterial puncture was determined using combined information from palpation, ultrasound, and fluoroscopy over the middle of the medial third of the femoral head. Local anesthesia was administered. Femoral artery access was obtained using (_)-gauge [type] needle and the Seldinger technique, single-wall entry under direct ultrasound visualization/by palpation. Once good pulsatile arterial flow was detected, a (_)-inch [type] guidewire was advanced through the needle, up the femoral artery, into the aorta under direct fluoroscopic visualization and a (_)-French vascular sheath was placed.

Subsequently, a (_)-French, (_) cm long [type] radiofrequency catheter was advanced into the abdominal aorta over a (_)-inch [hydrophilic/type] guidewire under direct fluoroscopic visualization and the right/left renal artery was selected. Digital subtraction views of the renal artery were obtained by injecting (_) mL of contrast media manually/using automated injector at a rate of (_) mL/sec, showing [specify findings]. Following this, the catheter was advanced into the distal renal artery and radiofrequency was applied to the endothelial lining for (_) minutes then the catheter was drawn back (_) mm and circumferentially rotated, and radiofrequency was applied to the endothelial lining for (_) minutes and this was repeated (number) times, with intravenous use of analgesia prophylaxis.

Following the procedure the right/left femoral artery sheath was removed and adequate hemostasis was achieved by (_) minute-compression/using [type] vascular closure device.

The femoral pulses were checked following the procedure and were [comparable to the pre-procedure pulses/specify if otherwise needed]. The patient was transferred to the floor/recovery room for close monitoring following the procedure in a stable condition. Staff was present for the entire procedure.

Intra-Procedure Findings: List all relevant findings.

Immediate Complications: None encountered during or directly after the procedure. List complications if any.

Post-Procedure Plan:

Standard post-angiogram management plan

- Keep patient in complete bed rest with the right/left leg extended for 6 h *[adjust depending on the puncture site]*.
- Check the right/left groin/[specify the puncture site if different] for any bleeding or hematoma formation every 15 min for 1 h, then every 30 min for 1 h, then every hour for 4 h; inform interventional radiology team if any signs of bleeding are observed *[adjust depending on the puncture site]*.
- Check and document lower extremity pulses every 30 min for 2 h then every 1 h for 4 h *[adjust depending on the puncture site]*.
- Monitor vital signs every 15 min for 1 h, then every 30 min for 4 h; notify interventional radiology team if systolic blood pressure <95 mmHg, or heart rate > 110 beats/min.
- Resume diet and previous orders as needed and if otherwise not contraindicated.
- Continue adequate intravenous hydration and monitor fluid (intake–output) status.
- Check complete blood count and creatinine on the day following the procedure or as clinically indicated.
- Perform regular neurological examination when the procedure includes manipulation in the ascending thoracic aorta, aortic arch or brachiocephalic arteries.

Procedure-specific management plan:

- Follow-up physical examination and laboratory studies closely for signs of hemorrhage.
- Perform cross sectional imaging (e.g., CT or MR angiography) if clinically indicated to evaluate the presence of pseudoaneurysm formation and recurrent bleeding caused by delayed rupture.
- Follow-up blood pressure closely and change antihypertensive medications accordingly.

Impression:

- Catheter directed renal sympathetic denervation, as described above.
- The patient tolerated the procedure well and left the interventional unit in a stable condition.
- The patient was unstable and the procedure was canceled/terminated prematurely.
- List any other relevant or important information/finding.

References

1. Esler MD, Krum H, Sobotka PA, Schlaich MP, Schmieder RE, Böhm M. Renal sympathetic denervation in patients with treatment-resistant hypertension (The Symplicity HTN-2 Trial): a randomized controlled trial. Lancet. 2010;376(9756):1903–9.
2. Bhatt DL, Kandzari DE, O'Neill WW, D'Agostino R, Flack JM, Katzen BT, et al. A controlled trial of renal denervation for resistant hypertension. N Engl J Med. 2014;370(15):1393–401.
3. Doumas M, Faselis C, Papademetriou V. Renal sympathetic denervation and systemic hypertension. Am J Cardiol. 2010;105(4):570–6.
4. Symplicity HTN-1 Investigators. Catheter-based renal sympathetic denervation for resistant hypertension: durability of blood pressure reduction out to 24 months. Hypertension. 2011;57(5):911–7.
5. Taslakian B, Sebaaly MG, Al-Kutoubi A. Patient evaluation and preparation in vascular and interventional radiology: what every interventional radiologist should know (part 1: patient assessment and laboratory tests). Cardiovasc Intervent Radiol. 2016;39(3):325–33.
6. Taslakian B, Sebaaly MG, Al-Kutoubi A. Patient evaluation and preparation in vascular and interventional radiology: what every interventional radiologist should know (part 2: patient preparation and medications). Cardiovasc Intervent Radiol. 2016;39(4):489–99. doi: 10.1007/s00270-015-1239-4. [Epub 2015 Nov 25].

Renal Venography

103

Mikhael Georges Sebaaly

INTRODUCTION

Renal venography is a simple but an important fluoroscopic guided diagnostic procedure. Renal venography has been proposed for the evaluation of the venous bed in several clinical scenarios. In addition, it can be used to enhance the precision of renal vein renin collection.

COMMON INDICATIONS [1, 2]

- Renal vein thrombosis
- Unknown cause of hematuria
- Tumors: retroperitoneal, renal pelvic carcinoma, renal cell carcinoma, avascular tumors
- Renovascular hypertension
- Differentiation of renal agenesis from small kidneys
- Renal vein renin determination
- Preoperative evaluation of the renal vein
- Pre-renal transplant donor with no opacification on arteriography or inconclusive CT
- Post-operative evaluation of the renal vein
- Evaluation in patients with portal hypertension before splenorenal shunt operation
- Renal vein varices

M.G. Sebaaly (✉)
Department of Diagnostic Radiology, American University of Beirut Medical Center (AUBMC), Riad El-Solh, Beirut 1107 2020, Lebanon
e-mail: ms246@aub.edu.lb

COMMON CONTRAINDICATIONS

Absolute contraindications:
- Severe venous thrombosis of the inferior vena cava

Relative contraindications (benefits of venography should be weighed against risks of management):
- Past history of allergy to intravenous contrast media
- Pregnancy
- Impaired renal function
- Severe compromise of cardiopulmonary status

POSSIBLE COMPLICATIONS

- Hemorrhage *(puncture-site hematoma)*
- Arteriovenous fistula
- Thrombosis of the renal vein
- Embolization of a thrombus from renal vein
- Contrast-induced allergic reaction
- Contrast-induced nephropathy
- Venous perforation or dissection
- Catheter or guidewire breakage

PREPROCEDURAL ASSESSMENT AND PLANNING [3–5]

- History, indications, and physical examination *(Appendix 1* in Chap. 149*)*

B. Taslakian et al. (eds.), *Procedural Dictations in Image-Guided Intervention*,
DOI 10.1007/978-3-319-40845-3_103

- Periprocedural management of coagulation status *(Appendices 2* in Chap. 150 *and 3* in Chap. 151*)*
- Antibiotic prophylaxis: Not routinely recommended [3] *(Appendices 4* in Chap. 152 *and 5* in Chap. 153*)*
- Imaging modality for guidance: Fluoroscopy
- Positioning: Supine
- Start intravenous fluids the night before venography in order to ensure adequate hydration, combined with effective monitoring of fluid status
- Insert a urinary catheter or ask the patient to void before the procedure depending on the estimated time of the procedure
- Considerations for patient with specific diseases or conditions, patients on specific medications or patients with history of multiple comorbidities: consult with the referring clinician, anesthesia, cardiology, nephrology, endocrinology, and pulmonary specialist as needed. These conditions include but are not limited to heparinized patient, patients on Coumadin, thrombocytopenic patients, patients with known renal or hepatic dysfunction, history of allergic reaction to contrast media or local anesthesia, seizure, cardiac and pulmonary diseases, sickle cell anemia, and pheochromocytoma.
- Venous access:
  - Transfemoral route for the majority of cases
  - Transjugular or antecubital route can be useful if contraindications of transfemoral access are present

PROCEDURE NOTE

Procedure: Right/left/bilateral renal venography
Staff: [_]
Fellow: [_]
Resident: [_]
Clinical Information: Describe history and list indications
Allergies: None known/Allergic to [specify/type of allergy]
Anesthesia: Local anesthesia/Conscious sedation
Medications: *List any relevant medications used*
Contrast Used: (_) mL of [type] contrast media was used for venography
Field: Sterile
Procedure Classification: Clean
Position: Supine
Monitoring: Intravenous access line was secured and vital signs were continuously monitored by nursing staff/anesthesia team throughout the procedure
Total fluoroscopy time: (_) minutes
Cumulative radiation dose: (_) mGy

Description of Procedure:

The risks, benefits, alternatives, and the procedure itself were explained to the patient/patient's Power of Attorney/patient's legal guardian, and informed written consent was obtained. The site of the puncture was identified and marked. Time out was performed to confirm the correct patient, procedure and site.

The skin of both groins/neck and upper chest was shaved, prepped, and draped in the usual sterile fashion. The right/left femoral/jugular vein was located by palpation/ultrasound and marked. The site of venous puncture was determined using combined information from palpation and ultrasound. Local anesthesia was administered. Femoral/Jugular venous access was obtained using a (_)-gauge [type] needle and the Seldinger technique, double-/single-wall entry under direct ultrasound visualization/by palpation. Once good venous flow was detected, a (_)-inch [type] guidewire was advanced through the needle, into the inferior/superior vena cava under direct fluoroscopic visualization and a (_)-French vascular sheath was placed.

Subsequently, a (_)-French, (_) cm-long [type] catheter was advanced into the inferior vena cava over a (_)-inch [hydrophilic/type] guidewire, under direct fluoroscopic visualization, and the left/right renal vein ostium was selectively catheterized. Once the catheter was positioned within the renal vein, (_) mL of contrast was injected to rule out renal vein thrombosis. The guidewire was then reintroduced and the catheter was advanced within the renal vein to the hilum of the kidney and venography was performed showing [specify findings].

Following the procedure, the venous sheath was removed and adequate hemostasis was achieved by (_) minute-compression. The patient was transferred to the floor/recovery room for close monitoring/discharged home following the procedure in a stable condition. Staff was present and scrubbed for the entire procedure.

Intra-Procedure Findings: List all relevant findings.

Immediate Complications: None encountered during or directly after the procedure. List complications if any..

Post-Procedure Plan:

- Keep patient in complete bed rest for (_) hours *[adjust depending on the access site]*.
- Check the access site for any bleeding or hematoma formation every 15 min for 1 h, then every 30 min for 1 h, then every hour; inform interventional radiology team if any observed.
- Monitor vital signs and notify interventional radiology team if systolic blood pressure < 95 mmHg, or heart rate > 110 beats/min.
- Resume diet and previous orders as needed and if otherwise not contraindicated.
- Heparin can be restarted within 2 h after removal of the catheter and puncture-site compression, and documenting absence of puncture-site-related problems, if not otherwise contraindicated.
- Continue adequate intravenous hydration and monitor fluid (intake-output) status.
- Check complete blood count, creatinine, and blood urea nitrogen on the day following the procedure or as clinically indicated.

Impression:

- Right/left/bilateral renal venography, as described above.
- The patient tolerated the procedure well and left the interventional unit in a stable condition.
- The procedure was canceled/terminated prematurely.
- List any other relevant or important information/finding.

References

1. Myers GH Jr, Fehrenbaker LG, Kelalis PP. Prognostic significance of renal vein invasion by hypernephroma. J Urol. 1968;100(4):420â€“3.
2. Perez CA, Kaiman HA, Keith J, Mill WB, Vietti TJ, Powers WE. Treatment of Wilmsâ€™ tumor and factors affecting prognosis. Cancer. 1973;32(3):609–17.
3. Venkatesan AM, Kundu S, Sacks D, Wallace MJ, Wojak JC, Rose SC, et al. Practice guidelines for adult antibiotic prophylaxis during vascular and interventional radiology procedures. J Vasc Interv Radiol. 2010;21(11):1611–30.
4. Taslakian B, Sebaaly MG, Al-Kutoubi A. Patient evaluation and preparation in vascular and interventional radiology: what every interventional radiologist should know (part 1: patient assessment and laboratory tests). Cardiovasc Intervent Radiol. 2016;39(3):325–33.
5. Taslakian B, Sebaaly MG, Al-Kutoubi A. Patient evaluation and preparation in vascular and interventional radiology: what every interventional radiologist should know (part 2: patient preparation and medications). Cardiovasc Intervent Radiol. 2016;39(4):489–99. doi: 10.1007/s00270-015-1239-4. [Epub 2015 Nov 25].

Transcatheter Embolization for the Treatment of Renal Trauma

104

Jonathan S. Gross

Abbreviations

CT	Computed tomography
AAST	American Association for the Surgery of Trauma

INTRODUCTION

Mechanical injury to the kidney may occur in the setting of either blunt or penetrating abdominal trauma and is associated with varying degrees of parenchymal and vascular injury. In the past, surgical exploration was commonly performed in the setting of suspected severe kidney injury. However, as the availability, speed, and accuracy of computed tomography (CT) have increased, there has been a trend toward less invasive management of kidney trauma [1, 2].

While treatment protocols differ, most institutions rely on the American Association for the Surgery of Trauma (AAST) grading system, which classifies kidney injury according to extent of laceration and proximity of the injury to the renal hilum. It is generally agreed that hemodynamically stable patients with lower grade injuries may be treated conservatively without the need for invasive intervention [3–5]. However, there is controversy regarding the relative benefits of angiography and embolization versus conservative management for the treatment of grade 4 and 5 renal injuries in hemodynamically *stable* patients [1, 2, 4–6] and regarding the relative benefits of endovascular therapy versus emergent surgery for the treatment of high grade injuries in hemodynamically *unstable* patients [7, 8].

The goal of embolization in the setting of high grade trauma to the kidney is to stop flow through the injured vessel while minimizing injury to the renal parenchyma. Hemostasis is usually achieved using coils, though in select settings, a temporary occlusive agent, such as Gelfoam or Avitene, may be used instead. Regardless of the type of embolic material used, it is important to perform good angiographic imaging, including CT angiography and abdominal aortography, prior to embolization. This can help to determine the presence of any relevant accessory renal arteries, the presence of injury to the main renal artery which might require covered stent placement or surgical intervention, and the presence of injury in adjacent vessels, such as the lumbar arteries.

J.S. Gross (✉)
Department of Radiology, New York University Langone Medical Center, 660 First Avenue, 7th Floor, New York, NY 10016, USA
e-mail: jonathan.gross@nyumc.org

B. Taslakian et al. (eds.), *Procedural Dictations in Image-Guided Intervention*,
DOI 10.1007/978-3-319-40845-3_104

COMMON INDICATIONS [3–5, 7–9]

Generally accepted:

- Hemodynamically stable patient with blunt or penetrating renal trauma and evidence of active hemorrhage on CT angiography
- Grade 4 renal injury which has failed conservative non-invasive management

Varying acceptance:

- Hemodynamically unstable patient with grade 4 or 5 renal injury
- Grade 5 renal injury which has failed conservative non-invasive management

COMMON CONTRAINDICATIONS [5, 6]

Absolute:

- Uncorrected coagulopathy
- Hemorrhage from venous rather than arterial injury
- Avulsion of the renal pedicle

Relative:

- Patient with multifocal trauma who requires emergent surgery for other injuries
- History of severe allergy to intravenous contrast media
- Pregnancy
- Acute or chronic infection of the kidney

POSSIBLE COMPLICATIONS

General (angiography-related) complications:

- Hemorrhage *(puncture-site hematoma, retroperitoneal hematoma if "high" puncture above inguinal ligament)*
- Pseudoaneurysm *(superficial femoral artery "low" puncture)*
- Arteriovenous fistula *(puncture-site artery)*
- Thrombosis of the femoral artery
- Distal embolization
- Contrast-induced allergic reaction
- Contrast-induced nephropathy
- Arterial perforation or dissection
- Catheter or guidewire breakage
- Limb amputation *(rare)*
- Risks related to any minimally invasive procedure performed under conscious sedation *(e.g., allergy to medications)*

Renal artery embolization (procedure-specific) complications [8]:

- Post-embolization syndrome *(fever, nausea, pain)*
- Partial or complete infarction of the kidney
- Arterial dissection
- Decreased renal function
- Non-target embolization
- Pyelonephritis/formation of renal abscess
- Hypertension

PREPROCEDURAL ASSESSMENT AND PLANNING [10–12]

- Review relevant medical history, including mechanism and anatomic site of trauma, hemodynamic status, and recent need for blood products and vasopressors
- Evaluate diagnostic CT to determine relevant vascular anatomy and to identify sites of injury
- Review coagulation status; if necessary, transfuse to platelets >50,000 and INR 1.5 *(Appendices 2* in Chap. 150 *and 3* in Chap. 151*)*
- Antibiotic prophylaxis: It is unclear whether the administration of prophylactic antibiotics is helpful prior to embolization in the setting of trauma. However, given the high risk for infarction of renal parenchyma following embolization, a single pre-procedure dose of a broad spectrum antibiotic, such as ceftriaxone, is commonly administered [10] *(Appendices 4* in Chap. 152 *and 5* in Chap. 153*)*.
- Imaging modality for guidance: Fluoroscopy; sometimes combined with ultrasound for arterial puncture
- Positioning: Supine
- Arterial access: Common femoral artery *(preferred)*, left radial, left brachial, or left axillary artery

PROCEDURE NOTE

Procedure: Catheter-directed abdominal aortography and left/right renal arteriography; subselective embolization of injured renal vessel
Staff: [_]
Fellow: [_]
Resident: [_]
Clinical History and Indications: Describe history and list indications
Allergies: None known/Allergic to [specify/type of allergy]
Anesthesia: Local anesthesia/Conscious sedation/General anesthesia
Medications: List any relevant medications used, including antibiotic
Contrast Material: (_) mL [type of contrast], intra-arterial
Field: Sterile
Procedure classification: Clean
Position: Supine
Monitoring: Intravenous access line was secured and vital signs were continuously monitored by nursing staff/anesthesia team throughout the procedure
Total fluoroscopy time: (_) minutes
Cumulative radiation dose: (_) mGy

Description of Procedure:

The risks and benefits of the procedure were discussed with the patient, and informed consent was obtained. Time out was performed to confirm the correct patient, procedure, and planned site of arterial access.

The right/left groin was prepped and draped in sterile fashion. The right/left common femoral artery was accessed using a (_) gauge needle under fluoroscopic/sonographic guidance. Using Seldinger technique, the needle was exchanged over a (_)-inch guidewire for a (_) French sheath.

A (_) French flush catheter was advanced over a wire into the suprarenal portion of the abdominal aorta, and an abdominal aortogram was performed. The flush catheter was then exchanged over a wire for a (_) French [Cobra, Sos, Simmons] catheter, and the right/left renal artery was selected. A right/left renal arteriogram was performed.

A (_) French [type] microcatheter was advanced through the (_) French catheter, and the injured branch [specify segmental branch] of the renal artery was selected. A subselective right/left renal arteriogram was performed. Based on the angiographic findings, the abnormal branch of the right/left renal artery was embolized using (number) (_) mm × (_) cm [type] coils (or Gelfoam/Avitene).

Post-embolization subselective right/left renal arteriogram was performed through the microcatheter. The microcatheter was removed, and a selective post-embolization right/left renal arteriogram was performed through the (_) French catheter.

Based on the post-embolization findings, the catheter and sheath were removed, and hemostasis was achieved using manual compression/[type] vascular closure device. Post-procedure physical examination demonstrated no change in lower extremity pulses [specify if otherwise]. The patient was transferred to the floor/recovery room/ICU in stable condition. Staff was present for the entire procedure.

Intra-Procedure Findings: List all relevant findings.
Immediate Complications: No immediate complications. List complications if any.

Post-Procedure Plan:
Standard post-angiogram management plan

- Keep patient in complete bed rest with the right/left leg extended for 6 h *[adjust depending on the puncture site]*.
- Check the right/left groin/[specify the puncture site if different] for any bleeding or hematoma formation every 15 min for 1 h, then every 30 min for 1 h, then every hour for 4 h; inform interventional radiology team if any signs of bleeding are observed *[adjust depending on the puncture site]*.
- Check and document lower extremity pulses every 30 min for 2 h then every 1 h for 4 h *[adjust depending on the puncture site]*.
- Monitor vital signs every 15 min for 1 h, then every 30 min for 4 h; notify interventional

radiology team if systolic blood pressure <95 mmHg, or heart rate >110 beats/min.

- Resume diet and previous orders as needed and if otherwise not contraindicated.
- Continue adequate intravenous hydration and monitor fluid (intake–output) status.
- Check complete blood count and creatinine on the day following the procedure or as clinically indicated.
- Perform regular neurological examination when the procedure includes manipulation in the ascending thoracic aorta, aortic arch or brachiocephalic arteries.

Procedure-specific management plan:

- Administer narcotics/analgesics/antiemetics/antipyretics if needed for post-embolization pain, nausea, fever.
- For hemodynamically stable patients: Monitor vital signs every 15 min × 4, then every 30 min × 2, then every hour × 4, then per routine. Check complete blood count 4 h following embolization then on the morning after embolization.
- Resume diet and previous orders (if not contraindicated).
- For hemodynamically unstable patients: Continuous monitoring in ICU setting. Check complete blood count immediately following embolization then every 4 h. Administer blood products, vasopressors, as needed.
- If hemoglobin does not rise appropriately or if patient remains hemodynamically unstable, consider repeat CT to evaluate for additional/untreated sites of vascular injury.
- In the setting of high grade injury, consider long-term follow-up to evaluate for development of renovascular hypertension.

Impression:

- Selective and subselective right/left renal arteriograms demonstrating [pseudoaneurysm, extravasation, dissection, truncation, etc.] from [intraparenchymal] branch of the right/left renal artery.
- Subselective embolization of injured branch of right/left renal artery using (coil/Gelfoam/Avitene).

References

1. Chow SJ, Thompson KJ, Hartman JF, Wright ML. A 10 year review of blunt renal injuries at an urban level I trauma center. Injury. 2009;40(8):844–50.
2. Santucci RA, Fisher MB. The literature increasingly supports expectant (conservative) management of renal trauma—a systematic review. J Trauma. 2005;59(2):493–503.
3. Mani NB, Kim L. The role of interventional radiology in urologic tract trauma. Semin Intervent Radiol. 2011;28(4):415–23.
4. Morey AF, Brandes S, Dugi DD, Armstrong JH, Breyer BN, Broghammer JA, et al. Urotrauma: AUA guideline. J Urol. 2014;192(2):327–35.
5. Shoobridge JJ, Corcoran NM, Martin KA, Koukounaras J, Royce PL, Bultitude MF. Contemporary management of renal trauma. Rev Urol. 2011;13 (2):65–72.
6. Hagiwara A, Sakaki S, Goto H, Takenega K, Fukushima H, Matuda H, et al. The role of interventional radiology in the management of blunt renal injury: a practical protocol. J Trauma. 2001;51 (3):526–31.
7. Stewart AF, Brewer ME, Daley BJ, Klein FA, Kim ED. Intermediate term follow up of patients with percutaneous embolization for grade 5 blunt renal trauma. J Trauma. 2010;69(2):468–70.
8. Breyer BN, McAninch JW, Elliott SP, Master VA. Minimally invasive endovascular techniques to treat acute renal hemorrhage. J Urol. 2008;179(6):2248–52 (discussion 2253).
9. Sarani B, Powell E, Taddeo J, Carr B, Patel A, Seamon M, et al. Contemporary comparison of surgical and interventional arteriography management of blunt renal injury. J Vasc Interv Radiol. 2011;22 (5):723–8.
10. Venkatesan AM, Kundu S, Sacks D, Wallace MJ, Wojak JC, Rose SC, et al. Practice guidelines for adult antibiotic prophylaxis during vascular and interventional radiology procedures. J Vasc Interv Radiol. 2010;21:1611–30.
11. Taslakian B, Sebaaly MG, Al-Kutoubi A. Patient evaluation and preparation in vascular and interventional radiology: what every interventional radiologist should know (part 1: patient assessment and laboratory tests). Cardiovasc Intervent Radiol. 2016;39 (3):325–33.
12. Taslakian B, Sebaaly MG, Al-Kutoubi A. Patient evaluation and preparation in vascular and interventional radiology: what every interventional radiologist should know (part 2: patient preparation and medications). Cardiovasc Intervent Radiol. 2016;39 (4):489–99. doi: 10.1007/s00270-015-1239-4. [Epub 2015 Nov 25].

105 Transjugular Renal Biopsy

Mikhael Georges Sebaaly

INTRODUCTION

Renal tissue histopathological examination started in the 1950 with percutaneous renal biopsy, and it became an essential diagnostic utility for many kidney diseases. Percutaneous image-guided renal biopsy is a fast, relatively safe, high yield, and the gold standard for renal biopsies. However, the risk of hematoma increases to more than 70 % in high risk individuals who are on blood thinners. Hence transjugular renal biopsy was developed for high bleeding risk patients, since it decreases the risk of perirenal hematoma tremendously. The right kidney is preferred for biopsy due to favorable anatomy of the right renal vein. In case of single left kidney, or difficult right renal vein anatomy, the left kidney is biopsied.

COMMON INDICATIONS [1]

- Nephrotic syndrome
- Permanent proteinuria with or without microhematuria
- Rapidly progressive nephropathies
- Systemic lupus erythematosus
- Acute renal failure of unknown origin
- Isolated microhematuria and intermittent proteinuria
- Renal involvement accompanying systemic diseases

Specific Indications of transjugular Biopsy [2–5]

- Known case of renal micro-aneurysms
- Morbidly obese patients
- Failed percutaneous biopsy
- Single functioning kidney
- Severe uncorrectable coagulopathy
- Uncooperative patients and patients on mechanical ventilation
- Acute renal failure patients undergoing placement of dialysis catheter
- When other diagnostic studies are needed, such as transvenous liver biopsy, and venography

COMMON CONTRAINDICATIONS

Relative contraindications:

- Past history of allergy to intravenous contrast media
- Pregnancy
- Superior vena cava obstruction
- Congenital absence or occlusion of right internal jugular vein
- Inferior vena cava or renal vein thrombosis
- Recurrent course of the renal vein

M.G. Sebaaly (✉)
Department of Diagnostic Radiology, American University of Beirut Medical Center (AUBMC), Riad El-Solh, Beirut 1107 2020, Lebanon
e-mail: ms246@aub.edu.lb

B. Taslakian et al. (eds.), *Procedural Dictations in Image-Guided Intervention*,
DOI 10.1007/978-3-319-40845-3_105

POSSIBLE COMPLICATIONS [5–7]

Access-site-related complications:
- Hemorrhage *(neck hematoma)*
- Accidental carotid puncture
- Transient Horner's syndrome
- Cardiac arrhythmias
- Pneumothorax
- Contrast-induced allergic reaction
- Contrast-induced nephropathy
- Catheter or guidewire breakage
- Risks related to any minimally invasive procedure performed under conscious sedation *(e.g., allergy to medications)*

Procedure-specific complications:
- Transient microscopic hematuria
- Perforation of the renal capsule
- Perirenal hemorrhage
- Pelvicalyceal system hemorrhage
- Fistula between blood vessels and renal pelvicalyceal system
- Arteriovenous fistula
- Renal pseudoaneurysm

PREPROCEDURAL ASSESSMENT AND PLANNING [8–10]

- History, indications, and physical examination *(Appendix 1* in Chap. 149*)*
- Evaluation of diagnostic imaging studies and physiologic tests to determine the relevant vascular anatomy, anatomic relations, physiologic, and pathologic conditions
- Periprocedural management of coagulation status *(Appendices 2* in Chap. 150 *and 3* in Chap. 151*)*
- Antibiotic prophylaxis: Not routinely recommended [8] *(Appendices 4* in Chap. 152 *and 5* in Chap. 153*)*
- Imaging modality for guidance: Fluoroscopy; combined with ultrasound for venous access
- Positioning: Supine
- Venous access:
  - Transjugular route through the right internal jugular vein, for the majority of cases
  - Left internal jugular vein, the external jugular veins, or femoral veins are rarely used

PROCEDURE NOTE

Procedure: Transjugular biopsy of the right/left kidney
Staff: [_]
Fellow: [_]
Resident: [_]
Clinical Information: Describe history and list indications
Allergies: None known/Allergic to [specify/type of allergy]
Anesthesia: Local anesthesia/Conscious sedation
Medications: List any relevant medications used
Contrast Used: (_) mL of [type] contrast media was used for venography
Field: Sterile
Procedure classification: Clean
Position: Supine
Monitoring: Intravenous access line was secured and vital signs were continuously monitored by nursing staff/anesthesia team throughout the procedure
Total fluoroscopy time: (_) minutes
Cumulative radiation dose: (_) mGy

Description of Procedure:
The risks, benefits, alternatives, and the procedure itself were explained to the patient/patient's Power of Attorney/patient's legal guardian, and informed written consent was obtained. The site of the puncture was identified and marked. Time out was performed to confirm the correct patient, procedure and site.

The skin of the neck was prepped and draped in the usual sterile fashion. The right internal jugular vein was located and the site of venous puncture was determined using combined information from palpation, ultrasound, and fluoroscopy. Local anesthesia was administered. Jugular venous access was obtained using a (_)-gauge [type] needle and the Seldinger technique, under direct ultrasound visualization/by palpation with the table placed in a moderate Trendelenburg position. Once good venous flow was detected, a (_)-inch [type] guidewire was advanced through the needle under direct fluoroscopic visualization and a (_) French [vascular/type] sheath was placed into the right internal jugular vein in an antegrade fashion. Subsequently, a (_)-inch [hydrophilic/type] guidewire was advanced through the sheath into the inferior vena cava. A (_)-French, multipurpose curved [type] catheter was introduced through the sheath and guided into the right renal vein over the guidewire. The catheter was then manipulated into the posterior lower branch of the right renal vein.

The inserted hydrophilic wire was then exchanged for a (_)-cm long, (_)-inch [Amplatz Super-stiff/type] guidewire. Then a (7)-French, (_)-cm long [type] catheter was advanced over the extra stiff guidewire into the right renal vein under fluoroscopic guidance. The transvenous (_)-gauge [type] core biopsy needle was then advanced through the catheter gently as distally as possible into the cortical vein of the lower pole of the right kidney. (_) mL of contrast media was flushed into the catheter and optimal peripheral position was confirmed by enhancement of a wedge of the cortical parenchyma. The straight catheter was then withdrawn and (number) samples were obtained by releasing the fire mechanism of the core biopsy needle and sent for histopathologic interpretation. Venography was performed by the manual injection of (_) mL of contrast media through the catheter and showed no evidence of renal capsule perforation.

Following the procedure, the catheter and jugular sheath were removed and adequate hemostasis was achieved by (_) minutes manual compression. The patient was transferred to the floor/recovery room for close monitoring following the procedure in a stable condition. Staff was present and scrubbed for the entire procedure.

Intra-Procedure Findings: List all relevant findings.

Immediate Complications: None encountered during or directly after the procedure. List complications if any.

Post-Procedure Plan:

- Keep patient in complete bed rest for (_) hours.
- Check the right neck *(access site)* for any bleeding or hematoma formation every 15 min for 1 h, then every 30 min for 1 h, then every hour; inform interventional radiology team if any observed.
- Monitor vital signs every 15 min for 1 h, then every 30 min; notify interventional radiology team if systolic blood pressure < 95 mmHg, or heart rate > 110 beats/min.
- Resume diet and previous orders as needed and if otherwise not contraindicated.
- Continue adequate intravenous hydration and monitor fluid (intake–output) status.
- Check complete blood count, creatinine, and blood urea nitrogen on the day following the procedure or as clinically indicated.

Impression:

- Transjugular right/left renal biopsy, as described above.
- The patient tolerated the procedure well and left the interventional unit in a stable condition.
- The procedure was canceled/terminated prematurely.
- List any other relevant or important information/finding.

References

1. Ahmed MS, Patel A, Borge MA, Picken MM, Leehey DJ. Simultaneous transjugular renal biopsy and haemodialysis catheter placement in patients with ARF. Am J Kidney Dis. 2004;44:429–36.
2. Mal F, Meyrier A, Callard P, Kleinknecht D, Altmann JJ, Beaugrand M. The diagnostic yield of transjugular renal biopsy: experience in 200 cases. Kidney Int. 1992;41:445–9.
3. Mal F, Meyrier A, Callard P, Altman JJ, Kleinknecht D, Beaugrand M, et al. Transjugular Ren Biopsy. Lancet. 1990;335:1512–3.
4. Thompson BC, Kingdon E, Johnston M, Tibballs J, Watkinson A, Jarmulowicz M, et al. Transjugular kidney biopsy. Am J Kidney Dis. 2004;43:651–62.
5. Cluzel P, Martinez F, Bellin MF, Michalik Y, Beaufils H, Jouanneau C, et al. Transjugular versus percutaneous renal biopsy for the diagnosis of parenchymal disease: comparison of sampling effectiveness and complications. Radiology. 2000;215:689–93.
6. Abbott KC, Musio FM, Chung EM, Lomis NN, Lane JD, Yuan CM. Transjugular renal biopsy in

high-risk patients: an American case series. BMC Nephrol. 2002;3:5.
7. Sam R, Leehey DJ, Picken MM, Borge MA, Yetter EM, Ing TS, et al. Transjugular renal biopsy in patients with liver disease. Am J Kidney Dis. 2001;37:1144–51.
8. Venkatesan AM, Kundu S, Sacks D, Wallace MJ, Wojak JC, Rose SC, et al. Practice guidelines for adult antibiotic prophylaxis during vascular and interventional radiology procedures. J Vasc Interv Radiol. 2010;21(11):1611–30.
9. Taslakian B, Sebaaly MG, Al-Kutoubi A. Patient evaluation and preparation in vascular and interventional radiology: what every interventional radiologist should know (part 1: patient assessment and laboratory tests). Cardiovasc Intervent Radiol. 2016;39(3):325–33.
10. Taslakian B, Sebaaly MG, Al-Kutoubi A. Patient evaluation and preparation in vascular and interventional radiology: what every interventional radiologist should know (part 2: patient preparation and medications). Cardiovasc Intervent Radiol. 2016;39 (4):489–99. doi: 10.1007/s00270-015-1239-4. [Epub 2015 Nov 25].

Part XVI

Vascular Interventional Procedures: Hepatic Vascular System

Aghiad Al-Kutoubi and Karen T. Brown, Section Reviewers

Transarterial therapies have been used for the past 3–4 decades to treat hepatocellular carcinoma (HCC) and metastatic disease to the liver. Methods of transarterial therapy exploit the dual blood supply to the liver, with the primary trophic blood supply to the liver arising from portal venous blood flow whereas the primary blood supply to tumors, even so-called "hypo-vascular" tumors, arises from the hepatic arteries. This allows a variety of agents to be delivered into the tumor arterial blood supply with relative sparing of the underlying hepatic parenchyma. These methods were originally explored to treat HCC since there was no effective systemic therapy for this tumor, and primitive surgical techniques made hepatic resection untenable in most cases. Most patients with HCC have underlying cirrhosis and thus physicians treating these patients must remember that patients have two diseases, HCC and cirrhosis. The idea is to "kill" the tumor without "killing" the liver.

It is important to recognize that imaging, interventional techniques and tools, systemic chemotherapies, and surgical techniques have evolved in parallel so that indications and outcomes have changed over the years and we understand these methods differently. Indications have evolved so that transarterial treatment may be used in patients who are resectable or transplantable, either as a "test of time" (use a minimally invasive method of controlling disease while waiting to see if other lesions develop) or an effort to maintain the patient on a transplant list. Better imaging and screening protocols allow detection of hepatic disease at earlier stages so that tumors may be treated with "curative" rather than only "palliative" intent. Systemic therapies for metastases from many different primary tumors, in particular colorectal cancer, are more effective and have kept even patients with extra-hepatic disease alive longer, so that we are sometimes asked to treat a single lesion growing in the liver in the face of disease elsewhere that is controlled with systemic therapy. At the same time, these patients have often been exposed to multiple lines of chemotherapy and, as a result, their liver function is not normal. Once again, we are treating patients with two diseases, liver tumor(s) and underlying liver disease.

Each patient is different. It is important to be clear about the indication for the procedure and understand how "success" will be measured. It is important that the patient understands that these treatments are not curative, although they may be able to be repeated if/when hepatic disease progresses. Most importantly, it is important to recognize when these transarterial therapies are unlikely to be helpful, or may even be harmful. We do not use hepatic embolization to treat imaging findings; we use it to treat patients.

In patients with complicated portal hypertension, a thorough knowledge of the indications, contraindications, and limitations of several interventional therapies, and in-depth understanding of individual vascular anatomy and flow dynamics are necessary. Transjugular intrahepatic portosystemic shunt (TIPS) placement has an established role in the management of intractable ascites and recurrent variceal hemorrhage. Venous occlusive disease presents a continuing challenge.

This section provides a comprehensive list of procedural reports that covers the vast majority of image-guided procedures performed in the hepatic vascular system with up-to-date explanatory notes, synopsis of the indications and contraindications, and potential complications in an organized and practical format. In addition, pre- and post-procedure issues are addressed, as well as methods of follow-up.

Section Chapters

Embolization of Hepatic Tumors—Part 1: Bland and Chemoembolization

106

Nadim Muallem

Abbreviations

TAE	Transarterial embolization
TACE	Transarterial chemoembolization
cTACE	Conventional chemoembolization
DEB	Drug-eluting beads
TARE	Transarterial radio-embolization
HCC	Hepatocellular carcinoma
GIST	Gastrointestinal stromal tumors
ECOG	Eastern Cooperative Oncology Group

INTRODUCTION [1, 2]

Transarterial embolization (TAE) is a well-recognized locoregional therapy used in the treatment of primary and secondary liver tumors. Over the years, several different techniques were developed but the basis of therapy remains essentially the same whether the technique consists of TAE, transarterial chemoembolization (TACE), conventional with lipiodol (cTACE), or using drug-eluting beads (DEB-TACE), or transarterial radio-embolization (TARE). Based on fundamental observations by Breedis et al. back in 1954, we know that 80–100 % of hepatic tumor blood supply arises from the hepatic artery, while only 0–20 % of the supply is provided by the portal vein. In contrast, the majority of the trophic blood supply to the normal liver is supplied by the portal vein. This allows for targeting the arterial supply of hepatic tumors ensuring treatment delivery to the tumor while sparing normal liver parenchyma. The pre-procedure preparation and procedural details of these techniques are very similar, with only minor but important differences. In this chapter, we will review the procedural details and notes related to TAE and TACE.

COMMON INDICATIONS [2–6]

Patients considered for embolization should be carefully reviewed by a multidisciplinary team, preferably including a hepatobiliary surgeon,

N. Muallem (✉)
Department of Radiology, Division of Interventional Radiology, Memorial Sloan Kettering Cancer Center, 1275 York Ave, New York, NY 10065, USA
e-mail: nadim.muallem@gmail.com

B. Taslakian et al. (eds.), *Procedural Dictations in Image-Guided Intervention*,
DOI 10.1007/978-3-319-40845-3_106

gastrointestinal oncologist, and interventional oncologist.

- Primary treatment in combination with percutaneous ablation has shown comparable long-term results to partial hepatectomy in Okuda 1 patients with solitary HCC <7 cm [5]
- Prolong patient survival by treatment of unresectable liver tumors, both primary such as in hepatocellular carcinoma (HCC) and secondary, such as in neuroendocrine, gastrointestinal stromal tumors (GIST), certain sarcomas, ocular melanoma, breast, and renal cancer metastases, where the liver is the only site of disease with an appropriate disease free interval. Tumors that are considered the best candidates for TAE are those that are deemed "hypervascular" *(i.e., demonstrate enhancement on the arterial phase acquisition of a CT or MRI).*
- Palliation of symptoms as in hormonally active neuroendocrine metastases [6]
- Bridge to liver transplant by preventing progression outside of Milan criteria
- Downstage patients to allow for resection or to meet transplant criteria

Special considerations:

- In patients with underlying liver disease, Child C patients are not embolized as their survival is determined primarily by underlying liver disease, not tumor
- Eastern Cooperative Oncology Group (ECOG) performance status 0–2

COMMON CONTRAINDICATIONS [2, 3, 7, 8]

Absolute contraindication:

- Decompensated baseline liver function such as in Child C cirrhosis and following constellation of laboratory findings: LDH >425 IU/L, AST >100 IU/L, Bilirubin >2 mg/dL—survival is more likely determined by liver disease
- Cardiac insufficiency, in case of TACE when using cardiotoxic chemotherapeutic agents or significant renal insufficiency

Relative contraindication:

- Patients with well-compensated Child C cirrhosis—selective TACE may be performed but in this case, should be reserved for transplant candidates
- ECOG 3–4
- Asymptomatic metastases with progressive extrahepatic disease—locoregional treatment is unlikely to prolong survival
- Thrombocytopenia in the setting of cirrhosis—can be counteracted with transfusion of 1 unit of platelets
- INR >2—should be corrected
- Treatment of metastatic disease involving more than 75 % of liver best staged with treatment of individual segments or divisions at separate sessions allowing the patient to recover from each treatment session
- Creatinine >1.5 ng/dL—nephroprotective measures can be taken such as adequate hydration before and after the procedure and administration of sodium bicarbonate 1 h before and maintained infusion for 6 h after the procedure
- Contrast allergy—premedicate with 50 mg oral prednisone 13, 8 and 1 h prior to the procedure
- Portal vein tumor—hepatic artery embolization can be performed safely if preserved liver function with collateral flow to the liver
- Elevated bilirubin—if due to obstruction this does not contraindicate hepatic artery embolization. Might consider stent placement first, depending on bilirubin level

POSSIBLE COMPLICATIONS [4, 9–12]

Angiography-related complications: Please refer to Chap. 75.

Procedure-specific complications

- Postembolization syndrome (80 %)—believed to be a type of tumor lysis syndrome, more common following ischemic necrosis of tumor from bland embolization when compared with chemo and radio-embolization. It is characterized by some or all of the following symptoms:

pain, fever, nausea/vomiting, fatigue, hypertension. Symptoms are managed with analgesics, antipyretics, and antiemetics. The acute phase can last 24–72 h with lingering mild symptoms that can take weeks to completely subside. Most patients can be discharged after the acute phase and any residual symptoms can typically be managed conservatively with oral medication on an outpatient basis.

- Nontarget embolization (<10 %)—complications depend on location and include:
  - Gallbladder (most common)—may result in prolonged postembolization syndrome but rarely requires surgical intervention
  - Spleen, pancreas, and stomach are less common; can result in splenic infarct, pancreatitis, or gastric ulcer.
  - Lungs—pulmonary hypertension from particles passing through tumor into hepatic vein and then pulmonary arteries (<1 %). Irreversible pulmonary artery blockade and respiratory failure can occur and is often fatal [11].
- Hepatic abscess/biloma (0.2–4 %)—does not usually occur earlier than 7–10 days post-procedure. It is seen almost exclusively in patients with prior biliary interventions [12] where the sphincter of Oddi has been compromised including bilioenteric anastomosis, sphincterotomy, stent across sphincter, presence of pneumobilia. Risk factors when present may be mitigated by use of prophylactic antibiotics.
- Hepatic infarct or necrosis (2 %)—can be segmental, or sectoral, and are usually associated with underlying portal vein compromise with no collateralization
- Liver failure (<5 %)
- Death—30 day mortality is approximately 1 % as reported by several TAE and TACE studies [4, 9, 10]

PREPROCEDURAL ASSESSMENT AND PLANNING

- History, and physical examination *(Appendix 1* in Chap. 149*)*.
- Evaluation of diagnostic imaging studies (Multiphasic CT, PET-CT, MRI) within 1 month of the procedure to assess indications and radiologically stage the tumor, determine the location of the lesion(s), the relevant arterial anatomy, and develop an embolization strategy. It also serves as a baseline for follow-up.
- Histopathologic diagnosis of the lesion should be generally obtained before the embolization, unless the lesion fulfills clinical diagnostic criteria for HCC or the patient is considered to be at very high risk, in which case biopsy and embolization can be performed concomitantly. Embolization immediately prior to the biopsy has not been shown to affect the pathologic diagnosis and may in fact be protective and decrease any bleeding risk related to the biopsy. Baseline tumor markers in case of HCC can be helpful in assessing response and monitoring for recurrence.
- Periprocedural management of coagulation status *(Appendices 2* in Chap. 150 *and 3* in Chap. 151*)*
- Antibiotic prophylaxis *(Appendices 4* in Chap. 152 *and 5* in Chap. 153*)*: Pre-procedure antibiotic usually tailored to cover skin flora such as cefazolin. However, choice of antibiotic should be changed to cover enteric organisms in patients with compromised biliary sphincters since they have a 300-fold increased risk of intrahepatic abscess formation. Prophylactic antibiotic use before the procedure includes cefotetan which is continued during the hospital stay followed by a 1 week course of metronidazole and ciprofloxacin [13]. Some authors advocate the use of moxifloxacin [14].
- Imaging modality for guidance: High resolution fluoroscopy. Fluoroscopic detectors equipped with cone beam functionality are preferred in order to assess technical success of the treatment. Combined multi-detector CT and flat panel fluoroscopic setup is ideal but not essential.
- Positioning: Supine

- Vascular access: choice of vascular access site is dependent on operator preference. Traditionally, the right femoral artery is catheterized, but embolization through a transradial approach is becoming popular since this allows for immediate ambulation following the procedure [15].
- Pneumatic venous compression stockings and Foley catheterization may be used for prolonged procedure and recovery times where the patient is expected to remain supine throughout

PROCEDURE NOTE

Procedure: Visceral angiography and hepatic artery bland/chemoembolization
Staff: [_]
Fellow: [_]
Resident: [_]
Clinical Information: Specify existing diagnosis; describe history and list indications
Allergies: No known allergic disorders/Allergic to [specify/type of allergy]
Anesthesia and Monitoring: General anesthesia/conscious sedation
Medications: List any relevant medications used (sedation, antibiotics)/specify dose
Contrast Material: (_) mL of [type] nonionic contrast material
Field: Sterile
Procedure classification: Clean, clean-contaminated
Position: Supine
Monitoring: Intravenous access line was secured and vital signs were continuously monitored by nursing staff/anesthesia team throughout the procedure
Total fluoroscopy time: (_) minutes
Cumulative radiation dose: (_) mGy

Description of Procedure:

The risks, benefits, alternatives and procedure itself were explained to the patient/patient's Power of Attorney/patient's legal guardian, and informed written consent was obtained. The site of the procedure was identified and marked. Time out was performed to confirm the correct patient, procedure, and site.

Bilateral lower extremity pulses were evaluated and the skin over where they were best felt was marked immediately prior to the procedure. The patient was placed in supine position on the procedure table. The right/left groin area was prepped and draped in the usual sterile fashion.

Using manual palpation/ultrasound guidance, the right/left common femoral artery and site of puncture were located. Subcutaneous infiltration of local anesthetic was performed using a thin gauge needle and a small skin incision was made at the localized site. Under manual palpation/ultrasound guidance, the right/left common femoral artery was accessed using a single-wall puncture/double-wall puncture/micropuncture needle. The needle was exchanged over guidewire for a (6)-French vascular sheath using the Seldinger technique. The vascular sheath was then connected to a running heparinized saline bag in a pressure infuser. The pressure and rate of infusion was titrated until the infusion line was cleared from the refluxed blood. All additional catheter manipulations and exchanges were subsequently performed over guidewire and through the vascular sheath.

EMBOLIZATION TECHNIQUE

A (5) French [Cobra/Simmons 2/Sos 2] catheter in combination with a hydrophilic glidewire was used for the catheterization of the following vessels: Celiac artery, superior mesenteric artery, common hepatic artery.

A (2.4)-French microcatheter was used coaxially via the (5)-French catheter in combination with a single angle/double angle/shapeable tip microwire for the superselective catheterization of the following vessels: Anterior and posterior divisions of the right hepatic artery, left hepatic artery, segment 4 artery, phrenic artery, falciform artery.

Catheter positions and pre-embolization angiographic imaging: Angiography was performed in the right common femoral artery,

Celiac artery, superior mesenteric artery, common hepatic artery, right/left hepatic artery, selective branches, segment 4 artery, etc…

Embolization catheter positions: Embolization was performed in the anterior division of the right hepatic artery/segment 3 branch of the left hepatic artery, etc.

Embolization was performed using bland particles/Oil-Based emulsion/Drug-eluting beads/combination of oil-based emulsion and bland particles/combination of drug-eluting beads and bland particles

Embolization material: It is important to mention volume of material delivered and size of particles as well as brand/type used. e.g., 1–10 ml, 40–120/100–300 micron of Embospheres/Bead Block/Embozene/LC Bead/Oncozene/Hepaspheres/PVA (Bland) or Emulsion of Lipiodol/Ethiodol and doxorubicin/epirubicin/cisplatin/oxaliplatin (Oil-based emulsion) or LC/DC Bead/Oncozene/Hepaspheres (drug-eluting beads)

Catheter positions and postembolization angiographic imaging: Right hepatic artery, common hepatic artery, celiac artery, etc…

CT performed: Yes/No [specify findings]

Groin Hemostasis: Manual Compression/[-type] vascular closure device

Brachial/radial hemostasis: Manual compression for (_) minutes

Intra-Procedure Findings: List all relevant findings.

- The hepatic arterial anatomy was evaluated with conventional digital subtraction angiography/3D rotational angiography/CT angiography performed at the level of the celiac artery/CHA/SMA/PHA/RHA/LHA/Gastric artery/etc…
- Pre-embolization angiography demonstrated conventional hepatic arterial anatomy/variant hepatic arterial anatomy consisting of replaced/accessory left/right hepatic artery/extrahepatic vascular supply/extrahepatic shunting/etc…
- Replaced/accessory right/left hepatic/extrahepatic vasculature originated from the SMA/left gastric artery/right phrenic artery/right renal artery/intercostal artery/etc…
- Digital subtraction angiography performed at the level of the SMA/splenic artery with delayed image acquisition demonstrates a patent portal vein with hepatopetal/hepatofugal/mixed flow.
- Tumor supply: Vascular supply to the tumor was seen to arise from the right/left hepatic arteries/phrenic arteries/intercostal arteries/left gastric replaced/accessory hepatic artery/etc…
- Postembolization findings: Following particle embolization/drug-eluting bead embolization/chemoembolization, stasis was achieved in the right/left hepatic artery/selective branch/replaced branch/etc… Blood flow to the remainder of the vessels including the common hepatic artery, cystic artery, gastroduodenal artery, left gastric artery, SMA, celiac artery was preserved.
- Post-procedural CT scan (if performed) demonstrates static contrast material deposited throughout the tumor(s) in segment(s) 1–8.
- Distal pulse examination was unchanged compared to pre-procedure.

Immediate Complications: None encountered during or directly after the procedure. List complications if any.

Post-Procedure Plan

Assuming successful procedure with no evidence of bleeding/dissection/desaturation:

- Transfer patient to recovery unit and plan for potential admission for management of postembolization syndrome and monitoring of liver function tests.
- Observe in recovery unit for 1–4 h with continuous vital signs and pulse oximeter monitoring.
- Complete bedrest ×4 h and clear liquids only for the duration of observation.
- Maintain patient in supine position with right/left leg straight 1–4 h depending on whether a vascular closure device was used and whether it was successfully deployed with observation of puncture site for signs of

bleeding/hematoma every 15 min × 1 h then every 30 min × 1 h then every 1 h × 2 h.

- Post-procedure pain control as needed *(consider starting patient controlled analgesia as soon as patient gets to the recovery unit).*
- Administer supplemental nasal oxygen as needed *(O_2 saturation less than baseline/patient still sedated).*
- Administer post procedural antibiotics only if there has been prior bilioenteric anastomosis or biliary interventions, because of the increased risk of infection. Continued oral antibiotics for up to 10 days are believed to be helpful.
- If the patient's condition deteriorates during recovery, depending on symptoms, hepatic infarct, bleeding, pancreatitis, nontarget embolization, and pulmonary aspiration should be considered and appropriate imaging obtained immediately. Do not disregard other potential complications as well. Hepatic abscess typically occurs 7–10 days following procedure, not in immediate post-procedure time period.
- If the patient experiences little or no postembolization syndrome, and pain, if present, is controlled with oral analgesics, it is possible for the patient to be discharged home the same day as long as his liver function tests are repeated within the following week. If not, the patient will be admitted to the inpatient service with standing orders of analgesics or patient controlled analgesia using morphine, hydromorphone, meperidine, or fentanyl if needed and transition slowly to oral analgesics once oral intake of solid food is tolerated.
- Discharge home once the patient is able to tolerate oral intake, oral analgesics, and moving bowels.
- Discharge instructions:
  - Abstain from strenuous activities for 3 days.
  - Call the Interventional oncologist who performed the procedure for fever, chills, or worsening pain not controlled by oral medication.
  - Start clear liquid diet after discharge from observation, then slowly advances diet thereafter if tolerated and no complications occur.
  - Take prescribed pain medications as needed and take prescribed antibiotic medications as prescribed (only for patients with contaminated biliary tree).
- Follow-up imaging [16]:
  - Obtain first follow-up multiphase contrast-enhanced CT scan or MRI within 1–3 months of the procedure.
  - Most surveillance schedules suggest follow-up imaging every 3 months for the first 2 years for patients with HCC.
  - Similar follow-up protocols could be designed to monitor recurrences for other tumors types. Including the baseline scan, the optimal schedule for HCC suggested by one study would be 2, 4, 6, 8, 11, 14, 18, and 24 months.

Impression:

- Bland particle/Chemo/Drug-eluting bead embolization of [specify location/segment/lobe] tumor via the right/left/accessory/replaced/branch hepatic artery with delivery of a total of [specify volume, type, and size of embolic used].
- The patient tolerated the procedure well and left the interventional unit in a stable condition.
- List any other relevant or important information/finding.
- The primary operator [specify name] was present for the entire/key parts of the procedure.

References

1. Breedis C, Young G. The blood supply of neoplasms in the liver. Am J Pathol. 1954;30(5):969–77.
2. Kritzinger J, Klass D, Ho S, Lim H, Buczkowski A, Yoshida E, et al. Hepatic embolotherapy in interventional oncology: technology, techniques, and applications. Clin Radiol. 2013;68(1):1–15.
3. Brown KT. Bland embolization for hepatic malignancies. In: Mauro MA, Murphy KPJ, Thomson KR, Venbrux AC, Morgan RA, editors. Image-guided interventions. 2nd ed. Philadelphia: Saunders Elsevier; 2014. p. 467–75.
4. Brown DB, Geschwind J-FH, Soulen MC, Millward SF, Sacks D. Society of interventional radiology

position statement on chemoembolization of hepatic malignancies. J Vasc Interv Radiol. 2006;17(2 Pt 1):217–23.
5. Elnekave E, Erinjeri JP, Brown KT, Thornton RH, Petre EN, Maybody M, et al. Long-term outcomes comparing surgery to embolization-ablation for treatment of solitary HCC < 7 cm. Ann Surg Oncol. 2013;20:2881–6.
6. Brown KT, Koh BY, Brody LA, Getrajdman GI, Susman J, Fong Y, et al. Particle embolization of hepatic neuroendocrine metastases for control of pain and hormonal symptoms. J Vasc Interv Radiol. 1999;10(4):397–403.
7. Sofocleous CT, Aguado AS. Embolotherapy for the management of liver malignancies other than hepatocellular carcinoma. In: Mauro MA, Murphy KPJ, Thomson KR, Venbrux AC, Morgan RA, editors. Image-guided interventions. 2nd ed. Philadelphia: Saunders Elsevier; 2014. p. 450–9.
8. Soulen MC. Chemoembolization for hepatocellular carcinoma. I. In: Mauro MA, Murphy KPJ, Thomson KR, Venbrux AC, Morgan RA, editors. Image-guided interventions. 2nd ed. Philadelphia: Saunders Elsevier; 2014. p. 436–40.
9. Maluccio MA, Covey AM, Porat LB, Schubert J, Brody LA, Sofocleous CT, et al. Transcatheter arterial embolization with only particles for the treatment of unresectable hepatocellular carcinoma. J Vasc Interv Radiol. 2008;19(6):862–9.
10. Llovet JM, Real MI, Montaña X, Planas R, Coll S, Aponte J, et al. Arterial embolisation or chemoembolisation versus symptomatic treatment in patients with unresectable hepatocellular carcinoma: a randomised controlled trial. Lancet. 2002;359(9319):1734–9.
11. Brown KT. Fatal pulmonary complications after arterial embolization with 40–120-micro m tris-acryl gelatin microspheres. J Vasc Interv Radiol. 2004;15(2 Pt 1):197–200.
12. Woo S, Chung JW, Hur S, Joo SM, Kim HC, Jae HJ, et al. Liver abscess after transarterial chemoembolization in patients with bilioenteric anastomosis: frequency and risk factors. AJR Am J Roentgenol. 2013;200(6):1370–7.
13. Venkatesan AM, Kundu S, Sacks D, Wallace MJ, Wojak JC, Rose SC, et al. Practice guideline for adult antibiotic prophylaxis during vascular and interventional radiology procedures. J Vasc Interv Radiol. 2010;21(11):1611–30.
14. Khan W, Sullivan KL, McCann JW, Gonsalves CF, Sato T, Eschelman DJ, et al. Moxifloxacin prophylaxis for chemoembolization or embolization in patients with previous biliary interventions: a pilot study. AJR Am J Roentgenol. 2011;197(2):W343–5.
15. Fischman AM, Swinburne NC, Patel RS. A technical guide describing the use of transradial access technique for endovascular interventions. Tech Vasc Interv Radiol. 2015;18(2):58–65.
16. Boas FE, Do B, Louie JD, Kothary N, Hwang GL, Kuo WT, et al. Optimal imaging surveillance schedules after liver-directed therapy for hepatocellular carcinoma. J Vasc Interv Radiol. 2015;26(1):69–73.

Embolization of Hepatic Tumors—Part 2: Radioembolization

107

Nadim Muallem

Abbreviations

TARE	Transarterial radioembolization
TAE	Transarterial embolization
cTACE	Conventional transarterial chemoembolization
DEB-TACE	Drug eluting bead chemoembolization
HCC	Hepatocellular carcinoma
LSF	Lung shunt fraction
RILD	Radioembolization-induced liver disease

INTRODUCTION [1]

Transarterial radioembolization (TARE) is a transarterial therapy used in the treatment of primary and secondary liver tumors that is growing in popularity for a variety of reasons. Unlike transarterial embolization (TAE) and conventional transarterial chemoembolization (cTACE) or drug eluting bead chemoemboliza-tion (DEB-TACE), although delivered via the hepatic artery, the therapeutic effect is not embolic, but results instead from the delivery of internal radiation in the form of Yttrium 90. Essentially, targeting the arterial supply of hepatic tumors ensures the deposition of radioactive particles into the tumor resulting in a high local dose of radiation-a form of brachytherapy. The tumoricidal effect of the treatment agent is mediated through direct radiation injury [2]. Since complications of radiation exposure to nontarget organs are difficult to treat and can be fatal, dosimetry needs to be performed, and lung shunt fraction (LSF) calculated, therefore, TARE is typically performed in two stages. The first stage consists of a pretreatment mapping arteriogram which involves a careful and aggressive search for hepatic artery branches that supply nontarget organs (e.g., the right gastric artery) and these vessels are coil occluded. At the same time, unification of hepatic blood flow can be effected by occluding any accessory hepatic vessels. Once this is completed Tc99m-MAA radiotracer is injected in the vessel to be treated, simulating patient dose delivery and allowing for calculation of LSF, as well as confirming the

N. Muallem (✉)
Department of Radiology, Division of Interventional Radiology, Memorial Sloan Kettering Cancer Center, 1275 York Ave, New York, NY 10065, USA
e-mail: nadim.muallem@gmail.com

B. Taslakian et al. (eds.), *Procedural Dictations in Image-Guided Intervention*,
DOI 10.1007/978-3-319-40845-3_107

absence of flow to nontarget organs. Based on this initial procedure the Yttrium-90 dose is calculated and prepared. The second stage occurs within a few weeks, delivering the prepared radioembolic dose in the vessel that was previously prepared and mapped. Should any extrahepatic perfusion or a collateral vessel be identified either during the SPECT-CT or during the second stage of the procedure, the vessel supplying extrahepatic flow can be embolized at that time, immediately prior to dose delivery. Ideally, a TARE procedure is performed in collaboration with a nuclear medicine specialist. The most commonly used radioembolic agents in the United States both carry Yttrium-90. One, SIR-spheres (Sirtex Medical INC, Woburn MA, USA), is resin based and approved for the treatment of unresectable colorectal hepatic metastases. The other, TheraSphere (Biocompatibles, UK Ltd) is glass based, and approved by the FDA under a Humanitarian Device Exemption (HDE) for treatment of primary liver cancer.

COMMON INDICATIONS [3–6]

Patient selection for embolization should be carefully reviewed by a multidisciplinary team, preferably including a hepatobiliary surgeon, gastrointestinal oncologist, and interventional oncologist.

- Primary treatment of potentially resectable solitary tumors in patients who are not surgical candidates, or in the case of hepatocellular carcinoma (HCC), as a bridge to transplant
- Treatment of unresectable primary HCC as well as cholangiocarcinoma and metastatic tumors such as colorectal metastases in patients who have failed conventional chemotherapy, in an effort to prolong overall survival
- Palliation of symptoms, as in hormonally active neuroendocrine metastases
- In an attempt to downstage patient with HCC to transplant

COMMON CONTRAINDICATIONS [1, 7, 8]

Prior to mapping angiography:

- Decompensated baseline liver function such as in Child C cirrhosis and elevated liver function tests (AST, ALT, alkaline phosphatase > 5 × normal limit and baseline bilirubin > 2 mg/dL)—patients are at high risk of developing radiation induced liver injury
- Eastern Cooperative Oncology Group (ECOG) performance score 3–4
- Large tumor burden—more than 70 % of liver replaced with adequate albumin level or more than 50 % of liver replaced and albumin level < 3 g/dL
- Significant extrahepatic disease
- Compromised pulmonary function—increased risk of radiation pneumonitis
- Prior external beam radiation therapy
- Prior chemotherapy or TACE within 2 months of planned treatment
- Renal insufficiency—Creatinine > 2 mg/dL
- Untreated coagulopathy
- Contrast allergy—premedicate with 50 mg prednisone 13, 8 and 1 h prior to the procedure

At the time of mapping angiography any of the following contraindications may be discovered:

- Increased hepatopulmonary shunting with lung shunt fraction >20 %
- Uncorrectable perfusion of extrahepatic regions
- Predicted treatment dose >30 Gy from a single treatment session or >50 Gy of accumulated dose to be delivered to the lungs

POSSIBLE COMPLICATIONS [1, 7, 9]

Complications similar to those encountered with TAE and TACE are also seen following TARE due to similar technique of vascular access, catheterization and delivery of particles. The difference lies in the fact that the primary mechanism of action in TARE is caused by radiation exposure and with minimal embolic or ischemic effects from the particles.

Angiography-related complications: Please refer to Chap. 75.

Procedure-related complications:

- Postembolization syndrome, when it occurs (20–70 %)—is a much milder form than what is encountered from bland and chemoembolization. This is likely because tumor death and necrosis occur over a more prolonged period of time, and as a result the tumor-lysis effect is not as pronounced. The constellation of symptoms that may occur include fever, nausea, vomiting, fatigue, abdominal pain, and discomfort but in contrast to TAE and TACE, hospitalization is rarely required and recovery is much faster.
- Biliary complications (<10 %) can occur, related to the embolic effect of the microspheres, similar to what is seen after TAE and TACE but compounded by radiation induced injury to the biliary system. Other potential complications include radiation cholecystitis (minimized by temporary or permanent cystic artery embolization [10]), and radiation-induced cholangitis in addition to abscesses and biloma formation.
- Risk of liver abscess is increased in patients with prior biliary interventions where the sphincter or ampulla has been compromised resulting in a contaminated biliary tree. Prior interventions include bilioenteric anastomosis, sphincterotomy, and stent across sphincter or presence of pneumobilia. Use of antibiotics in these circumstances is advocated.
- Non-target radioembolization is the most feared complication from TARE as it frequently results in irreversible radiation injury to nontarget organs. This can be avoided by careful pre-embolization mapping angiography and aggressive prophylactic embolization of extrahepatic collaterals and parasitized vasculature. Potential nontarget radiation complications include:
  - Intractable gastrointestinal ulcers (<5 %) refractory to medical therapy
  - Radioembolization induced liver disease (RILD) (0–4 %)—results from exposure of normal liver parenchyma to radiation, the embolic effect of the microspheres being negligible. Risk is increased in patients with poor baseline liver function, baseline bilirubin >2 mg/dL, prior treatment with chemotherapy, or either intra-arterial chemo-infusion or TACE within 2 months, whole liver TARE and sequential treatment with TARE in an interval less than 6 weeks. Risk can be mitigated by avoiding whole liver treatments and sparing as much normal liver as possible by sequential superselective treatments at intervals of 6 weeks.
  - Radiation pneumonitis (<1 %)—results from excessive exposure of normal pulmonary parenchyma to radiation. It is for that reason that LSF is calculated and cumulative radiation dose is kept below 50 Gy in multiple treatments and below 30 Gy in one treatment. In the event of LSF between 10 and 20 %, the delivered dose can be reduced to minimize the risk of pneumonitis. A lung shunt fraction above 20 % is a contraindication to TARE due to the high risk of radiation pneumonitis. Treatment may involve steroid administration [8].
- Death—30 day mortality has been reported as 2–3 % by several studies. This can be further decreased by appropriate patient selection since in most cases, and with the proper precautions, TARE-related toxicities can be kept to a minimum [5, 11].

PREPROCEDURAL ASSESSMENT AND PLANNING [1, 12, 13]

- History, indications, and physical examination *(Appendix 1* in Chap. 149*)*
- Evaluation of diagnostic imaging studies (Multiphase CT, PET-CT, MRI) is crucial to assess indications and radiologically stage the tumor, and to determine the location of the lesion, the relevant anatomy, and develop a treatment strategy. It also serves as a baseline for follow-up.
- Histopathologic diagnosis of the lesion should be sought before the embolization if there is any doubt about the diagnosis. In the appropriate clinical scenario when lesion(s) fulfill imaging criteria for HCC or when patients with known malignancy develop new lesions typical for metastases, biopsy is probably not warranted. Baseline tumor markers in case of HCC can be helpful in both assessing response and monitoring for recurrence.
- Periprocedural management of coagulation status *(Appendices 2* in Chap. 150 *and 3* in Chap. 151*)*
- Antibiotic prophylaxis: Pre-procedure antibiotic usually tailored to cover skin flora such as Cefazolin. However, choice of antibiotic should be changed to cover enteric organisms in patients with compromised biliary sphincters, particularly during the treatment stage or radioembolization, since they are at increased risk of developing intrahepatic abscess formation. Prophylactic antibiotic use before the procedure includes Cefotetan which is continued during their hospital stay followed by a 1 week course of metronidazole and ciprofloxacin.
- Imaging modality for guidance: High resolution fluoroscopy. Fluoroscopic detectors equipped with cone beam CT or rotational angiography functionality can improve detection of vessels supplying the tumor. A SPECT-CT should be performed immediately following angiographic mapping and injection of Tc99m-MAA radiotracer in order to calculate Yttrium-90 dose and assess LSF. A SPECT-CT should also be performed following Yttrium-90 dose delivery to assess for proper deposition within the liver tumor and exclude nontarget radioembolization.
- Positioning: Supine
- Vascular access: choice of site is dependent on operator preference. Traditionally, the right femoral artery is catheterized, but embolization through a transradial approach [14] is becoming popular since as it allows for immediate ambulation following the procedure.
- Pneumatic venous compression may be used for prolonged procedure and recovery times where the patient is expected to remain supine throughout.
- Since Y90 is excreted in the urine, Foley catheters are recommended (and mandatory at many institutions) to prevent radiation spillage until the patients are able to void normally.

PROCEDURE NOTE [15, 16]

The procedure note for the pretreatment mapping angiography closely follows that of the treatment angiography—as well it should—since the radioembolization should closely if not identically reproduce the findings of a successful mapping procedure.

The overall structure remains the same and most details are relevant to both procedures with key differences highlighted by a single asterisk sign [*] to indicate information relevant to the mapping angiography and a double asterisk sign [**] to indicate what should be included in the radioembolization or treatment procedure note.

Procedure:

[*] Mapping visceral angiography and selective coil embolization and radiotracer injection.

[**] Visceral angiography and hepatic artery radioembolization

Clinical Information: Specify existing diagnosis, describe history, and list indications

Staff: [_]

Fellow: [_]
Resident: [_]
Allergies: No known allergic disorders/Allergic to [specify/type of allergy]
Anesthesia and Monitoring: General anesthesia/conscious sedation
Medications: List any relevant medications used (sedation, antibiotics)/specify dose
Contrast Material: (_) mL of [type] nonionic contrast material
Field: Sterile
Procedure classification: Clean
Position: Supine
Monitoring: Intravenous access line was secured and vital signs were continuously monitored by nursing staff/anesthesia team throughout the procedure
[*] **Radiotracer:** (_) mCi of Tc-99m MAA
[**] **Radioembolic dose administered:** (_) mCi Yttrium-90 SIRspheres/Theraspheres
Total fluoroscopy time: (_) minutes
Cumulative radiation dose: (_) mGy

Description of Procedure:
The risks, benefits, alternatives, and procedure itself were explained to the patient/patient's Power of Attorney/patient's legal guardian, and informed written consent was obtained. The site of the procedure was identified and marked. Time out was performed to confirm the correct patient, procedure, and site.

Using manual palpation/ultrasound guidance, the right/left common femoral artery and site of puncture were located. The relationship to the right/left femoral head was determined using fluoroscopy. Subcutaneous infiltration of local anesthetic was performed using a thin gauge needle and a small skin incision was made at the localized site. Under manual palpation/ultrasound guidance, the right/left common femoral artery was accessed using a single-wall puncture/double-wall puncture/micropuncture needle. The needle was exchanged over guide-wire for a (_)-French vascular sheath using the Seldinger technique. The vascular sheath was then connected to heparinized saline in a pressure infuser. The pressure and rate of infusion of the heparinized saline was titrated until the infusion line was cleared. All additional catheter manipulations and exchanges were subsequently performed over guide-wire and through the vascular sheath.

ANGIOGRAPHIC AND EMBOLIZATION TECHNIQUE

A (5)-French Cobra/Simmons 2/Sos 2 catheter in combination with a hydrophilic glide-wire was used for the catheterization of the following vessels: Celiac artery, superior mesenteric artery, common hepatic artery.

A (2.4) French microcatheter was used coaxially via the (5)-French catheter in combination with a single angle/double angle/shapeable tip microwire for the superselective catheterization of the following vessels: Anterior and posterior divisions of the right hepatic artery; left hepatic artery, segment 4 artery, falciform artery.

Catheter positions and angiographic imaging: Angiography was performed in the right common femoral artery, Celiac artery, superior mesenteric artery, common hepatic artery, right/left hepatic artery, selective branches, segment 4 artery, etc…

Following evaluation of the hepatic arterial anatomy, no embolization was required/coil embolization was performed of extrahepatic directed artery/of accessory artery to correct intrahepatic flow.

Embolization materials and vessels embolized: It is important to mention number/type/length of coils used, e.g., one 2 mm × 3 mm Nester microcoil, two 5 mm figure of eight microcoils were delivered in the GDA/falciform artery/right inferior phrenic artery/accessory hepatic artery/etc…

Catheter positions and postembolization angiographic imaging: Right hepatic artery, common hepatic artery, celiac artery, etc…

[**] (Although unusual, if additional collaterals or vessels with extrahepatic course are detected on the treatment angiography, then completion or repeat embolization can be performed prior to Yttrium-90 administration, in which case, details should be noted as in the preceding example)

[*] Once the location of the desired future administration of Yttrium-90 was decided, the microcatheter was positioned in the targeted location and selective administration of Tc-99m MAA radiotracer was performed as follows:

[*] Catheter position and tracer administration: 2.3 mCi in the proximal right hepatic artery; 2.3 mCi in the proximal left hepatic artery.

[**] The planned location of radioembolic delivery was again selected and the Yttrium-90 spheres, delivery blocks, and delivery set were prepared in standard fashion corresponding to the manufacturer's instructions. In conjunction with a Nuclear Medicine specialist, the prepared dose of radioactive microspheres were administered in multiple small aliquots into the hepatic tumor bed with repeatedly monitored flow by contrast injection.

[**] Catheter position and Yttrium-90 radioembolic administration: 16 mCi in the proximal right hepatic artery; 14 mCi in the proximal left hepatic artery

[**] Subsequently all contaminated catheters and material were removed and disposed of in compliance with local/national radiation safety measures.

Groin Hemostasis: Manual Compression/[-type] vascular closure device

Brachial/Radial hemostasis: Manual compression for (_) minutes

[*] The patient was then transferred to the scintigraphic imaging suite and a SPECT-CT was performed for evaluation of Lung-Shunt Fraction and calculation of radioembolic treatment dose. Findings of the scintigraphic imaging will be reported separately.

[**] The patient was then transferred to the scintigraphic imaging suite and a SPECT-CT was performed for evaluation of treatment delivery. Findings of the scintigraphic imaging will be reported separately.

Intra-Procedure Findings: List all relevant findings.

- Digital subtraction angiography demonstrated [*] conventional hepatic arterial anatomy/variant hepatic arterial anatomy consisting of replaced/accessory left/right hepatic artery/extrahepatic vascular supply/extrahepatic shunting/etc…//[**] no change in hepatic arterial anatomy from the mapping angiography performed on (Date)/persistent occlusion of extrahepatic directed arteries following embolization during pretreatment and mapping angiography/satisfactory internal collateralization of tumor vascular supply following embolization of extrahepatic collateral for flow redirection.
- Tumor supply: [*] Vascular supply to the tumor was seen to arise from the right/left hepatic arteries/phrenic arteries/intercostal arteries/left gastric replaced/accessory hepatic artery/etc.… [**] Vascular supply to the tumor remains unchanged from the mapping study/redirected supply is seen from intrahepatic collaterals
- [*] Extrahepatic directed vessels identified requiring embolization: None/GDA/right gastric artery/falciform artery/etc.…
- [*] Collateral tumor supply/variant anatomy requiring flow redirection: None/Right inferior phrenic artery/replaced hepatic artery/accessory hepatic artery/etc…
- [**] Additional extrahepatic directed vessels identified requiring embolization: None/falciform artery/etc…
- [**] Additional collateral tumor supply/variant anatomy requiring flow redirection: None/Right inferior phrenic artery/etc…
- Digital subtraction angiography performed at the level of the SMA/splenic artery with delayed image acquisition demonstrates a patent portal vein with hepatopetal flow.
- Postembolization findings (if performed): Following embolization, there was complete cessation of extrahepatic/collateral flow. The rest of the vessels including the common hepatic artery, SMA, celiac artery, etc… remain widely patent.
- [*] Treatment plan and desired location of radioembolic administration and current location radiotracer administration: Proximal left hepatic artery and proximal right hepatic

artery/proximal left hepatic artery with additional treatment to the right side planned after treatment of the left lobe.

- [**] Location of radioembolic administration: Proximal left hepatic artery and proximal right hepatic artery/proximal left hepatic artery with additional treatment to the right side planned after treatment of the left lobe.
- Distal pulse examination was unchanged compared to pre-procedure.

Immediate Complications: None encountered during or directly after the procedure. List complications if any.

Post-Procedure Plan

Assuming successful procedure with no evidence of bleeding/dissection/desaturation:

- Transfer patient to the scintigraphic imaging suite and then to the recovery unit and plan for discharge (This applies for both mapping angiography and radioembolization since in the latter, postembolization syndrome is relatively mild and most patient go home the same day).
- Observe in recovery unit for 1–4 h with continuous vital signs and pulse oximeter monitoring and IV fluids at 75–100 mL/h
- Complete bed rest ×2–4 h with clear liquids allowed when patient is awake and alert.
- Maintain patient in supine position with right/left leg straight 1–4 h depending on whether a vascular closure device was used and whether it was successfully deployed with observation of puncture site for signs of bleeding/hematoma q15 min × 1 h then q30 min × 1 h then q1 h × 2 h.
- Check pedal pulses q30 min × 2 h.
- Post-procedure pain control is often not required or limited to mild analgesics in mapping angiography, and usually, oral analgesics are sufficient to control most pain symptoms following radioembolization.
- Administer supplemental nasal oxygen as needed (O_2 saturation less than baseline/patient still sedated…)

[**] For radioembolization, the following additional instructions apply:

- Most serious complications from radiation induced injury following radioembolization are delayed. If the patient's condition was to deteriorate during recovery (which would be quite unusual), things such as oversedation, puncture site bleeding, nontarget embolization, and aspiration should all be considered and appropriate imaging obtained to assess.
- Patients typically experience little or no postembolization syndrome and can be discharged home the same day. Patients rarely experience symptoms requiring overnight admission such as pain, nausea, or urinary retention, but typically recover quickly and are discharged the following day.
- *Discharge instructions*
  - Abstain from strenuous activities for 3 days.
  - Call the Interventional Radiologist who treated patient for fevers, chills, shortness of breath, severe fatigue, or worsening pain not controlled by PO medication.
  - Take prescribed pain medications as needed.
  - Take prescribed antibiotic medications as prescribed (only for patients with contaminated biliary tree).
- *Follow-up imaging*
  - [*] For mapping angiography, if SPECT-CT and treatment dose calculation fulfills the safety criteria for administration of radioembolics, then radioembolization should be performed within the next 1–4 weeks.
  - [**] Following radioembolization, immediate postembolization SPECT-CT is performed to confirm radioembolic deposition within the tumor and to exclude non-target embolization.
  - Standard follow-up imaging schedules apply, with baseline triphasic contrast-enhanced CT scan or MRI within 1–3 months after the procedure.

Follow-up with imaging (Multiphase CT/MRI or PET/CT) every 3 months for the first 2 years. Scheduling can be optimized based on tumor type and imaging modality [17].

Impression:

- Hepatic angiography demonstrates standard hepatic arterial anatomy with no extrahepatic directed artery or collateral vascular supply to the tumor/variant anatomy/collateral tumor supply from accessory left hepatic artery/extrahepatic directed flow from the gastroduodenal/etc.
- Coil embolization was not needed/was performed with successful occlusion of gastroduodenal/phrenic artery/accessory hepatic artery/etc…
- [*] Treatment was planned and Technetium-99m MAA radiotracer was administered in the*: target vessel (name).*
- [**] Successful radioembolization with Yttrium-90 microspheres administered in the target vessel (name).
- The patient tolerated the procedure well and left the interventional unit in a stable condition.
- List any other relevant or important information/finding.
- The primary operator (specify Dr name) was present for the entire/key parts of the procedure.

References

1. Denys A, Pracht M, Duran R, Guiu B, Adib S, Boubaker A, et al. How to prepare a patient for transarterial radioembolization? A practical guide. Cardiovasc Interv Radiol. 2015;38:794–805.
2. Wang LM, Jani AR, Hill EJ, Sharma RA. Anatomical basis and histopathological changes resulting from selective internal radiotherapy for liver metastases. J Clin Pathol. 2013;66:205–11.
3. Murthy R, Nunez R, Szklaruk J, et al. Yttrium-90 microsphere therapy for hepatic malignancy: devices, indications, technical considerations, and potential complications. Radiographics. 2005;25(Suppl 1):S41–55.
4. Geschwind J-FH, Salem R, Carr BI, et al. Yttrium-90 microspheres for the treatment of hepatocellular carcinoma. Gastroenterology. 2004;127(5 Suppl 1):S194–205.
5. Saxena A, Meteling B, Kapoor J, Golani S, Morris DL, Bester L. Is yttrium-90 radioembolization a viable treatment option for unresectable, chemorefractory colorectal cancer liver metastases? A large single-center experience of 302 patients. Ann Surg Oncol. 2015;22(3):794–802.
6. Hyder O, Marsh JW, Salem R, et al. Intra-arterial therapy for advanced intrahepatic cholangiocarcinoma: a multi-institutional analysis. Ann Surg Oncol. 2013;20(12):3779–86.
7. Riaz A, Lewandowski RJ, Kulik LM, et al. Complications following radioembolization with Yttrium-90 microspheres: a comprehensive literature review. J Vasc Interv Radiol. 2009;20(9):1121–30.
8. Wright CL, Werner JD, Tran JM, et al. Radiation pneumonitis following Yttrium-90 radioembolization: case report and literature review. J Vasc Interv Radiol. 2012;23(5):669–74.
9. Salem R, Thurston KG. Radioembolization with 90 Yttrium microspheres: a state-of-the-art brachytherapy treatment for primary and secondary liver malignancies. Part 2: special topics. J Vasc Interv Radiol. 2006;17:1425–39.
10. Theysohn JM, Müller S, Schlaak JF, et al. Selective internal radiotherapy (SIRT) of hepatic tumors: how to deal with the cystic artery. Cardiovasc Interv Radiol. 2013;36(4):1015–22. doi:10.1007/s00270-012-0474-1.
11. Salem R, Lewandowski RJ, Mulcahy MF, et al. Radioembolization for hepatocellular carcinoma using Yttrium-90 microspheres: a comprehensive report of long-term outcomes. Gastroenterology. 2010;138(1):52–64.
12. Kim W, Clark TW, Baum RA, Soulen MC. Risk factors for liver abscess formation after hepatic chemoembolization. J Vasc Interv Radiol. 2001;12(8):965–8.
13. Venkatesan AM, Kundu S, Sacks D, et al. Practice guideline for adult antibiotic prophylaxis during vascular and interventional radiology procedures. J Vasc Interv Radiol. 2010;21(11):1611–30.
14. Fischman AM, Swinburne NC, Patel RS. A technical guide describing the use of transradial access technique for endovascular interventions. Tech Vasc Interv Radiol. 2015;18(2):58–65.
15. Salem R, Lewandowski RJ, Gates VL, et al. Research reporting standards for radioembolization of hepatic malignancies. J Vasc Interv Radiol. 2011;22(3):265–78.
16. Brown DB, Gould JE, Gervais DA, et al. Transcatheter therapy for hepatic malignancy: standardization of terminology and reporting criteria. J Vasc Interv Radiol. 2007;18(12):1469–78.
17. Boas FE, Do B, Louie JD, et al. Optimal imaging surveillance schedules after liver-directed therapy for hepatocellular carcinoma. J Vasc Interv Radiol. 2015;26(1):69–73.

108 Embolization of the Hepatic Artery in Traumatic Liver Injury

Amy Deipolyi and Bedros Taslakian

INTRODUCTION

During the past decade, there has been a major shift in the management of blunt liver trauma toward endovascular management, attributed to the use of helical computed tomography (CT) in the diagnosis and grading of liver trauma. The most widely used CT-based grading system for blunt hepatic injury is the one established by the American Association for the Surgery of Trauma (AAST).

COMMON INDICATIONS [1–5]

Penetrating hepatic trauma:

- Evidence of recurrent hemorrhage following surgical management
- Focal penetrating wounds isolated to the liver, with absence of signs and symptoms of peritonitis or bowel injury

Blunt hepatic trauma:

- Imaging evidence of contrast material extravasation within the liver, along the hepatic capsule or into the peritoneum
- Evidence of recurrent hemorrhage following initial surgical management
- Evidence of recurrent hemorrhage following initial successful embolization
- Patients with liver laceration or hematoma and evidence of continuous hemorrhage *(e.g., patient remains hemodynamically unstable after adequate resuscitation or greater than 4 units of packed red blood cell transfusion requirements over 24 h)*
- Posttraumatic hepatic pseudoaneurysm, arteriovenous fistulas, arterioportal fistulas *(because of their relatively high risk of delayed bleeding)*
- Posttraumatic arteriobiliary fistula causing persistent hemobilia *(biliary colic, gastrointestinal bleeding, and obstructive jaundice)*
- Hemodynamically stable patient with CT grade 4 or 5 liver injury associated with major hepatic vascular involvement *(angiography is recommended)*

COMMON CONTRAINDICATIONS [1, 2, 5]

Absolute contraindications:

- Hemodynamic instability despite adequate resuscitation, requiring emergent surgical exploration
- Associated injuries such as bowel perforation, requiring emergent surgical exploration

A. Deipolyi (✉)
Department of Radiology, Division of Interventional Radiology, Memorial Sloan Kettering Cancer Center, 1275 York Ave, New York, NY 10065, USA
e-mail: amy.deipolyi@nyumc.org

B. Taslakian
Department of Radiology, New York University Langone Medical Center, 660 First Ave, New York, NY 10016, USA
e-mail: btaslakian@gmail.com

B. Taslakian et al. (eds.), *Procedural Dictations in Image-Guided Intervention*,
DOI 10.1007/978-3-319-40845-3_108

Relative contraindications (benefits should be weighed against risks of continued hemorrhage or surgical management):

- Past history of allergy to intravenous contrast media or renal dysfunction *(consider CO_2 or gadolinium)*
- Patients with known severe liver disease or impaired portal venous supply *(selective and superselective embolization can minimize deterioration of the liver function)*

POSSIBLE COMPLICATIONS [1, 2, 6]

General (angiography-related) complications:

- Hemorrhage *(puncture-site hematoma, retroperitoneal hematoma if "high" puncture above inguinal ligament)*
- Pseudoaneurysm *(superficial femoral artery "low" puncture)*
- Arteriovenous fistula *(puncture-site artery)*
- Thrombosis of the femoral artery
- Distal embolization
- Contrast-induced allergic reaction
- Contrast-induced nephropathy
- Arterial perforation or dissection
- Catheter or guidewire breakage
- Limb amputation *(rare)*
- Risks related to any minimally invasive procedure performed under conscious sedation *(e.g., allergy to medications)*

Embolization (procedure-specific) related complications:

- Liver infarction, necrosis, or failure in patients with preexisting liver diseases, portal vein thrombosis, or severe hypotension
- Nontarget embolization causing nontarget organ infarction, such as gallbladder necrosis
- Biliary ischemia, leading to biloma, bile fistula, and biliary cyst formation
- Postembolization syndrome *(fever, nausea, pain)*
- Hepatic abscess formation
- Continued or recurrent hemorrhage requiring additional management

PREPROCEDURAL ASSESSMENT AND PLANNING [7–9]

- History, indications, and physical examination *(Appendix 1* in Chap. 149*)*. Document indications of the procedure, lower or upper extremity pulses, and vital signs.
- Evaluation of diagnostic imaging studies to determine the relevant vascular anatomy and identify all potential sites of injury and occult sources of bleeding
- Periprocedural management of coagulation status *(Appendices 2* in Chap. 150 *and 3* in Chap. 151*)*
- Antibiotic prophylaxis: Routinely recommended if intent to create infarction or high likelihood of solid organ infarction. Remains controversial in the setting of embolization for the purposes of controlling bleeding, such as in the setting of trauma [7] *(Appendices 4* in Chap. 152 *and 5* in Chap. 153*)*
- Imaging modality for guidance: Fluoroscopy, combined with ultrasound for arterial puncture
- Positioning: Supine
- Arterial access: Common femoral artery *(preferred)*, left brachial artery, left radial artery

PROCEDURE NOTE

Procedure: Catheter-directed hemostatic hepatic arteriography and embolization
Staff: [_]
Fellow: [_]
Resident: [_]
Clinical History and Indications: Describe history and list indications
Allergies: None known/Allergic to [specify/type of allergy]
Anesthesia: Local anesthesia/conscious sedation/general anesthesia
Medications: List any relevant medications used
Contrast Material: (_) mL of [type] contrast material was used for intra-arterial injection

Field: Sterile
Procedure classification: Clean
Position: Supine
Monitoring: Intravenous access line was secured and vital signs were continuously monitored by nursing staff/anesthesia team throughout the procedure
Total fluoroscopy time: (_) minutes
Cumulative radiation dose: (_) mGy

Description of Procedure *(front-door and backdoor "sandwich" embolization of hepatic pseudoaneurysm):*
The risks, benefits, alternatives, and procedure itself were explained to the patient/patient's Power of Attorney/patient's legal guardian, and informed written/verbal consent was obtained. Time out was performed to confirm the correct patient, procedure, and site. The site of the procedure was identified and marked.

The skin of both groins were shaved, prepped, and draped in the usual sterile fashion. The right/left common femoral artery as well as the inguinal ligament were located by palpation/ultrasound and marked. The site of arterial puncture was determined using combined information from palpation, ultrasound, and fluoroscopy over the middle of the medial third of the femoral head. Local anesthesia was administered. Common femoral artery access was obtained using (_)-gauge [type] needle and the Seldinger technique under direct ultrasound visualization/by palpation. Once good pulsatile arterial flow was detected, a (_)-inch [type] guidewire was advanced through the needle into the aorta under direct fluoroscopic visualization and a (_)-French vascular sheath was placed.

Subsequently, a (_)-French, (_) cm-long [type] catheter was advanced into the abdominal aorta over a (0.035)-in. [hydrophilic/type] guidewire under direct fluoroscopic visualization and the superior mesenteric artery was selectively catheterized. Selective superior mesenteric artery angiography through the venous phase was performed by injecting (_) mL of contrast manually/using the injector at a flow rate of (_) mL/s demonstrating portal vein patency and absence of portal vein injuries, accessory or aberrant hepatic artery.

Then, the catheter was advanced over the guidewire and the celiac trunk was selectively catheterized. Digital subtraction views of the liver were obtained by injecting (_) mL of contrast media manually/using automated injector at a rate of (_) mL/s, showing [*specify findings*]. Following this, a microcatheter was advanced into the [name the artery/arterial branch] and angiography was performed. Embolization of the pseudoaneurysm/aneurysm was performed by occluding the distal outflow first and then the proximal inflow/feeding arteries. The distal outflow hepatic artery was canalized beyond the pseudoaneurysm neck using a (_)-French [type] catheter which was advanced over a (_)-inch [type] guidewire and was embolized by deploying (number) [type] detachable coils {(_) cm length/(_) mm diameter}/(_) mm [type] Amplatzer plug. Complete occlusion of the outflow vessel was documented and the catheter was withdrawn and placed proximal to the pseudoaneurysm neck. The inflow artery was then embolized by deploying (number) [type] detachable coils {(_) cm length/(_) mm diameter}/(_) mm [type] Amplatzer plug.

Following this, completion digital subtraction views of the [_] were obtained by manual injection of (_) mL contrast media confirming adequate occlusion, and absence of contrast extravasation.

Following the procedure, the right/left femoral artery sheath was removed and adequate hemostasis was achieved by compression for (_) minutes/using [type] vascular closure device. The lower extremity pulses were checked following the procedure and were [comparable to the pre-procedure pulses/specify if otherwise needed]. The patient was transferred to the floor/recovery room/ICU for close monitoring following the procedure in a stable/critical condition. Staff was present for the entire procedure.

Description of Procedure *(multiple points of extravasation):*
The risks, benefits, alternatives, and procedure itself were explained to the patient/patient's Power of Attorney/patient's legal guardian, and informed written/verbal consent was obtained. Time out was performed to confirm the correct patient, procedure, and site. The site of the procedure was identified and marked.

The skin of both groins were shaved, prepped, and draped in the usual sterile fashion. The right/left common femoral artery as well as the inguinal ligament were located by palpation/ultrasound and marked. The site of arterial puncture was determined using combined information from palpation, ultrasound, and fluoroscopy over the middle of the medial third of the femoral head. Local anesthesia was administered. Common femoral artery access was obtained using (_)-gauge [type] needle and the Seldinger technique under direct ultrasound visualization/by palpation. Once good pulsatile arterial flow was detected, a (_)-inch [type] guidewire was advanced through the needle into the aorta under direct fluoroscopic visualization and a (_)-French vascular sheath was placed.

Subsequently, a (_)-French, (_) cm-long [type] catheter was advanced into the abdominal aorta over a (0.035)-in. [hydrophilic/type] guidewire under direct fluoroscopic visualization and the superior mesenteric artery was selectively catheterized. Selective superior mesenteric artery angiography through the venous phase was performed by injecting (_) mL of contrast manually/using the injector at a flow rate of (_) mL/s demonstrating portal vein patency and absence of portal vein injuries, accessory or aberrant hepatic artery.

Then, the catheter was advanced over the guidewire and the celiac trunk was selectively catheterized. Digital subtraction views of the liver were obtained by injecting (_) mL of contrast media manually/using automated injector at a rate of (_) mL/s, showing [specify findings]. Following this, the catheter was advanced into the common hepatic artery/hepatic artery proper and selective angiography was performed, demonstrating [list findings]. Due to the presence of multiple points of arterial extravasation in the hepatic parenchyma, embolization of the left and right hepatic artery was performed using gelfoam pledgets/(number) [type] detachable coils {(_) cm length/(_) mm diameter} placed in the [name the anatomic location] hepatic artery, distal to the cystic artery to avoid nontarget embolization.

Following this, completion digital subtraction views of the [_] were obtained by manual injection of (_) mL contrast media confirming adequate occlusion, and absence of contrast extravasation.

Following the procedure, the right/left femoral artery sheath was removed and adequate hemostasis was achieved by compression for (_) minutes/using [type] vascular closure device. The lower extremity pulses were checked following the procedure and were [comparable to the pre-procedure pulses/specify if otherwise needed]. The patient was transferred to the floor/recovery room/ICU for close monitoring following the procedure in a stable/critical condition. Staff was present for the entire procedure.

Description of Procedure *(single point of extravasation, arteriovenous fistula, arterioportal fistula, and arteriobiliary fistula):*
The risks, benefits, alternatives, and procedure itself were explained to the patient/patient's Power of Attorney/patient's legal guardian, and informed written/verbal consent was obtained. Time out was performed to confirm the correct patient, procedure, and site. The site of the procedure was identified and marked.

The skin of both groins were shaved, prepped, and draped in the usual sterile fashion. The right/left common femoral artery as well as the inguinal ligament were located by palpation/ultrasound and marked. The site of arterial puncture was determined using combined information from palpation, ultrasound, and fluoroscopy over the middle of the medial third of the femoral head. Local anesthesia was administered. Common femoral artery access was obtained using (_)-gauge [type] needle and the Seldinger technique under direct ultrasound visualization/by palpation. Once good pulsatile arterial flow was detected, a (_)-inch [type] guidewire was advanced through the needle into the aorta under direct fluoroscopic visualization and a (_)-French vascular sheath was placed.

Subsequently, a (_)-French, (_) cm-long [type] catheter was advanced into the abdominal aorta over a (0.035)-in. [hydrophilic/type] guidewire under direct fluoroscopic visualization and the superior mesenteric artery was selectively catheterized. Selective superior mesenteric artery angiography through the venous phase was performed by injecting (_) mL of contrast manually/using the injector at a flow rate of (_) mL/s demonstrating portal vein patency and absence of portal vein injuries, accessory or aberrant hepatic artery.

Then, the catheter was advanced over the guidewire and the celiac trunk was selectively catheterized. Digital subtraction views of the liver were obtained by injecting (_) mL of contrast media manually/using automated injector at a rate of (_) mL/s. A focal area of contrast extravasation from [name the artery/arterial branch] was detected. A microcatheter was advanced to the feeding vessel and selective embolization was performed using a (_)-French [type] coaxial microcatheter and (number) [type] detachable microcoils {(_) cm length/(_) mm diameter}/gelfoam pledgets completely occluding the affected arterial branch/isolating the conduit [name] artery from the fistula.

Following this, completion digital subtraction angiography was performed by manual injection of (_) mL contrast media confirming adequate occlusion, and absence of contrast extravasation.

Following the procedure, the right/left femoral artery sheath was removed and adequate hemostasis was achieved by compression for (_) minutes/using [type] vascular closure device. The femoral pulses were checked following the procedure and were [comparable to the pre-procedure pulses/specify if otherwise needed]. The patient was transferred to the floor/recovery room for close monitoring following the procedure in a stable condition. Staff was present for the entire procedure.

Intra-Procedure Findings: List all relevant findings.

Immediate Complications: None encountered during or directly after the procedure. List complications if any.

Post-Procedure Plan:

Standard post-angiogram management plan

- Keep patient complete bed rest with the right/left leg extended for 6 h *[adjust depending on the puncture site]*.
- Check the right/left groin/[specify the puncture site if different] for any bleeding or hematoma formation every 15 min for 1 h, then every 30 min for 1 h, then every hour for 4 h; inform interventional radiology team if any signs of bleeding are observed *[adjust depending on the puncture site]*.
- Check and document lower extremity pulses every 30 min for 2 h then every 1 h for 4 h *[adjust depending on the puncture site]*.
- Monitor vital signs every 15 min for 1 h, then every 30 min for 4 h; notify interventional radiology team if systolic blood pressure <95 mmHg, or heart rate >110 beats/min.
- Resume diet and previous orders as needed and if otherwise not contraindicated.
- Continue adequate intravenous hydration and monitor fluid (intake–output) status.
- Check complete blood count and creatinine on the day following the procedure or as clinically indicated.
- Perform regular neurological examination when the procedure includes manipulation in the ascending thoracic aorta, aortic arch or brachiocephalic arteries.

Procedure-specific management plan:

- Follow-up physical examination and laboratory studies closely for signs of persistent or delayed hemorrhage.

- Start adequate antibiotic and deep venous thrombosis prophylaxis as needed.
- Perform cross-sectional imaging prior to discharge or as clinically indicated to evaluate the presence of pseudoaneurysm formation and recurrent bleeding caused by delayed rupture.
- Manage postembolization syndrome conservatively using appropriate antiemetic and analgesic medication and adequately hydrate the patient.

Impression:

- Celiac and hepatic arteriography, demonstrating [list findings].
- Catheter-directed hepatic arterial embolization, with resolutions of [*abnormality*].
- The patient tolerated the procedure well and left the interventional unit in stable condition.
- The patient was unstable and the procedure was canceled/terminated prematurely.
- List any other relevant or important information/finding.

References

1. Mathur VV, Sclafani SJA. Trauma management. In: Kandarpa K, Machan L, editors. Handbook of interventional radiologic procedures. 4th ed. Philadelphia: Lippincott Williams & Wilkins; 2011. p. 245–57.
2. Dondelinger RF. Management of trauma to the liver and spleen. In: Mauro MA, Murphy KPJ, Thomson KR, Venbrux AC, Morgan RA, editors. Image-guided interventions. 2nd ed. Philadelphia: Saunders Elsevier; 2014. p. 491–502.
3. Kong YL, Zhang HY, He XJ, Zhao G, Liu CL, Xiao M, et al. Angiographic embolization in the treatment of intrahepatic arterial bleeding in patients with blunt abdominal trauma. Hepatobiliary Pancreat Dis Int. 2014;13(2):173–8.
4. Poletti PA, Mirvis SE, Shanmuganathan K, Killeen KL, Coldwell D. CT criteria for management of blunt liver trauma: correlation with angiographic and surgical findings. Radiology. 2000;216(2):418–27.
5. Hommes M, Navsaria PH, Schipper IB, Krige JE, Kahn D, Nicol AJ. Management of blunt liver trauma in 134 severely injured patients. Injury. 2014 Nov 26. pii: S0020-1383(14)00605-6
6. Lopera JE. Embolization in trauma: principles and techniques. Semin Interv Radiol. 2010;27(1):14–28.
7. Venkatesan AM, Kundu S, Sacks D, Wallace MJ, Wojak JC, Rose SC, et al. Practice guidelines for adult antibiotic prophylaxis during vascular and interventional radiology procedures. J Vasc Interv Radiol. 2010;21(11):1611–30.
8. Taslakian B, Sebaaly MG, Al-Kutoubi A. Patient evaluation and preparation in vascular and interventional radiology: what every interventional radiologist should know (part 1: patient assessment and laboratory tests). Cardiovasc Intervent Radiol. 2016;39(3):325–33.
9. Taslakian B, Sebaaly MG, Al-Kutoubi A. Patient evaluation and preparation in vascular and interventional radiology: what every interventional radiologist should know (part 2: patient preparation and medications). Cardiovasc Intervent Radiol. 2016;39(4):489–99. doi: 10.1007/s00270-015-1239-4. [Epub 2015 Nov 25].

Management of Budd–Chiari Syndrome

109

Hearns W. Charles

Abbreviations

BCS	Budd–Chiari syndrome
MOVC	Membranous occlusion of the inferior vena cava
IVC	Inferior vena cava
TIPS	Transjugular intrahepatic portosystemic shunt
DIPS	Direct intrahepatic portocaval shunt
IJ	Internal jugular
SMA	Superior mesenteric artery
PV	Portal vein
SMV	Superior mesenteric vein
IMV	Inferior mesenteric vein
RA	Right atrium
CBC	Complete blood count
CMP	Complete metabolic profile
INR	International normalized ratio

INTRODUCTION

Budd–Chiari syndrome (BCS) is characterized by obstruction of hepatic venous outflow, anywhere from the hepatic venules to the inferior atriocaval junction, as a result of various mechanisms [1]. Regardless of the etiology, the resulting increase in hepatic sinusoidal pressure and portal hypertension leads to predictable clinical sequelae. Etiologies differ according to the region of the world, with hypercoagulable states comprising the most common underlying disorders in the western hemisphere, while extrahepatic venous outflow obstruction, membranous occlusion of the inferior vena cava (MOVC), is the major, albeit secondary cause in the eastern hemisphere.

The triad of hepatomegaly, abdominal pain, and ascites is a common presentation of patients with BCS. Lower extremity edema is also a manifestation. Langlet's classification scheme of

H.W. Charles (✉)
Division of Interventional Radiology,
Department of Radiology, New York University
Langone Medical Center, 660 First Avenue,
7th Floor, New York, NY 10016, USA
e-mail: hearns.charles@nyumc.org

B. Taslakian et al. (eds.), *Procedural Dictations in Image-Guided Intervention*,
DOI 10.1007/978-3-319-40845-3_109

the disease offers prognostic value. In this classification system, patients are divided into three categories: type I, acute injury only, corresponding to onset of hepatic outflow obstruction; type II, chronic lesions only, corresponding to the sequelae of remote hepatic outflow obstruction; and type III, acute injury superimposed on chronic. Patients with type III have the worst prognosis [2]. Nausea, vomiting, and jaundice occur more often in those with the fulminant and acute forms. Signs of portal hypertension, such as esophageal varices and splenomegaly, are more commonly seen in the chronic form. In some instances, the hepatic sinusoids may be sufficiently decompressed by large portosystemic and intrahepatic collaterals so that patients are completely asymptomatic. The diagnosis of BCS should be considered in patients with known hypercoagulable states who present with abnormalities of liver function tests, upper abdominal pain, and ascites [3].

CT and MRI are the most useful tools in imaging diagnosis of BCS. Liver congestion and edema leading to global organ enlargement are seen in acute BCS, with regional heterogeneity of hepatic parenchymal enhancement [4]. In subacute disease, intra- and extrahepatic venous collateral circulation may relieve hepatic congestion and edema [5]. With chronic BCS, caudate lobe hypertrophy, myriad regenerative nodules, and an irregular liver contour are visible [6].

On venography, with investigation of the inferior vena cava (IVC) and the hepatic veins, the degree of hepatic vein obstruction is variable, dependent on the etiology of the disease. Smooth, regional tapering stenosis of the intrahepatic IVC can be seen, rarely with more proximal endoluminal caval thrombus. Myriad intrahepatic collateral venous channels ("spider webs") are a venographic hallmark of BCS and are secondary to rich collateral circulation between the tributaries of the obstructed, more distal hepatic veins.

Medical management of BCS concentrates on the underlying cause, with control of ascites and preventing progression of venous thrombosis with anticoagulation therapy. Liver transplantation is the mainstay of surgical treatment. Surgical shunt procedures, with inherent significant risk of morbidity and mortality, have largely been supplanted by the creation of transjugular intrahepatic portosystemic shunt (TIPS). This latter procedure is a great treatment option for patients who present with acute, subacute, and chronic symptoms. It is associated with less morbidity and mortality compared with open surgical procedures [7, 8]. Like mesoatrial shunts, TIPS provides outflow into the suprahepatic IVC, bypassing intrahepatic caval stenosis or thrombus. In cases where there is significant technical challenge by unavailable, occluded or thrombosed, hepatic veins for access, a direct intrahepatic portocaval shunt (DIPS) between the IVC and portal vein is an alternative approach [9]. A created portosystemic shunt can also serve as a bridge to liver transplantation.

Lesser percutaneous procedures such as venous angioplasty and stent placement of isolated hepatic vein(s) and caval angioplasty may be considered, depending on the cause of BCS. These are treatment options for BCS patients in the acute presentation and venous anatomy amenable to such treatment modality. Eradicating the thrombus or providing a bypass sufficient to decrease hepatic congestion may be achieved through percutaneous interventional management. Restoration of outflow through just one of the main three hepatic veins is usually sufficient to resolve symptoms. For patent hepatic vein segments with central and focal stenosis or occlusion, thrombolysis and angioplasty procedures, with possible stent placement, constitute the best forms of management. A short stenosis or occlusion in the common outflow tract of the left and middle hepatic veins provides the opportunity to restore normal drainage to more than half the liver if the obstruction is relieved [3]. Potential accesses for venoplasty include jugular and femoral venous accesses. For ultrasound-guided transhepatic needle puncture access to the hepatic vein, a wire is inserted at the access site, passed through the venous obstruction, and then snared and pulled through the jugular venous access site. Angioplasty and potential stent placement are then accomplished from the jugular site to avoid enlarging the liver capsule puncture site [10]. Stent insertion may be indicated if there is inadequate response to balloon dilatation or venous recoiling or recurrent stenosis or occlusion [11–13]. Hepatic venous interventions (thrombolysis, angioplasty, and stent placement) are particularly suited for transplanted organs with appropriately treatable venous outflow pathology, short-length stenosis, or occlusion. Such lesions typically reflect intimal hyperplasia and fibrosis at the anastomotic sites or compression and twisting of the anastomosis caused by graft regeneration [14]. However, if flow dynamics remain unfavorable following adequate venous treatment, TIPS creation can be considered as this would lead to the alteration of flow to the liver. TIPS also has this advantage in non-transplant recipients, with acute or chronic clinical presentation [15, 16].

COMMON INDICATIONS [3]

- Ascites
- Lower extremity edema
- Abdominal pain
- Gastroesophageal varices
- Gastroesophageal variceal bleeding

COMMON CONTRAINDICATIONS

Absolute contraindications:
- Active infection
- Acute hepatic dysfunction

Relative contraindications:
- Coagulopathy (INR > 1.5)
- Thrombocytopenia (platelet count < 50–100 k)
- Anemia (hemoglobin < 8)
- History of allergic reaction to iodinated contrast
- Significant renal insufficiency

POSSIBLE COMPLICATIONS [17]

- Access site complications *(e.g., bleeding, hematoma)*
- Radiation injury to skin
- Intrahepatic arterial injury and pseudoaneurysm formation
- Malpositioned stent placement
- Contrast-induced nephropathy
- Contrast-induced allergic reaction
- Biliary fistula formation
- Extrahepatic needle injury *(bloody ascites; injury to gallbladder, duodenum, colon, right kidney)*
- Hemoperitoneum
- Hepatic encephalopathy
- Acute hepatic dysfunction
- Stent stenosis and occlusion
- Rare *(cardiac injury; extrahepatic portal vein access)*

PREPROCEDURAL ASSESSMENT AND PLANNING

- History and physical examination *(assess the need for Anesthesia)*
- Evaluation of diagnostic imaging studies (CT or MRI) for anatomic delineation
- Order blood analysis, dated <30 days from the procedure: complete blood count (CBC), complete metabolic profile (CMP), international normalized ratio (INR)
- Periprocedural management of hemoglobin, platelet, and coagulation status *(Appendices 2* in Chap. 150 *and 3* in Chap. 151*)*
- Antibiotic (broad-spectrum) prophylaxis *(Appendices 4* in Chap. 152 *and 5* in Chap. 153*)*
- Imaging modality for guidance: Fluoroscopy; combined with ultrasound for access
- Positioning: Supine
- Venous access: Right common femoral artery; right internal jugular vein

PROCEDURE NOTE

Procedure:

- Mesenteric angiogram
- Transjugular intrahepatic portosystemic shunt (TIPS)
- Right internal jugular (IJ) central venous catheter placement

Staff: [_]
Fellow: [_]
Resident: [_]
Clinical Information: Describe history and list indications
Allergies: None known/Allergic to [specify/type of allergy]
Anesthesia: General anesthesia
Medications: List any relevant medications used
Contrast Material: (_) mL of [type] nonionic contrast material
Field: Sterile
Procedure classification: Clean
Position: Supine
Total fluoroscopy time: (_) minutes
Cumulative radiation dose: (_) mGy

Description of Procedure: *(TIPS)*
Informed consent was obtained where the risks, benefits, and alternatives to the procedure were explained to the patient.

I. Sterile technique and fluoroscopic guidance were used to catheterize the right common femoral artery using a (_)-French introducer sheath. Through this, a (_)-French catheter was used to catheterize the superior mesenteric artery (SMA).

Contrast examination shows:

1. SMA: widely patent, leading to faint opacification of the portal vein
2. Splenic artery and vein: both, widely patent, leading to normal opacification of the portal vein. No apparent varices.
3. Portal vein (PV): wide patency, with antegrade flow. Left main branch, more prominent than the right
4. Coronary vein and gastroesophageal varices: None.

II. Sterile technique, sonographic and fluoroscopic guidance were used to catheterize the right internal jugular vein using a (10)-French long introducer sheath. Through this, a (5)-French catheter was advanced and used to catheterize the main hepatic vein. Measured pressures were as follows:

1. Wedged hepatic vein pressure: (_) mmHg
2. Free hepatic vein pressure: (_) mmHg

Wedged hepatogram shows: truncation of the main hepatic vein, with no dominant branches. Myriad tortuous intrahepatic hepatic venous collateral branches, reflective of BCS, without propagation to any dominant hepatic venous branch.

Exchange was then made over a guide wire for a (_)-French transjugular liver access [type] set. The (18)-gauge Colapinto needle was used to gain needle access to the portal vein bifurcation. Over a guide wire, a (5)-French catheter was inserted, with the distal tip left within the proximal portal vein. Contrast examination shows:

1. Splenic vein: minimal distal reflux opacification. More was seen in the superior (SMV) and inferior mesenteric (IMV) veins
2. Portal vein: as aforementioned.
3. Coronary vein and varices: very small burden, opacified.
4. Mean portal vein pressure: (_) mmHg; right atrium (RA): (_) mmHg.

The portosystemic tract was dilated with an (8)-mm balloon catheter, allowing the deployment of a (10)-mm × (8)-cm [type/Viatorr] stent. This was then dilated with an (8)-mm balloon catheter.

Repeat portography shows:

1. TIPS stent: properly positioned, with excellent flow.
2. Portal vein: no new abnormality.
3. Coronary vein: no longer visualized. Resolution of retrograde flow into the SMV and IMV.
4. Smooth tapering of the intrahepatic inferior vena cava (IVC).
5. Portosystemic gradient was measured to be (_) mmHg; [PV: (_) mmHg; RA: (_) mmHg]

Contrast examination of the right external iliac and common femoral arteries was performed, showing no disease. The catheter and introducer sheath were then removed, with simultaneous deployment of an extravascular [type] arterial closure device, with supplemental manual compression applied to effect hemostasis.

III. The catheter and introducer sheath were then removed from the right internal jugular vein, over a guide wire, and an (8.5)-French short introducer sheath was left in place, with the distal tip left within the superior vena cava. The sheath was secured in place and flushed with heparinized saline solution.

Patient tolerated the procedure well and was transferred to the recovery room/ICU/floor in a stable/critical condition.

Intra-Procedure Findings: List all the relevant findings.

Immediate Complications: None were encountered during or directly after the procedure. List the complications if any.

Post-Procedure Plan [1–3]:

- Keep patient in complete bed rest with the right/left leg extended for (2) h.
- Check the (right groin) access site for any bleeding or hematoma formation every 15 min × 4, then every 30 min × 2, then every 1 h × 2.
- Check neurovascular exam: (right groin) access and popliteal, and ankle arterial pulses; every 15 min × 4, then every 30 min × 2, then every 1 h × 2.
- Inform interventional radiology team for any access site bleeding or hematoma formation.
- Monitor vital signs every 15 min × 4, then every 30 min × 2, then every 1 h × 2.
- Notify Interventional Radiology team if systolic blood pressure ≥130 mmHg or ≤90 mmHg; or diastolic BP >100 mmHg.
- Notify Interventional Radiology team if heart rate ≥100 BPM or ≤60 BPM, at extension (_). If not during regular work hours, page beeper number (_).
- Remove Foley catheter when patient is ambulatory.
- Resume diet and previous orders as needed and if not otherwise contraindicated.
- Encourage fluid intake and continue routine monitoring (intake/output) status.
- Immediate post-procedure labs: CBC, CMP, INR, Ammonia.
- 2-h post-procedure labs: CBC, CMP, INR.
- 4-h post-procedure labs: CBC, CMP, INR.
- Post-procedure day 1 labs: CBC, CMP, INR, Ammonia.

Impression:

- Angiographic findings consistent with Budd–Chiari syndrome—dominant hepatic vein, with no major branches—narrowed intrahepatic IVC.
- Creation of a portosystemic shunt using a 10-mm Viatorr stent, with final portosystemic gradient of (_) mmHg.
- Central venous introducer sheath left in place via the right IJ vein.

References

1. Ludwig J, Hashimoto E, McGill DB, van Heerden JA. Classification of hepatic venous outflow obstruction: ambiguous terminology of the Budd-Chiari syndrome. Mayo Clin Proc. 1990;65:51–5.
2. Langlet P, Escolano S, Valla D, Coste-Zeitoun D, Denie C, Mallet A, et al. Clinicopathological forms and prognostic index in Budd-Chiari syndrome. J Hepatol. 2003;39(4):496–501.
3. Copelan A, Remer EM, Sands M, Nghiem H, Kapoor B. Diagnosis and management of Budd-Chiari syndrome: an update. Cardiovasc Interv Radiol. 2015;38(1):1–12.
4. Noone TC, Semelka RC, Woosley JT, Pisano ED. Ultrasound and MR findings in acute Budd-Chiari syndrome with histopathologic correlation. J Comput Assist Tomogr. 1996;20(5):819–22.
5. Miller WJ, Federle MP, Straub WH, Davis PL. Budd-Chiari syndrome: imaging with pathologic correlation. Abdom Imaging. 1993;18(4):329.
6. Bolondi L, Gaiani S, Li Bassi S, Zironi G, Bonino F, Brunetto M, et al. Diagnosis of Budd-Chiari syndrome by pulsed Doppler ultrasound. Gastroenterol. 1991;100:1324–31.
7. Michl P, Bilzer M, Waggershauser T, Gülberg V, Rau HG, Reiser M, et al. Successful treatment of chronic Budd-Chiari syndrome with a transjugular intrahepatic portosystemic shunt. J Hepatol. 2000;32 (3):516–20.
8. Ochs A, Sellinger M, Haag K, Nöldge G, Herbst EW, Walter E, et al. Transjugular intrahepatic portosystemic stent-shunt (TIPS) in the treatment of

Budd-Chiari syndrome. J Hepatol. 1993;18(2): 217–25.
9. Soares GM, Murphy TP. Transcaval TIPS: indications and anatomic considerations. J Vasc Interv Radiol. 1999;10:1233–8.
10. Cooper S, Olliff SP, Elias E. Recanalisation of hepatic veins by a combined transhepatic, transjugular approach in three cases of Budd Chiari syndrome. J Interv Radiol. 1996;11:9–13.
11. Valla D, Hadengue A, el Younsi M, Azar N, Zeitoun G, Boudet MJ, et al. Hepatic venous outflow block caused by short length hepatic vein stenoses. Hepatology. 1997;25(4):814–9.
12. Griffith JF, Mahmoud AE, Cooper S, Elias E, West RJ, Olliff SP. Radiological intervention in Budd-Chiari syndrome: techniques and outcome in 18 patients. Clin Radiol. 1996;51:775–84.
13. Pelage JP, Denvs A, Valla D, Sibert A, Sauvanet A, Belghiti J, et al. Budd-Chiari syndrome due to prothrombotic disorder: mid-term patency and efficacy of endovascular stents. Eur Radiol. 2003;13 (2):286–93.
14. Umehara M, Narumi S, Sugai M, Toyoki Y, Ishido K, Kudo D, et al. Hepatic venous outflow obstruction in living donor liver transplantation: balloon angioplasty or stent placement? Transp Proc. 2012;44:711–69.
15. Walser EM, DeLa Pena R, Villanueva-Meyer J, Ozkan O, Soloway R. Hepatic perfusion before and after the transjugular intrahepatic portosystemic shunt procedure: impact on survival. J Vasc Interv Radiol. 2000;11:913–8.
16. Walser EM, Nguyen M. Hepatic perfusion and hemodynamic effects of transjugular intrahepatic portosystemic shunts. Semin Interv Radiol. 2005;22 (4):271–7.
17. Gaba RC, Khiatani VL, Knuttinen MG, Omene BO, Carrillo TC, Bui JT, et al. Comprehensive review of TIPS technical complications and how to avoid them. AJR. 2011;196:675–85.

Preoperative Portal Vein Embolization

110

Debkumar Sarkar and Anne M. Covey

Abbreviations

FLR	Future liver remnant
PVE	Portal vein embolization

INTRODUCTION

Portal vein embolization (PVE) is a neoadjuvant procedure to increase the number of patients eligible for curative hepatic resection by causing hypertrophy of the future liver remnant (FLR) [1]. Major liver resection, however, can only safely be performed when there is sufficient FLR. The right hepatic lobe is typically larger in volume than the left. Therefore, left hepatectomy or even trisegmentectomy uncommonly results in insufficient FLR.

The liver has considerable regenerative capacity. In patients with normal underlying liver parenchyma, the FLR should be > 20–25 % of the total liver volume. In patients with hepatitis, steatosis, or exposure to hepatotoxic chemotherapy, a larger FLR is required, in the range of 30–40 %. In patients with cirrhosis FLR > 40 % is optimal. In the weeks following portal vein embolization, contralateral hypertrophy occurs in the majority of patients. This may be due in part to increased blood flow and/or release of growth factors like hepatocyte growth factor as well as interleukin 6 and tumor necrosis factor alpha. In approximately 5 % of patients, contralateral hypertrophy fails to occur. These patients are usually not given further consideration for resection having failed to regenerate.

Percutaneous ipsilateral or contralateral portal vein access is typically used for the procedure. PVE can be performed with a variety of agents including particles, coils, and liquid embolic agents such as glue and ethanol [1–3]. In normal livers, sufficient hypertrophy typically occurs within 2–4 weeks. In patients with chemotherapy associated steatohepatitis or cirrhosis regeneration may take longer.

INDICATIONS [1, 2]

- Pre-resection primary or metastatic liver malignancy in patients with insufficient FLR

D. Sarkar (✉)
Department of Radiology, Richard L. Roudebush VA Medical Center, Indianapolis, IN, USA
e-mail: debkumarsarkar@gmail.com

A.M. Covey
Department of Radiology, Division of Interventional Radiology, Memorial Sloan Kettering Cancer Center, 1275 York Ave, New York, NY 10065, USA
e-mail: coveya@mskcc.org

B. Taslakian et al. (eds.), *Procedural Dictations in Image-Guided Intervention*,
DOI 10.1007/978-3-319-40845-3_110

CONTRAINDICATIONS [1–3]

- Coagulopathy
- Massive ascites
- Severe portal hypertension
- Portal vein occlusion
- Extrahepatic disease precluding resection

POSSIBLE COMPLICATIONS [4]

- Hemorrhage
- Hemobilia
- Vascular injury *(e.g., pseudoaneurysm)*
- Pneumothorax
- Nontarget embolization
- Symptomatic portal hypertension

PREPROCEDURAL ASSESSMENT AND PLANNING [5]

- History, indications, and physical examination *(Appendix 1* in Chap. 149*)*
- Evaluation of diagnostic imaging studies to determine the relevant anatomy of the portal vein and presence of biliary obstruction or bilioenteric bypass, assess liver volume, and calculate FLR
- Review with surgeon the planned surgery to determine which portal vein branches should be embolized and which should be spared
- Periprocedural management of coagulation status *(Appendices 2* in Chap. 150 *and 3* in Chap. 151*)*
- Antibiotic prophylaxis: Not routinely recommended, unless there is biliary obstruction or history of biliary intervention or surgery
- Imaging modality for guidance: Fluoroscopy; combined with ultrasound
- Positioning: Supine

PROCEDURE NOTE

Procedure: Portal venogram and right/left/segment IV portal vein embolization
Staff: [_]
Fellow: [_]
Resident: [_]
Clinical History and Indications: Describe history and list indications
Allergies: None known/Allergic to [specify/type of allergy]
Anesthesia: Local anesthesia/Moderate sedation/Monitored anesthesia care/General anesthesia
Medications: List any relevant medications used
Contrast Material: (_) mL of [type] contrast material was used for venography before, during, and after embolization
Field: Sterile
Procedure classification: Clean-contaminated (unless bactibilia is expected in which case the procedure is contaminated)
Position: Supine
Monitoring: Intravenous access line was secured and vital signs were continuously monitored by nursing staff/anesthesia team throughout the procedure
Total fluoroscopy time: (_) minutes
Cumulative radiation dose: (_) mGy

Description of Procedure:

The risks, benefits, alternatives, and procedure itself were explained to the patient/patient's Power of Attorney/patient's legal guardian, and informed written consent was obtained. Time out was performed to confirm the correct patient, procedure, and site. The site of the procedure was identified and marked.

The right abdomen/left epigastrium was prepped and draped in the usual sterile fashion. Local anesthesia was administered. A small skin incision was made.

A (_) gauge needle was advanced into the liver under ultrasound/fluoroscopic guidance until a target portal vein was accessed. The needle was exchanged over a wire for a coaxial dilator and subsequently a short (_) French sheath. Through the sheath, a (_) French multi-sidehole catheter was advanced over a wire into the main portal vein. Digital venography in the AP/RAO/LAO projection(s) was performed. The catheter was exchanged over a wire for a Kumpe/Cobra/Sos/Simmons catheter. The same catheter was advanced into each branch of the portal vein targeted for embolization. Venography was performed. Each branch of the target portal vein was embolized to stasis. At the end the procedure, the left/right portal vein and main portal veins remained widely patent.

The patient was transferred to the floor/recovery room following the procedure in a stable condition. Staff was present for the entire procedure.

Technique:

Patient position: Supine.

Image guidance: Fluoroscopy (+/− ultrasound).

Access site: Segment II–VIII portal vein.

Laterality of access: Ipsilateral/Contralateral.

Access system: Jeff/Neff.

Access sheath: [Name the sheath used].

Catheter used for portal venogram: [Name the catheter used].

Projections used for portal venography: AP/RAO/LAO.

Catheter used to select target branches: [Name the catheter used].

Embolic agent: [List embolic agent(s) used, the size and volume if applicable].

Intra-Procedure Findings: List all relevant findings.

- **Portal vein anatomy:** Standard/variant.
- **Portal venous flow prior to embolization:** Hepatopedal/hepatofugal.
- **Portal venous flow following embolization:** Cessation of flow in right/left portal vein, patent main and left/right portal vein branches.

Immediate Complications: None encountered during or directly after the procedure. List complications if any.

Post-Procedure Plan:

- Bed rest for 2–4 h and abstain from strenuous activities.
- Start fluid diet for the first hour, then regular diet thereafter if tolerated and otherwise not contraindicated.
- Check vital signs every 15 min for 1 h, every 30 min for 1 h and then every 60 min for up to 2 h.
- Inform interventional radiology team if systolic blood pressure < 95 mmHg, heart rate > 100 beats per minute, or if abdominal pain develops.
- If the patient is asymptomatic at 4 h, without pain, signs, or symptoms of bleeding, consider discharging home.
- Assessment of response with cross-sectional volumentric analysis can be performed as soon as 2–4 weeks postembolization. The degree of hypertrophy expected after PVE differs depending on the presence of underlying liver disease. In normal livers, sufficient hypertrophy typically occurs within 2–4 weeks, whereas regeneration in patients with significant steatohepatitis or cirrhosis can take $\geq$ 4 weeks [6].

Impression:

- Preoperative embolization of the right/left portal vein.
- The patient tolerated the procedure well and left the interventional unit in stable condition.
- The patient was unstable and the procedure was canceled/terminated prematurely.
- List any other relevant or important information/finding.

References

1. May BJ, Talenfeld AD, Madoff DC. Update on portal vein embolization: evidence-based outcomes, controversies, and novel strategies. J Vasc Interv Radiol JVIR. 2013;24(2):241–54.
2. May BJ, Madoff DC. Portal vein embolization: rationale, technique, and current application. Semin Interv Radiol. 2012;29(2):81–89.
3. Avritscher R, Duke E, Madoff DC. Portal vein embolization: rationale, outcomes, controversies and future directions. Expert Rev Gastroenterol Hepatol. 2010;4(4):489–501.
4. Di Stefano DR1, de Baere T, Denys A, Hakime A, Gorin G, Gillet M, et al. Preoperative percutaneous

portal vein embolization: evaluation of adverse events in 188 patients. Radiology. 2005;234(2):625–30.
5. Covey AM, Brody LA, Getrajdman GI, Sofocleous CT, Brown KT. Incidence, patterns, and clinical relevance of variant portal vein anatomy. AJR Am J Roentgenol. 2004;183(4):1055–1064.
6. Covey AM, Brown KT, Jarnagin WR, Brody LA, Schwartz L, Tuorto S, et al. Combined portal vein embolization and neoadjuvant chemotherapy as a treatment strategy for resectable hepatic colorectal metastases. Ann Surg. 2008;247(3):451–5.

Transjugular Intrahepatic Portosystemic Shunt (TIPS)

111

Bedros Taslakian

Abbreviations

TIPS	Transjugular intrahepatic portosystemic shunt
MELD	Model of end-stage liver disease
CBC	Complete blood count
CMP	Complete metabolic profile
INR	International Normalized Ratio

INTRODUCTION

Transjugular intrahepatic portosystemic shunt (TIPS) is an effective percutaneous image-guided method of reducing portal vein pressure by creating a decompressive channel between a hepatic vein and an intrahepatic branch of the portal vein. It has proven benefit in the treatment of patients who have complications of portal hypertension such as acute and chronic esophageal, gastric, intestinal, and stomal variceal bleeding; severe or refractory ascites; and hepatic hydrothorax; as well as Budd–Chiari syndrome in selected cases. However, TIPS is not a replacement for endoscopic therapy or surgery. The major disadvantages of the TIPS procedure are deterioration of hepatic function caused by diversion of portal venous blood flow and shunt dysfunction, requiring routine imaging surveillance and shunt maintenance procedures.

B. Taslakian (✉)
Department of Radiology, New York University Langone Medical Center, 660 First Ave, New York, NY 10016, USA
e-mail: btaslakian@gmail.com

COMMON INDICATIONS [1–5]

- Secondary prevention of recurrent variceal bleeding in high-risk patients *(Level of evidence: 1A)*
- Refractory ascites defined as ascites that cannot be mobilized or early recurrence of ascites that cannot be adequately prevented by medical therapy *(Level of evidence: 1A)*
- Refractory or uncontrollable acute variceal bleeding *(Level of evidence: 1B)*
- Portal hypertensive gastropathy *(Level of evidence: 2B)*
- Hepatorenal syndromes (types 1 and 2) *(Level of evidence: 2B)*
- Budd–Chiari syndrome with refractory ascites, liver failure, and upper gastrointestinal bleeding *(Level of evidence: 4)*
- Hepatic hydrothorax: significant pleural effusion *(>500 mL)* in a patient with cirrhosis but

B. Taslakian et al. (eds.), *Procedural Dictations in Image-Guided Intervention*,
DOI 10.1007/978-3-319-40845-3_111

no primary cardiopulmonary disease *(Level of evidence: 4)*
- Hepatic venoocclusive disease *(Level of evidence: 4)*
- Hepatopulmonary syndrome *(Level of evidence: 4)*
- Decompression of portosystemic collaterals prior to abdominal surgeries

Levels of evidence: 1A = systematic review of randomized controlled trials, 1B = individual randomized control trial, 2B = individual cohort study, and 4 = case series.

COMMON CONTRAINDICATIONS [1–5]

Absolute contraindications:
- Unproved portal hypertension
- Severe pulmonary arterial hypertension *(mean pulmonary artery pressure > 45 mmHg)*
- Congestive heart failure
- Severe tricuspid regurgitation

Relative contraindications (conditions likely to increase the rates of procedural or TIPS-related complications):
- APACHE II score, especially in Child C patients *(significant post-procedure mortality)*
- Irreversible phase of hemorrhagic shock
- Child-Pugh score > 12 *(significant post-procedure mortality)*
- Model of end-stage liver disease (MELD) score > 18 *(significant post-procedure mortality)*
- Right-sided heart failure with elevation of the central venous pressure *(mean right atrium pressure > 15 mmHg)*
- Rapidly progressive liver failure *(listed as absolute contraindications in Ref.* [5]*)*
- Severe or uncontrolled hepatic encephalopathy, especially in patients older than 60, patients with diabetes, and patients receiving hemodialysis *(listed as absolute contraindications in reference 5)*
- Thrombosis of the portal vein and its branches, inferior vena cava or hepatic veins
- Extensive primary or metastatic hepatic malignancy
- Severe, uncorrectable coagulopathy
- Polycystic liver disease
- Active intrahepatic infection
- Uncontrolled systemic infection or sepsis
- Unrelieved biliary obstruction

POSSIBLE COMPLICATIONS [1–5]

- Access-site-related complications *(e.g., neck hematoma ~ 2 %; inadvertent carotid puncture; transient Horner's syndrome; transient dysphonia; and pneumothorax)*
- Contrast-induced allergic reaction
- Cardiac arrhythmias
- Abdominal pain
- Perforation of the liver capsule; *5–30 %*
- Stent misplacement too far into the inferior vena cava or the right atrium at the cranial end or far into the main portal vein at the caudal end of the shunt in up to *20 % (major stent malposition and migration in 1 %)*
- New or worsened controlled encephalopathy; *5–35 % (refractory encephalopathy, 2–8 % —rates variable and dependent on patient selection)*
- Deterioration of hepatic function; *10 %*
- Recurrence of portal hypertension *(TIPS dysfunction)* secondary to stent stenosis and occlusion *(resulting from intimal hyperplasia, 18–78 % for bare-metal stents, 15 % for PTFE-covered stents)*
- Gallbladder puncture; < *10 %*
- Biliary duct puncture; < *5 %*
- Transient renal failure; *2 % (severe renal failure requiring dialysis, 0.25 %)*
- Fever; *2 %*
- Clinically significant hemobilia; *2 %*
- Significant intraperitoneal hemorrhage; *1–2 %*
- Right kidney puncture; *1.5 %*
- Transient pulmonary edema; *1 %*
- Intrahepatic arterial injury and pseudoaneurysm formation; *1 %*
- Radiation induced skin injury; *0.1 %*
- Hepatic infarction; *0.5 %*
- Mortality; *1 %*

PREPROCEDURAL ASSESSMENT AND PLANNING

- History, indications, and physical examination *(Appendix 1* in Chap. 149*)*. Assess hemodynamic stability in acutely bleeding patients.
- Evaluation of recent (<1 month) diagnostic imaging studies to determine the relevant vascular anatomy and assess portal vein patency. Perform new Doppler ultrasound examination of the liver if there is a recent deterioration in hepatic function.
- Perform an echocardiogram in patients with known cardiac or pulmonary diseases, to exclude pulmonary hypertension
- Ascites drainage in patients with large volume ascites
- Periprocedural management of coagulation status *(Appendices 2* in Chap. 150 *and 3* in Chap. 151*)*
- Obtain laboratory studies within 24 h of a TIPS procedure *(complete blood count, coagulation panel, and a comprehensive metabolic panel including serum electrolyte levels, creatinine level, and liver function tests)*
- Prepare cross-matched blood products
- Antibiotic prophylaxis: Routinely recommended *(Appendices 4* in Chap. 152 *and 5* in Chap. 153*)* [5, 6]
- Imaging modality for guidance: Fluoroscopy; combined with ultrasound for venous access
- Positioning: Supine
- Venous access: Right internal jugular vein *(preferred);* left internal jugular vein, external jugular veins or femoral veins are rarely used for catheterization [5]

PROCEDURE NOTE

Procedure: Transjugular Intrahepatic portosystemic shunt
Staff: [_]
Fellow: [_]
Resident: [_]
Clinical History and Indications: Describe history and list indications
Allergies: None known/Allergic to [specify/type of allergy]
Anesthesia: Monitored conscious sedation/general anesthesia
Medications: List any relevant medications used
Contrast Material: (_) mL of [type] contrast material was used for venography
Field: Sterile
Procedure classification: Clean/clean contaminated
Position: Supine
Monitoring: Intravenous access line was secured and vital signs were continuously monitored by nursing staff/anesthesia team throughout the procedure
Total fluoroscopy time: (_) minutes
Cumulative radiation dose: (_) mGy

Description of Procedure:

The risks, benefits, alternatives, and procedure itself were explained to the patient/patient's Power of Attorney/patient's legal guardian, and informed written consent was obtained. Time out was performed to confirm the correct patient, procedure, and site. The site of the procedure was identified and marked.

The patient was positioned supine, with the neck turned to the contralateral side. The patient's cervical and upper thoracic regions were prepped and draped in the usual sterile fashion. Ultrasound examination was performed to determine the site of venous puncture. Local anesthesia was administered. The right internal jugular vein was punctured under ultrasound guidance using a (_)-gauge [type] needle. Once good venous flow was detected, a (_)-inch [type] guidewire was advanced through the needle under direct fluoroscopic visualization and placed in the inferior vena cava. A small skin incision was made and a (_)-French, (_) cm-long vascular TIPS sheath was advanced over the guidewire into the right atrium, and initial arterial pressures were recorded. The sheath was then advanced and its tip was positioned in the upper aspect of the inferior vena cava.

Subsequently, a (_)-French, curved [type] catheter was introduced through the sheath over a (_)-inch [hydrophilic/type] guidewire and the right/middle hepatic vein was selectively catheterized. Venography was performed by the manual injection of (_) mL of contrast media and showed [specify findings]. The diagnostic catheter was then wedged/exchanged for an occlusion [type] balloon. The balloon was inflated with (1-3) mL of diluted contrast/air, followed by a gentle injection of a small amount of contrast/carbon dioxide to ensure adequate wedge position. Wedge hepatic venous pressure and free hepatic venous pressure were obtained and documented. Views of the portal vein were obtained during the wedged injection.

Following pressure measurement, a (_)-inch [Amplatz extra stiff/type] guidewire was inserted through the catheter into the selected hepatic vein to provide adequate support. The diagnostic catheter was removed, and the sheath was advanced into the selected vein. A [type] transjugular puncture needle was advanced through the sheath. The needle was rotated anteriorly and moved centrally within the vein to within approximately 2 cm of the hepatic vein ostium. The needle was then gently withdrawn while aspirating the attached contrast-filled syringe. After confirming intraportal position of the needle tip with gentle contrast injection, a (_)-inch portal entry wire was manipulated through needle and the punctured portal vein into the main portal/splenic/superior mesenteric vein to provide adequate support. The needle was then removed and a (_)-French diagnostic catheter was advanced over the guidewire into the main portal/splenic/superior mesenteric vein. A second (_)-inch [type] stiff guidewire was advanced through the catheter and the first wire was left in place as a safety wire in a stable position. Portography was performed and the portal pressure was recorded from the main portal vein. In addition, vessels supplying the varices were selected and venography was performed showing [specify findings]. A (_) × (_) mm balloon catheter was advanced over the stiff wire and the tract was dilated to an adequate size. A (_)-French radiopaque marker catheter was then inserted into the portal vein and simultaneous injection was performed through the intravenous sheath and intraportal catheter to measure the length of the tract and identify the lending zones of the stent. Then, a (_) × (_) mm [Viatorr/other] stent was advanced over the guidewire and deployed at the level of the tract, extending from the portal entry site several millimeters into the inferior vena cava/specify other location if needed.

Post-shunting pressures were obtained and trans-TIPS portal venography was performed.

Postdilatation of the stent was performed using a (_) × (_) mm balloon to document patency and adequate size/blood flow and for future reference. Postdilatation pressures were obtained and trans-TIPS portal venography was performed for documentation and future reference.

The catheter and introducer sheath were then removed from the right internal jugular vein, over a guide wire, and an (8.5)-French short introducer sheath was left in place, with the distal tip left within the superior vena cava. The sheath was secured in place and flushed with heparinized saline solution. Sterile dressing was applied and the patient was transferred to the floor/recovery room/intensive care unit following the procedure in a stable/critical condition. Staff was present for the entire procedure.

Intra-Procedure Findings: List all relevant findings.

Pre-shunting portal vein flow: *hepatofugal/hepatopetal*

Pre-shunting pressures:
Mean Portal Pressure: (_) mmHg
Mean Central Venous Pressure: (_) mmHg
Mean Portosystemic Pressure Gradient: (_) mmHg

Post-shunting pressures:
Mean Portal Pressure: (_) mmHg
Mean Central Venous Pressure: (_) mmHg
Mean Portosystemic Pressure Gradient: (_) mmHg
Mean Intrashunt Pressure: (_) mmHg

Postdilatation pressures:
Mean Portal Pressure: (_) mmHg
Mean Central Venous Pressure: (_) mmHg

Mean Portosystemic Pressure Gradient:
(_) mmHg
Mean Intrashunt Pressure: (_) mmHg

Immediate Complications: None encountered during or directly after the procedure. List complications if any.

Post-Procedure Plan [1, 5]:

- Keep patient in complete bed rest for (_) hours *[adjust depending on the venostomy site]*.
- Check the puncture site for any bleeding or hematoma formation every 15 min for 1 h, then every 30 min for 2 h; inform interventional radiology team if any complications are observed.
- Monitor vital signs every 15 min for 1 h, then every 30 min for 2 h; notify interventional radiology team if systolic blood pressure < 95 mmHg, or heart rate > 110 beats/min.
- Inform interventional radiology team if any severe abdominal pain, chest pain, or shortness of breath develops.
- Resume diet and previous orders as needed and if not otherwise contraindicated.
- Immediate post-procedure labs: CBC, CMP, INR, Ammonia.
- 2-h post-procedure labs: CBC, CMP, INR.
- 4-h post-procedure labs: CBC, CMP, INR.
- Post-procedure day 1 labs: CBC, CMP, INR, Ammonia.
- Monitor for signs of pulmonary edema and hepatic encephalopathy and manage accordingly.
- Monitor right atrial pressures; overnight diuresis as clinically appropriate if pressure > 10 mmHg.
- Perform post-procedure baseline TIPS sonography prior to discharge (in case of bare mesh Wallstents) and within 1–2 weeks if Viatorr graft was used.
- Perform urgent Doppler examination of the liver in patient with recurrence or worsening portal hypertension symptoms.
- Follow up TIPS sonography at 3, 6, and 12 months in the first year and then every 3–6 months.
- Perform TIPS venography in cases of suspected shunt dysfunction as clinically indicated.

Impression:

- Transjugular intrahepatic portosystemic shunt, as described above.
- The patient tolerated the procedure well and left the interventional unit in stable condition.
- The patient was unstable and the procedure was canceled/terminated prematurely.
- List any other relevant or important information/finding.

References

1. Fidelman N, Kwan SW, LaBerge JM, Gordon RL, Ring EJ, Kerlan RK Jr. The transjugular intrahepatic portosystemic shunt: an update. AJR Am J Roentgenol. 2012;199(4):746–55.
2. Krajina A, Hulek P, Fejfar T, Valek V. Quality improvement guidelines for transjugular intrahepatic portosystemic shunt (TIPS). Cardiovasc Interv Radiol. 2012;35(6):1295–300.
3. Haskal ZJ, Martin L, Cardella JF, Cole PE, Drooz A, Grassi CJ, et al. Quality improvement guidelines for transjugular intrahepatic portosystemic shunts. J Vasc Interv Radiol. 2003;14(9 Pt 2):S265–70.
4. Amended 2014 (Resolution 39)* ACR–SIR–SPR Practice parameter for the creation of a transjugular intrahepatic portosystemic shunt (TIPS).
5. Haskal ZJ. transjugular intrahepatic portosystemic shunts. In: Kandarpa K, Machan L, editors. Handbook of interventional radiologic procedures. 4th ed. Philadelphia: Lippincott Williams & Wilkins; 2011. p. 390–7.
6. Venkatesan AM, Kundu S, Sacks D, Wallace MJ, Wojak JC, Rose SC, et al. Practice guidelines for adult antibiotic prophylaxis during vascular and interventional radiology procedures. J Vasc Interv Radiol. 2010;21(11):1611–30.

Transjugular Liver Biopsy

112

Amy Deipolyi and Bedros Taslakian

INTRODUCTION

Despite enormous advancement in clinical medicine, diagnostic imaging and laboratory testing, harvesting liver specimens is often mandatory to enable histopathologic characterization and staging of hepatic disease. Although percutaneous image-guided liver biopsy allows fast, safe, and adequate tissue sampling, there is a significant risk for intrahepatic and perihepatic hematoma. Transjugular liver biopsy offers well-accepted first-line alternative approach to hepatic tissue sampling in patients with contraindications to percutaneous biopsy and also allows for the collection of additional information such as portal manometry.

COMMON INDICATIONS [1–5]

To obtain samples of liver tissue in diffuse liver disease *(see Chap.* 32*)* associated with:

- Massive ascites *(contraindication to percutaneous biopsy)*
- Severe uncorrectable coagulopathy *(contraindication to percutaneous biopsy)*
- Failure of percutaneous liver biopsy *(e.g., massive obesity)*
- Suspected conditions associated with high risk of bleeding *(e.g., diffuse hypervascular tumor, peliosis hepatic, amyloidosis, cardiac liver, hemodialysis and chronic renal insufficiency, and hereditary hemorrhagic telangiectasia)*
- Liver transplant patients in early postoperative period with ascites and coagulopathy
- When other concurrent vascular procedures are planned *(e.g., transvenous renal biopsy, transjugular intrahepatic portosystemic shunting, venography and hepatic venous pressure gradient measurement)*

COMMON CONTRAINDICATIONS [1–3]

- Past history of allergy to intravenous contrast media and impaired renal function *(consider use of CO_2 for venography)*
- Pregnancy
- Severe uncontrolled coagulopathy *(take corrective measures)*
- Need for focal biopsy of hepatic lesion
- Absence of venous access *(i.e., thrombosis of the right internal jugular vein, inferior vena cava, or hepatic veins)*
- Suspected or confirmed hydatid cyst in the liver
- Cholangitis

A. Deipolyi (✉)
Department of Radiology, Division of Interventional Radiology, Memorial Sloan Kettering Cancer Center, 1275 York Ave, New York, NY 10065, USA
e-mail: amy.deipolyi@nyumc.org

B. Taslakian
Department of Radiology, New York University Langone Medical Center, 660 First Ave, New York, NY 10016, USA
e-mail: btaslakian@gmail.com

B. Taslakian et al. (eds.), *Procedural Dictations in Image-Guided Intervention*,
DOI 10.1007/978-3-319-40845-3_112

POSSIBLE COMPLICATIONS [1–4]

- Access-site related complications *(e.g., neck hematoma, inadvertent carotid puncture, transient Horner's syndrome, transient dysphonia, and pneumothorax)*
- Cardiac arrhythmias
- Abdominal pain
- Perforation of the liver capsule
- Hepatic hematoma
- Intraperitoneal hemorrhage
- Fistula formation between the hepatic vein, hepatic artery, portal vein, or biliary tree
- Hepatic artery pseudoaneurysm
- Inferior vena cava and renal vein perforation
- Death

PREPROCEDURAL ASSESSMENT AND PLANNING

- History, indications, and physical examination *(Appendix 1* in Chap. 149*)*
- Evaluation of diagnostic imaging studies to determine the relevant vascular anatomy
- Periprocedural management of coagulation status *(Appendices 2* in Chap. 150 *and 3 in* Chap. 151*)*
- Antibiotic prophylaxis: Not routinely recommended [2, 4]
- Imaging modality for guidance: Fluoroscopy, combined with ultrasound for venotomy
- Positioning: Supine
- Venous access: Right internal jugular vein *(preferred);* left internal jugular vein, external jugular veins or femoral veins are rarely used for catheterization [1–3]

PROCEDURE NOTE

Procedure: Transjugular random liver biopsy
Staff: [_]
Fellow: [_]
Resident: [_]
Clinical History and Indications: Describe history and list indications
Allergies: None known/Allergic to [specify/type of allergy]
Anesthesia: Local anesthesia with conscious sedation/general anesthesia
Medications: List any relevant medications used
Contrast Material: (_) mL of [type] contrast material
Field: Sterile
Procedure classification: Clean
Position: Supine
Monitoring: Intravenous access line was secured and vital signs were continuously monitored by nursing staff/anesthesia team throughout the procedure
Total fluoroscopy time: (_) minutes
Cumulative radiation dose: (_) mGy

Description of Procedure:
The risks, benefits, alternatives, and procedure itself were explained to the patient/patient's Power of Attorney/patient's legal guardian, and informed written/verbal consent was obtained. Time out was performed to confirm the correct patient, procedure, and site. The site of the procedure was identified and marked.

The patient was positioned supine, with the neck turned to the contralateral side. The patient's left/right cervical and upper thoracic regions were prepped and draped in the usual sterile fashion. Ultrasound examination was performed to determine the site of venous puncture. Local anesthesia was administered. The left/right internal jugular vein was punctured under ultrasound guidance using a (_)-gauge [type] needle. Once good venous flow was detected, a (_)-inch [type] guidewire was advanced through the needle under direct fluoroscopic visualization and placed in the inferior vena cava. A small skin incision was made and a (_)-French vascular sheath was advanced over the guidewire into the inferior vena cava.

Subsequently, (_)-French, multipurpose curved [type] catheter was introduced through the sheath over a (_)-inch [hydrophilic/type] guidewire and the right/middle hepatic vein was selectively catheterized. Venography was performed by the manual injection of (_) mL of contrast media and showed [specify findings].

The diagnostic catheter was then exchanged for an occlusion [type] balloon, which was placed within the hepatic vein. The balloon was inflated with (1–3) mL of diluted contrast/air, followed by a gentle injection of a small amount of contrast to ensure adequate wedge position. Wedge hepatic venous pressure and free hepatic venous pressure were obtained and documented.

Following pressure measurement, a (_)-cm long, (_)-inch [Amplatz extra stiff/type] guidewire was inserted through the catheter into the hepatic vein to provide adequate support. Then a (_)-French, (_)-cm long [type] guiding catheter was advanced over the stiff guidewire into the selected hepatic vein. Correct position [3–5 cm from the inferior vena cava] was documented by the manual injection of (_) mL of contrast media through the catheter. The transvenous (_)-gauge [type] core biopsy needle was then advanced through the guiding catheter, the tip of the catheter was turned out of the axis of the hepatic vein and the biopsy needle was advanced into the parenchyma. (number) samples were obtained from peripheral and central locations of the liver and sent for histopathologic interpretation. Venography was performed by the manual injection of (_) mL of contrast media through the catheter and showed no evidence of hepatic capsule perforation or contrast extravasation.

The catheter and sheath were removed and adequate hemostasis was achieved at the venotomy site by compression for (_) minutes. Sterile dressing was applied and the patient was transferred to the floor/recovery room following the procedure in a stable condition. Staff was present for the entire procedure.

Intra-Procedure Findings: List all relevant findings, especially wedged and free hepatic pressures.

Immediate Complications: None encountered during or directly after the procedure. List complications if any.

Post-Procedure Plan [1–3]:

- Keep patient in complete bed rest for (_) hours *[adjust depending on the venotomy site, typically 2 h for jugular access]*.
- Check the puncture site for any bleeding or hematoma formation every 15 min for 1 h, then every 30 min for 2 h; inform interventional radiology team if any complications are observed.
- Monitor vital signs every 15 min for 1 h, then every 30 min for 2 h; notify interventional radiology team if systolic blood pressure <95 mmHg, or heart rate >110 beats/min.
- Inform interventional radiology team if any severe abdominal pain, chest pain, or shortness of breath develops.
- Resume diet and previous orders as needed and if not otherwise contraindicated.
- Continue adequate intravenous hydration and monitor fluid (intake-output) status.
- Check complete blood count, creatinine, and blood urea nitrogen on the day following the procedure or as clinically indicated.

Impression:

- Transjugular random liver biopsy, as described above.
- The patient tolerated the procedure well and left the interventional unit in stable condition.
- The patient was unstable and the procedure was canceled/terminated prematurely.
- List any other relevant or important information/finding.

References

1. Behrens G, Ferral H. Transjugular liver biopsy. Semin Interv Radiol. 2012;29(2):111–7.
2. Kos S, Bilecen D, Jacob AL, Heim MH. Transjugular liver biopsy. In: Mauro MA, Murphy KPJ, Thomson KR, Venbrux AC, Morgan RA, editors. Image-guided interventions. 2nd ed. Philadelphia: Saunders Elsevier; 2014. p. 431–5.
3. Dohan A, Guerrache Y, Boudiaf M, Gavini JP, Kaci R, Soyer P. Transjugular liver biopsy: indications, technique and results. Diagn Interv Imaging. 2014;95(1):11–5.
4. Kalambokis G, Manousou P, Vibhakorn S, Marelli L, Cholongitas E, Senzolo M, et al. Transjugular liver biopsy—indications, adequacy, quality of specimens,

and complications—a systematic review. J Hepatol. 2007;47(2):284–94.
5. Gorriz E, Reyes R, Lobrano MB, Pulido-Duque JM, San Roman JL, Lonjedo E, et al. Transjugular liver biopsy: a review of 77 biopsies using a spring-propelled cutting needle (biopsy gun). Cardiovasc Interv Radiol. 1996;19(6):442–5.
5. Gorriz E, Reyes R, Lobrano MB, Pulido-Duque JM, San Roman JL, Lonjedo E, et al. Transjugular liver biopsy: a review of 77 biopsies using a spring-propelled cutting needle (biopsy gun). Cardiovasc Interv Radiol. 1996;19(6):442–5.

Part XVII

Vascular Interventional Procedures: Genital Organs

Introduction by Aghiad Al-Kutoubi, Section Reviewer

Varicocele embolization has long been established although the available devices have influenced the approach. Pelvis congestion syndrome however is still under-diagnosed and under-treated when endovascular methods of treatment are simple and frequently performed as “outpatient” procedures.

Uterine artery embolization (UAE) for fibroids is one of a number of methods helping in affecting nonsurgical management of this common condition. There are sufficient data in the literature proving the safety and effectiveness of UAE compared to surgical management. Pain management is an essential component of establishing a UAE service. Some of the uncommon complications such as nerve injury and fibroid expulsion should be kept in mind and efforts made to minimize these through careful planning and meticulous technique.

This section provides a comprehensive list of procedural reports that covers the vast majority of the currently performed vascular procedures for the management of varicocele, pelvic congestion syndrome and uterine leiomyomas with up-to-date explanatory notes, synopsis of the indications and contraindications, and potential complications in an organized and practical format.

Section Chapters

Interventional Therapy for Varicoceles

113

Sahar Semaan

INTRODUCTION

Dilatation of the internal spermatic veins, also known as varicocele, is seen in up to 10 % of males. The incidence increases to up to 30 % when screening infertile couples. Varicoceles are associated with pain, infertility, and in advanced cases may lead to testicular atrophy. Testicular vein embolization is a common nonsurgical procedure for the treatment of varicoceles. Unlike the surgical approach, the patient does not undergo scrotal incision, and the procedure does not need general anesthesia or hospital admission. In addition, the associated risk of infection is significantly reduced. Another advantage is the ability to treat bilateral varicoceles through one puncture, rather than bilateral scrotal incisions. The success rates are comparable to those of surgical treatment in terms of improvement of sperm count and fertility rates.

COMMON INDICATIONS [1–3]

- Scrotal pain
- Infertility
- Failure of surgical therapy
- Testicular atrophy in a child

COMMON CONTRAINDICATIONS [1–3]

- Reactions to contrast media
- Uncorrectable coagulopathy
- Impaired renal function

POSSIBLE COMPLICATIONS [1–3]

General (angiography-related) complications:
- Access site complications *(e.g., hematoma, retroperitoneal hemorrhage, arterial injury, thrombosis)*
- Contrast-induced allergic reaction
- Contrast-induced nephropathy
- Catheter or guidewire breakage
- Risks related to any minimally invasive procedure performed under conscious sedation *(e.g., allergy to medications)*

Procedure-specific complications:
- Depending on the embolization material used:
  - *Coils*-may be misplaced or may migrate into the central venous system, may cause venous perforation
  - *Balloons*-may migrate
  - *Hot contrast and sclerosing agents*-may cause phlebitis of the pampiniform plexus and paresthesias of the thigh

S. Semaan (✉)
Department of Radiology, Icahn School of Medicine at Mount Sinai, One Gustave L. Levy Place, New York, NY 10029-6574, USA
e-mail: saharsemaan@gmail.com

B. Taslakian et al. (eds.), *Procedural Dictations in Image-Guided Intervention*,
DOI 10.1007/978-3-319-40845-3_113

PREPROCEDURAL ASSESSMENT AND PLANNING [4–6]

- History, indications, and physical examination *(Appendix 1* in Chap. 149*)*
- Evaluation of diagnostic imaging studies: Testicular ultrasound and Doppler to assess the severity and bilaterality of varicocele and testicular size
- Periprocedural management of coagulation status *(Appendices 2* in Chap. 150 *and 3 in* Chap. 151*)*
- Antibiotic prophylaxis: Not routinely recommended [4] *(Appendices 4* in Chap. 152 *and 5* in Chap. 153*)*
- Imaging modality for guidance: Fluoroscopy ± ultrasound *(to guide venous puncture in difficult cases and obese patients)*
- Positioning of the patient: Supine

PROCEDURE NOTE

Procedure: Left/right/bilateral testicular vein embolization for varicocele
Staff: [_]
Fellow: [_]
Resident: [_]
Clinical Information: Describe history and list indications
Allergies: None known/Allergic to [specify/type of allergy]
Anesthesia: Local anesthesia/Monitored conscious sedation
Medications: List any relevant medications used (sedation)
Contrast Used: (_) mL of [type] contrast media was used for intravenous injection
Field: Sterile
Procedure classification: Clean
Position: Supine
Monitoring: Intravenous access line was secured and vital signs were continuously monitored by nursing staff/anesthesia team throughout the procedure
Total fluoroscopy time: (_) minutes
Cumulative radiation dose: (_) mGy

Description of Procedure:
The risks, benefits, alternatives, and the procedure itself were explained to the patient/patient's Power of Attorney/patient's legal guardian, and informed written consent was obtained. The site of the procedure was identified and marked. Time out was performed to confirm the correct patient, procedure and site.

The skin of both groins was shaved, prepped, and draped in the usual sterile fashion. The right/left femoral vein was located by palpation/ultrasound and marked. The site of venous puncture was determined using combined information from palpation and ultrasound. Local anesthesia was administered. Femoral venous access was obtained using a (_)-gauge [type] needle and the Seldinger technique, double-/single-wall entry under direct ultrasound visualization/by palpation. Once good venous flow was detected, a (_)-inch [type] guidewire was advanced through the needle, up the femoral vein into the inferior vena cava under direct fluoroscopic visualization and a (_)-French vascular sheath was placed.

Once access was secured, a (_)-French [type] catheter was advanced to reach the left renal vein. Contrast was injected and a venogram was performed demonstrating reflux down to the left spermatic vein. The catheter was then advanced into the spermatic vein and 15 cc of contrast was injected, while the patient performed Valsalva maneuver, showing retrograde flow into the vein, which measured (_) mm in diameter.

- *If metallic coils were used:*
  A (_)-French hydrophilic catheter was advanced into the spermatic vein and a (0.018/0.025/0.038)-in. coil(s) was/were placed at the level of the superior pubic ramus. Subsequently a venogram was performed showing no local collateral vessels. The catheter was withdrawn to the level of the upper third of the pelvis, where two (0.018/0.025/0.038)-in. coils were deployed. The catheter was then withdrawn to the proximal portion of the internal spermatic vein and another (0.018/0.025/0.038)-in. coil was placed. A venogram was again

performed confirming spermatic vein occlusion and the presence of prominent collateral vessels, which were each catheterized and occluded using (0.018/0.025/0.038)-in. coils.

- *If detachable balloons were used:*
  A (_)-French hydrophilic catheter was advanced into the spermatic vein and a [type/size] balloon was inflated and detached at its distal aspect. A second balloon was placed along the proximal portion of the internal spermatic vein with 70 % glucose solution sandwiched between the two balloons. A venogram was again performed confirming spermatic vein occlusion.
- *If hot contrast or sclerosing agents were used:*
  A (_)-French catheter was advanced into the spermatic vein to reach the mid to upper level of the sacroiliac joint. With firm compression of the distal part of the vein at the level of the superior pubic ramus, (_) mL of body temperature contrast was injected followed by (_) of lidocaine. The vein was then aspirated and emptied of blood. Subsequently, (_) mL of boiling hyperosmolar contrast material was injected into the internal spermatic vein. This was repeated (_) times.
- *If the right side was also embolized.*
  The catheter was withdrawn from the left renal vein and its tip was moved to the inferior vena cava. Contrast was injected and a venogram was performed demonstrating reflux down to the right spermatic vein. The catheter was then advanced into the right spermatic vein and 15 cc of contrast was injected, while the patient performed Valsalva maneuver, showing retrograde flow into the vein, which measured (_) mm in diameter.
  **Describe embolization procedure as above.*

After confirmation of spermatic vein occlusion, the catheters and venous sheath were withdrawn and hemostasis was attained. The patient was transferred to the floor/recovery room following the procedure in a stable condition. Staff was present for the entire procedure.

Intra-Procedure Findings: List all relevant findings.

Immediate Complications: None encountered during or directly after the procedure. List complications if any.

Post-Procedure Plan:

- Monitor patient in recovery room for (_) hours before discharge.
- Keep patient complete bed rest with the right/left leg extended for (_) hours *[adjust depending on the puncture site]*.
- Analgesic use such as acetaminophen for possible back pain as needed.
- Chest radiography if there is suspicion of coil or balloon migration.
- Follow up with urologist.

Impression:

- Embolization of right/left spermatic vein, as described above.
- The patient tolerated the procedure well and left the interventional unit in stable condition.
- The procedure was canceled/terminated prematurely [reason].
- List any other relevant or important information/finding.

References

1. Vanlangenhove P, Dhondt E, Everaert K, Defreyne L. Pathophysiology, diagnosis and treatment of varicoceles: a review. Minerva Urol Nefrol. 2014;66(4):257–82.
2. Kwak N, Siegel D. Imaging and interventional therapy for varicoceles. Curr Urol Rep. 2014;15(4):399.
3. Grieme B, Venbrux A. Management of male varicocele. In: Mauro MA, Murphy KPJ, Thomson KR, Venbrux AJ, Zollikofer CL, editors. Image-guided interventions. Philadelphia: Saunders Elsevier; 2008.
4. Moon E, Tam MD, Kikano RN, Karuppasamy K. Prophylactic antibiotic guidelines in modern interventional radiology practice. Semin Interv Radiol. 2010;27(4):327–37.
5. Taslakian B, Sebaaly MG, Al-Kutoubi A. Patient evaluation and preparation in vascular and interventional radiology: what every interventional radiologist should know (part 1: patient assessment and laboratory tests). Cardiovasc Intervent Radiol. 2016;39(3):325–33.
6. Taslakian B, Sebaaly MG, Al-Kutoubi A. Patient evaluation and preparation in vascular and interventional radiology: what every interventional radiologist should know (part 2: patient preparation and medications). Cardiovasc Intervent Radiol. 2016;39(4):489–99. doi: 10.1007/s00270-015-1239-4. [Epub 2015 Nov 25].

Ovarian Vein Embolization

114

Arwa Zaghal

Abbreviations

PCS	Pelvic congestion syndrome
PVI	Pelvic venous incompetence

INTRODUCTION

Pelvic congestion syndrome (PCS) or pelvic venous incompetence (PVI) is defined as the presence of ovarian and pelvic varicose veins associated with chronic pelvic pain persisting for more than 6 months that increases with prolonged standing, coitus, and menstruation. Minimally invasive embolization is the current standard treatment for PCS and is considered as one of the main procedures in "Women's Health Intervention." Once ovarian vein reflux and pelvic varicosities are demonstrated in symptomatic patients, the ovarian veins are then occluded. Peripheral occlusion of the uterine and pelvic veins is the most frequently reported method. Materials used include an absorbable gelatin sponge and a sclerosing agent followed by mechanical occlusion. Sometimes concomitant occlusion of the internal iliac vein tributaries is also performed to increase success rates.

A. Zaghal (✉)
Department of Diagnostic Radiology, American University of Beirut Medical Center, Riad El-Solh, Beirut 1107 2020, Lebanon
e-mail: aa200@aub.edu.lb

INDICATIONS [1, 2]

- Women with chronic non-cyclic pelvic pain for 6 months or more that is not relieved by medical therapies, in whom enlargement of the ovarian veins is documented. Pelvic vein embolization is the standard of treatment (grade 2B evidence)

CONTRAINDICATIONS [1]

- Active infection *(e.g., bacteremia, pelvic inflammatory disease,* etc.*)*
- Allergy to contrast
- Severe coagulopathy
- Pregnancy

COMPLICATIONS [1, 3]

General (angiography-related) complications:

- Access site complications *(e.g., hematoma, retroperitoneal hemorrhage, arterial injury, thrombosis)*
- Contrast-induced allergic reaction
- Contrast-induced nephropathy

B. Taslakian et al. (eds.), *Procedural Dictations in Image-Guided Intervention*,
DOI 10.1007/978-3-319-40845-3_114

- Catheter or guidewire breakage
- Risks related to any minimally invasive procedure performed under conscious sedation *(e.g., allergy to medications)*

Procedure-specific complications: Complications of embolotherapy for PVI are rare (less than 2 %)

- Non-target embolization including coil embolization to the pulmonary circulation
- Cardiac arrhythmias
- Vessel perforation
- Ovarian vein thrombophlebitis
- Recurrence of varices
- Radiation exposure to the ovaries

Outcome [1, 3, 4]:

- Procedural technical success rates for pelvic vein embolization are as high as 65–99 % [1, 4]
- Kim et al. reported significant clinical improvement in 89 % of patients; 13 % reported no change, and 4 % experienced worsening of symptoms [3]
- Limited long-term data has not demonstrated negative effects on menstrual cycle or fertility from transcatheter embolotherapy. Kim et al. [3] reported a 50 % pregnancy rate in premenopausal women who would otherwise become infertile with other medical or surgical techniques
- Most patients return to normal activity within 3–5 days

PREPROCEDURAL ASSESSMENT AND PLANNING

- Clinical history and indications *(Appendix 1* in Chap. 149*)*
- Evaluation of diagnostic imaging studies to determine the relevant vascular anatomy, document presence of pelvic varices, and to exclude other potential causes of pelvic pain such as endometriosis, adhesions, fibroids, atypical urological or menstrual pain, and irritable bowel syndrome
- Periprocedural management of coagulation status *(Appendices 2* in Chap. 150 *and 3 in* Chap. 151*)*
- Antibiotic prophylaxis: Single dose of antibiotic is routinely administered intravenously on the day of the procedure [1, 5]
- Imaging modality for guidance: Fluoroscopy ± ultrasound *(to guide venous puncture in difficult cases and obese patients)*
- Positioning: Supine.
- Venous access: Femoral vein, internal jugular vein
- Counseling the patient in an appropriate clinical setting, to discuss the risks, benefits, potential complications, outcomes, and specific details of the procedure
- Patient should be informed that she might experience significant pain following the procedure requiring admission for a "short stay" for pain management
- Negative pregnancy test should be documented *(medical-legal requirement)*

PROCEDURE NOTE

Procedure: Ovarian vein embolization
Staff: [_]
Fellow: [_]
Resident: [_]
Clinical History and Indications: Describe history and list indications
Allergies: None known/Allergic to [specify/type of allergy]
Anesthesia: Local anesthesia/Monitored conscious sedation
Medications: List any relevant medications used
Contrast Material: (_) mL of [type] contrast material was used for venography
Field: Sterile
Procedure classification: Clean
Position: Supine
Monitoring: Intravenous access line was secured and vital signs were continuously monitored by

nursing staff/anesthesia team throughout the procedure.

Total fluoroscopy time: (_) minutes
Cumulative radiation dose: (_) mGy

Description of Procedure:

The risks, benefits, alternatives, and procedure itself were explained to the patient/patient's Power of Attorney/patient's legal guardian, and informed written/verbal consent was obtained. Time out was performed to confirm the correct patient, procedure, and site. The site of the procedure was identified and marked.

Jugular Approach

The patient was positioned supine, with the neck turned to the contralateral side. The patient's cervical and upper thoracic regions were prepped and draped in a sterile fashion. Ultrasound examination was performed to determine the site of venous puncture. Local anesthesia was administered. The right internal jugular vein was punctured under ultrasound guidance using a (_)-gauge [type] needle. Once good venous flow was detected, a (_)-inch [type] guidewire was advanced through the needle under direct fluoroscopic visualization and placed in the superior vena cava. A small skin incision was made and a (_)-French vascular sheath was advanced over the guidewire.

Femoral Approach

The skin of both groins were shaved, prepped, and draped in the usual sterile fashion. The right/left common femoral vein was located by palpation/ultrasound and marked. Local anesthesia was administered and a small skin incision was made. Femoral venous access was obtained using a (_)-gauge [type] needle under direct ultrasound visualization/by palpation. Once good venous flow was detected, a (_)-inch [type] guidewire was advanced through the needle, up through the femoral vein into the inferior vena cava under direct fluoroscopic visualization and a (_)-French vascular sheath was advanced over the guidewire.

Then, a (_)-French [type] guiding catheter was used to select the left renal vein. A (_)-French coaxially directed hydrophilic [type] microcatheter was subsequently advanced over a guidewire into the left ovarian vein and down into the pelvis. An ovarian venogram was performed.

At that point, the embolic agent was prepared by mixing Gelfoam and 5 % sodium morrhuate: multiple small 3–4 mm pieces of Gelfoam were compressed in a 20 mL syringe. The sclerosant was placed in another 20 mL horizontal syringe. Using a three-way stopcock interposed between the syringes, the two materials were mixed until they formed thick paste.

The sclerosant and Gelfoam slurry mixture was then injected through the catheter. After an interval of 3–5 min, the left ovarian vein was selectively embolized using (number) coils [specify size/type].

Then selective catheterization of the right ovarian vein from the inferior vena cava was performed using a (_)-French [type] guiding catheter. A (_)-French coaxially directed hydrophilic [type] microcatheter was used to advance access down the right ovarian vein. A right ovarian venography was performed and the embolization procedure was repeated using the Gelfoam and morrhuate slurry mixture. After an interval of 3–5 min, the right ovarian vein was embolized using (number) coils [specify size/type].

After ovarian vein embolization, the anterior division of the internal iliac vein was selectively catheterized using a (_)-French [type] catheter and a (_)-inch [type] guidewire. Venography was performed to confirm location, and the diagnostic catheter was exchanged for a (_)-French occlusion [type/size] balloon catheter. The balloon was inflated at the anterior division of the internal iliac vein. A venogram was repeated to confirm location and the absence of reflux. The Gelfoam–sodium morrhuate slurry was injected with the occlusion balloon in place to prevent non-target embolization. After an interval period of 5–10 min the balloon was deflated. Completion venography was performed to exclude complications.

The vascular sheath was removed and adequate hemostasis was achieved at the puncture site by compression for (_) minutes. Sterile dressing was applied and the patient was transferred to the floor/recovery room following the procedure in a stable condition. Staff was present for the entire procedure.

Intra-Procedure Findings: List all relevant findings.

Immediate Complications: None encountered during or directly after the procedure. List complications if any.

Post-Procedure Plan [2, 3]:

- Keep patient complete bed rest with the right/left leg extended for (2–3) h *[adjust depending on the puncture site]*.
- Check the puncture site for any bleeding or hematoma formation every 15 min for 1 h, then every 30 min for 2 h; inform interventional radiology team if any complications are observed.
- Provide adequate pain control in the recovery room.
- If severe pain persists, the patient should be admitted to an inpatient service with access to patient-controlled analgesia (PCA) pump.
- Monitor vital signs every 15 min for 1 h, then every 30 min for 4 h; notify interventional radiology team if systolic blood pressure <95 mmHg, or heart rate >110 beats/min.
- Resume diet and previous orders as needed and if not otherwise contraindicated.
- Continue adequate intravenous hydration and monitor fluid (intake-output) status.
- Check complete blood count, creatinine, and blood urea nitrogen on the day following the procedure or as clinically indicated.
- At discharge, prescribe pain medication, short course of oral antibiotic, and an antiemetic.
- Schedule follow-up in clinic after 3–6 weeks to assess pelvic pain and decide if further endovascular therapy is needed.

Impression:

- Embolization of pelvic (ovarian/internal iliac) veins as described above.
- The patient tolerated the procedure well and left the interventional unit in stable condition.
- The procedure was canceled/terminated prematurely.
- List any other relevant or important information/finding.

References

1. Venbrux AC, Sharma GK, Jackson ET, Harper AP, Hover L. Pelvic varices embolization. In: Ignacio E, Venbrux AC, editors. Women's health in interventional radiology. New York: Springer; 2012. p. 37–59.
2. Smith PC. The outcome of treatment for pelvic congestion syndrome. Phlebology. 2012;27(Suppl 1):74–7.
3. Kim HS, Malhotra AD, Rowe PC, Lee JM, Venbrux AC. Embolotherapy for pelvic congestion syndrome: long-term results. J Vasc Interv Radiol. 2006;17(2 Pt 1):289–97.
4. Women's health interventions. In: Singh H, Neutze J, Enterline JR, editors. Radiology fundamentals. New York: Springer; 2015. p. 149–53.
5. Bittles MA, Hoffer EK. Gonadal vein embolization: treatment of varicocele and pelvic congestion syndrome. Semin Interv Radiol. 2008;25(3):261–70.

Uterine Artery Embolization

115

Sahar Semaan

INTRODUCTION

First reported in the late 1990s and derived from interventions to reduce posttraumatic or postpartum pelvic hemorrhage; transcatheter embolization of the uterine arteries for the management of uterine fibroids has become a widely accepted substitute to hysterectomy and myomectomy, especially in patients who desire fertility or are high-risk candidates for surgery. The procedure is associated with a high success rate primarily for the treatment of symptomatic leiomyomas, with symptoms including bleeding and pelvic pain, and also has been reported in the management of symptomatic adenomyosis. Transcatheter embolization generally has a low rate of postprocedural complications and has been associated with high patient satisfaction rates.

COMMON INDICATIONS [1–3]

- Symptomatic uterine leiomyomas:
  - Severe bleeding and secondary anemia
  - Pelvic pain and pressure symptoms
  - Mass effect on the urinary bladder with associated urinary frequency
  - Constipation
- Less commonly, adenomyosis with associated bleeding and pain

COMMON CONTRAINDICATIONS [1–3]

- History of reaction to contrast media
- Uncorrectable coagulopathy
- Impaired renal function
- Pregnancy
- Gynecologic malignancy
- Active pelvic inflammatory disease
- Endometritis
- Prior pelvic radiation
- Connective tissue disease

POSSIBLE COMPLICATIONS [1–3]

General (angiography-related) complications:

- Access site complications *(e.g., hematoma, retroperitoneal hemorrhage, arterial injury/pseudoaneurysm/arteriovenous fistula, thrombosis)*
- Contrast-induced allergic reaction
- Contrast-induced nephropathy
- Catheter or guidewire breakage
- Risks related to any minimally invasive procedure performed under conscious sedation *(e.g., allergy to medications)*

S. Semaan (✉)
Department of Radiology, Icahn School of Medicine at Mount Sinai, One Gustave L. Levy Place, New York, NY 10029-6574, USA
e-mail: saharsemaan@gmail.com

B. Taslakian et al. (eds.), *Procedural Dictations in Image-Guided Intervention*,
DOI 10.1007/978-3-319-40845-3_115

Procedure-specific complications:

- Amenorrhea
- Vaginal discharge
- Fibroid expulsion
- Pelvic pain
- Fever and chills

PREPROCEDURAL ASSESSMENT AND PLANNING [4–6]

- History, indications, and physical examination *(Appendix 1* in Chap. 149*)*
- Evaluation of diagnostic imaging studies: Pelvic ultrasound to assess uterine volume and size of fibroid(s), pelvic MRI with Gadolinium
- Periprocedural management of coagulation status *(Appendices 2* in Chap. 150 *and 3 in* Chap. 151*)*
- Antibiotic prophylaxis: Recommended, but no consensus for first choice. Common antibiotics used include: *1 g cefazolin IV, 2 g ampicillin IV, 900 mg clindamycin plus 1.5 mg/kg gentamicin IV, 1.5–3 g ampicillin/sulbactam* [4] *(Appendices 4* in Chap. 152 *and 5* in Chap. 153*)*
- Imaging modality for guidance: Fluoroscopy ± ultrasound *(to guide arterial puncture in difficult cases and obese patients)*
- Positioning of the patient: Supine

PROCEDURE NOTE

Procedure: Uterine artery embolization
Staff: [_]
Fellow: [_]
Resident: [_]
Clinical Information: Describe history and list indications
Allergies: None known/Allergic to [specify/type of allergy]
Anesthesia: Local anesthesia/conscious sedation
Medications: List any relevant medications used (sedation, antibiotics)
Contrast Used: (_) mL of [type] contrast media was used for intra-arterial injection
Field: Sterile
Procedure classification: Clean/Clean contaminated
Position: Supine
Monitoring: Intravenous access line was secured and vital signs were continuously monitored by nursing staff/anesthesia team throughout the procedure
Total fluoroscopy time: (_) minutes
Cumulative radiation dose: (_) mGy

Description of Procedure:
The risks, benefits, alternatives, and the procedure itself were explained to the patient/patient's Power of Attorney/patient's legal guardian, and informed written consent was obtained. The site of the procedure was identified and marked. Time out was performed to confirm the correct patient, procedure, and site.

The skin of both groins was shaved, prepped, and draped in the usual sterile fashion. The right/left femoral artery as well as the inguinal ligament were located by palpation/ultrasound and marked. The site of arterial puncture was determined using combined information from palpation, ultrasound, and fluoroscopy over the middle of the medial third of the femoral head. Local anesthesia was administered. Femoral artery access was obtained using a (_)-gauge [type] needle and the Seldinger technique, double-/single-wall entry under direct ultrasound visualization/by palpation. Once good pulsatile arterial flow was detected, a (_)-inch [type] guidewire was advanced through the needle, up the femoral artery, into the aorta under direct fluoroscopic visualization and a (_)-French vascular sheath was placed. Following this, a (_)-French [type] catheter was advanced over a guidewire into the aorta. With the tip of the catheter caudal to the renal arteries, contrast was injected and pelvic arteriography was performed to assess the uterine artery anatomy. Then, a (_)-French hydrophilic [type] catheter was used to selectively catheterize the right/left uterine artery and selective angiogram was performed. A (_)-French hydrophilic [type] microcatheter was then advanced to the transverse portion of the uterine artery and (_) mL of (size) polyvinyl alcohol embolization particles was injected until stasis of blood flow was achieved.

The catheter was then advanced to the opposite uterine artery and the procedure was repeated. A pelvic flush arteriogram was performed to evaluate the outcome and the catheter was then withdrawn. Following the procedure the right/left femoral artery sheath was removed and adequate hemostasis was achieved by (_) minute-compression/using [type] vascular closure device.

The femoral pulses were checked following the procedure and were comparable to the pre-procedure pulses/specify if otherwise needed.

The patient was transferred to the floor/recovery room/discharged home following the procedure in a stable condition. Staff was present for the entire procedure.

Intra-Procedure Findings: List all relevant findings.

Immediate Complications: None encountered during or directly after the procedure. List complications if any.

Post-Procedure Plan:

- Keep patient complete bed rest with the right/left leg extended for (_) hours.
- Check the right/left groin for any bleeding or hematoma formation every 15 min for 1 h, then every 30 min for 1 h, then every hour for 4 h; inform interventional radiology team if any observed.
- Check lower extremity pulses every 30 min for 2 h then every 1 h for 4 h and document in medical chart.
- Monitor vital signs every 15 min for 1 h, then every 30 min for 4 h; notify interventional radiology team if systolic blood pressure <95 mmHg, or heart rate >110 beats/min.
- Vigorous hydration (3 L of normal saline/24 h) until oral intake is optimal, unless otherwise contraindicated.
- Intravenous morphine 1–4 mg per hour by patient controlled anesthesia (PCA) pump.
- Antiemetic therapy as needed.
- Remove Foley catheter the next morning.
- Discharge patient home when oral intake is adequate and intravenous narcotics are no longer required.
- Follow up with gynecologist after 1–4 weeks.
- Follow up pelvic ultrasound in 3 and 6 months. Repeat MRI with Gadolinium at 6 months.
- Repeat FSH level on day 3 of next menstrual period or randomly if amenorrhea occurs.

Impression:

- Embolization of right/left/bilateral uterine artery(ies), as described above.
- The patient tolerated the procedure well and left the interventional unit in stable condition.
- The procedure was canceled/terminated prematurely.
- List any other relevant or important information/finding.

References

1. Stokes LS, Wallace MJ, Godwin RB, Kundu S, Cardella JF. Quality Improvement guidelines for uterine artery embolization for symptomatic leiomyomas. J Vasc Interv Radiol. 2010;21(8):1153–63.
2. Vilos GA, Allaire C, Laberge PY, Leyland N, Vilos AG, Murji A, et al. The management of uterine leiomyomas. J Obstet Gynaecol Can. 2015;37(2):157–81.
3. Marshburn PB, Matthews ML, Hurst BS. Uterine artery embolization as a treatment option for uterine myomas. Obstet Gynecol Clin North Am. 2006;33(1):125–44.
4. Venkatesan AM, Kundu S, Sacks D, Wallace MJ, Wojak JC, Rose SC, et al. Practice guidelines for adult antibiotic prophylaxis during vascular and interventional radiology procedures. J Vasc Interv Radiol. 2010;21(11):1611–30.
5. Taslakian B, Sebaaly MG, Al-Kutoubi A. Patient evaluation and preparation in vascular and interventional radiology: what every interventional radiologist should know (part 1: patient assessment and laboratory tests). Cardiovasc Intervent Radiol. 2016;39(3):325–33.
6. Taslakian B, Sebaaly MG, Al-Kutoubi A. Patient evaluation and preparation in vascular and interventional radiology: what every interventional radiologist should know (part 2: patient preparation and medications). Cardiovasc Intervent Radiol. 2016;39(4):489–99. doi: 10.1007/s00270-015-1239-4. [Epub 2015 Nov 25].

Part XVIII

Vascular Interventional Procedures: Pulmonary and Bronchial Arteries

Introduction by Aghiad Al-Kutoubi, Section Reviewer

Percutaneous transcatheter treatment for hemoptysis and transcatheter embolization of pulmonary arteriovenous malformations (AVM), aneurysms, and pseudoaneurysms were first reported in the 1970s. Intervention on the pulmonary arteries can vary from the elective management of pulmonary AVMs to the emergency treatment of acute pulmonary embolism. Catheter-based thrombolysis with intrapulmonary artery infusion of thrombolytic drugs, percutaneous thrombectomy, or embolus fragmentation can be performed in the patients with life-threatening pulmonary embolism.

Bronchial artery intervention is almost exclusively required in cases of hemoptysis. However, awareness of the various anatomical variants and the potential connection with spinal arterial supply, as well as supply from non-bronchial arteries such as the inferior phrenic arteries or branches of the axillary arteries, is a prerequisite for safe and effective management.

These minimally invasive procedures are well established, safe, and effective when performed by experienced interventionalists and may obviate open surgery.

This section provides a comprehensive list of procedural reports that covers the vast majority of the currently performed procedures in the pulmonary and bronchial arteries, with up-to-date explanatory notes, synopsis of the indications and contraindications, and potential complications in an organized and practical format.

Section Chapters

116 Bronchial Artery Embolization

Sean Farquharson

INTRODUCTION

Massive hemoptysis has been defined as expectoration of more than 200–600 mL of blood over a 24-h period [1, 2].

Although massive hemoptysis accounts for only 5 % of cases, mortality from massive hemoptysis can be as high as 80 % and these patients usually die from asphyxiation not exsanguination. The lung has blood flow from both the pulmonary and bronchial arteries, and although hemoptysis can result from pathology affecting either system, the bronchial arteries are the source of 90 % of massive hemoptysis encountered. Historically, many of these patients underwent bronchoscopy to localize the site of bleeding and attempt treatment with iced saline lavage, topical agents, or balloon tamponade. If the source of bleeding could not be visualized on bronchoscopy, or if bronchoscopic treatment failed, then the next step was bronchial artery angiography with embolization. Bronchial artery embolization has proven to be a very effective treatment to control massive hemoptysis with reported success rates ranging from 64 to 100 % [3] and in many institutions it has become the first line treatment. Despite the high success in initial control of bleeding, depending on the etiology, recurrent hemoptysis can be seen in 23 % of patients at 5 years [4]. In most cases, recurrent bleed can be managed with repeat embolization. Due to the extreme variability in pulmonary artery anatomy, preprocedural chest CT angiography is recommended to localize the side/lobe of the hemorrhage and possibly localize the origin of the target bronchial artery to assist in cannulation during angiography.

COMMON INDICATIONS [5, 6]

- Massive hemoptysis *(not related to pulmonary artery)*
  - Common causes include:
    Bronchogenic carcinoma
    Chronic inflammatory lung diseases due to bronchiectasis, cystic fibrosis, or aspergillosis
    Tuberculosis
    Lung abscess
    Pneumonia
    Pulmonary interstitial fibrosis
    Pneumoconiosis

COMMON CONTRAINDICATIONS [5, 6]

- Past history of allergy to intravenous contrast media *(steroid preparation)*

S. Farquharson (✉)
Department of Radiology, New York University Langone Medical Center, 660 First Ave, 7th Floor, New York, NY 10016, USA
e-mail: sean.farquharson@nyumc.org

B. Taslakian et al. (eds.), *Procedural Dictations in Image-Guided Intervention*,
DOI 10.1007/978-3-319-40845-3_116

- Impaired renal function *(Hydration, non-ionic contrast, mycomyst)*
- Uncorrected coagulopathy *(FFP, Vitamin K, Kcentra)*
- Spinal artery originating from target bronchial artery *(embolize distal to spinal artery)*

POSSIBLE COMPLICATIONS [5, 6]

Angiography-related complications:

- Access site complications *(e.g., hematoma, retroperitoneal hemorrhage, arterial injury, thrombosis)*
- Contrast-induced allergic reaction
- Contrast-induced nephropathy
- Catheter or guidewire breakage
- Risks related to any minimally invasive procedure performed under conscious sedation *(e.g., allergy to medications)*

Procedure-specific complications:

- Lower extremity paralysis *(due to off target spinal arterial embolization, 1.4–6.5 %)* [5, 6]
- Chest pain; *24–91 %*
- Dysphagia, *0.7–18.2 %*
- Subintimal dissection of the aorta
- Stroke
- Transient cortical blindness
- Pulmonary infarcts

PREPROCEDURAL ASSESSMENT AND PLANNING

- History, indications, and physical examination *(Appendix 1* in Chap. 149*)*. Document indications of the procedure, lower or upper extremity pulses and vital signs
- Evaluation of diagnostic imaging studies, especially chest CT angiography to localize side of hemorrhage and level of origin of target bronchial arteries
  - *Most common configuration, seen in 40 % of patients—two left bronchial arteries, one right bronchial artery which arises from an intercostobronchial trunk*
  - *80 % of bronchial arteries arise from aorta between the T5 and T6 level [7]*
  - *20 % of bronchial arteries have anomalous origins not from the aorta; these can include the subclavian, thyrocervical, internal mammary, innominate, pericardiophrenic, superior intercostals, abdominal aorta, and inferior phrenic arteries* [7–9]
- Periprocedural management of coagulation status *(Appendices 2* in Chap. 150 *and 3 in* Chap. 151*)*
- Antibiotic prophylaxis: Not routinely recommended [10] *(Appendices 4* in Chap. 152 *and 5* in Chap. 153*)*
- Imaging modality for guidance: Fluoroscopy; combined with ultrasound for arterial puncture
- Positioning: Supine
- Arterial access: Common femoral artery
- Anesthesia: Conscious sedation/Monitored Anesthesia Care *(general anesthesia with Double-lumen endotracheal tube placement may be needed to protect unaffected lung and decreased respiratory motion in the lung being studied)*
- Low-osmolar contrast preferred
- Embolic agent:
  - 300–500 micron particles (Embospheres or Polyvinyl alcohol) or larger
  - Consider n-BCA glue embolization if significant shunting is present
- Consider somatosensory evoked potentials (SEP) monitoring, especially if patient is going to be under general anesthesia and neurologic status cannot be assessed intra-procedurally

PROCEDURE NOTE

Procedure: Thoracic aortogram, (right/left) subclavian artery angiogram, (right/left/bilateral) bronchial artery angiogram and (right/left/bilateral) bronchial artery embolization

Staff: [_]

Fellow: [_]

Resident: [_]

Clinical History and Indications: Describe history and list indications

Allergies: None known/Allergic to [specify/type of allergy]
Anesthesia: Local anesthesia/Conscious sedation/General anesthesia
Medications: List any relevant medications used
Contrast Material: (_) mL of [type] contrast material was used for intra-arterial injection
Field: Sterile
Procedure classification: Clean
Position: Supine
Monitoring: Intravenous access line was secured and vital signs were continuously monitored by nursing staff/anesthesia team throughout the procedure
Total fluoroscopy time: (_) minutes
Cumulative radiation dose: (_) mGy

Description of Procedure *(particle embolization of (right/left/bilateral) bronchial artery):*
The risks, benefits, alternatives, and procedure itself were explained to the patient/patient's Power of Attorney/patient's legal guardian, and informed written/verbal consent was obtained. Time out was performed to confirm the correct patient, procedure, and site. The site of the procedure was identified and marked.

The skin of right/left groin was shaved, prepped, and draped in the usual sterile fashion. The right/left common femoral artery was located by palpation/ultrasound and marked. After the administration of (_) subcutaneous local anesthesia, the right/left common femoral artery was accessed using (Modified) Seldinger technique (and direct ultrasound guidance) using a (_)-gauge needle. Once good pulsatile arterial flow was detected, a (_)-inch [type] guidewire was advanced through the needle (and exchange made for a (_) French coaxial dilator which was used to place a 0.035-in. wire), up through the common femoral artery, into the aorta under direct fluoroscopic visualization. A (_)-French vascular sheath was placed over the wire and the side port was attached to heparinized saline infusion. A (_)-French, (_) cm-long [type] flush catheter was advanced through the sheath, over the wire up to the origin of the descending thoracic aorta, just distal to the origin of the left subclavian artery. Descending thoracic aortogram was then performed by injecting [type] contrast, at a rate of (20–30 mL/s) for a total of (40–60) mL and digital subtraction imaging was performed at (4–8) frames per second during suspended respiration in anterior-posterior projection. The [type] flush catheter was exchanged over a (0.035)-in. guidewire for a (_)-French [Mikaelson/Cobra/Simmons-1/headhunter/other] catheter which was formed in the aorta and used to cannulate the right/left bronchial artery. Angiography of the selected bronchial artery was performed by injecting (5–10) mL of contrast, at a rate of (1–3 mL/s) and digital subtraction imaging was performed. Superselective catheterization of the bronchial artery was performed using a (_)-French [type] coaxial microcatheter advanced further into the selected bronchial artery, past the origin of the spinal artery/intercostal artery and selective digital subtraction angiography was repeated followed by superselective embolization of the bronchial artery using a mixture of [type] contrast and (_) micron (Embospheres/Polyvinyl alcohol/other particles). The embolic mixture was injected in a controlled fashion under real-time fluoroscopic monitoring of flow and reflux, until near stasis in the artery was achieved. The microcatheter was cleared of embolic material and removed. Controlled hand injection of contrast through the main catheter in the proximal bronchial artery was performed to assess patency; then the catheter was repositioned into the aorta and exchanged over a (0.035)-in. wire for a (_)-French selective catheter which was used to cannulate the ipsilateral subclavian artery. Angiography of the right/left subclavian artery was performed by injecting [type] contrast, at a rate of (3–5 mL/s) for a total of (10–15) mL and digital subtraction imaging was performed during suspended respiration in anterior-posterior projection.

An anomalous bronchial artery originating from the (_) branch of the (right/left) subclavian artery was cannulated with the [type] catheter advanced over a [type] (0.035)-in. wire. Superselective catheterization of the bronchial artery was performed using the (_)-French [type] coaxial microcatheter and selective digital subtraction angiography was performed followed by superselective embolization of the bronchial artery using a mixture of [type] contrast and (_) micron (Embospheres/Polyvinyl alcohol/other particle). The embolic mixture was injected in a controlled fashion under real-time fluoroscopic monitoring of flow and reflux, until near stasis of the artery was achieved. The microcatheter was cleared of embolic material and removed; controlled hand injection through the main catheter in the origin of the bronchial artery was performed. The catheter was pulled back into the right/left subclavian artery and digital subtraction angiography performed.

The catheter was then pulled back into the aorta where it was exchanged over a (0.035)-in. wire for a (_) French [type] flush catheter which was placed at the origin of the descending thoracic aorta, just distal to the origin of the left subclavian artery. Descending thoracic aortography was then performed by injecting [type] contrast, at a rate of (20–30 mL/s) for a total of (40–60) mL and digital subtraction imaging was performed at (4–8) frames per second during suspended respiration in anterior-posterior projection. The catheter was then removed over a wire.

Following the procedure, the right/left femoral artery sheath was removed and adequate hemostasis was achieved by compression for (_) minutes/using [type] vascular closure device. The femoral pulses were checked following the procedure and were [comparable to the preprocedure pulses/specify if otherwise needed]. The patient was able to move (right/left/bilateral) lower extremities at the end of the procedure and was transferred to the floor/recovery room for close monitoring following the procedure in a stable condition. Staff was present for the entire procedure.

Intra-Procedure Findings: List all relevant findings.

Immediate Complications: None encountered during or directly after the procedure. List complications if any.

Post-Procedure Plan [1, 2]:

Standard post-angiogram management plan:

- Keep patient complete bed rest with the right/left leg extended for (_) hours *[adjust depending on the puncture site]*.
- Check the right/left groin/[specify the puncture site if different] for any bleeding or hematoma formation every 15 min for 1 h, then every 30 min for 1 h, then every hour for 4 h; inform interventional radiology team if any observed *[adjust depending on the puncture site]*.
- Check and document lower extremity pulses every 30 min for 2 h then every 1 h for 4 h *[adjust depending on the puncture site]*.
- Monitor vital signs every 15 min for 1 h, then every 30 min for 4 h; notify interventional radiology team if systolic blood pressure <95 mmHg, or heart rate >110 beats/min.
- Resume diet and previous orders as needed and if otherwise not contraindicated.
- Heparin can be restarted within 2 h after removal of the vascular sheath and documenting the absence of puncture site-related complication.
- Continue adequate intravenous hydration and monitor fluid (intake-output) status.
- Check complete blood count, creatinine, and blood urea nitrogen on the day following the procedure or as clinically indicated.

Impression:

- Catheter-directed [right/left/bilateral bronchial artery embolization, as described above.
- The patient tolerated the procedure well and left the interventional unit in stable condition.
- The patient was unstable and the procedure was canceled/terminated prematurely.
- List any other relevant or important information/finding.

References

1. Knott-Craig CJ, Oostuizen JG, Rossouw G, Joubert JR, Barnard PM. Management and prognosis of massive hemoptysis: recent experience with 120 patients. J Thorac Cardiovasc Surg. 1993;105(3):394–7.
2. Crocco JA, Rooney JJ, Fankushen DS, DiBenedetto RJ, Lyons HA. Massive hemoptysis. Arch Intern Med. 1968;121(6):495–8.
3. Dweik RA1, Stoller JK. Role of bronchoscopy in massive hemoptysis. Clin Chest Med. 1999;20(1):89–105.
4. Rabkin JE, Astafjev VI, Gothman LN, Grigorjev YG. Transcatheter embolization in the management of

pulmonary hemorrhage. Radiology. 1987;163 (2):361–5.
5. Ramakantan R, Bandekar VG, Gandhi MS, Aulakh BG, Deshmukh HL. Massive hemoptysis due to pulmonary tuberculosis: control with bronchial artery embolization. Radiology. 1996;200(3):691–4.
6. Tonkin IL, Hanissian AS, Boulden TF, Baum SL, Gavant ML, Gold RE, et al. Bronchial arteriography and embolotherapy for hemoptysis in patients with cystic fibrosis. Cardiovasc Interv Radiol. 1991;14 (4):241–6.
7. Burke CT, Mauro MA. Bronchial artery embolization. Semin Interv Radiol. 2004;21(1):43–8.
8. McPherson S, Routh WD, Nath H, Keller FS. Anomalous origin of bronchial arteries: potential pitfall of embolotherapy for hemoptysis. J Vasc Interv Radiol. 1990;1(1):86–8.
9. Cohen AM, Antoun BW, Stern RC. Left thyrocervical trunk bronchial artery supplying right ling: source of recurrent hemoptysis in cystic fibrosis. AJR Am J Roentgenol. 1992;158(5):1131–3.
10. Venkatesan AM, Kundu S, Sacks D, Wallace MJ, Wojak JC, Rose SC, et al. Practice guidelines for adult antibiotic prophylaxis during vascular and interventional radiology procedures. J Vasc Interv Radiol. 2010;21(11):1611–30.

Embolization of Pulmonary Arteriovenous Malformations

117

Jonathan S. Gross

Abbreviations

AVMS	Arteriovenous malformations
HHT	Hereditary hemorrhagic telangiectasia

INTRODUCTION

Pulmonary arteriovenous malformations (AVMs) are of special concern, because they are foci of right to left shunting and may be complicated by hypoxia, solid organ abscess, and stroke. Because they are associated with high morbidity and mortality, they require aggressive management, and treatment is recommended for all pulmonary AVMs with feeding arteries greater than 3 mm in diameter [1]. The standard treatment for pulmonary AVMs is endovascular embolization with coils, which is reportedly technically successful in 97 % of cases [2]. The most feared complication of embolization is passage of a coil through the AVM into the systemic arterial circulation, a complication which may be prevented by oversizing the embolization coil, by deploying the tip of the coil in a small side branch artery which anchors the coil in position, using detachable coils, or using a vascular plug. Because there is a risk of recanalization following embolization, patients should have routine follow up with imaging to evaluate the need for further treatment [3].

While they may occur due to entities such as trauma, hepatopulmonary syndrome, or cardiac surgery, at least 60 % of pulmonary AVMs occur in the setting of the autosomal dominant hereditary hemorrhagic telangiectasia (HHT) [4]. Therefore, in the absence of another obvious etiology, it is recommended that patients found to have one or more pulmonary AVMs be screened for HHT [5].

INDICATIONS

- Pulmonary AVM with feeding artery ≥ 3 mm in diameter [5]
- Pulmonary AVM with feeding artery <3 mm in diameter in symptomatic patients *(hypoxia due to diffuse AVMS; history of stroke, transient ischemic attack, brain abscess, or other symptoms of right to left embolism)* [6]

Possible Indications:

- Pulmonary AVM with feeding artery <3 mm in diameter, even in asymptomatic adults in effort to reduce risk of right to left embolism [2, 4]
- Pulmonary AVM in asymptomatic children <12 years of age [6]

J.S. Gross (✉)
Department of Radiology, New York University Langone Medical Center, 660 First Avenue, 7th Floor, New York, NY 10016, USA
e-mail: jonathan.gross@nyumc.org

B. Taslakian et al. (eds.), *Procedural Dictations in Image-Guided Intervention*,
DOI 10.1007/978-3-319-40845-3_117

CONTRAINDICATIONS

Absolute contraindications:
- Uncorrected coagulopathy
- Active, untreated pneumonia

Relative contraindications:
- History of severe allergic reaction to intravenous contrast media
- Pregnancy
- Renal insufficiency which may be exacerbated by contrast exposure
- Pulmonary arterial hypertension [7]
- Left bundle branch block: If a patient has left bundle branch block, external pacing equipment should be available in case patient develops right bundle branch block during passage of the catheter through the atrium [8]

POSSIBLE COMPLICATIONS

General (angiography-related) complications:
- Access site complications *(e.g., hematoma, retroperitoneal hemorrhage, arterial injury, thrombosis)*
- Contrast-induced allergic reaction
- Contrast-induced nephropathy
- Catheter or guidewire breakage
- Risks related to any minimally invasive procedure performed under conscious sedation *(e.g., allergy to medications)*

Procedure-specific complications:
- Hemorrhage
- Arrhythmias, including right bundle branch block [8]
- Embolization of coil through the AVM into the systemic circulation [9, 10]
- Pleurisy [9]
- Myocardial ischemia due to embolization of air bubbles into the coronary arteries [4]
- Pulmonary infarction
- Non-target embolization of normal pulmonary vessels
- Pulmonary arterial hypertension [4, 10]

PREPROCEDURAL ASSESSMENT AND PLANNING

- Review relevant medical history
  - Screen for history of hypoxia, stroke/transient ischemic attack, unusual systemic infection or solid organ abscess which might be attributable to the presence of pulmonary AVM
  - Screen for any signs/personal or family history suggestive of HHT
  - Screen for signs/symptoms of pulmonary arterial hypertension
- Evaluate diagnostic CT or MR pulmonary angiogram to determine number, location, and anatomy of AVM(s)
- Evaluate electrocardiogram for arrhythmia, especially left bundle branch block
- Review coagulation status; if necessary, transfuse to platelets >50,000 and INR < 1.6
- Antibiotic prophylaxis: No consensus, though some groups routinely administer cefazolin [2, 9] *(Appendices 4* in Chap. 152 *and 5* in Chap. 153*)*
- Immediate preprocedure heparin bolus 3000–5000 units
- Imaging modality for guidance: Fluoroscopy *(± ultrasound for venous puncture)*
- Positioning: Supine
- Venous access: Ipsilateral or contralateral common femoral vein *(preferred)* or internal jugular vein

PROCEDURE NOTE

Procedure: Selective and subselective pulmonary arteriograms; embolization of pulmonary arteriovenous malformation
Staff: [_]
Fellow: [_]
Resident: [_]
Clinical History and Indications: Describe history and list indications
Allergies: None known/Allergic to [specify/type of allergy]

Anesthesia: Local anesthesia/Conscious sedation/General anesthesia
Medications: List any relevant medications used, including antibiotic
Contrast Material: (_) mL [type] contrast
Field: Sterile
Procedure classification: Clean
Position: Supine
Monitoring: Intravenous access line was secured and vital signs were continuously monitored by nursing staff/anesthesia team throughout the procedure. Air filters were applied to intravenous tubing to minimize risk of paradoxical embolization of air bubbles.
Total fluoroscopy time: (_) minutes
Cumulative radiation dose: (_) mGy

Description of Procedure:

The risks, benefits, alternatives, and procedure itself were explained to the patient/patient's Power of Attorney/patient's legal guardian, and informed written/verbal consent was obtained. Time out was performed to confirm the correct patient, procedure, and site. The patient was positioned supine on the angiographic table. The site of the venous access was identified and marked.

The right/left groin was prepped and draped in sterile fashion. The right/left common femoral vein was accessed using a (_) gauge needle under sonographic guidance. Using Seldinger technique, the needle was exchanged over a (_)-inch guidewire for a (_) French sheath.

A (_) French flush catheter was advanced over a wire through the sheath into the main pulmonary artery and the pulmonary arterial pressure was measured. The catheter was then advanced into the right/left pulmonary artery, and a pulmonary arteriogram was performed. Based on the angiographic findings, a branch of the left/right/upper/middle/lower lobe pulmonary artery was selected. A subselective pulmonary arteriogram was performed.

A (_) mm × (_) cm coil was deployed in the artery just proximal to the pulmonary arteriovenous malformation. A post-embolization subselective pulmonary arteriogram was performed. The catheter was then directed into a second/third/,etc., arterial branch supplying the AVM. A subselective pulmonary arteriogram was performed, and a (_) mm × (_) cm coil was deployed in the artery just proximal to the pulmonary arteriovenous malformation.

The catheter was positioned in the right/left pulmonary artery, and a post-embolization pulmonary arteriogram was performed. The catheter was then positioned in the main pulmonary artery, and post-embolization pulmonary artery pressure was measured.

The catheter and sheath were removed, and pressure was held over the access site to achieve hemostasis. The patient was transferred to the floor/recovery room/ICU in a stable condition. Staff was present for the entire procedure.

Intra-Procedure Findings: List all relevant findings.

Immediate Complications: No immediate complications. List complications if any.

Post-Procedure Plan:

Standard post-venogram management:

- Complete bed rest with the right/left leg extended for 2 h *[adjust depending on the puncture site]*.
- Check the right/left groin [specify the puncture site if different] for any bleeding every 15 min for 1 h, then every 30 min for 1 h; inform interventional radiology team if patient develops any signs of bleeding.
- Administer adequate intravenous hydration and monitor fluid intake and output.

Procedure-specific management plan:

- Administer narcotics/analgesics if needed for pain.
- Monitor vital signs every 15 min × 4, then every 30 min × 2, then per routine.
- Resume diet and previous orders (if not otherwise contraindicated).

Impression:

- Subselective coil embolization of the right/left upper/middle/lower lobe pulmonary arteriovenous malformation.
- The patient tolerated the procedure well and left the interventional unit in stable condition.

- The patient was unstable and the procedure was canceled/terminated prematurely.
- List any other relevant or important information/finding.

References

1. White RI, Pollak JS, Wirth JA. Pulmonary arteriovenous malformations: diagnosis and transcatheter embolotherapy. J Vasc Interv Radiol. 1996;7(6):787–804.
2. Pollak JS, Saluja S, Thabet A, Henderson KJ, Denbow N, White RI Jr. Clinical and anatomic outcomes after embolotherapy of pulmonary arteriovenous malformations. J Vasc Interv Radiol. 2006;17(1):35–44; quiz 45.
3. Pollak JS, White RI. Distal cross sectional occlusion is the key to treating pulmonary arteriovenous malformations. J Vasc Interv Radiol. 2012;23(12):1578–80.
4. Meek ME, Meek JC, Beheshti MV. Management of pulmonary arteriovenous malformations. Semin Interv Radiol. 2011;28(1):24–31.
5. Faughnan ME, Palda VA, Garcia-Tsao G, Geisthoff UW, McDonald J, Proctor DD, et al. International guidelines for the diagnosis and management of hereditary hemorrhagic telangiectasias. J Med Genet. 2011;48(2):73–87.
6. Trerotola SO, Pyeritz RE. PAVM embolization: an update. AJR Am J Roentgenol. 2010;195(4):837–45.
7. Shovlin CL, Tighe HC, Davies RJ, Gibbs JSR, Jackson JE. Embolization of pulmonary arteriovenous malformations: no consistent effect on pulmonary artery pressure. Eur Respir J. 2008;32(1):162–9.
8. Sprung CL, Elser B, Schein RM, Marcial EH, Schrager BR. Risk of right bundle branch block and complete heart block during pulmonary artery catheterization. Crit Care Med. 1989;17(1):1–3.
9. Narsinh KH, Ramaswamy R, Kinney TB. Management of pulmonary arteriovenous malformations in hereditary hemorrhagic telangiectasia patients. Semin Interv Radiol. 2013;30(4):408–12.
10. Haitjema T, ten Berg J, Overtoom J, Ernst J, Westermann CJ. Unusual complications after embolization of a pulmonary arteriovenous malformation. Chest. 1996;109(5):1401–4.

Pulmonary Angiography

118

Sean Farquharson

Abbreviations

PE	Pulmonary embolism
CTA	CT angiography
AVM	Arteriovenous malformations

INTRODUCTION

Pulmonary angiography, long held as the gold standard for diagnosing pulmonary embolism (PE) has been eclipsed by noninvasive helical pulmonary artery CT angiography (CTA) as the diagnostic study of choice when PE is suspected. However, there is still a role for conventional pulmonary angiography in patients with a high clinical suspicion of PE and equivocal CTA results due to its greater sensitivity and specificity at detecting small peripheral emboli [1]. During diagnostic pulmonary angiography, direct pressure measurements of right heart and pulmonary artery can be obtained and these can be important in determining the degree of compromise in the acute setting and the degree of pulmonary hypertension in patients with chronic PE.

Probably the most common indication for diagnostic pulmonary angiography is for intra-procedural planning prior to proceeding directly to catheter directed therapy in the setting of pulmonary arteriovenous malformations (AVM), acute PE (pulmonary thrombectomy or thrombosis) or as part of the work up for planned surgical embolectomy in patients with chronic PE [2].

COMMON INDICATIONS [1, 2]

- High clinical suspicion of PE in a patient with discordant noninvasive imaging (ventilation/perfusion scan and /or CTA)
- Intra-procedural planning prior to proceeding directly to catheter directed therapy in the setting of pulmonary AVM or PE
- Pre-operative workup for planned surgical embolectomy in patients with chronic PE
- Intra-procedure planning prior to catheter directed retrieval of a foreign body from the pulmonary artery

S. Farquharson (✉)
Department of Radiology, New York University Langone Medical Center, 660 First Avenue, 7th Floor, New York, NY 10016, USA
e-mail: sean.farquharson@nyumc.org

B. Taslakian et al. (eds.), *Procedural Dictations in Image-Guided Intervention*,
DOI 10.1007/978-3-319-40845-3_118

CONTRAINDICATIONS

Absolute contraindications:

- Hemodynamically too unstable to come to interventional radiology suite

Relative contraindications:

- Contrast allergy *(should receive pre-medication)*
- Severe pulmonary hypertension—systolic pulmonary artery pressure ≥60 mm Hg [3] *(re-assess need for the study, use non-ionic low osmolality contrast and more selective injections with less contrast)*
- Left bundle-branch block *(place transvenous pacing leads or have external pacing pads in place in case of complete heart block)*

POSSIBLE COMPLICATIONS

General (angiography-related) complications:

- Access site complications *(e.g., hematoma, retroperitoneal hemorrhage, arterial injury, thrombosis)*
- Contrast-induced allergic reaction
- Contrast-induced nephropathy
- Catheter or guidewire breakage
- Risks related to any minimally invasive procedure performed under conscious sedation *(e.g., allergy to medications)*

Procedure-specific complications:

- Cardiac arrhythmia, most notably complete heart block in patients with pre-existing left bundle-branch block
- Fatal cardiac arrest due to right ventricular failure *(in patients with severe pulmonary hypertension)* [3]

PREPROCEDURAL ASSESSMENT AND PLANNING

- History, indications and physical examination
- Evaluation of diagnostic imaging studies:
  - Pulmonary CTA, to determine the relevant vascular anatomy and location of any suspected pulmonary emboli, foreign body, or vascular malformation to be evaluated
  - Echocardiogram to determine degree of right heart dysfunction and gauge degree of pulmonary hypertension
  - Lower extremity Doppler to access for presence of deep venous thrombosis which could influence choice of access site
- Review EKG to look for left bundle-branch block
- Consider the need for inferior vena cava filter which can be placed concurrently via the same access
- Periprocedural management of coagulation status *(Appendices 2* in Chaps. 150 *and 3* in 151*)*; these patients are often on intravenous heparin drip which can be held in the periprocedure period
- Antibiotic prophylaxis: Not routinely recommended [4] *(Appendices 4* in Chaps. 152 *and 5* in 153*)*
- Imaging modality for guidance: Fluoroscopy; combined with ultrasound for access
- Positioning: Supine
- Venous access: Common femoral vein, internal jugular vein

PROCEDURE NOTE

Procedure: Bilateral/Right/Left pulmonary angiogram with pressure measurements
Staff: [_]
Fellow: [_]
Resident: [_]
Clinical History and Indications: Describe history and list indications
Allergies: None known/Allergic to [specify/type of allergy]
Anesthesia: Local anesthesia/Conscious sedation/Monitored anesthesia care
Medications: List any relevant medications used
Contrast Material: (_) mL of [type] contrast material was used for pulmonary angiogram. *[Preferably non-ionic low osmolality contrast]*
Field: Sterile
Procedure classification: Clean
Position: Supine
Monitoring: Intravenous access line was secured, vital signs, including continuous cardiac

monitoring followed by nursing staff/anesthesia team throughout the procedure
Total Fluoroscopy time: (_) minutes
Cumulative radiation dose: (_) mGy

Description of Procedure:
The risks, benefits, alternatives, and procedure itself were explained to the patient/patient's Power of Attorney/patient's legal guardian, and informed written/verbal consent was obtained. Time out was performed to confirm the correct patient, procedure and site. The patient was positioned supine on the angiographic table. The site of the procedure was identified and marked.

Femoral approach {Preferred}- The skin of the right/left groin was shaved, prepped and draped in the usual sterile fashion. The right/left common femoral vein was located by palpation/ultrasound and marked. Local anesthesia was administered and a small skin incision was made. Femoral venous access was obtained using a (_)-gauge [type] needle under direct ultrasound visualization/by palpation. Once good venous flow was detected, a (_)-inch [type] guidewire was advanced through the needle, and exchange made for a (_)-French co-axial dilator which was used to place a 0.035-in. wire which was advanced up through the femoral vein into the inferior vena cava under direct fluoroscopic visualization and a (_)-French, (_)-cm-long vascular sheath was placed.

Jugular approach {If femoral approach is not possible due to thrombus or other reasons}- With the neck turned to the contralateral side, the patient's left/right cervical and upper thoracic regions were prepped and draped in the usual sterile fashion. Ultrasound examination was performed to determine the site of venous puncture. Local anesthesia was administered. The left/right internal jugular vein was punctured under ultrasound guidance using an (_)-gauge [type] needle. Once good venous flow was detected, a (_)-inch [type] guidewire was advanced through the needle under direct fluoroscopic visualization and exchange made for a (_)-French co-axial dilator which was used to place a 0.035-in. wire into the superior vena cava. A small skin incision was made and a (_)-French vascular sheath was advanced over the guidewire.

A (_)-French [type] flush catheter was advanced through the sheath into the superior/inferior vena cava over the (_)-inch [type] guidewire. The wire and catheter were advanced in a stepwise fashion trough the right atrium and into the right ventricle where right ventricle pressure measurements were obtained through the catheter. The wire was then re-introduced through the catheter and in a stepwise fashion the wire and catheter were advanced into the main pulmonary artery. Catheter position was confirmed with hand injection of contrast followed by obtaining pulmonary artery pressure measurements through the catheter. The catheter was then advanced over the wire into the left/right pulmonary artery where angiography was performed by injecting (20–30) mL of [type] contrast, at a rate of (15–25 mL/s) and digital subtraction angiography imaging was performed at (6) frames per second during suspended respiration in both anterior-posterior, and 45° ipsilateral posterior-oblique projections [specify if sub-selective injections of pulmonary artery branches or other projections were obtained]. The Catheter was then repositioned into the right/left pulmonary artery where angiography was performed by injecting (20–30) mL of [type] contrast, at a rate of (15–25 mL/s) and digital subtraction angiography imaging was performed at (6) frames per second during suspended respiration in both anterior-posterior, and 45° ipsilateral posterior-oblique projections [specify if sub-selective injections of pulmonary artery branches or other projections are obtained].

The catheter was then removed followed by the sheath and adequate hemostasis was achieved at the venotomy site by compression for (_) minutes. Sterile dressing was applied and the patient was transferred to the floor/recovery room following the procedure in a stable/critical condition. Staff was present for the entire procedure.
Intra-Procedure Findings: List all relevant findings, including measured right atrial and pulmonary artery pressures.

Immediate Complications: None encountered during or directly after the procedure. List complications if any.

Post-Procedure Plan

- Keep patient complete bed rest with the right/left leg extended for (2–3) h. *{Femoral approach}*
- Keep patient on bed rest with head of bed greater than 45° for 2 h.*{jugular approach}*
- Check the puncture site for any bleeding or hematoma formation every 15 min for 1 h, then every 30 min for 2 h; inform interventional radiology team if any complications are observed.
- Monitor vital signs every 15 min for 1 h, then every 30 min for 2 h; notify interventional radiology team if systolic blood pressure <95 mm Hg, or heart rate >110 beats/min.
- Resume diet and previous orders as needed and if not otherwise contraindicated.
- Continue adequate intravenous hydration and monitor fluid (intake–output) status.
- Check complete blood count, creatinine and blood urea nitrogen on the day following the procedure or as clinically indicated.

Impression:

- Bilateral/Right/Left pulmonary angiogram with pressure measurements.
- The patient tolerated the procedure well and left the interventional unit in stable condition.
- The patient was unstable and the procedure was canceled/terminated prematurely.
- List any other relevant or important information/finding.

References

1. Goldhaber SZ. Pulmonary embolism. N Engl J Med. 1998;339:93–104.
2. Auger WR, Fedullo PF, Moser KM, Buchbinder M, Peterson KL. Chronic major-vessel thromboembolic pulmonary artery obstruction: appearance at angiography. Radiology. 1993;182:393–8.
3. Hofmann LV, Lee DS, Gupta A, Arepally A, Sood S, Girgis R, Eng J. Safety and Hemodynamic Effects of Pulmonary Angiography in Patients with Pulmonary Hypertension: 10-Year Single-Center Experience. AJR Am J Roentgenol. 2004;183(3):779–86.
4. Venkatesan AM, Kundu S, Sacks D, Wallace MJ, Wojak JC, Rose SC, et al. Practice guidelines for adult antibiotic prophylaxis during vascular and interventional radiology procedures. J Vasc Interv Radiol. 2010;21(11):1611–30.

Pulmonary Artery Thrombectomy and Thrombolysis

119

Sean Farquharson

Abbreviations

PE	Pulmonary embolism
tPA	tissue plasminogen activator

INTRODUCTION

Venous thromboembolism is the third most frequent cardiovascular disease after myocardial infarction and stroke [1, 2] with an estimated 530,000 cases per year of symptomatic pulmonary embolism (PE) in the United States alone [3]; and resulting in approximately 300,000 deaths every year from acute PE [4]. There are multiple treatment options available ranging from simple anticoagulation to systemic thrombolytic to surgical embolectomy with the catheter directed therapies falling somewhere in the middle. Catheter directed thrombolysis and catheter thrombectomy can be utilized together or separately depending on the patient's presentation and co-morbid factors. In patients with acute decompensation, who are not surgical candidates, catheter directed thrombectomy and catheter directed fragmentation can quickly improve flow and pressures in the pulmonary arteries by removing or fragmenting, and allowing distal embolization of, a portion of the obstructive thrombus. Catheter directed thrombolysis, although slower, allows lysis of the thrombus while using only a fraction of the systemic dose of thrombolytic possibly decreasing systemic bleeding complications [5].

COMMON INDICATIONS [6]

Catheter directed thrombolysis

- Submassive PE *(right heart strain/dysfunction without hemodynamic instability)*

Catheter thrombectomy

- Massive PE *(right heart strain/dysfunction with hemodynamic instability)* not eligible for open embolectomy
- Submassive PE *(right heart strain/dysfunction without hemodynamic instability)* with contradiction to lytic therapy

S. Farquharson (✉)
Department of Radiology, New York University
Langone Medical Center, 660 1st Avenue, 7th Floor,
New York, NY 10016, USA
e-mail: sean.farquharson@nyumc.org

B. Taslakian et al. (eds.), *Procedural Dictations in Image-Guided Intervention*,
DOI 10.1007/978-3-319-40845-3_119

CONTRAINDICATIONS

(a) ***Thrombectomy and thrombolysis***
- ***Absolute***
  - Hemodynamically too unstable to come to the interventional suite
- ***Relative***
  - Contrast allergy *(should receive premedication)*
  - Severe Pulmonary hypertension-systolic pulmonary artery pressure ≥60 mm Hg [7] *(re-assess indications, use non-ionic low osmolality contrast and more selective injections with less contrast)*
  - Left bundle-branch block *(place transvenous pacing leads or have external pacing pads in place in case of complete heart block)*

(b) ***Thrombolysis*** [8]
- ***Absolute***
  - Active internal bleeding
  - Recent (within 2 months) cerebrovascular accident or other active intracranial process *(aneurysm, vascular malformation, or neoplasm)*
  - Recent (within 3 months) intracranial or intraspinal surgery or trauma
- **Relative**
  - Recent (<10 days) Major surgery, obstetrical delivery, organ biopsy or puncture on non-compressible vessels
  - Recent Gastrointestinal bleeding (<10 days)
  - Major internal bleeding within the past 6 months
  - Recent major trauma
  - Severe arterial hypertension (≥200 mm Hg systolic or ≥110 mm Hg diastolic)
  - Hemorrhagic retinopathy

POSSIBLE COMPLICATIONS [5, 7]

General (angiography-related) complications:
- Access site complications *(e.g., hematoma, retroperitoneal hemorrhage, arterial injury, thrombosis)*
- Contrast-induced allergic reaction
- Contrast-induced nephropathy
- Catheter or guidewire breakage
- Risks related to any minimally invasive procedure performed under conscious sedation *(e.g., allergy to medications)*

Procedure-specific complications (thrombectomy and thrombolysis)
- Cardiac arrhythmia, most notably complete heart block in patients with pre-existing left bundle-branch block
- Fatal cardiac arrest due to right ventricular failure *(in patients with severe pulmonary hypertension)*

Procedure-specific complications (thrombolysis)
- External bleeding or hematoma from access site or any recent wound or puncture sites
- Internal bleeding, including intracranial hemorrhage, gastrointestinal bleed, retroperitoneal hemorrhage

PREPROCEDURAL ASSESSMENT AND PLANNING [9–11]

- History, indications, and physical examination
- Evaluation of diagnostic imaging studies:
  - Pulmonary CT angiography, to determine the relevant vascular anatomy and location of pulmonary emboli
  - Echocardiogram to determine degree of right heart dysfunction and gauge degree of pulmonary hypertension
  - Lower extremity Doppler to assess for presence and extent of deep venous thrombosis which could influence choice of access site
- Review EKG to look for left bundle-branch block
- Consider the need for IVC filter which can be placed concurrently via the same access
- Antibiotic prophylaxis: Not routinely recommended [9] *(Appendices 4* in Chaps. 152 *and 5* in 153*)*
- Imaging modality for guidance: Fluoroscopy; combined with ultrasound for access

venotomy *(if thrombolysis is planned, ultrasound guided access is recommended to ensure single wall puncture and avoid inadvertent arterial puncture)*

- Positioning: Supine
- Venous access: Common femoral vein (preferred), internal jugular vein; *bilateral common femoral access may be needed to lyse bilateral PE; Jugular approach is not recommended for thrombolysis.*
- ICU monitoring will be required if thrombolytic medications are going to be infused

PROCEDURE NOTE

Procedure: Bilateral/Right/Left pulmonary angiogram with pressure measurements and bilateral/right/left pulmonary artery (thrombectomy/thrombolysis)
Staff: [_]
Fellow: [_]
Resident: [_]
Clinical History and Indications: Describe history and list indications
Allergies: None known/Allergic to [specify/type of allergy]
Anesthesia: Local anesthesia/Conscious sedation/Monitored anesthesia care
Medications: List any relevant medications used
Contrast Material: (_) mL of [type] contrast material was used for pulmonary angiogram {preferably non-ionic low osmolality contrast}
Field: Sterile
Procedure classification: Clean
Position: Supine
Monitoring: Intravenous access line was secured, vital signs, including continuous cardiac monitoring followed by nursing staff/anesthesia team throughout the procedure
Total Fluoroscopy time: (_) minutes
Cumulative radiation Dose: (_) mGy

Description of Procedure *(Pulmonary artery thrombectomy/thrombus fragmentation}:*
The risks, benefits, alternatives, and procedure itself were explained to the patient/patient's Power of Attorney/patient's legal guardian, and informed written/verbal consent was obtained. Time out was performed to confirm the correct patient, procedure and site.

(Femoral vein access)- The patient was positioned supine on the angiographic table. The site of the procedure was identified and marked. The skin of the right/left groin was shaved, prepped and draped in the usual sterile fashion. The right/left common femoral vein was located by palpation/ultrasound and marked. Local anesthesia was administered and a small skin incision was made. The right/left common femoral vein was accessed using an (_)-gauge [type] needle under direct ultrasound visualization.

(Jugular vein access)- With the neck turned to the contralateral side, the patient's left/right cervical and upper thoracic regions were prepped and draped in the usual sterile fashion. Ultrasound examination was performed to determine the site of venous puncture. Local anesthesia was administered. The left/right internal jugular vein was punctured using an (_)-gauge [type] needle under direct ultrasound visualization.

Once good venous flow was detected, a (_)-inch [type] guidewire was advanced through the needle into the accessed vein, the needle was exchanged over the wire for a (_) French co-axial dilator which was used to place a (0.035)-in. wire into the cava under direct fluoroscopic visualization. A (_)-French, (_) cm-long vascular sheath was advanced over the wire into right atrium. A (_)-French [type] flush catheter was advanced through the sheath into right atrium over a (_)-inch [type] guidewire; the wire and catheter were advanced in a stepwise fashion trough the right atrium and into the right ventricle where right ventricle pressure measurements were obtained through the catheter. The wire was then re-introduced through the catheter and in a stepwise fashion the wire and catheter were advanced into the main pulmonary artery. Catheter position was confirmed with hand injection of contrast followed by obtaining pressure measurements through the catheter. The Catheter was then advanced over the wire into the (left/right) pulmonary artery where digital subtraction angiography was performed by injecting (10–30) mL of [type] contrast, at a rate of (10–25 mL/s) [titrate volume and rate based on pulmonary artery pressure] and digital subtraction angiography imaging was performed at (6) frames per second during suspended respiration in anterior–posterior, and 45° ipsilateral posterior-oblique [limit views based on pulmonary artery pressure] projection(s) [specify if sub-selective injections of pulmonary artery branches or other projections are obtained]. The catheter was removed over a stiff (0.035/0.038)-in. wire and the sheath was advanced over the stiff wire into the proximal (left/right) pulmonary artery.

A (_)-French directable [type] catheter was advanced through the sheath into the pulmonary artery. A (0.035)-in. [type] wire was advanced through the catheter and was used to probe and cross the thrombus in the (left/right) pulmonary artery. The catheter was removed over the wire and a (size) [angioplasty balloon/pigtail fragmentation device/type of other device] was advanced over the wire into the thrombus where it was used to disrupt and fragment the thrombus/a [type] thrombectomy device was introduced through the sheath and advanced into the thrombus in the (left/right) pulmonary artery where it was used to remove the thrombus. Following thrombectomy, the device was removed through the sheath. The flush catheter was re-inserted into the pulmonary artery and digital subtraction angiography was repeated to evaluate the pulmonary artery.

The catheter was then repositioned into the (right/left) pulmonary artery where angiography was performed by injecting (10–30) mL of [type] contrast, at a rate of (10–25 mL/s) [titrate volume and rate based on pulmonary artery pressure] and digital subtraction angiography imaging was performed at (6) frames per second during suspended respiration in anterior–posterior, and 45° ipsilateral posterior-oblique [limit views based on pulmonary artery pressure] projection(s) [specify if sub-selective injections of pulmonary artery branches or other projections are obtained]. The catheter was removed over a stiff (0.035/0.038)-in. wire and the sheath was advanced over the stiff wire into the proximal (right/left) pulmonary artery. A (_)-French directable [type] catheter was advanced through the sheath into the pulmonary artery. A (0.035)-in. [type] wire was advanced through the catheter and was used to probe and cross the thrombus in the (right/left) pulmonary artery. The catheter was removed over the wire and a (size) [angioplasty balloon/pigtail fragmentation device/type of other device] was advanced over the wire into the thrombus where it was used to disrupt and fragment the thrombus/a [type] thrombectomy device was introduced through the sheath and advanced into the thrombus in the (left/right) pulmonary artery where it was use to remove the thrombus. Following thrombectomy the device was then removed through the sheath. The flush catheter was re-inserted into the pulmonary artery and digital subtraction angiography was repeated to evaluate the pulmonary artery.

The catheter was then removed followed by the sheath and adequate hemostasis was achieved at the venotomy site by compression for (_) minutes. Sterile dressing was applied and the patient was transferred to the ICU/recovery room following the procedure in a stable condition. Staff was present for the entire procedure.

Description of Procedure *(Pulmonary angiogram with catheter directed thrombolysis; femoral Approach):*
The risks, benefits, alternatives and procedure itself were explained to the patient/patient's Power of Attorney/patient's legal guardian, and informed written/verbal consent was obtained. Time out was performed to confirm the correct patient, procedure, and site.

The patient was positioned supine on the angiographic table. The site of the procedure was identified and marked. The skin of both groins was shaved, prepped and draped in the usual sterile fashion. Both common femoral veins were located by ultrasound and marked. Local anesthesia was administered and a small skin incision was made at each planned entry site. The right common femoral vein was accessed using an (_)-gauge [type] needle under direct ultrasound visualization. Once good venous flow was detected, a (_)-inch [type] guidewire was advanced through the needle into the accessed vein, the needle was exchanged over the wire for a (_) French co-axial dilator which was used to place a (0.035)-in. wire into the inferior vena cava under direct fluoroscopic visualization. A (_)-French, (_) cm-long vascular sheath was advanced over the wire into the inferior vena cava. Using the same technique a (_)-French, (_) cm-long vascular sheath was placed from the left common femoral vein.

A (_)-French [type] flush catheter was advanced through the right femoral sheath into right atrium over a (0.035)-in. [type] guidewire, The wire and catheter were advanced in a step-wise fashion trough the right atrium and into the right ventricle where right ventricle pressure measurements were obtained through the catheter. The wire was then re-introduced through the catheter and in a stepwise fashion the wire and catheter were advanced into the main pulmonary artery. Catheter position was confirmed with hand injection of contrast followed by obtaining pressure measurements through the catheter. The Catheter was then advanced over the wire into the left/right pulmonary artery where digital subtraction angiography was performed by injecting (10–30) mL of [type] contrast, at a rate of (10–25 mL/s) [titrate volume and rate based on pulmonary artery pressure] and digital subtraction angiography imaging was performed at (6) frames per second during suspended respiration in anterior-posterior, and 45 degree ipsilateral posterior-oblique [limit views based on pulmonary artery pressure] projection(s) [specify if sub-selective injections of pulmonary artery branches or other projections are obtained]. The catheter was then exchanged over a (_)-inch stiff wire for a (_)-French directable [type] catheter. A (0.035)-in. [type] wire was advanced through the catheter and was used to probe and cross the thrombus in the left/right pulmonary artery. The length of the thrombus was gauged with a measuring catheter, then the catheter was removed over the wire and a (_) French, (_) cm-long [ultrasound assisted/type] infusion catheter with (_) cm infusion length was advanced over the wire and though the thrombus in the (left/right) pulmonary artery. A hand injection of [type] contrast was performed through the infusion catheter to confirm proper positioning then the infusion catheter was flushed with saline.

A (_)-French [type] flush catheter was advanced through the left femoral sheath into right atrium over a (0.035)-in. [type] guidewire. The wire and catheter were advanced in a step-wise fashion trough the right atrium, into the right ventricle then into the main pulmonary artery. Catheter position was confirmed with hand injection of contrast followed by obtaining pressure measurements through the catheter. The Catheter was then advanced over the wire into the left/right pulmonary artery where digital subtraction angiography was performed by injecting (10–30) mL of [type] contrast, at a rate of (10–25 mL/s) [titrate volume and rate based on pulmonary artery pressure] and digital subtraction angiography imaging was performed at (6) frames per second during suspended respiration in anterior-posterior, and 45° ipsilateral posterior-oblique [limit views based on pulmonary artery pressure] projection(s) [specify if sub-selective injections of pulmonary artery branches or other projections are obtained]. The catheter was then exchanged over a stiff (_)-inch wire for a (_)-French directable [type] catheter. A (0.035)-in. [type] wire was advanced through the catheter and was used to probe and cross the thrombus in the (left/right) pulmonary artery. The length of the thrombus was gauged with a measuring catheter then the catheter was removed over the wire and a (_) French, (_) cm-long [ultrasound assisted/type] infusion catheter with (_) cm infusion length was advanced over the wire and though the thrombus in the left/right pulmonary artery. A hand injection of [type] contrast was performed.

An Infusion of tissue plasminogen activator (tPA) was started though both of the infusion catheters at a rate of (0.5–1 mg/h/catheter). Intravenous heparin infusion was started via bilateral femoral vein sheaths at 200 units/h/sheath. Bilateral femoral sheaths and catheters were secured at the access sites with sutures and dressings. Patient tolerated the procedure (with no immediate complications) and was taken to ICU for close monitoring during tPA infusion.

Intra-Procedure Findings: List all relevant findings including measured right atrial and pulmonary artery pressures.

Immediate Complications: None encountered during or directly after the procedure. List complications if any.

Post-Procedure Plan: ***(Thrombectomy)***

- Keep patient complete bed rest with the right/left leg extended for (_) hours *[adjust depending on the use of anticoagulation {Femoral approach}.*
- Keep patient on bed rest with head of bed greater than 45° for 2 h.*{jugular approach}*
- Check the puncture site for any bleeding or hematoma formation every 15 min for 1 h, then every 30 min for 4 h; inform interventional radiology team if any complications are observed.
- Monitor vital signs every 15 min for 1 h, then every 30 min for 2 h; notify interventional radiology team if systolic blood pressure <95 mmHg, or heart rate >110 beats/min.
- Resume diet and previous orders as needed and if not otherwise contraindicated.
- Continue adequate intravenous hydration and monitor fluid (intake–output) status.
- Check complete blood count, creatinine and blood urea nitrogen on the day following the procedure or as clinically indicated.

Post-Procedure Plan: (Thrombolysis)

- Admit to intensive care unit for monitoring during tPA infusion.
- Strict bed rest with legs extended and head of bed less than 15°.
- Check the puncture site for any bleeding or hematoma formation every 15 min for 1 h, then every 30 min for the entire procedure time; inform interventional radiology team if any complications are observed.
- Monitor serial neurologic exams, CBC, PT, PTT, INR, fibrinogen level every 4 h.
- Stop lytic infusion if patient develops neurologic symptoms, gross bleeding, evidence of internal bleeding, or fibrinogen drops below half its initial value or 150.
- Stop lytic infusion once a total of 24 mg tPA has been administered and either repeat pulmonary angiogram via existing access or remove catheters and sheaths at bedside and monitor improvement with repeat echocardiogram.

Impression:

- Bilateral/Right/Left pulmonary angiogram with pressure measurements and bilateral/right/left pulmonary artery thrombectomy/thrombolysis.
- The patient tolerated the procedure well and left the interventional unit in stable condition.
- The patient was unstable and the procedure was canceled/terminated prematurely.
- List any other relevant or important information/finding.

References

1. Heit JA. The epidemiology of venous thromboembolism in the community. Arterioscler Thromb Vasc Biol. 2008;28(3):370–2.
2. Cohen AT, Agnelli G, Anderson FA, Arcelus JI, Bergqvist D, Brecht JG, et al. Venous thromboembolism (VTE) in Europe. The number of VTE events and associated morbidity and mortality. Thromb Haemost. 2007;98(4):756–64.
3. Heit JA, Cohen AT, Anderson FA. Estimated annual number of incident and recurrent, non-fatal and fatal venous thromboembolism (VTE) events in the U.S. Blood. 2005;106:267a.
4. Tapson VF. Acute pulmonary embolism. N Engl J Med. 2008;358:1037–52.
5. Kennedy RJ, Kenney HH, Dunfee BL. Thrombus resolution and hemodynamic recovery using ultrasound-accelerated thrombolysis in acute pulmonary embolism. J Vasc Interv Radiol. 2013;24 (6):841–8.
6. Reza N, Dudzinski DM. Pulmonary embolism response teams. Curr Treat Options Cardiovasc Med. 2015;17(6):387.
7. Hofmann LV, Lee DS, Gupta A, Arepally A, Sood S, Girgis R, et al. Safety and hemodynamic effects of pulmonary angiography in patients with pulmonary hypertension: 10-year single-center experience. AJR Am J Roentgenol. 2004;183(3):779–86.

8. Sherry S, Bell WR, Duckert FH, Fletcher AP, Gurewich V, Long DM, et al. Thrombolytic therapy in thrombosis: A National Institutes of Health consensus development conference. Ann Intern Med. 1980;93:141–4.
9. Venkatesan AM, Kundu S, Sacks D, Wallace MJ, Wojak JC, Rose SC, et al. Practice guidelines for adult antibiotic prophylaxis during vascular and interventional radiology procedures. J Vasc Interv Radiol. 2010;21(11):1611–30.
10. Taslakian B, Sebaaly MG, Al-Kutoubi A. Patient evaluation and preparation in vascular and interventional radiology: what every interventional radiologist should know (part 1: patient assessment and laboratory tests). Cardiovasc Intervent Radiol. 2016;39(3):325–33.
11. Taslakian B, Sebaaly MG, Al-Kutoubi A. Patient evaluation and preparation in vascular and interventional radiology: what every interventional radiologist should know (part 2: patient preparation and medications). Cardiovasc Intervent Radiol. 2016;39 (4):489–99. doi: 10.1007/s00270-015-1239-4. [Epub 2015 Nov 25].

Part XIX

Vascular Interventional Procedures: Upper Extremities

Introduction by Jamal J. Hoballah, Section Reviewer

Endovascular therapy has become a valuable and indispensable addition to the armamentarium of physicians caring for patients with occlusive or thrombotic pathology in the upper extremities.

In the venous system, thrombolytic therapy to treat effort axillary vein thrombosis (Paget Schroetter syndrome) became an essential component in the initial management of this pathology. Special devices were developed to incorporate a mechanical thrombectomy to the thrombolytic therapy. This pharmaco-mechanical thrombectomy is intended to provide faster and more complete resolution of the thrombus, setting the stage for addressing the thoracic outlet obstruction via surgical first rib resection.

In the arterial system, digital subtraction angiography remains irreplaceable when trying to delineate the detailed anatomy of occlusive disease in the hand. Such technique can be supplemented by thrombolytic therapy to address distal emboli or thrombotic occlusions. Angioplasty and stenting for treatment of subclavian artery stenosis or occlusion has replaced the traditional open carotid subclavian bypasses that used to address such pathology.

This section provides a comprehensive list of procedural reports that covers the vast majority of the currently performed vascular procedures in the upper extremities, with up-to-date explanatory notes, synopsis of the indications and contraindications, and potential complications in an organized and practical format.

Section Chapters

Subclavian Artery Balloon Angioplasty and Stenting

120

Maen Aboul Hosn

INTRODUCTION

Subclavian artery occlusive disease is uncommon compared to extracranial carotid artery disease. Proximal lesions are predominantly due to atherosclerosis and spillover from aortic disease, whereas distal lesions can be affected by either atherosclerosis or other disease processes, including arteritis, trauma and thoracic outlet obstruction. Surgical management traditionally included a transthoracic approach and/or carotid subclavian bypass/transposition. More recently, endovascular management including angioplasty and stenting has become more popular with excellent technical success, patency rate and minimal periprocedural morbidity.

COMMON INDICATIONS [1–3]

- Upper extremity ischemia
- Subclavian artery stenosis/occlusion

M. Aboul Hosn (✉)
Department of Vascular Surgery, University of Iowa Hospitals and Clinics, 200 Hawkins Dr, Iowa City, IA 52242, USA
e-mail: maen-aboulhosn@uiowa.edu

COMMON CONTRAINDICATIONS [1, 2]

- Coagulopathy
- Contrast allergy
- Hemodynamic instability

POSSIBLE COMPLICATIONS [1, 2]

General (angiography-related) complications:
- Hemorrhage *(puncture-site hematoma, retroperitoneal hematoma if "high" puncture above inguinal ligament)*
- Pseudoaneurysm *(superficial femoral artery "low" puncture)*
- Arteriovenous fistula *(puncture-site artery)*
- Thrombosis of the femoral artery
- Distal embolization
- Contrast-induced allergic reaction
- Contrast-induced nephropathy
- Arterial perforation or dissection
- Catheter or guide-wire breakage
- Limb amputation *(rare)*
- Risks related to any minimally invasive procedure performed under conscious sedation *(e.g., allergy to medications)*

Procedure-specific complications:
- Stroke
- Distal embolization
- Arterial injury/thrombosis

B. Taslakian et al. (eds.), *Procedural Dictations in Image-Guided Intervention*,
DOI 10.1007/978-3-319-40845-3_120

PREPROCEDURAL ASSESSMENT AND PLANNING

- History, indications and physical examination *(Appendix 1* in Chap. 149*)*. Document indications of the procedure, lower and upper extremity pulses and vital signs.
- Evaluation of diagnostic imaging studies to determine the relevant vascular anatomy
- Periprocedural management of coagulation status *(Appendices 2* in Chaps. 150 *and 3* in 151*)*
- Antibiotic prophylaxis: Not routinely recommended *(Appendices 4* in Chaps. 152 *and 5* in 153*)*
- Imaging modality for guidance: Fluoroscopy, combined with ultrasound for arterial puncture
- Positioning: Supine with arm abducted
- Arterial access: Femoral artery, brachial artery, axillary artery
- Patient preparation:
  - Start intravenous fluids the night before angiography in order to ensure adequate hydration, combined with effective monitoring of fluid status.
  - Insert a urinary catheter or ask the patient to void before the procedure depending on the estimated time of the procedure.
  - Considerations for patients with specific diseases or conditions, patients on specific medications or patients with history of multiple comorbidities: consult with the referring clinician, and obtain subspecialty consultation as needed.

PROCEDURE NOTE

Procedure: Left/right subclavian artery balloon angioplasty and stenting
Staff: [_]
Fellow: [_]
Resident: [_]
Clinical Information: Describe history and list indications
Allergies: No known drug allergy/Allergic to (specify)
Anesthesia: Local anesthesia/Monitored conscious sedation
Medications: List any relevant medications used (sedation, heparin)
Contrast Material: (_) mL of [type] contrast material was used for intra-arterial injection
Field: Sterile
Procedure Classification: Clean
Position: Supine with arm abducted
Monitoring: Intravenous access was secured and vitals were continuously monitored by nursing staff/anesthesia team throughout the procedure
Total fluoroscopy time: (_) minutes
Cumulative radiation dose: (_) mGy

Description of Procedure:
The risks, benefits, alternatives, and the procedure itself were explained to the patient/patient's Power of Attorney/legal guardian, and informed written consent was obtained. The site of the procedure was identified and marked. Time out was performed to confirm the correct patient, procedure and site.

The groin area was prepped and draped in the usual sterile manner. After infiltrating the skin with 1 % Lidocaine, and using ultrasound guidance, the right/left common femoral/brachial artery was accessed with a micropuncture kit and the position of the microwire was confirmed by fluoroscopy. A small nick in the skin was done using an 11 blade and the microsheath was exchanged with a (_)-French vascular sheath over an exchange wire.

For femoral approach: A Glidewire was advanced into the abdominal aorta and followed into the aortic arch. A (_)-French pigtail/Omni flush catheter was advanced over the wire to the aortic arch and an arch aortogram was performed delineating the anatomy of the great vessels. Next, the pigtail catheter was removed and using a (_)-French [type] glide catheter; the hydrophilic wire was maneuvered into the left/right subclavian/axillary artery.

For brachial approach: A glide multipurpose catheter was advanced over a hydrophilic wire to the level of the stenosis.

Selective upper extremity angiography was performed delineating the area of stenosis/

occlusion. The patient was given systemic unfractionated heparin at this point. A (_)-inch [type] wire was advanced through the catheter into the proximal left/right subclavian artery and the short sheath was exchanged with a (_)-French, (_)-cm long [Flexor/Ansel] sheath. Using a glide catheter, the glide wire was maneuvered across the subclavian/axillary stenosis/occlusion. A repeat angiogram was performed through the sheath and the dimensions of the diseased segment were measured. A low profile (4–6) mm angioplasty balloon was then advanced to the level of the lesion and inflated to its nominal pressure. It was deflated at 1 min. Follow up angiography showed resolution/persistence of the stenosis. The decision was made to deploy a stent across the lesion. A (_) × (_) mm [type] bare metal/drug eluting/covered stent was advanced and positioned across the lesion and deployed successfully with repeat angiography showing complete resolution of the stenosis.

Following the procedure, the vascular sheaths were removed and hemostasis was achieved by compression/using [type] occlusion device. The patient was transferred to the floor/recovery room after the procedure in a stable condition. Staff was present during the entire procedure.

Intra-Procedure Findings: List all relevant radiologic findings.

Immediate Complications: None encountered during or directly after the procedure. List the complications if any.

Post-Procedure Plan [3]:

Standard post-angiogram management plan

- Keep patient complete bed rest with the right/left leg extended for 6 h *[adjust depending on the puncture site]*.
- Check the right/left groin/[specify the puncture site if different] for any bleeding or hematoma formation every 15 min for 1 h, then every 30 min for 1 h, then every hour for 4 h; inform interventional radiology team if any signs of bleeding are observed *[adjust depending on the puncture site]*.
- Check and document lower extremity pulses every 30 min for 2 h then every 1 h for 4 h *[adjust depending on the puncture site]*.
- Monitor vital signs every 15 min for 1 h, then every 30 min for 4 h; notify interventional radiology team if systolic blood pressure <95 mmHg, or heart rate >110 beats/min.
- Resume diet and previous orders as needed and if otherwise not contraindicated.
- Continue adequate intravenous hydration and monitor fluid (intake-output) status.
- Check complete blood count and creatinine on the day following the procedure or as clinically indicated.
- Perform regular neurological examination when the procedure includes manipulation in the ascending thoracic aorta, aortic arch or brachiocephalic arteries.

Procedure-specific management plan:

- Check for chest pain, dyspnea, focal neurologic deficits and bleeding.

Impression:

- Left/right subclavian artery angioplasty and stenting, as described above.
- The patient tolerated the procedure well and left the interventional unit in a stable condition.
- The patient was unstable and the procedure was cancelled/terminated prematurely.
- List any other relevant of important information/finding.

References

1. Sullivan TM, Gray BH, Bacharach JM, Perl J 2nd, Childs MB, Modzelewski L, et al. Angioplasty and primary stenting of the subclavian, innominate, and common carotid arteries in 83 patients. J Vasc Surg. 1998;28(6):1059–65.
2. De Vries JP, Jager LC, van den Berg JC, Overtoom TT, Ackerstaff RG, Van de Pavoordt ED, et al. Durability of percutaneous transluminal angioplasty for obstructive lesions of proximal subclavian artery: long term results. J Vasc Surg. 2005;41(1):19–23.
3. Patel SN, White CJ, Collins TJ, Daniel GA, Jenkins JS, Reilly JP, et al. Catheter-based treatment of the subclavian and innominate arteries. Catheter Cardiovasc Interv. 2008;71(7):963–8.

121 Subclavian Vein Thrombolysis

Maen Aboul Hosn

Abbreviations

TOS	Thoracic outlet syndrome
rtPA	Recombinant tissue plasminogen activator

INTRODUCTION

Subclavian vein thrombosis is an uncommon pathology mostly seen in the setting of thoracic outlet syndrome (TOS). Other contributing factors include instrumentation and catheter placement within the subclavian vein as well as hypercoagulability. Treatment depends on the underlying cause and ranges from anticoagulation and physical therapy to thrombolysis and angioplasty. A first rib resection may also be indicated for TOS.

COMMON INDICATIONS [1–3]

- Thoracic outlet syndrome (Paget-von Schrötter syndrome)
- Catheter-associated subclavian vein thrombosis

M. Aboul Hosn (✉)
Department of Vascular Surgery, University of Iowa Hospitals and Clinics, 200 Hawkins Dr, Iowa City, IA 52242, USA
e-mail: maen-aboulhosn@uiowa.edu

COMMON CONTRAINDICATIONS [1–3]

- Active internal bleeding
- Coagulopathy
- Recent cerebrovascular event
- Neurosurgical intervention within 3 months
- Major trauma
- Organ biopsy

POSSIBLE COMPLICATIONS [3]

- Access site bleeding
- Pulmonary embolism
- Intracranial hemorrhage
- Stroke *(in the presence of patent foramen ovale)*
- Iatrogenic injury to nearby neurovascular structures

PREPROCEDURAL ASSESSMENT AND PLANNING

- History, indications and physical examination *(Appendix 1* in Chap. 149*)*. Document

B. Taslakian et al. (eds.), *Procedural Dictations in Image-Guided Intervention*,
DOI 10.1007/978-3-319-40845-3_121

indications of the procedure and vital signs. Rule out any contraindications to lytic therapy.

- Evaluation of diagnostic imaging studies to determine the relevant vascular anatomy and assess the access site
- Periprocedural management of coagulation status *(Appendices 2* in Chaps. 150 *and 3* in 151*)*
- Antibiotic prophylaxis: Not routinely recommended *(Appendices 4* in Chaps. 152 *and 5* in 153*)*
- Imaging modality for guidance: Fluoroscopy; combined with ultrasound for venous puncture
- Positioning: Supine

PROCEDURE NOTE

Procedure: Catheter-directed thrombolysis of right/left subclavian vein thrombosis
Staff: [_]
Fellow: [_]
Resident: [_]
Clinical Information: Describe history and list indications
Allergies: No known drug allergy/Allergic to (specify)
Anesthesia: Local anesthesia/Monitored conscious sedation
Medications: List any relevant medications used
Contrast Material: (_) mL of [type] contrast material was used for venography
Field: Sterile
Procedure Classification: Clean
Position: Supine with arm abducted
Monitoring: Intravenous access was secured and vitals were continuously monitored by nursing staff/anesthesia team throughout the procedure
Total fluoroscopy time: (_) minutes
Cumulative radiation dose: (_) mGy

Description of Procedure:

The risks, benefits, alternatives and the procedure itself were explained to the patient/patient's Power of Attorney/legal guardian, and informed written/consent was obtained. The site of the procedure was identified and marked. Time out was performed to confirm the correct patient, procedure and site. The patient was fully anticoagulated and maintained on an unfractionated heparin drip.

The left/right upper extremity, chest and neck were prepped and draped in the usual sterile manner. Under ultrasound guidance, the ipsilateral basilic vein was accessed with a micropuncture kit. A small nick in the skin was done using an 11 blade and the microsheath was exchanged with a (_)-French sheath over an exchange wire. A venogram was then performed and the location of the thrombosis was confirmed. A hydrophilic wire was advanced across the thrombosed vein using a (_)-French glide catheter and wire tip was parked at the level of the superior vena cava/right atrium. The hydrophilic wire was exchanged for a *Bentson wire/stiff Glidewire/ Amplatz wire* and the (_)-French Angiojet catheter was advanced and positioned across the thrombosed region. Recombinant tissue plasminogen activator (rtPA) was pulse injected into the thrombus for a total of (_) mg of rtPA and multiple passes of the Angiojet catheter were performed. A venogram was done next showing a decrease in the clot burden. The Angiojet catheter was then exchanged for a (_) French multi-sidehole catheter for delivery of the lytic solution and it was positioned across the remaining thrombus. rtPA infusion was started at a rate of (0.5) mg/h and the catheter was secured to the skin with a 3-0 Nylon suture for a planned repeat venogram in 24 h. A dry dressing was applied over the catheter exit site.

The patient was transferred to the recovery room in a stable condition. Staff was present for the entire procedure.

Intra-Procedure Findings: List all relevant radiologic findings.
Immediate Complications: None encountered during or directly after the procedure. List the complications if any.

Post-Procedure Plan [4]:

- Patient observation for 24 h in a monitored unit.

- Check for chest pain, dyspnea, weakness, focal neurologic deficits and bleeding.
- Continue rtPA infusion for 24 h.
- Serial Fibrinogen and D-dimer levels
- Repeat venogram in 24–48 h.

Impression:

- Catheter-directed thrombolysis of thrombosed left/right subclavian vein as described above.
- The patient tolerated the procedure well and left the interventional unit in a stable condition.
- The patient was unstable and the procedure was canceled/terminated prematurely.
- List any other relevant or important information/finding.

References

1. Klitfod L, Broholm R, Baekgaard N. Deep venous thrombosis of the upper extremity. A review. Int Angiol. 2013;32(5):447–52.
2. Thompson JF, Winterborn RJ, Bays S, White H, Kinsella DC, Watkinson AF. Venous thoracic outlet compression and the Paget-Schroetter syndrome: a review and recommendations for management. Cardiovasc Intervent Radiol. 2011;34(5):903–10.
3. Vik A, Holme PA, Singh K, Dorenberg E, Nordhus KC, Kumar S, et al. Catheter-directed thrombolysis for treatment of deep venous thrombosis in the upper extremities. Cardiovasc Intervent Radiol. 2009;32 (5):980–7.
4. Molina JE, Hunter DW, Dietz CA. Paget-Schroetter syndrome treated with thrombolytics and immediate surgery. J Vasc Surg. 2007;45(2):328–34.

Subclavian/Brachial Artery Thrombolysis

122

Maen Aboul Hosn

Abbreviations

rt-PA Recombinant tissue plasminogen activator

INTRODUCTION

Upper extremity angiography is the preferred diagnostic imaging modality especially when a concomitant endovascular intervention is contemplated. Among these interventions is subclavian/axillary thrombolysis which is utilized for subacute upper extremity ischemia when a proximal thrombosis/occlusion is identified or for runoff vessel recanalization for future bypass.

COMMON INDICATIONS [1–3]

- Subacute upper extremity ischemia
- Subclavian/axillary artery thrombosis
- Brachial artery thrombosis

M. Aboul Hosn (✉)
Department of Vascular Surgery, University of Iowa Hospitals and Clinics, 200 Hawkins Dr, Iowa City, IA 52242, USA
e-mail: maen-aboulhosn@uiowa.edu

COMMON CONTRAINDICATIONS [2–4]

- Active internal bleeding
- Coagulopathy
- Recent cerebrovascular event
- Neurosurgical intervention within 3 months
- Major trauma
- Organ biopsy

POSSIBLE COMPLICATIONS [1–4]

General (angiography-related) complications:

- Hemorrhage *(puncture-site hematoma, retroperitoneal hematoma if "high" puncture above inguinal ligament)*
- Pseudoaneurysm *(superficial femoral artery "low" puncture)*
- Arteriovenous fistula *(puncture-site artery)*
- Thrombosis of the femoral artery
- Distal embolization
- Contrast-induced allergic reaction
- Contrast-induced nephropathy
- Arterial perforation or dissection
- Catheter or guide-wire breakage
- Limb amputation *(rare)*

B. Taslakian et al. (eds.), *Procedural Dictations in Image-Guided Intervention*,
DOI 10.1007/978-3-319-40845-3_122

- Risks related to any minimally invasive procedure performed under conscious sedation *(e.g., allergy to medications)*

Procedure-specific complications:
- Stroke
- Intracranial hemorrhage
- Distal embolization
- Arterial injury

PREPROCEDURAL ASSESSMENT AND PLANNING

- History, indications and physical examination *(Appendix 1* in Chap. 149*)*. Document indications of the procedure and vital signs. Rule out any contraindications to lytic therapy.
- Evaluation of diagnostic imaging studies to determine the relevant vascular anatomy and assess the access site
- Periprocedural management of coagulation status *(Appendices 2* in Chap. 150 *and 3* in Chap. 151*)*
- Antibiotic prophylaxis: Not routinely recommended *(Appendices 4* in Chap. 152 *and 5* in Chap. 153*)*
- Imaging modality for guidance: Fluoroscopy, combined with ultrasound for arterial puncture
- Positioning: Supine

PROCEDURE NOTE

Procedure: Right/Left subclavian/brachial artery thrombolysis
Staff: [_]
Fellow: [_]
Resident: [_]
Clinical Information: Describe history and list indications
Allergies: No known drug allergy/Allergic to (specify)
Anesthesia: Local anesthesia/Monitored conscious sedation
Medications: List any relevant medications used (sedation, thrombolytic agent, heparin)
Contrast Material: (_) mL of [type] contrast material was used for intra-arterial injection
Field: Sterile
Procedure Classification: Clean
Position: Supine with arm abducted
Monitoring: Intravenous access was secured and vitals were continuously monitored by nursing staff/anesthesia team throughout the procedure
Total fluoroscopy time: (_) minutes
Cumulative radiation dose: (_) mGy

Description of Procedure:
The risks, benefits, alternatives and the procedure itself were explained to the patient/patient's Power of Attorney/legal guardian, and informed written consent was obtained. The site of the procedure was identified and marked. Time out was performed to confirm the correct patient, procedure and site.

The patient was fully anticoagulated and maintained on an unfractionated heparin drip. The groin area was prepped and draped in the usual sterile manner. After infiltrating the skin with 1 % Lidocaine, and using ultrasound guidance, the right/left common femoral artery was accessed with a micropuncture kit and the position of the microwire was confirmed by fluoroscopy. A small nick in the skin was done using an 11 blade and the microsheath was exchanged with a (_)-French sheath over an exchange wire. A glidewire was advanced into the abdominal aorta and followed into the aortic arch. A (_)-French pigtail/Omni flush catheter was advanced over the wire to the aortic arch and an arch aortogram was performed delineating the anatomy of the great vessels. Next, the pigtail catheter was removed and using a (_)-French [type] glide catheter; the glide wire was maneuvered into the left/right subclavian/axillary artery. The catheter was then advanced over the wire into the subclavian/axillary artery. Selective upper extremity angiography was performed, showing the area of occlusion [specify location]. After obtaining all the necessary images, the glidewire was advanced across the thrombosed segment using the glide catheter. The glidewire was then exchanged for a Bentson wire/stiff Glidewire/Amplatz wire and the short sheath was exchanged with a (_)-French, (_) cm-long Balkan/Ansel sheath with its tip parked in the proximal subclavian artery. A (_)-French Angiojet catheter was advanced and positioned across the thrombosed region. Recombinant tissue plasminogen activator (rt-PA) was pulse injected into the thrombus for a total of (_) mg and multiple passes of the Angiojet catheter were performed. An angiogram was done next showing a decrease in the clot burden. The thrombectomy catheter was then exchanged with a (_)-French, (_) cm-long multi-sidehole catheter for delivery of the lytic solution and it was positioned across the remaining thrombus. An initial bolus of (_) mg of rt-PA was administered into the clot and then an infusion of (0.5 to 1.5) mg/hour was started. The catheter was secured to the skin with a 3–0 Nylon suture for a planned repeat angiogram in 24 h and a dry dressing was applied over the catheter exit site.

The patient was transferred to the recovery room in a stable condition. Staff was present for the entire procedure.

Intra-Procedure Findings: List all relevant radiologic findings.

Immediate Complications: None encountered during or directly after the procedure. List the complications if any.

Post-Procedure Plan [3]:

Standard post-angiogram management plan

- Keep patient complete bed rest with the right/left leg extended.
- Check the right/left groin/[specify the puncture site if different] for any bleeding or hematoma formation every 15 min for 1 h, then every 30 min for 1 h, then every hour for the entire observation period; inform interventional radiology team if any signs of bleeding are observed *[adjust depending on the puncture site]*.
- Check and document lower extremity pulses every 30 min for 2 h then every 1 h for the entire observation period *[adjust depending on the puncture site]*.
- Monitor vital signs every 15 min for 1 h, then every 30 min for 4 h; notify interventional radiology team if systolic blood pressure <95 mmHg, or heart rate >110 beats/minute.
- Continue adequate intravenous hydration and monitor fluid (intake–output) status.
- Check complete blood count and creatinine on the day following the procedure or as clinically indicated.

Procedure-specific management plan:

- Patient observation for 24 h in a monitored unit.
- Check for chest pain, dyspnea and bleeding.
- Perform regular neurological examination.
- Serial fibrinogen and D-dimer levels.
- Repeat angiogram in 24 h.

Impression:

- Right/left subclavian/brachial artery thrombolysis as described above.
- The patient tolerated the procedure well and left the interventional unit in a stable condition.
- The patient was unstable and the procedure was canceled/terminated prematurely.
- List any other relevant of important information/finding.

References

1. Leung DA, Blitz LR, Nelson T, Amin A, Soukas PA, Nanjundappa A, et al. Rheolytic pharmacomechanical thrombectomy for the management of acute limb ischemia: results from the PEARL registry. J EndovascTher. 2015;22(4):546–57.
2. Byrne RM, Taha AG, Avgerinos E, Marone LK, Makaroun MS, Chaer RA. Contemporary outcomes of endovascular interventions for acute limb ischemia. J Vasc Surg. 2014;59(4):988–95 Epub 2013 Dec 17.
3. Knuttinen MG, Emmanuel N, Isa F, Rogers AW, Gaba RC, Bui JT, et al. Review of pharmacology and physiology in thrombolysis interventions. Semin Intervent Radiol. 2010;27(4):374–83.
4. Malgor RD, Gasparis AP. Pharmaco-mechanical thrombectomy for early thrombus removal. Phlebology. 2012;27(Suppl 1):155–62.

Upper Extremity Angiogram

123

Hiba Ezzeddine and Maen Aboul Hosn

INTRODUCTION

Upper extremity angiography has long been considered the gold standard for imaging of upper extremity vasculature. However, with the advent of computed tomography angiography (CTA), magnetic resonance angiography (MRA) and high resolution duplex ultrasonography, its use has become limited. However, it is still utilized when detailed visualization of the distal forearm, palmar arch or digital vessels is needed or when an alternative imaging modalities cannot be obtained or a therapeutic modality is required.

COMMON INDICATIONS [1–3]

- Upper extremity ischemia/arteritis
- Upper extremity injury/bleeding
- Arterial thoracic outlet syndrome
- Dialysis fistula assessment

H. Ezzeddine
Department of General Surgery, American University in Beirut Medical Center, Riad El Solh, Beirut 1107 2020, Lebanon
e-mail: he52@aub.edu.lb

M. Aboul Hosn (✉)
Department of Vascular Surgery, University of Iowa Hospitals and Clinics, 200 Hawkins Dr, Iowa City, IA 52242, USA
e-mail: maen-aboulhosn@uiowa.edu

COMMON CONTRAINDICATIONS [1, 2]

- Coagulopathy
- Contrast allergy
- Hemodynamic instability

POSSIBLE COMPLICATIONS [1, 2]

- Hemorrhage *(puncture site hematoma, retroperitoneal hematoma if "high" puncture above inguinal ligament)*
- Pseudoaneurysm *(superficial femoral artery "low" puncture)*
- Arteriovenous fistula *(puncture site artery)*
- Thrombosis of the femoral artery
- Distal embolization
- Contrast-induced allergic reaction
- Contrast-induced nephropathy
- Arterial perforation or dissection
- Catheter or guide-wire breakage
- Limb amputation *(rare)*
- Risks related to any minimally invasive procedure performed under conscious sedation *(e.g., allergy to medications)*

PREPROCEDURAL ASSESSMENT AND PLANNING

- History, indications and physical examination *(Appendix 1* in Chap. 149*)*. Document

B. Taslakian et al. (eds.), *Procedural Dictations in Image-Guided Intervention*,
DOI 10.1007/978-3-319-40845-3_123

indications of the procedure, lower and upper extremity pulses and vital signs.

- Evaluation of diagnostic imaging studies to determine the relevant vascular anatomy
- Periprocedural management of coagulation status *(Appendices 2* in Chap. 150 *and 3* in Chap. 151*)*
- Antibiotic prophylaxis: Not routinely recommended [4] *(Appendices 4* in Chap. 152 *and 5* in Chap. 153*)*
- Imaging modality for guidance: Fluoroscopy; combined with ultrasound for arterial puncture
- Positioning: Supine with arm abducted
- Arterial access: Femoral artery, left brachial artery, left axillary artery
- Patient preparation:
  - Start intravenous fluids the night before angiography in order to ensure adequate hydration, combined with effective monitoring of fluid status
  - Insert a urinary catheter or ask the patient to void before the procedure depending on the estimated time of the procedure
  - Considerations for patients with specific diseases or conditions, patients on specific medications or patients with history of multiple comorbidities: consult with the referring clinician, and obtain subspecialty consultation as needed

PROCEDURE NOTE

Procedure: Left/Right upper extremity angiography
Staff: [_]
Fellow: [_]
Resident: [_]
Clinical Information: Describe history and list indications
Allergies: No known drug allergy/Allergic to (specify)
Anesthesia: Local anesthesia/Monitored conscious sedation
Medications: List any relevant medications used
Contrast Material: (_) mL of [type] contrast material was used for intra-arterial injection
Field: Sterile
Procedure Classification: Clean
Position: Supine with arm abducted
Monitoring: Intravenous access was secured and vitals were continuously monitored by nursing staff/anesthesia team throughout the procedure.
Total fluoroscopy time: (_) minutes
Cumulative radiation dose: (_) mGy

Description of Procedure:

The risks, benefits, alternatives and the procedure itself were explained to the patient/patient's Power of Attorney/legal guardian, and informed written/verbal consent was obtained. The site of the procedure was identified and marked. Time out was performed to confirm the correct patient, procedure and site.

The groin area was prepped and draped in the usual sterile manner. After infiltrating the skin with 1 % Lidocaine, and using ultrasound guidance, the right/left common femoral artery was accessed with a micropuncture kit and the position of the microwire was confirmed by fluoroscopy. A small nick in the skin was done using an 11 blade and the microsheath was exchanged with a (_)-French sheath over an exchange wire. A glidewire was advanced into the abdominal aorta and followed into the aortic arch. A (_)-French pigtail/Omni flush catheter was advanced over the wire to the aortic arch and an arch aortogram was performed delineating the anatomy of the great vessels. Next, the pigtail catheter was removed and using a (_)-French [type] glide catheter; the glidewire was maneuvered into the left/right subclavian/axillary artery. The catheter was then advanced over the wire into the subclavian/axillary artery. Selective upper extremity angiography was performed by injecting contrast through the catheter and performing sequential imaging of the entire upper extremity arterial system down to the hand. After obtaining all necessary images, the procedure was concluded. The catheter was removed over the wire and the sheath was pulled out. Manual compression was held for 10–15 min and then a dry compression dressing was applied.

The patient was transferred to the recovery room in a stable condition. Staff was present for the entire procedure.

Intra-Procedure Findings: List all relevant radiologic findings.

Immediate Complications: None encountered during or directly after the procedure. List the complications if any.

Post-Procedure Plan [3]:

- Keep patient complete bed rest with the right/left leg extended for 6 h *[adjust depending on the puncture site]*.
- Check the right/left groin/[specify the puncture site if different] for any bleeding or hematoma formation every 15 min for 1 h, then every 30 min for 1 h, then every hour for 4 h; inform interventional radiology team if any signs of bleeding are observed *[adjust depending on the puncture site]*.
- Check and document lower extremity pulses every 30 min for 2 h then every 1 h for 4 h *[adjust depending on the puncture site]*.
- Monitor vital signs every 15 min for 1 h, then every 30 min for 4 h; notify interventional radiology team if systolic blood pressure <95 mmHg, or heart rate >110 beats/min.
- Resume diet and previous orders as needed and if otherwise not contraindicated.
- Continue adequate intravenous hydration and monitor fluid (intake–output) status.
- Check complete blood count and creatinine on the day following the procedure or as clinically indicated.
- Perform regular neurological examination when the procedure includes manipulation in the ascending thoracic aorta, aortic arch or brachiocephalic arteries.

Impression:

- Selective right/left upper extremity angiography as described above.
- The patient tolerated the procedure well and left the interventional unit in a stable condition.
- The patient was unstable and the procedure was canceled/terminated prematurely.
- List any other relevant of important information/finding.

References

1. Islam A, Edgerton C, Stafford JM, Koman A, Li Z, Smith BP, et al. Anatomic findings and outcomes associated with upper extremity arteriography and selective thrombolysis for acute finger ischemia. J Vasc Surg. 2014;60(2):410–7.
2. Capers Q 4th, Phillips J. Advances in percutaneous therapy for upper extremity arterial disease. Cardiol Clin. 2011;29(3):351–61.
3. Halpin DP, Moran KT, Jewell ER. Arm ischemia secondary to giant cell arteritis. Ann Vasc Surg. 1998;2 (4):381–4.
4. Venkatesan AM, Kundu S, Sacks D, Wallace MJ, Wojak JC, Rose SC, et al. Practice guidelines for adult antibiotic prophylaxis during vascular and interventional radiology procedures. J Vasc Interv Radiol. 2010;21(11):1611–30.

Part XX

Vascular Interventional Procedures: Lower Extremities

Introduction by Jamal J. Hoballah, Section Reviewer

Endovascular therapy is an essential component of the treatment of lower extremity arterial and venous disease.

In the venous system, thrombolytic therapy to treat iliofemoral deep venous thrombosis has gained a wider popularity especially in the young patients. Mechanical thrombectomy has been incorporated in the treatment providing a pharmaco-mechanical approach intended to provide faster and more complete resolution of the thrombus. This treatment is often combined with the placement of a temporary inferior vena cava filter that is later removed once the thrombus is cleared and any residual mechanical obstruction is addressed with angioplasty stenting.

In the arterial system, the "endovascular approach first" is now the standard approach as long as no bridges are burned towards future other interventions. All the vessels of the lower extremity down to the foot are amenable to endovascular interventions. These include angioplasty, stenting, recanalization, and atherectomy. Thrombolytic therapy can often save the day and avoid major repeat open surgical interventions on critically ill patients with acute limb ischemia. Even aneurysmal disease of the lower extremities, especially popliteal artery aneurysms, are now amenable to endovascular treatment with stent grafts.

This section provides a comprehensive list of procedural reports that covers the vast majority of the currently performed vascular procedures in the lower extremities, with up-to-date explanatory notes, synopsis of the indications and contraindications, and potential complications in an organized and practical format.

Section Chapters

Endovascular Treatment of Popliteal Aneurysm

124

Maen Aboul Hosn

Abbreviations

PAAs Popliteal Artery Aneurysms

INTRODUCTION

Popliteal Artery Aneurysms (PAAs) are the most prevalent type of peripheral arterial aneurysms, accounting for 70–80 % of all peripheral aneurysms. The current gold standard of PAA repair is ligation or resection of the aneurysm along with saphenous vein bypass. In high-risk patients or in those with no suitable vein conduit, another treatment option is endovascular exclusion of the aneurysm with covered stents. This approach provides shorter operative times, shorter hospital stays, and lower perioperative morbidity with a reported patency rate approximating 70 % at 6 years.

COMMON INDICATIONS [1–4]

- Popliteal aneurysm >2 cm in diameter
- Popliteal aneurysm with distal embolization
- Popliteal aneurysm with large mural thrombus

COMMON CONTRAINDICATIONS [1–4]

- Poor runoff to the foot
- Lack of proximal and/or distal landing zones
- Coagulopathy
- Contrast allergy
- Hemodynamic instability

POSSIBLE COMPLICATIONS [1]

- Access site bleeding
- Arterial injury
- Access vessel thrombosis
- Distal embolization
- Worsening limb ischemia
- Contrast induced nephropathy
- Iatrogenic injury to nearby neurovascular structures

PREPROCEDURAL ASSESSMENT AND PLANNING

- History, indications, and physical examination *(Appendix 1* in Chap. 149*)*. Document indications of the procedure, lower extremity pulses, and vital signs.

M. Aboul Hosn (✉)
Department of Vascular Surgery, University of Iowa Hospitals and Clinics, 200 Hawkins Dr, Iowa City, IA 52242, USA
e-mail: maen-aboulhosn@uiowa.edu

B. Taslakian et al. (eds.), *Procedural Dictations in Image-Guided Intervention*,
DOI 10.1007/978-3-319-40845-3_124

- Evaluation of diagnostic imaging studies to determine the relevant vascular anatomy and assess the access site
- Periprocedural management of coagulation status *(Appendices 2* in Chap. 150 *and 3* in Chap. 151*)*
- Antibiotic prophylaxis: Perioperative antibiotics are recommended [5] *(Appendices 4* in Chap. 152 *and 5* in Chap. 153*)*
- Imaging modality for guidance: Fluoroscopy; combined with ultrasound for arterial puncture
- Positioning: Supine
- Patient preparation:
  - Start intravenous fluids the night before angiography in order to ensure adequate hydration, combined with effective monitoring of fluid status
  - Insert a urinary catheter or ask the patient to void before the procedure depending on the estimated time of the procedure
  - Considerations for patients with specific diseases or conditions, patients on specific medications or patients with history of multiple comorbidities: consult with the referring clinician, and obtain subspecialty consultation as needed

PROCEDURE NOTE

Procedure: Endovascular Treatment of right/left popliteal aneurysm
Staff: [_]
Fellow: [_]
Resident: [_]
Clinical Information: Describe history and list indications
Allergies: No known drug allergy/Allergic to (specify)
Anesthesia: Local anesthesia/Monitored conscious sedation
Medications: List any relevant medications used
Contrast Material: (_) mL of [type] contrast material was used for intra-arterial injection
Field: Sterile
Procedure Classification: Clean
Position: Supine
Monitoring: Intravenous access was secured and vitals were continuously monitored by nursing staff/anesthesia team throughout the procedure
Total fluoroscopy time: (_) minutes
Cumulative radiation dose: (_) mGy

Description of Procedure:
The risks, benefits, alternatives, and the procedure itself were explained to the patient/patient's Power of Attorney/legal guardian, and informed written consent was obtained. The site of the procedure was identified and marked. Time out was performed to confirm the correct patient, procedure, and site.

The groin area was prepped and draped in the usual sterile manner. After infiltrating the skin with 1 % Lidocaine, and using ultrasound guidance, the right/left common femoral artery was accessed retrogradely with a micropuncture kit and the position of the microwire was confirmed by fluoroscopy. A small nick in the skin was done using an 11 blade and the microsheath was exchanged with a (_)-French sheath over an exchange wire. A (_)-inch glidewire was advanced into the abdominal aorta. A (_)-French pigtail catheter/Omni flush catheter was advanced over the wire to the abdominal aorta and angiographic runs of the aorto-iliac and bilateral proximal femoral arteries were then performed. Next, a (_)-French [type] catheter was used to maneuver the glide wire into the contralateral common iliac artery down to the femoral artery and the catheter was advanced over it and parked in the distal external iliac artery. Selective contralateral lower extremity angiography was performed confirming the presence and location of the popliteal aneurysm. The glidewire was advanced to the level of the aneurysm and down to the tibio-peroneal trunk and was then exchanged with a (_)-French Bentson wire/stiff Glidewire/Amplatz wire over the catheter. Unfractionated heparin was infused to achieve a therapeutic ACT level and then the short (_)-French sheath was exchanged for a long (_) cm, (_)-French Flexor/Ansel Sheath with its tip parked in the distal superficial femoral artery.

Alternatively a small cutdown under local anesthesia was used to expose the proximal superficial femoral artery. The artery was punctured antegradely and a size 8–9 French sheath was introduced.

Another angiogram was done through the sheath allowing for measurement of the aneurysm dimensions. Over the stiff wire, a (_) mm diameter-(_) mm long Viabahn/Fluency covered stent was advanced and positioned across the aneurysm. The self-expanding stent was deployed allowing for a 2 cm landing zone. A follow up angiogram showed complete exclusion of the aneurysm with adequate runoff to the foot (*alternatively, if the measured length to be stented exceeds the length of one stent graft, another stent is placed with an overlap zone between stent grafts of at least 3 cm*). After obtaining all the necessary images, the procedure was concluded. The long sheath was exchanged for a short one. An ACT level was measured and then the sheath was pulled and manual compression held for 20 min/a [type] closure device was used to achieve adequate hemostasis. A dry compression dressing was applied. The patient had palpable pulses/Doppler signals over the pedal vessels.

The patient was then transferred to the recovery room in a stable condition. Staff was present for the entire procedure.

Intra-Procedure Findings: List all relevant radiologic findings.

Immediate Complications: None encountered during or directly after the procedure. List the complications if any.

Post-Procedure Plan [3]:

- Keep patient complete bed rest with the right/left leg extended for (_) hours.
- Check the puncture site for any bleeding or hematoma formation every 15 min for 1 h, then every 30 min for 4 h; inform interventional radiology team if any complications are observed.
- Lower extremity neurovascular checks every hour.
- Resume diet and previous orders as needed and if not otherwise contraindicated.
- Continue adequate intravenous hydration and monitor fluid (intake-output) status.
- Check complete blood count, creatinine and blood urea nitrogen on the day following the procedure or as clinically indicated.

Impression:

- Endovascular treatment of left/right popliteal aneurysm as described above.
- The patient tolerated the procedure well and left the interventional unit in a stable condition.
- The patient was unstable and the procedure was canceled/terminated prematurely.
- List any other relevant of important information/finding.

References

1. Trinidad-Hernandez M, Ricotta JJ 2nd, Gloviczki P, Kalra M, Oderich GS, Duncan AA, et al. Results of elective and emergency endovascular repairs of popliteal artery aneurysms. J Vasc Surg. 2013;57(5):1299–305.
2. Garg K, Rockman CB, Kim BJ, Jacobowitz GR, Maldonado TS, Adelman MA, et al. Outcome of endovascular repair of popliteal artery aneurysm using the Viabahn Endoprosthesis. J Vasc Surg. 2012;55(6):1647–53.
3. Pulli R, Dorigo W, Fargion A, Pratesi G, Innocenti AA, Angiletta D, et al. Comparison of early and midterm results of open and endovascular treatment of popliteal artery aneurysms. Ann Vasc Surg. 2012;26(6):809–18.
4. Midy D, Berard X, Ferdani M, Alric P, Brizzi V, Ducasse E, et al. A retrospective multicenter study of endovascular treatment of popliteal artery aneurysm. J Vasc Surg. 2010;51(4):850–6.
5. Venkatesan AM, Kundu S, Sacks D, Wallace MJ, Wojak JC, Rose SC, et al. Practice guidelines for adult antibiotic prophylaxis during vascular and interventional radiology procedures. J Vasc Interv Radiol. 2010;21(11):1611–30.

Lower Extremity Angiogram

125

Hiba Ezzeddine and Maen Aboul Hosn

INTRODUCTION

Despite the advancements in noninvasive vascular imaging modalities such as duplex ultrasonography, computed tomography angiography (CTA) and magnetic resonance angiography (MRA), digital subtraction angiography remains the gold standard for delineating the lower extremity arterial anatomy especially when an intervention is contemplated.

COMMON INDICATIONS [1–4]

- Lower extremity ischemia/arteritis
- Lower extremity injury/bleeding
- Assessment of a lower extremity arterial bypass
- Preoperative planning for a distal bypass

COMMON CONTRAINDICATIONS [2, 3]

- Coagulopathy
- Contrast allergy
- Hemodynamic instability
- Chronic renal insufficiency approaching dialysis

POSSIBLE COMPLICATIONS [2–4]

- Hemorrhage *(puncture-site hematoma, retroperitoneal hematoma if "high" puncture above inguinal ligament)*
- Pseudoaneurysm *(superficial femoral artery "low" puncture)*
- Arteriovenous fistula *(puncture-site artery)*
- Thrombosis of the femoral artery
- Distal embolization
- Contrast-induced allergic reaction
- Contrast-induced nephropathy
- Arterial perforation or dissection
- Catheter or guide-wire breakage
- Limb amputation *(rare)*
- Risks related to any minimally invasive procedure performed under conscious sedation *(e.g., allergy to medications)*

H. Ezzeddine
Department of General Surgery, American University in Beirut Medical Center, Riad El Solh, Beirut 1107 2020, Lebanon
e-mail: he52@aub.edu.lb

M. Aboul Hosn (✉)
Department of Vascular Surgery, University of Iowa Hospitals and Clinics, 200 Hawkins Dr, Iowa City, IA 52242, USA
e-mail: maen-aboulhosn@uiowa.edu

B. Taslakian et al. (eds.), *Procedural Dictations in Image-Guided Intervention*,
DOI 10.1007/978-3-319-40845-3_125

PREPROCEDURAL ASSESSMENT AND PLANNING

- History, indications, and physical examination *(Appendix 1* in Chap. 149*)*. Document indications of the procedure, lower extremity pulses, and vital signs.
- Evaluation of diagnostic imaging studies to determine the relevant vascular anatomy and assess the access site
- Periprocedural management of coagulation status *(Appendices 2* in Chap. 150 *and 3* in Chap. 151*)*
- Antibiotic prophylaxis: Not routinely recommended *(Appendices 4* in Chap. 152 *and 5* in Chap. 153*)*
- Imaging modality for guidance: Fluoroscopy; combined with ultrasound for arterial puncture
- Positioning: Supine
- Patient preparation:
  - Start intravenous fluids the night before angiography in order to ensure adequate hydration, combined with effective monitoring of fluid status
  - Insert a urinary catheter or ask the patient to void before the procedure depending on the estimated time of the procedure
  - Considerations for patients with specific diseases or conditions, patients on specific medications or patients with history of multiple comorbidities: consult with the referring clinician, and obtain subspecialty consultation as needed

PROCEDURE NOTE

Procedure: Lower extremity angiography
Staff: [_]
Fellow: [_]
Resident: [_]
Clinical Information: Describe history and list indications
Allergies: No known drug allergy/Allergic to (specify)
Anesthesia: Local anesthesia/Monitored conscious sedation
Medications: List any relevant medications used
Contrast Material: (_) mL of [type] contrast material was used for intra-arterial injection
Field: Sterile
Procedure Classification: Clean
Position: Supine
Monitoring: Intravenous access was secured and vitals were continuously monitored by nursing staff/anesthesia team throughout the procedure
Total fluoroscopy time: (_) minutes
Cumulative radiation dose: (_) mGy

Description of Procedure *(Retrograde Angiography):*
The risks, benefits, alternatives, and the procedure itself were explained to the patient/patient's Power of Attorney/legal guardian, and informed written/verbal consent was obtained. The site of the procedure was identified and marked. Time out was performed to confirm the correct patient, procedure, and site.

The groin area was prepped and draped in the usual sterile manner. After infiltrating the skin with 1 % Lidocaine, and using ultrasound guidance, the right/left common femoral artery was accessed retrogradely with a micropuncture kit and the position of the microwire was confirmed by fluoroscopy. A small nick in the skin was done using an 11 blade and the microsheath was exchanged with a (_)-French sheath over an exchange wire. A glidewire was advanced into the abdominal aorta. A pigtail catheter/Omni flush catheter was advanced over the wire to the abdominal aorta and angiographic runs of the aorto-iliac and bilateral proximal femoral arteries were then performed. Next, a (_)-French [type] catheter was used to maneuver the glidewire into the contralateral common iliac artery down to the femoral artery and the catheter was advanced over it and parked in the distal external iliac artery. Selective contralateral lower extremity angiography was performed by injecting contrast through the catheter and performing sequential imaging of the entire lower extremity arterial system down to the foot. After obtaining all the necessary images, the procedure was concluded. The catheter was removed over the wire and the sheath was pulled out. Adequate hemostasis was achieved at the puncture site by compression for (_) minutes/using a vascular closure device and then a dry compression dressing was applied. The patient was transferred to the recovery room in a stable condition. Staff was present for the entire procedure.

Description of Procedure *(Antegrade Angiography):*
The risks, benefits, alternatives, and the procedure itself were explained to the patient/patient's Power of Attorney/legal guardian, and informed written consent was obtained. The site of the procedure was identified and marked. Time out was performed to confirm the correct patient, procedure, and site.

The groin area was prepped and draped in the usual sterile manner. After infiltrating the skin with 1 % Lidocaine, and using ultrasound guidance, the right/left common femoral artery was accessed antegradely with a micropuncture kit and the position of the microwire was confirmed by fluoroscopy to be in the ipsilateral superficial femoral artery. A small nick in the skin was done using an 11 blade and the microsheath was exchanged with a (_)-French sheath over an exchange wire. Selective ipsilateral lower extremity angiography was performed by injecting contrast through the sheath and performing sequential imaging of the entire lower extremity arterial system down to the foot. After obtaining all the necessary images, the procedure was concluded and the sheath was pulled out. Manual compression was held for 10–15 min and then a dry compression dressing was applied.

The patient was transferred to the recovery room in a stable condition. Staff was present for the entire procedure.

Intra-Procedure Findings: List all relevant radiologic findings.

Immediate Complications: None encountered during or directly after the procedure. List the complications if any.

Post-Procedure Plan [3]

- Keep patient complete bed rest with the right/left leg extended for 6 h *[adjust depending on the puncture site]*.
- Check the right/left groin/[specify the puncture site if different] for any bleeding or hematoma formation every 15 min for 1 h, then every 30 min for 1 h, then every hour for 4 h; inform interventional radiology team if any signs of bleeding are observed *[adjust depending on the puncture site]*.
- Check and document lower extremity pulses every 30 min for 2 h then every 1 h for 4 h *[adjust depending on the puncture site]*.
- Monitor vital signs every 15 min for 1 h, then every 30 min for 4 h; notify interventional radiology team if systolic blood pressure <95 mmHg, or heart rate >110 beats/min.
- Resume diet and previous orders as needed and if otherwise not contraindicated.
- Continue adequate intravenous hydration and monitor fluid (intake-output) status.
- Check complete blood count and creatinine on the day following the procedure or as clinically indicated.
- Perform regular neurological examination when the procedure includes manipulation in the ascending thoracic aorta, aortic arch, or brachiocephalic arteries.

Impression:

- Selective right/left lower extremity angiography as described above.
- The patient tolerated the procedure well and left the interventional unit in a stable condition.
- The patient was unstable and the procedure was canceled/terminated prematurely.
- List any other relevant of important information/finding.

References

1. Pollak AW, Kramer CM. MRI in lower extremity peripheral arterial disease: recent advancements. Curr Cardiovasc Imaging Rep. 2013;6(1):55–60.
2. Pomposelli F. Arterial imaging in patients with lower extremity ischemia and diabetes mellitus. J Vasc Surg. 2010;52(3 Suppl):81S–91S.
3. Chan D, Anderson ME, Dolmatch BL. Imaging evaluation of lower extremity infrainguinal disease: role of the noninvasive vascular laboratory, computed tomography

angiography, and magnetic resonance angiography. Tech Vasc Interv Radiol. 2010;13(1):11–22.
4. Quinn SF, Sheley RC, Semonsen KG, Leonardo VJ, Kojima K, Szumowski J. Aortic and lower-extremity arterial disease: evaluation with MR angiography versus conventional angiography. Radiology. 1998;206(3):693–701.

Superficial Femoral, Popliteal and Tibial Artery Angioplasty, and Stenting

126

Maen Aboul Hosn

INTRODUCTION

Percutaneous angioplasty and stenting is a minimally invasive therapy for the treatment of patients with peripheral artery disease who suffer from intermittent claudication or critical limb ischemia. It carries a low complication rate ranging between 0.5 and 4 %, and a high technical success rate approaching 90 %. In many centers, it is considered the treatment option of choice for aortoiliac, femoropopliteal, and tibial disease even in the presence long segment occlusion/stenosis. Tibial interventions are typically carried for critical limb ischemia

COMMON INDICATIONS [1–4]

- Lifestyle limiting claudication
- Chronic lower extremity ischemia with multilevel infra-inguinal/infra-popliteal disease
- TASC A and B lesions in the superficial femoral and popliteal artery
- Superficial femoral/popliteal in-stent stenosis

COMMON CONTRAINDICATIONS [2–4]

- Coagulopathy
- Contrast allergy
- Hemodynamic instability

POSSIBLE COMPLICATIONS [1–4]

- Hemorrhage *(puncture-site hematoma, retroperitoneal hematoma if "high" common femoral artery puncture above inguinal ligament)*
- Pseudoaneurysm *(superficial femoral artery "low" puncture)*
- Arteriovenous fistula *(puncture-site artery)*
- Thrombosis of the artery
- Distal embolization
- Contrast-induced allergic reaction
- Contrast-induced nephropathy
- Arterial perforation or dissection
- Catheter or guide-wire breakage
- Limb amputation *(rare)*
- Risks related to any minimally invasive procedure performed under conscious sedation *(e.g., allergy to medications)*

M. Aboul Hosn (✉)
Department of Vascular Surgery, University of Iowa Hospitals and Clinics, 200 Hawkins Dr, Iowa City, IA 52242, USA
e-mail: maen-aboulhosn@uiowa.edu

B. Taslakian et al. (eds.), *Procedural Dictations in Image-Guided Intervention*,
DOI 10.1007/978-3-319-40845-3_126

PREPROCEDURAL ASSESSMENT AND PLANNING

- History, indications, and physical examination *(Appendix 1* in Chap. 149*)*. Document indications of the procedure, lower extremity pulses, and vital signs.
- Evaluation of diagnostic imaging studies to determine the relevant vascular anatomy
- Periprocedural management of coagulation status *(Appendices 2* in Chap. 150 *and 3* in Chap 151*)*
- Antibiotic prophylaxis: Routinely recommended [5] *(Appendices 4* in Chap. 152 *and 5* in Chap. 153*)*
- Imaging modality for guidance: Fluoroscopy; combined with ultrasound for arterial puncture
- Positioning: Supine
- Arterial access: Femoral artery

PROCEDURE NOTE

Procedure: Right/Left superficial femoral/popliteal/tibial artery angioplasty and stenting
Staff: [_]
Fellow: [_]
Resident: [_]
Clinical Information: Describe history and list indications
Allergies: No known drug allergy/Allergic to (specify)
Anesthesia: Local anesthesia/Monitored conscious sedation
Medications: List any relevant medications used
Contrast Material: (_) mL of [type] contrast material was used for intra-arterial injection
Field: Sterile
Procedure Classification: Clean
Position: Supine
Monitoring: Intravenous access was secured and vitals were continuously monitored by nursing staff/anesthesia team throughout the procedure
Total fluoroscopy time: (_) minutes
Cumulative radiation dose: (_) mGy

Description of Procedure:
The risks, benefits, alternatives, and the procedure itself were explained to the patient/patient's Power of Attorney/legal guardian, and informed written consent was obtained. The site of the procedure was identified and marked. Time out was performed to confirm the correct patient, procedure, and site.

Retrograde puncture: The groin area was prepped and draped in the usual sterile manner. After infiltrating the skin with 1 % Lidocaine, and using ultrasound guidance, the right/left common femoral artery was accessed retrogradely with a micropuncture kit and the position of the microwire was confirmed by fluoroscopy. A small nick in the skin was done using an 11 blade and the microsheath was exchanged with a (_)-French sheath over an exchange wire. A pigtail/Omni flush catheter was advanced over a wire to the abdominal aorta and angiographic runs of the aortoiliac and bilateral proximal femoral arteries were then performed. Next, a (_)-French [type] glide catheter was used to maneuver the glidewire into the contralateral common iliac artery down to the femoral artery and the catheter was advanced over it and parked in the distal external iliac artery.

Antegrade puncture: The groin area was prepped and draped in the usual sterile manner. After infiltrating the skin with 1 % Lidocaine, and using ultrasound guidance, the right/left common femoral artery was accessed antegradely with a micropuncture kit and the position of the microwire was confirmed by fluoroscopy to be in the ipsilateral superficial femoral artery. A small nick in the skin was done using an 11 blade and the microsheath was exchanged with a (_)-French sheath over an exchange wire.

Selective right/left lower extremity angiography was performed delineating the area of stenosis/occlusion. The patient was given systemic unfractionated heparin at this point. Next, a (_)-inch *Bentson wire/stiff Glidewire/Amplatz wire* was advanced to the level of the common femoral artery and the short sheath was exchanged with a long (_)-French, (_) cm-long Flexor/Ansel sheath. Using an angled-tip glide catheter, the glidewire was maneuvered across the femoral/popliteal stenosis/occlusion. A repeat angiogram was performed through the sheath and the dimensions of the diseased segments were measured. A low profile (_) mm angioplasty balloon was then advanced to the level of the lesion and inflated to its nominal pressure. It was deflated at 1 min and the process was repeated until the entire lesion was covered. Follow-up angiography showed resolution/persistence of the stenosis. The decision was made to deploy a stent across the lesion. A (_) mm diameter, (_) mm long bare metal/drug eluting/covered stent was advanced and positioned across the area in question and deployed successfully with repeat angiography showing complete resolution of the stenosis.

(*Alternatively, for a tibial lesion, the 0.035 wire was exchanged for a 0.014 floppy tip wire, which was passed through the tibial stenosis down to the ankle joint. A long 2 mm balloon was then used to angioplasty the affected segment*)

With the completion angiogram showing resolution of the stenosis and adequate runoff to the foot, the procedure was concluded. The long sheath was exchanged with a short one over a stiff wire. An ACT level was checked and the sheath was pulled and manual compression held for 15–20 min/a vascular closure device was used to achieve adequate hemostasis. A dry compressive dressing was applied over the puncture site. The patient had palpable/Doppler signals over his pedal vessels at the end of the procedure. He was transferred to the recovery room in a stable condition. Staff was present for the entire procedure.

Intra-Procedure Findings: List all relevant radiologic findings.

Immediate Complications: None encountered during or directly after the procedure. List the complications if any.

Post-Procedure Plan [3]:

- Keep patient complete bed rest with the right/left leg extended for 6 h *[adjust depending on the puncture site]*.
- Check the right/left groin/[specify the puncture site if different] for any bleeding or hematoma formation every 15 min for 1 h, then every 30 min for 1 h, then every hour for 4 h; inform interventional radiology team if any signs of bleeding are observed *[adjust depending on the puncture site]*.
- Check and document lower extremity pulses every 30 min for 2 h then every 1 h for 4 h *[adjust depending on the puncture site]*.
- Monitor vital signs every 15 min for 1 h, then every 30 min for 4 h; notify interventional radiology team if systolic blood pressure <95 mmHg, or heart rate >110 beats/min.
- Resume diet and previous orders as needed and if otherwise not contraindicated.
- Continue adequate intravenous hydration and monitor fluid (intake-output) status.
- Check complete blood count and creatinine on the day following the procedure or as clinically indicated.
- Perform regular neurological examination when the procedure includes manipulation in the ascending thoracic aorta, aortic arch, or brachiocephalic arteries.

Impression:

- Right/left superficial femoral/popliteal/tibial artery angioplasty and stenting as described above.
- The patient tolerated the procedure well and left the interventional unit in a stable condition.
- The patient was unstable and the procedure was canceled/terminated prematurely.
- List any other relevant of important information/finding.

References

1. Tepe G, Laird J, Schneider P, Brodmann M, Krishnan P, Micari A, et al. Drug-coated balloon versus standard percutaneous transluminal angioplasty for the treatment of superficial femoral and popliteal peripheral artery disease: 12-month results from the IN.PACT SFA randomized trial. Circulation. 2015;131(5):495–502.

2. Chowdhury MM, McLain AD, Twine CP. Angioplasty versus bare metal stenting for superficial femoral artery lesions. Cochrane Database Syst Rev. 2014; 6:CD006767.
3. Bradbury AW, Adam DJ, Bell J, Forbes JF, Fowkes FG, Gillespie I, et al. Bypass versus angioplasty in severe ischaemia of the leg (BASIL) trial: a description of the severity and extent of disease using the bollinger angiogram scoring method and the trans atlantic inter-society consensus II classification. J Vasc Surg. 2010;51(5 Suppl):32S–42S.
4. Surowiec SM, Davies MG, Eberly SW, Rhodes JM, Illig KA, Shortell CK, et al. Percutaneous angioplasty and stenting of the superficial femoral artery. J Vasc Surg. 2005;41(2):269–78.
5. Venkatesan AM, Kundu S, Sacks D, Wallace MJ, Wojak JC, Rose SC, et al. Practice guidelines for adult antibiotic prophylaxis during vascular and interventional radiology procedures. J Vasc Interv Radiol. 2010;21(11):1611–30.

Thrombectomy for Management of Acute Limb Ischemia

127

Maen Aboul Hosn

INTRODUCTION

Acute limb ischemia has traditionally been managed with urgent open thromboembolectomy and revascularization in order to restore flow in a timely fashion and prevent irreversible tissue damage and ultimately limb loss. Recently, endovascular techniques utilizing percutaneous mechanical thrombectomy have been used to reduce the thrombus burden as well as expose more surface area to adjunct thrombolytic therapy. These modalities offer a minimally invasive alternative especially in high risk patients who cannot tolerate an open surgical procedure and can also serve as adjuncts to open revascularization.

COMMON INDICATIONS [1–4]

- Mild/moderate limb ischemia *(Rutherford category I and IIA)*
- Acute limb ischemia in the setting of chronic atherosclerotic disease
- Clots < 14 days old

COMMON CONTRAINDICATIONS [1–4]

- Severe limb ischemia requiring immediate revascularization (Rutherford Category IIB and III)
- Active bleeding
- Intracranial hemorrhage
- Recent neurovascular intervention
- Recent cerebrovascular event
- Hemodynamic instability

POSSIBLE COMPLICATIONS [1, 2]

- Hemorrhage *(puncture site hematoma, retroperitoneal hematoma if "high" common femoral puncture above inguinal ligament)*
- Pseudoaneurysm *(superficial femoral artery "low" puncture)*
- Arteriovenous fistula *(puncture site artery)*
- Distal embolization
- Contrast-induced allergic reaction
- Contrast-induced nephropathy
- Arterial perforation or dissection
- Catheter or guide-wire breakage
- Limb amputation *(rare)*
- Risks related to any minimally invasive procedure performed under conscious sedation *(e.g., allergy to medications)*

M. Aboul Hosn (✉)
Department of Vascular Surgery, University of Iowa Hospitals and Clinics, 200 Hawkins Dr, Iowa City, IA 52242, USA
e-mail: maen-aboulhosn@uiowa.edu

B. Taslakian et al. (eds.), *Procedural Dictations in Image-Guided Intervention*,
DOI 10.1007/978-3-319-40845-3_127

Procedure-specific complications
- Intracranial hemorrhage
- Retroperitoneal bleeding

PREPROCEDURAL ASSESSMENT AND PLANNING

- History, indications, and physical examination *(Appendix 1* in Chap. 149*)*. Document indications of the procedure and vital signs. Rule out any contraindications to lytic therapy.
- Evaluation of diagnostic imaging studies to determine the relevant vascular anatomy and assess the access site
- Periprocedural management of coagulation status *(Appendices 2* in Chap. 150 *and 3* in Chap. 151*)*
- Antibiotic prophylaxis: Not routinely recommended *(Appendices 4* in Chap. 152 *and 5* in Chap. 153*)*
- Imaging modality for guidance: Fluoroscopy; combined with ultrasound for arterial puncture
- Positioning: Supine

PROCEDURE NOTE

Procedure: Lower extremity mechanical thrombectomy and thrombolysis
Staff: [_]
Fellow: [_]
Resident: [_]
Clinical Information: Describe history and list indications
Allergies: No known drug allergy/Allergic to (specify)
Anesthesia: Local anesthesia/Monitored conscious sedation
Medications: List any relevant medications used
Contrast Material: (_) mL of [type] contrast material was used for intra-arterial injection
Field: Sterile
Procedure Classification: Clean
Position: Supine
Monitoring: Intravenous access was secured and vitals were continuously monitored by nursing staff/anesthesia team throughout the procedure
Total fluoroscopy time: (_) minutes
Cumulative radiation dose: (_) mGy

Description of Procedure:
The risks, benefits, alternatives and the procedure itself were explained to the patient/patient's Power of Attorney/legal guardian, and informed written consent was obtained. The site of the procedure was identified and marked. Time out was performed to confirm the correct patient, procedure and site.

The groin area was prepped and draped in the usual sterile manner. After infiltrating the skin with 1 % Lidocaine, and using ultrasound guidance, the right/left common femoral artery was accessed with a micropuncture kit and the position of the microwire was confirmed by fluoroscopy. A small nick in the skin was done using an 11 blade and the microsheath was exchanged with a (_)-French sheath over an exchange wire. A pigtail/Omni flush catheter was advanced over the wire to the abdominal aorta and angiographic runs of the aorto-iliac and bilateral proximal femoral arteries were then performed. Next, the catheter was used to maneuver a glidewire into the contralateral common iliac artery down to the femoral artery and the catheter was advanced over it and parked in the distal external iliac artery. Selective contralateral lower extremity angiography was performed and the area of arterial occlusion was identified. A glidewire was advanced across the thrombosed segment using a glide catheter. The glidewire was then exchanged for a Bentson wire/stiff Glidewire/Amplatzwire and the short sheath was exchanged with a long (_)-French, (_) cm-long Balkan/Ansel sheath. The Angiojet thrombectomy catheter/Ekosonic catheter/Trellis infusion catheter was advanced and positioned across the thrombosed region. Multiple passes of the thrombectomy catheter were performed and clot fragments were aspirated. An angiogram was done next showing a decrease in the clot burden. The thrombectomy catheter was then exchanged with a (_)-French,

(_) cm multi-sidehole catheter for delivery of the lytic solution and it was positioned across the remaining thrombus. An initial bolus of (5–10) mg of recombinant tissue plasminogen activator (rt-PA) was administered into the clot and then an infusion of (0.5–1.5) mg/h was started. The catheter was secured to the skin with a 3–0 Nylon suture for a planned repeat angiogram in 24 h and a dry dressing was applied over the catheter exit site.

The patient was transferred to the recovery room in a stable condition. Staff was present for the entire procedure.

Intra-Procedure Findings: List all relevant radiologic findings.

Immediate Complications: None encountered during or directly after the procedure. List the complications if any.

Post-Procedure Plan [3]:

Standard post-angiogram management plan

- Keep patient complete bed rest with the right/left leg extended.
- Check the right/left groin/[specify the puncture site if different] for any bleeding or hematoma formation every 15 min for 1 h, then every 30 min for 1 h, then every hour for the entire observation period; inform interventional radiology team if any signs of bleeding are observed *[adjust depending on the puncture site]*.
- Check and document lower extremity pulses every 30 min for 2 h then every 1 h for the entire observation period *[adjust depending on the puncture site]*.
- Monitor vital signs every 15 min for 1 h, then every 30 min for 4 h; notify interventional radiology team if systolic blood pressure < 95 mmHg, or heart rate > 110 beats/min.
- Continue adequate intravenous hydration and monitor fluid (intake-output) status.
- Check complete blood count and creatinine on the day following the procedure or as clinically indicated.

Procedure-specific management plan:

- Patient observation for 24 h in a monitored unit.
- Check for chest pain, dyspnea and bleeding.
- Perform regular neurological examination.
- Serial fibrinogen and D-dimer levels.
- Repeat angiogram in 24 h.

Impression:

- Percutaneous lower extremity mechanical thrombectomy and thrombolysis as described above
- The patient tolerated the procedure well and left the interventional unit in a stable condition
- The patient was unstable and the procedure was canceled/terminated prematurely.
- List any other relevant of important information/finding.

References

1. Karnabatidis D, Spiliopoulos S, Tsetis D, Siablis D. Quality improvement guidelines for percutaneous catheter-directed intra-arterial thrombolysis and mechanical thrombectomy for acute lower-limb ischemia. Cardiovasc Interv Radiol. 2011;34(6):1123–36.
2. Lyden SP. Endovascular treatment of acute limb ischemia: review of current plasminogen activators and mechanical thrombectomy devices. Perspect Vasc Surg Endovasc Ther. 2010;22(4):219–22.
3. Ouriel K. Endovascular techniques in the treatment of acute limb ischemia: thrombolytic agents, trials, and percutaneous mechanical thrombectomy techniques. Semin Vasc Surg. 2003;16(4):270–9.
4. Ouriel K. Current status of thrombolysis for peripheral arterial occlusive disease. Ann Vasc Surg. 2002;16 (6):797–804.

128 Thrombolytic Therapy for Lower Extremity Deep Vein Trombosis

Maen Aboul Hosn

Abbreviations

DVT	Deep vein thrombosis
rt-PA	Recombinant tissue plasminogen activator

INTRODUCTION

The cornerstone for management of acute lower extremity deep vein thrombosis (DVT) has always been anticoagulation therapy and compressing stockings. However, up to 50 % of patients with proximal DVTs develop what is known as the post thrombotic syndrome which is characterized by valvular dysfunction resulting in chronic limb pain, heaviness, swelling, and possible skin ulcerations. As such, many physicians have advocated the early treatment of large lower extremity DVT, mainly ilio-femoral ones, with thrombolytic therapy attempting to preserve the valves and prevent valvular reflux therefore avoid the significant long-term complications and morbidity.

M. Aboul Hosn (✉)
Department of Vascular Surgery, University of Iowa Hospitals and Clinics, 200 Hawkins Dr, Iowa City, IA 52242, USA
e-mail: maen-aboulhosn@uiowa.edu

COMMON INDICATIONS [1–3]

- Ilio-femoral deep vein thrombosis in a young individual
- Acute proximal deep vein thrombosis < 2 weeks
- Limb threatening venous thrombosis (Phlegmasia Cerulea Dolens)

COMMON CONTRAINDICATIONS [1, 2, 4]

- Active internal bleeding
- Coagulopathy
- Recent cerebrovascular event
- Neurosurgical intervention within 3 months
- Major trauma
- Recent organ biopsy
- Pregnancy

POSSIBLE COMPLICATIONS [1, 2, 4]

- Access site bleeding; *5–10 %*
- Intracranial hemorrhage; *1–2 %*
- Pulmonary embolism; *1–5 %*

B. Taslakian et al. (eds.), *Procedural Dictations in Image-Guided Intervention*,
DOI 10.1007/978-3-319-40845-3_128

- Stroke *(in the presence of patent Foramen Ovale)*
- Iatrogenic injury to nearby neurovascular structures

REPROCEDURAL ASSESSMENT AND PLANNING

- History, indications and physical examination *(Appendix 1* in Chap. 149*)*. Document indications of the procedure and vital signs. Rule out any contraindications to lytic therapy.
- Evaluation of diagnostic imaging studies to determine the relevant vascular anatomy and assess the access site
- Periprocedural management of coagulation status *(Appendices 2* in Chap. 150 *and 3* in Chap. 151*)*
- Antibiotic prophylaxis: Not routinely recommended *(Appendices 4* in Chap. 152 *and 5* in Chap. 153*)*
- Imaging modality for guidance: Fluoroscopy; combined with ultrasound for venous puncture
- Positioning: Prone

PROCEDURE NOTE

Procedure: Catheter-directed thrombolysis of lower extremity deep vein thrombosis
Staff: [_]
Fellow: [_]
Resident: [_]
Clinical Information: Describe history and list indications
Allergies: No known drug allergy/Allergic to (specify)
Anesthesia: Local anesthesia/Monitored conscious sedation
Medications: List any relevant medications used (sedation, thrombolytic agent)
Contrast Material: (_) mL of [type] contrast material was used for venography
Field: Sterile
Procedure Classification: Clean
Position: Prone
Monitoring: Intravenous access was secured and vitals were continuously monitored by nursing staff/anesthesia team throughout the procedure
Total fluoroscopy time: (_) minutes
Cumulative radiation dose: (_) mGy

Description of Procedure

The risks, benefits, alternatives and the procedure itself were explained to the patient/patient's Power of Attorney/legal guardian, and informed written consent was obtained. The site of the procedure was identified and marked. Time out was performed to confirm the correct patient, procedure, and site.

The patient was fully anticoagulated and maintained on an unfractionated heparin drip. The patient was placed in a prone position and the left/right lower extremity was prepped and draped in the usual sterile manner. Under ultrasound guidance, the ipsilateral popliteal vein *(alternatively posterior tibial vein or saphenous vein)* was accessed with a micropuncture kit. A small nick in the skin was done using an 11 blade and the microsheath was exchanged with a (_)-French sheath over an exchange wire. A venogram was then performed and the location of the ilio-femoral venous thrombosis was confirmed. A (_)-inch glidewire was advanced across the thrombosed vein using a (_)-French [type] glide catheter and the glidewire was then exchanged for a Bentson wire/stiff Glidewire/Amplatz wire. A (_)-French Angiojet catheter was advanced and positioned across the thrombosed segment. The catheter was used in power pulse mode initially with (6–8) mg of recombinant tissue plasminogen activator (rt-PA) per segment for a total of (10–20) mg of rt-PA. It was then reactivated in regular thrombectomy mode after a 15-minute dwell time and multiple passes of the Angiojet catheter were performed. A venogram was done next showing a decrease in the clot burden. The Angiojet catheter was then exchanged with a (_)-French [type] multi-sidehole catheter for delivery of the lytic solution and it was positioned across the remaining thrombus. rt-PA infusion was started at a rate of (0.5) mg/h and the sheath was secured to the skin with a 3–0 Nylon suture for a planned repeat venogram in 24 h. A dry dressing was applied over the catheter exit site.

The patient was transferred to the recovery room in a stable condition. Staff was present for the entire procedure.

Note: If a temporary vena cava filter was inserted, refer to chapter on IVC filter.

Intra-Procedure Findings: List all relevant radiologic findings.

Immediate Complications: None encountered during or directly after the procedure. List the complications if any.

Post-Procedure Plan [1–3]:

- Keep patient complete bed rest with the right/left leg extended.
- Check the access site for any bleeding or hematoma formation every 15 min for 1 h, then every 30 min for 1 h, then every hour for the entire observation period; inform interventional radiology team if any signs of bleeding are observed.
- Monitor vital signs every 15 min for 1 h, then every 30 min for 4 h; notify interventional radiology team if systolic blood pressure < 95 mmHg, or heart rate > 110 beats/min.
- Continue adequate intravenous hydration and monitor fluid (intake–output) status.
- Check complete blood count and creatinine on the day following the procedure or as clinically indicated.

Procedure-specific management plan:

- Check for chest pain, dyspnea, weakness, focal neurologic deficits and bleeding.
- Lower extremity neurovascular checks every hour.
- Serial fibrinogen and D-dimer levels.
- Repeat venogram in 24–48 h.

Impression:

- Catheter-directed thrombolysis of lower extremity deep vein thrombosis as described above.
- The patient tolerated the procedure well and left the interventional unit in a stable condition.
- The patient was unstable and the procedure was canceled/terminated prematurely.
- List any other relevant of important information/finding.

References

1. Huang CY, Hsu HL, Kuo TT, Lee CY, Hsu CP. Percutaneous pharmacomechanical thrombectomy offers lower risk of post-thrombotic syndrome than catheter-directed thrombolysis in patients with acute deep vein thrombosis of the lower Limb. Ann Vasc Surg. 2015;29(5):995–1002.
2. Patterson BO, Hinchliffe R, Loftus IM, Thompson MM, Holt PJ. Indications for catheter-directed thrombolysis in the management of acute proximal deep venous thrombosis. Arterioscler Thromb Vasc Biol. 2010;30(4):669–74.
3. Gogalniceanu P, Johnston CJ, Khalid U, Holt PJ, Hincliffe R, Loftus IM, et al. Indications for thrombolysis in deep venous thrombosis. Eur J VascEndovasc Surg. 2009;38(2):192–8.
4. Nagarsheth KH, Sticco C, Aparajita R, Schor J, Singh K, Zia S, et al. Catheter directed therapy is safe and effective for the management of acute inferior vena cava thrombosis. Ann Vasc Surg. 2015;29(7):1373–9.

Part XXI

Vascular Interventional Procedures: Venous Sampling for Endocrine Disorders

Introduction by John A. Kaufman, Section Reviewer

When John L. Doppman, MD published the first report of transvenous sampling to localize an endocrine tumor in 1969, he changed the practice of endocrine surgery forever [1]. Rather than obtaining peripheral samples, he literally went right to the source, but through the venous system. What seems so obvious today was a major innovation at the time. With improvements in cross-sectional imaging these procedures have become less common. Nevertheless, they maintain a critical role in endocrine medicine today and likely for the foreseeable future.

Venous sampling is rarely performed without extensive prior clinical, laboratory, and imaging workup. Sometimes surgery has already been performed, with failure to localize the functional tumor. These data are essential to review prior to the procedure. During the procedure, great care is needed for precise labeling of samples, and recording the sampling locations. Verbal confirmation as each sample is handed off helps to minimize the risk of mislabeling. These may seem like rather mundane procedures, but there is no wiggle room; everyone involved has to have absolute confidence in the integrity of the samples.

This section provides a comprehensive list of procedural reports that covers a vast majority of venous sampling procedures, with up-to-date explanatory notes, synopsis of the indications and contraindications, and potential complications in an organized and practical format.

Reference

1. Doppman JL, Melson GL, Evens RG, Hammond WG. Selective superior and inferior thyroid vein catheterization. Invest Radiol. 1969;4:97–9.

Section Chapters

129 Adrenal Venous Sampling

Sandra Abi Fadel

Abbreviations

ACTH	Adrenocorticotropic hormone
CT	Computed tomography
DHEA	Dehydroepiandrosterone
MRI	Magnetic resonance imaging

INTRODUCTION

Adrenal venous sampling consists of simultaneous or sequential sampling of the bilateral adrenal veins, before and after the administration of adrenocorticotropic hormone (ACTH) intravenously, for localization of pathology before adrenalectomy in Conn, Cushing, and adrenogenital syndromes. Adrenal venous sampling has a high accuracy rate of nearly 100 %.

COMMON INDICATIONS [1–4]

- To localize the adenoma in patients with clinical and laboratory evidence of primary hyperaldosteronism and equivocal results of noninvasive imaging modalities
- To lateralize the adenoma in patients with clinical and laboratory evidence of primary hyperaldosteronism and apparent bilateral adrenal disease on noninvasive imaging modalities
- To localize the adenoma in patients with clinical and laboratory evidence of ACTH-independent Cushing syndrome with equivocal noninvasive imaging results
- To localize the adrenal adenoma in patients with clinical and laboratory evidence of virilization and equivocal noninvasive imaging results

COMMON CONTRAINDICATIONS [1]

- Increased bleeding diathesis
- Accelerated hypertension
- Significant ischemic heart disease
- Allergy to contrast

S. Abi Fadel (✉)
Department of Diagnostic Radiology, American University of Beirut Medical Center, Riad El-Solh, Beirut 1107 2020, Lebanon
e-mail: sa183@aub.edu.lb

B. Taslakian et al. (eds.), *Procedural Dictations in Image-Guided Intervention*,
DOI 10.1007/978-3-319-40845-3_129

POSSIBLE COMPLICATIONS [2, 4, 5]

- Infection of the puncture site
- Groin hematoma
- Venous spasm causing failure of the procedure
- Rupture of the adrenal vein
- Adrenal gland infarction
- Adrenal Hemorrhage
- Hypertensive crisis
- Adrenal insufficiency

PREPROCEDURAL ASSESSMENT AND PLANNING

- History, indications, and physical examination *(Appendix 1* in Chap. 149*)*
- Evaluation of diagnostic imaging studies (ultrasound, MRI, CT) to determine the location of the adrenal veins
- Periprocedural management of coagulation status *(Appendices 2* in Chap. 150 *and 3* in Chap. 151*)*
- Antibiotic prophylaxis: Not routinely recommended [6]
- Imaging modality for guidance: Fluoroscopy, ultrasound for localization of the femoral vein for puncture
- Positioning: Supine

PROCEDURE NOTE

Procedure: Fluoroscopic-guided percutaneous bilateral adrenal venous sampling with ACTH stimulation
Staff:: [_]
Fellow:: [_]
Resident:: [_]
Clinical Information: Describe history and list indications
Allergies: None known/Allergic to [specify/type of allergy]
Anesthesia: Local anesthesia/conscious sedation
Medications: List any relevant medications used (sedation, ACTH)
Contrast Used: (_) mL of [type] contrast media was used for intravenous injection
Field: Sterile
Procedure classification: Clean
Position: Supine
Monitoring: Intravenous access line was secured and vital signs were continuously monitored by nursing staff/anesthesia team throughout the procedure
Total fluoroscopy time: (_) minutes
Cumulative radiation dose: (_) mGy

Description of Procedure:
The risks, benefits, alternatives and the procedure itself were explained to the patient/patient's Power of Attorney/patient's legal guardian, and informed written/verbal consent was obtained. Time out was performed to confirm the correct patient and procedure.

The skin of both groins were shaved, prepped, and draped in the usual sterile fashion. The right/left femoral vein was located by palpation/ultrasound and marked. The site of venous puncture was determined using combined information from palpation and ultrasound. Local anesthesia was administered. Femoral venous access was obtained using an (_)-gauge [type] needle and the Seldinger technique, double-/single- wall entry under direct ultrasound visualization/by palpation. Once good venous flow was detected, a (_)-inch [type] guidewire was advanced through the needle into the inferior vena cava under direct fluoroscopic visualization and a (_)-French vascular sheath was placed.

Subsequently, a (_)-French [type] catheter was introduced in the left renal vein with the help of a tip-deflecting wire. A (_)-French [type] micro/catheter was directed toward the left adrenal vein and located after the confluence with the left phrenic vein. Small gentle hand injections of contrast material were used to verify the catheter position.

A (_)-French [type] micro/catheter was placed at the origin of the right adrenal vein. Small hand injections of contrast material were used to verify the catheter position.

[The right adrenal vein was not found, so samples were taken from the right renal vein/inferior vena cava above and below the expected location of the right adrenal vein].

After collection of simultaneous/consecutive baseline samples from both adrenal veins and the femoral vein, intravenous ACTH was administered in the form of 25 mcg bolus followed by an infusion of 25 mcg in 500 ml of normal saline at a rate of 150/200 mL per hour.

Repeat samples were obtained from the adrenal veins 15 min after the start of ACTH infusion, and the latter was discontinued.

All samples were sent to the lab for aldosterone and cortisol as well as testosterone/DHEA/androstenedione levels testing.

Following the procedure the right/left femoral venous sheath was removed and adequate hemostasis was achieved by compression for (_) minutes. The patient was transferred to the floor/recovery room following the procedure in a stable condition. Staff was present for the entire procedure.

Intra-Procedure Findings: List all relevant findings.

Immediate Complications: None encountered during or directly after the procedure. List complications if any.

Post-Procedure Plan [4]:

- Follow-up laboratory results.
- Keep complete bed rest for 2 h and abstain from strenuous activities.
- Check vital signs every 15 min for 1 h then every 30 min for 2 h.
- Inform interventional radiology team if blood pressure <95/65 mm Hg, heart rate >100 beats per minute, fever persisting more than 24 h after the procedure or severe persistent flank pain requiring large doses of analgesics.

Impression:

- Sampling of bilateral adrenal veins with ACTH stimulation, as described above.
- The patient tolerated the procedure well and left the interventional unit in stable condition.
- The patient was unstable during/unable to tolerate the procedure which was canceled/terminated prematurely.
- List any other relevant or important information/finding.

References

1. Georgia JD, Miler DL. Arteriography and venous sampling of the parathyroid glands, pancreas and adrenal glands. In: Curtis WB, James ES, Jacob C, Seymour S, editors. Vascular and interventional radiology-principles and practice. New York: Thieme; 2002. p. 434–9.
2. Adrenal vein sampling. In: Burke CT, Dixon RG, editors. High yield imaging: interventional. Philadelphia: Saunders; 2010. p. 328–30.
3. Endocrine, Exocrine and Reproductive Systems. In: Karim V, editor. The practice of interventional radiology. Philadelphia: Saunders; 2012:419–422.
4. Daunt N. Adrenal vein sampling: how to make it quick, easy and successful. RadioGraphics. 2005; 25:S143–S158.
5. Patel SM, Lingam RK, Beaconsfield TI, Tran TL, Brown B. Role of radiology in the management of primary aldosteronism. Radiographics. 2007;27 (4):1145–57.
6. Venkatesan AM, Kundu S, Sacks D, Wallace MJ, Wojak JC, Rose SC, et al. Practice guidelines for adult antibiotic prophylaxis during vascular and interventional radiology procedures. J Vasc Interv Radiol. 2010;21(11):1611–30.

130 Inferior Petrosal Vein Sampling

Sandra Abi Fadel

Abbreviations

CRH	Corticotropin-releasing hormone
ACTH	Adrenocorticotropic hormone

INTRODUCTION

Differentiating pituitary causes from ectopic causes of Adrenocorticotropic hormone (ACTH) secretion is somehow complex due to the cyclical and intermittent secretion of ACTH as well as the low sensitivity of cross-sectional imaging in detecting microadenomas of the pituitary. From these limitations rose the importance of inferior petrosal vein sampling as a way to confirm and lateralize a pituitary adenoma. Some studies reported improved accuracy and localization of pituitary adenomas with cavernous sinus sampling; however due to its increased neurologic complications rate, most centers continue to use bilateral inferior petrosal vein sampling for diagnosis of Cushing disease.

S. Abi Fadel (✉)
Department of Diagnostic Radiology, American University of Beirut Medical Center, Riad El-Solh, Beirut 10017 2020, Lebanon
e-mail: sa183@aub.edu.lb

COMMON INDICATIONS [1]

- Localize pituitary adenoma in Cushing disease with equivocal or negative noninvasive imaging results
- Diagnose Cushing disease with positive pituitary adenoma and equivocal peripheral ACTH results on corticotropin-releasing hormone (CRH) stimulation test
- Persistence of Cushing syndrome after trans-sphenoidal surgery
- Clinical need to resolve discrepancy between clinical, biochemical, and noninvasive imaging results

COMMON CONTRAINDICATIONS [2, 3]

- Patients who have undergone bilateral adrenalectomy *(a corticosteroid replacement regimen must be used during the week preceding the procedure)*
- Patients maintained on medications that suppress cortisol production *(the drug should be discontinued for as many weeks needed*

B. Taslakian et al. (eds.), *Procedural Dictations in Image-Guided Intervention*,
DOI 10.1007/978-3-319-40845-3_130

before the procedure, until patient reaches a hypercortisolemic state)

- Low levels of free cortisol in the urine or plasma in patients with periodic Cushing syndrome
- Bleeding diathesis
- Allergy to iodinated contrast
- Ischemic heart disease
- Orthopnea

POSSIBLE COMPLICATIONS [1, 4]

- Groin hematomas
- Acute renal insufficiency
- Headache
- Nausea
- Otalgia
- Tinnitus
- Venous subarachnoid hemorrhage
- Pulmonary thromboembolism
- Pontomedullary junction stroke
- Brainstem infarction
- Transient 6th cranial nerve palsy
- Obstructive hydrocephalus

PREPROCEDURAL ASSESSMENT AND PLANNING

- History, indications, and physical examination *(Appendix 1* in Chap. 149*)*
- Evaluation of diagnostic imaging studies to determine the location of the pituitary adenoma, if possible
- Periprocedural management of coagulation status *(Appendices 2* in Chap. 150 *and 3* in Chap. 151*)*
- Antibiotic prophylaxis: Not routinely recommended [5]
- Imaging modality for guidance: Fluoroscopy/ultrasound
- Positioning: Supine

PROCEDURE NOTE

Procedure: Fluoroscopy-guided bilateral inferior petrosal vein sampling with CRH stimulation
Staff: [_]
Fellow: [_]
Resident: [_]
Clinical Information: Describe history and list indications
Allergies: None known/Allergic to [specify/type of allergy]
Anesthesia: Local anesthesia/conscious sedation
Medications: List any relevant medications used
Contrast Used: (_) mL of [type] contrast media was used for intravenous injection
Field: Sterile
Procedure classification: Clean
Position: Supine
Monitoring: Intravenous access line was secured and vital signs were continuously monitored by nursing staff/anesthesia team throughout the procedure
Total fluoroscopy time: (_) minutes
Cumulative radiation dose: (_) mGy

Description of Procedure [6, 7]:
The risks, benefits, alternatives and the procedure itself were explained to the patient/patient's Power of Attorney/patient's legal guardian, and informed written consent was obtained. Time out was performed to confirm the correct patient and procedure.

The skin of both groins was shaved, prepped and draped in the usual sterile fashion. The right/left femoral vein was located by palpation/ultrasound and marked. The site of venous puncture was determined using combined information from palpation and ultrasound. Local anesthesia was administered. Right/left common femoral venous access was obtained using a (_)-gauge [type] needle and the Seldinger technique, double-/single- wall entry under direct ultrasound visualization/by palpation. A (_)-French femoral vascular sheath was then placed and connected via extension tubing and a three-way stop-cock to a continuous flush solution drip to allow peripheral vein sampling. (_) international units of heparin was injected as a bolus/drip during the entire procedure. Then a (_)-French [type] catheter was introduced through the femoral sheath and advanced into the right/left internal jugular vein using a (_)-inch [type] guidewire under direct fluoroscopic visualization. The catheter was rotated in the internal jugular vein at the level of C1–C2 vertebrae so that its tip pointed medially and anteriorly. Inferior petrosal, cavernous and intercavernous sinuses were outlined using gentle hand injection of (_) mL contrast material with digital subtraction techniques.

The catheter was then advanced superiorly till reaching the right/left inferior petrosal sinus. A second microcatheter was positioned in a similar manner on the opposite side, through a second femoral access. Catheter tip position was confirmed using gentle hand injection of (_) mL contrast material. The catheters were taped to the patient's skin to avoid withdrawal.

Two sets of (_) mL blood samples were obtained at baseline, each simultaneously from the right and left inferior petrosal sinuses and from the right/left femoral sheath.

Then CRH was diluted and administered at a dose of (1) microgram/kg as a slow peripheral intravenous bolus over 1 min. Desmopressin (10 µg) was administered as a slow peripheral intravenous infusion.

Simultaneous blood specimens were obtained at 3, 5, 10, and 15 min after CRH/desmopressin injection.

All the samples were immediately placed in marked, numbered lavender-top tubes on ice and transported to the laboratory.

Normal saline was infused continuously through the guiding catheter during the procedure as well as through the microcatheter when blood was not being withdrawn. Digital subtraction venography was performed at the end of procedure to document catheters' position.

Following the procedure, the catheters and venous sheaths were removed and adequate hemostasis was achieved by compression for (_) minutes. Sterile dressing was applied at the access site. The patient was transferred to the floor/recovery room following the procedure in a stable condition. Staff was present for the entire procedure.

Intra-Procedure Findings: List all relevant findings.

Immediate Complications: None encountered during or directly after the procedure. List complications if any.

Post-Procedure Plan:

- Follow-up laboratory results.
- Keep complete bed rest for 2–4 h and abstain from strenuous activities.
- Check vital signs and neurological exam every 15 min for 1 h, every 30 min for 1 h and then every 60 min for 2 h.
- Inform interventional radiology team if systolic blood pressure <95 mm Hg, heart rate >100 beats per minute, or if any severe headache or deterioration in the neurological exam develops.

Impression:

- Bilateral inferior petrosal vein sampling with CRH stimulation, as described above.
- The patient tolerated the procedure well and left the interventional unit in stable condition.
- The patient was unstable during/unable to tolerate the procedure which was canceled/terminated prematurely.
- List any other relevant or important information/finding.

References

1. Bonelli FS, Huston JT, Carpenter PC, Erickson D, Young WF, Meyer FB. Adrenocorticotropic hormone-dependent Cushing's syndrome: sensitivity and specificity of inferior petrosal sinus sampling. AJNR Am J Neuroradiol. 2000;21(4):690–696.
2. Kessel DO, Flood K. Principles of venous access. In: Mauro MA, Murphy KP, Thomson KR, Venbrux AC, Morgan RA, editors. Image guided interventions: Saunders; 2014. p. 135–143.
3. Miller DL, Doppman JL. Petrosal sinus sampling: technique and rationale. Radiology. 1991;178(1):37–47.

4. Oliverio PJ, Monsein LH, Wand GS, Debrun GM. Bilateral simultaneous cavernous sinus sampling using corticotropin-releasing hormone in the evaluation of cushing disease. AJNR Am J Neuroradiol 1996;17 (9):1669–1674.
5. Venkatesan AM, Kundu S, Sacks D, Wallace MJ, Wojak JC, Rose SC, et al. Practice guidelines for adult antibiotic prophylaxis during vascular and interventional radiology procedures. J Vasc Interv Radiol. 2010;21(11):1611–30.
6. Deipolyi AR, Hirsch JA, Oklu R. Bilateral inferior petrosal sinus sampling. J NeuroIntervent Surg. 2012;4 (3):215–218.
7. Deipolyi AR, Alexander B, Rho J, Hirsch JA, Oklu R. Bilateral inferior petrosal sinus sampling using desmopressin or corticotropic-releasing hormone: a single-center experience. J Neurointerv Surg. 2015;7 (9):690–3.

Parathyroid Venous Sampling

131

Sandra Abi Fadel

Abbreviations

PTH Parathyroid hormone

INTRODUCTION

Parathyroid venous sampling is a procedure during which venous blood draining the parathyroid glands is sampled for parathyroid hormone (PTH) to localize hypersecreting parathyroid adenomas. Noninvasive modalities suffer from high false-positive rates ranging from 5 to 25 % and may not exclude multifocal parathyroid disease. When noninvasive imaging techniques are inconclusive or fail to localize an adenoma, invasive localization with selective parathyroid angiography or, more commonly, parathyroid venous sampling may be useful. Parathyroid venous sampling has a reported sensitivity of 86 % and a positive predictive value of 93 %, when using a PTH gradient of >2 fold and super-selective sampling [1]. The success of invasive localization studies and interpretation of the results is highly dependent on the interventional radiologist's experience and understanding of the typical and unusual anatomic locations for enlarged parathyroid glands, and their blood supply and venous drainage.

COMMON INDICATIONS [1–3]

- Differentiation of diffuse hyperplasia from a single parathyroid adenoma
- Localization of the site of excess parathyroid hormone secretion before parathyroidectomy, when noninvasive imaging results are equivocal, non-concordant or show multiple parathyroid adenomas
- Identification of parathyroid adenoma in patients with familial hyperparathyroid syndromes
- Identification of parathyroid adenoma in patients with recurrent or persistent hyperparathyroidism after surgery

COMMON CONTRAINDICATIONS [4, 5]

- Severe allergy to iodinated contrast
- Bleeding diathesis
- Patients who are not surgical candidates for parathyroidectomy

S. Abi Fadel (✉)
Department of Diagnostic Radiology, American University of Beirut Medical Center, Riad El-Solh, Beirut 10017 2020, Lebanon
e-mail: sa183@aub.edu.lb

B. Taslakian et al. (eds.), *Procedural Dictations in Image-Guided Intervention*,
DOI 10.1007/978-3-319-40845-3_131

POSSIBLE COMPLICATIONS [5, 6]

- Access site complications, such as groin hematoma, pain, deep venous thrombosis
- Venous rupture
- Contrast-induced nephropathy and reaction
- Venous thrombosis

PREPROCEDURAL ASSESSMENT AND PLANNING

- History, indications, and physical examination *(Appendix 1* in Chap. 149*)*
- Evaluation of diagnostic imaging studies (CT, MRI, ultrasound, nuclear scan) to determine the location of the adenoma, and the possible variability in venous drainage
- Periprocedural management of coagulation status *(Appendices 2* in Chap. 150 *and 3* in Chap. 151*)*
- Antibiotic prophylaxis: Not routinely recommended [7]
- Imaging modality for guidance: Fluoroscopy, combined with ultrasound for venous access puncture
- Positioning: Supine

PROCEDURE NOTE

Procedure: Fluoroscopy-guided parathyroid venous sampling
Staff: [_]
Fellow: [_]
Resident: [_]
Clinical Information: Describe history and list indications
Allergies: None known/Allergic to [specify/type of allergy]
Anesthesia: Local anesthesia/conscious sedation
Medications: List any relevant medications used
Contrast Material: (_) mL of [type] contrast material was used for intravenous injection
Field: Sterile
Procedure classification: Clean
Position: Supine
Monitoring: Intravenous access line was secured and vital signs were continuously monitored by nursing staff/anesthesia team throughout the procedure
Total fluoroscopy time: (_) minutes
Cumulative radiation dose: (_) mGy

Description of Procedure:
The risks, benefits, alternatives, and the procedure itself were explained to the patient/patient's Power of Attorney/patient's legal guardian, and informed written consent was obtained. Time out was performed to confirm the correct patient and procedure.

The skin of both groins were shaved, prepped and draped in the usual sterile fashion. The right/left femoral vein was located by palpation/ultrasound and marked. The site of venous puncture was determined using combined information from palpation and ultrasound. Local anesthesia was administered. Femoral venous access was obtained using a (_)-gauge [type] needle and the Seldinger technique, double-/single- wall entry under direct ultrasound visualization/by palpation. Once good venous flow was detected, a (_)-inch [type] guidewire was advanced through the needle into the inferior vena cava under direct fluoroscopic visualization and a (_)-French vascular sheath was placed. A baseline peripheral blood sample was taken from the right/left common iliac vein at the beginning of the procedure.

Subsequently, a (_)-French [type] catheter was used to catheterize the relevant cervical and mediastinal veins. A small venous injection of contrast medium was performed to confirm location before sampling at each location. Subsequently samples were obtained from bilateral inferior thyroid veins/inferior thyroid trunk, right/left middle thyroid vein/superior thyroid vein/vertebral vein/thymic vein/internal mammary veins/innominate vein/internal jugular vein/superior vena cava/right hepatic vein [list any other veins sampled].

A repeat blood sample was taken from the right/left common iliac vein at the end of the procedure.

All samples were carefully labeled and transferred to the lab in iced container.

Following the procedure the right/left femoral venous sheath was removed and adequate hemostasis was achieved by compression for (_) minutes. The patient was transferred to the floor/recovery room following the procedure in a stable condition. Staff was present for the entire procedure.

Intra-Procedure Findings: List all relevant findings.

Immediate Complications: None encountered during or directly after the procedure. List complications if any.

Post-Procedure Plan [3, 5]:

- Follow-up laboratory results.
- Keep complete bed rest for 2 h and abstain from strenuous activities.
- Check vital signs every 15 min for 1 h, every 30 min for 2 h.
- Inform interventional radiology team if systolic blood pressure <95 mm Hg or heart rate >100 beats per minute.

Impression:

- Sampling of cervical/mediastinal veins for parathyroid adenoma localization, as described above.
- The patient tolerated the procedure well and left the interventional unit in stable condition.
- The patient was unstable during/unable to tolerate the procedure which was canceled/terminated prematurely.
- List any other relevant or important information/finding.

References

1. Lebastchi AH, Aruny JE, Donovan PI, Quinn CE, Callender GG, Carling T, et al. Real-time super selective venous sampling in remedial parathyroid surgery. J Am Coll Surg. 2015;220(6):994–1000.
2. Parathyroid venous sampling. In: Burke CT, Dixon RG, editors. High yield imaging: interventional. Philadelphia: Saunders; 2010:331–333.
3. Ogilvie CM, Brown PL, Matson M, Dacie J, Reznek RH, Britton K, et al. Selective parathyroid venous sampling in patients with complicated hyperparathyroidism. Eur J Endocrinol. 2006;155:813–21.
4. Kessel DO, Flood K. Principles of venous access. In: Mauro MA, Murphy KP, Thomson KR, Venbrux AC, Morgan RA, editors. Image guided interventions. Philadelphia: Saunders; 2014. p. 135–43.
5. Given M, Thomson KR. Parathyroid venous sampling. In: Mauro MA, Murphy KP, Thomson KR, Venbrux AC, Morgan RA, editors. Image guided interventions. Saunders; 2014. p. 1151–1154.
6. Witteveen JE, Kievit J, Erkel ARV, Morreau H, Romijn JA, Hamdy NAT. The role of selective venous sampling in the management of persistent hyperparathyroidism revisited. Eur J Endocrinol. 2010;163:945–52.
7. Venkatesan AM, Kundu S, Sacks D, Wallace MJ, Wojak JC, Rose SC, et al. Practice guidelines for adult antibiotic prophylaxis during vascular and interventional radiology procedures. J Vasc Interv Radiol. 2010;21(11):1611–30.

Renal Vein Renin Sampling

132

Sandra Abi Fadel

INTRODUCTION

Renin is a potent regulator of blood pressure via the renin-angiotensin-aldosterone system. It is produced in the juxtaglomerular apparatus of the kidney and in some tumors. Renal veins are sampled for blood renin levels to help determine whether a renal artery stenosis is a significant contributor to a patient's hypertension, and identify which kidney is responsible. In addition renal vein renin sampling helps determine whether patients with renal vascular hypertension may benefit from revascularization by percutaneous or surgical method.

COMMON INDICATIONS [1, 2]

- To determine which patients with renal vascular hypertension may benefit from revascularization
- To determine the physiologic significance of an anatomic renal stenosis that is of indeterminate grade
- To assess whether a renal tumor is secreting renin

COMMON CONTRAINDICATIONS [3, 4]

- Patients who are not candidates for revascularization by any means
- Patients with no access to the renal veins because of venous occlusion or anatomic abnormality
- Severe uncorrectable coagulopathy
- Severe allergy to contrast agent
- Patients on drug therapy that influences renin secretion *(withhold for 1–2 weeks before the procedure)*

POSSIBLE COMPLICATIONS [5]

- Access site-related complications, such as groin hematoma, pain, or infection
- Venous spasm causing failure of the procedure
- Damage to vena cava or branch veins
- Nephropathy induced by contrast material
- Allergic reaction to the contrast material

PREPROCEDURAL ASSESSMENT AND PLANNING

- History, indications, and physical examination *(Appendix 1* in Chap. 149*)*

S. Abi Fadel (✉)
Department of Diagnostic Radiology, American University of Beirut Medical Center, Riad El-Solh, Beirut 1107 2020, Lebanon
e-mail: sa183@aub.edu.lb

B. Taslakian et al. (eds.), *Procedural Dictations in Image-Guided Intervention*,
DOI 10.1007/978-3-319-40845-3_132

- Evaluation of diagnostic imaging studies to determine the location of the tumor/renal artery stenosis, its severity, and the relevant anatomy
- Periprocedural management of coagulation status *(Appendices 2* in Chap. 150 *and 3* in Chap. 151*)*
- Antibiotic prophylaxis: Not routinely recommended [6]
- Imaging modality for guidance: Fluoroscopy, combined with US for venous access puncture
- Positioning: Supine

PROCEDURE NOTE

Procedure: Fluoroscopy-guided percutaneous sampling of the right/left/both renal vein(s)
Staff: [_]
Fellow: [_]
Resident: [_]
Clinical Information: Describe history and list indications
Allergies: None known/Allergic to [specify/type of allergy]
Anesthesia: Local anesthesia/conscious sedation
Medications: List any relevant medications used
Contrast Material: (_) mL of [type] contrast material was used for intravenous injection.
Field: Sterile
Procedure classification: Clean
Position: Supine
Monitoring: Intravenous access line was secured and vital signs were continuously monitored by nursing staff/anesthesia team throughout the procedure.
Total fluoroscopy time: (_) minutes
Cumulative radiation dose: (_) mGy

Description of Procedure:
The risks, benefits, alternatives, and the procedure itself were explained to the patient/patient's Power of Attorney/patient's legal guardian, and informed written consent was obtained. Time out was performed to confirm the correct patient and procedure.

The skin of both groins were shaved, prepped, and draped in the usual sterile fashion. The right/left femoral vein was located by palpation/ultrasound and marked. The site of venous puncture was determined using combined information from palpation and ultrasound. Local anesthesia was administered. Femoral venous access was obtained using a (_)-gauge [type] needle and the Seldinger technique, double-/single- wall entry under direct ultrasound visualization/by palpation. Once good venous flow was detected, a (_)-inch [type] guidewire was advanced through the needle into the inferior vena cava under direct fluoroscopic visualization and a (_)-French vascular sheath was placed.

The catheter was advanced into the right main renal vein, and blood samples were drawn. The catheter was then positioned in the left renal vein, distal to the gonadal vein inflow and blood samples were drawn with simultaneous peripheral vein sampling from the femoral venous sheath.

Following the procedure the right/left femoral venous sheath was removed and adequate hemostasis was achieved by compression for (_) minutes. The patient was transferred to the floor/recovery room following the procedure in a stable condition. Staff was present for the entire procedure.
Intra-Procedure Findings: List all relevant findings.
Immediate Complications: None encountered during or directly after the procedure. List complications if any.

Post-Procedure Plan:
- Follow-up laboratory results.
- Keep complete bed rest for 2–4 h and abstain from strenuous activities.
- Check vital signs every 15 min for 1 h, every 30 min for 2 h.
- Inform interventional radiology team if systolic blood pressure <95 mm Hg or heart rate >100 beats per minute.

Impression:
- Sampling of the right/left/both renal vein(s), as described above.
- The patient tolerated the procedure well and left the interventional unit in stable condition.

- The patient was unstable during/unable to tolerate the procedure which was canceled/terminated prematurely.
- List any other relevant or important information/finding.

References

1. Renal vein renin sampling. In: Burke CT, Dixon RG, editors. High yield imaging: interventional. Philadelphia: Saunders;2010:327–327.
2. Balamuthusamy S, Kannan A, Thajudeen B, Ottley D, Jalandhara N. Mild renal artery stenosis can induce renovascular hypertension and is associated with elevated renal vein renin secretion. Semin Dial. 2015;28(3):93–298.
3. Trost DW, Sos TA. Renal vein renin sampling. In: Mauro MA, Murphy KP, Thomson KR, Venbrux AC, Morgan RA, editors. Image guided interventions. Philadelphia: Saunders; 2014. p. 1143–5.
4. Hasbak P, Jensen LT, Ibsen H. East danish study group on renovascular hypertension. Hypertension and renovascular disease: follow-up on 100 renal vein renin samplings. J Hum Hypertens. 2002;16(4):275–80.
5. Kaufman JA. Invasive vascular diagnosis. In: Mauro MA, Murphy KP, Thomson KR, Venbrux AC, Morgan RA, editors. Image guided interventions. Philadelphia: Saunders; 2014. p. 128–33.
6. Venkatesan AM, Kundu S, Sacks D, Wallace MJ, Wojak JC, Rose SC, et al. Practice guidelines for adult antibiotic prophylaxis during vascular and interventional radiology procedures. J Vasc Interv Radiol. 2010;21(11):1611–30.

Venous Sampling for Localizing Pancreatic Endocrine Tumors

133

Sandra Abi Fadel

Abbreviations

ASV	Sarterial stimulation and venous sampling
MEN	Multiple endocrine neoplasia

INTRODUCTION

Pancreatic endocrine tumors are subdivided into functional and nonfunctional based on whether the hormones they release produce a clinical syndrome or not. Pancreatic endocrine tumors other than gastrinoma and insulinoma are usually large at diagnosis and they can be diagnosed with noninvasive imaging. On the other hand, since hormonally active gastrinomas and insulinomas are highly symptomatic, they tend to be very small at time of diagnosis, thus warranting pancreatic venous sampling for localization. Pancreatic venous sampling is almost always associated with arteriography and arterial stimulation, giving rise to the term arterial stimulation and venous sampling (ASVS). ASVS consists of injecting a secretagogue into hepatic and pancreatic arteries and sampling for the appropriate hormone in the hepatic veins. The advantage of ASVS over anatomic imaging is that it is a functional study, therefore its sensitivity for detecting gastrinomas and insulinomas does not depend on tumor size.

S. Abi Fadel (✉)
Department of Diagnostic Radiology, American University of Beirut Medical Center, Riad El-Solh, Beirut 1107 2020, Lebanon
e-mail: sa183@aub.edu.lb

COMMON INDICATIONS [1, 2]

- Failure to identify gastrinoma with noninvasive imaging modalities
- Identify gastrinomas in surgical candidates with multiple pancreatic tumors, such as Zollinger–Ellison and multiple endocrine neoplasms (MEN) type 1 syndromes
- Failure to identify insulinoma with noninvasive imaging modalities
- Preoperative diagnosis of glucagonoma in patients with slightly elevated levels of basal glucagon values

COMMON CONTRAINDICATIONS [3, 4]

- Severe allergy to iodinated contrast
- Severe renal insufficiency
- Congestive heart failure
- Uncorrectable coagulopathy

B. Taslakian et al. (eds.), *Procedural Dictations in Image-Guided Intervention*,
DOI 10.1007/978-3-319-40845-3_133

- Uncontrolled hypertension
- Allergy to secretin *(in case of secretin ASVS)*
- Acute pancreatitis *(in case of secretin ASVS)*
- Intake of cardiac glycosides *(may cause severe arrhythmia in case of calcium ASVS)*
- Intake of diazoxide or other drugs that influence insulin secretion *(these should be discontinued prior to the procedure)*
- Infection at the puncture site

POSSIBLE COMPLICATIONS [4, 5]

- Access site complications (e.g., *hematoma, retroperitoneal hemorrhage, pseudoaneurysm, arteriovenous fistula, thrombosis)*
- Symptomatic hypoglycemia *(with calcium ASVS)*
- Pancreatitis *(with calcium ASVS)*
- Distal embolism
- Arterial thrombosis and dissection
- Venous injury

PREPROCEDURAL ASSESSMENT AND PLANNING

- History, indications and physical examination *(Appendix 1* in Chap. 149*)*
- Evaluation of diagnostic imaging studies (CT, MRI or scintigraphy) to determine the location of the tumors, if many are identified
- Periprocedural management of coagulation status *(Appendices 2* in Chap. 150 *and 3* in Chap. 151*)*
- Antibiotic prophylaxis: Not routinely recommended [6]
- Imaging modality for guidance: Fluoroscopy/Ultrasound (for femoral access)
- Positioning: Supine

PROCEDURE NOTE

Procedure: Fluoroscopy-guided percutaneous arteriography of the mid and proximal splenic/superior mesenteric/proper hepatic/proximal gastroduodenal arteries and calcium gluconate/secretin arterial stimulation with sampling of the right/left hepatic vein
Staff: [_]
Fellow: [_]
Resident: [_]
Clinical Information: Describe history and list indications
Allergies: None known/Allergic to [specify/type of allergy]
Anesthesia: Local anesthesia/conscious sedation
Medications: List any relevant medications used
Contrast Used: (_) mL of [type] contrast material was used for intra-arterial and intravenous injection
Field: Sterile
Procedure classification: Clean
Position: Supine
Monitoring: Intravenous access line was secured and vital signs were continuously monitored by nursing staff/anesthesia team throughout the procedure
Total fluoroscopy time: (_) minutes
Cumulative radiation dose: (_) mGy

Description of Procedure:
The risks, benefits, alternatives, and the procedure itself were explained to the patient/patient's Power of Attorney/patient's legal guardian, and informed written consent was obtained. Time out was performed to confirm the correct patient and procedure.

The skin of both groins were shaved, prepped and draped in the usual sterile fashion. The right/left femoral artery as well as the inguinal ligament were located by palpation/ultrasound and marked. The site of arterial puncture was determined using combined information from palpation, ultrasound, and fluoroscopy over the middle of the medial third of the femoral head. Local anesthesia was administered. Femoral artery access was obtained using a (_)-gauge [type] needle and the Seldinger technique, double-/single- wall entry under direct ultrasound visualization/by palpation. Once good pulsatile arterial flow was detected, a (_)-inch [type] guidewire was advanced through the needle into the aorta under direct fluoroscopic visualization and a (_)-French vascular sheath was placed.

The right/left femoral vein was also located by palpation/ultrasound and marked. The site of venous puncture was determined using combined information from palpation and ultrasound. Local anesthesia was administered. Femoral venous access was obtained using a (_)-gauge [type] needle and the Seldinger technique, double-/single- wall entry under direct ultrasound visualization/by palpation. Once good venous flow was detected, a (_)-inch [type] guidewire was advanced through the needle into the inferior vena cava under direct fluoroscopic visualization and a (_)-French vascular sheath was placed.

The right/left/right and left hepatic veins were catheterized using a (_)-French, (_) cm-long [type] catheter and 4 ml of blood was drawn from the right/left/right and left hepatic vein(s) and sent for baseline gastrin/insulin levels.

Subsequently, a (_)-French [type] catheter was advanced into the abdominal aorta over a (0.035)-in. [hydrophilic/type] guidewire under direct fluoroscopic visualization and the celiac artery was selectively catheterized. Selective celiac angiography was performed, followed by selective splenic/common hepatic/gastroduodenal/superior mesenteric arteriograms.

Tumor blush was visualized in the head and neck/body and tail of the pancreas/No tumor blush was visualized. The corresponding artery, the splenic/superior pancreaticoduodenal/inferior pancreaticoduodenal arteries, were selected for secretagogue test.

(_) international units of secretin/calcium gluconate diluted in (_) ml of normal saline were injected into the [name the artery].

Then through the venous catheters, samples from the right/left/right and left hepatic vein(s) were obtained at 20, 40, and 60s, and sent immediately to the laboratory.

Following the procedure the right/left femoral artery and venous sheaths were removed and adequate hemostasis was achieved by compression for (_) minutes/using [type] vascular closure device. The femoral pulses were checked following the procedure and were [comparable to the preprocedure pulses/specify if otherwise needed].

The patient was transferred to the floor/recovery room for close monitoring following the procedure in a stable condition. Staff was present for the entire procedure.

Intra-Procedure Findings: *List all relevant findings.*

Immediate Complications: None encountered during or directly after the procedure. *List complications if any.*

Post-Procedure Plan [5]:

- Follow-up laboratory results.
- Keep patient complete bed rest with the right/left leg extended for (6) h *[adjust depending on the puncture site]*.
- Check the right/left groin/[specify the puncture site if different] for any bleeding or hematoma formation every 15 min for 1 h, then every 30 min for 1 h, then every hour for 4 h; inform interventional radiology team if any signs of bleeding are observed *[adjust depending on the puncture site]*.
- Check and document lower extremity pulses every 30 min for 2 h then every 1 h for 4 h *[adjust depending on the puncture site]*.
- Monitor vital signs every 15 min for 1 h, then every 30 min for 4 h; notify interventional radiology team if systolic blood pressure <95 mmHg, or heart rate >110 beats/minute.
- Resume diet and previous orders as needed and if otherwise not contraindicated.
- Continue adequate intravenous hydration and monitor fluid (intake–output) status.
- Monitor blood dextrose level.

Impression:

- Arteriography and calcium/secretin ASVS, as described above
- The patient tolerated the procedure well and left the interventional unit in stable condition.
- The patient was unstable during/unable to tolerate the procedure which was canceled/terminated prematurely.
- List any other relevant or important information/finding.

References

1. Pancreatic sampling for neuroendocrine tumors. In: Burke CT, Dixon RG, editors. High Yield Imaging: Interventional. Philadelphia: Saunders; 2010:334–337.
2. Okabayashi T, Shima Y, Sumiyoshi T, Kozuki A, Ito S, Ogawa Y, et al. Diagnosis and management of insulinoma. World J Gastroenterol. 2013;19(6):829–37.
3. Wiesli P, Brändle M, Schmid C, Krähenbühl L, Furrer J, Keller U, et al. Selective arterial calcium stimulation and hepatic venous sampling in the evaluation of hyperinsulinemic hypoglycemia: potential and limitations. J Vasc Interv Radiol. 2004;15 (11):1251–6.
4. Kam AW, Wood BJ, Chang R. Arteriography and arterial stimulation with venous sampling for localizing pancreatic endocrine tumors. In: Mauro MA, Murphy KP, Thomson KR, Venbrux AC, Morgan RA, editors. Image guided interventions. Philadelphia: Saunders; 2014. p. 816–21.
5. Chun AK. Principles of arterial access. In: Mauro MA, Murphy KP, Thomson KR, Venbrux AC, Morgan RA, editors. Image guided interventions. Philadelphia: Saunders; 2014. p. 128–33.
6. Venkatesan AM, Kundu S, Sacks D, Wallace MJ, Wojak JC, Rose SC, et al. Practice guidelines for adult antibiotic prophylaxis during vascular and interventional radiology procedures. J Vasc Interv Radiol. 2010;21(11):1611–30.

Part XXII

Vascular Interventional Procedures: Miscellaneous

Introduction by Aghiad Al-Kutoubi, Section Reviewer

Since Dr. Charles Dotter, the father of interventional radiology, performed the first angioplasty on January 16, 1964, interventional radiologists pioneered with the invention of angioplasty and catheter-delivered stents. With recent and ongoing advances in imaging techniques and angiographic catheters, stents and guidewires, minimally invasive vascular procedures continue to evolve and play a pivotal role in modern medicine.

This section provides a comprehensive list of procedural reports that covers a vast majority of vascular procedures not included in the previous system-based sections, with up-to-date explanatory notes, synopsis of the indications and contraindications, and potential complications in an organized and practical format.

Section Chapters

134 Dialysis Access Interventions (Arteriovenous Fistulas and Grafts)

Divya Sridhar, David H. Hoffman, Nicole A. Lamparello and Mehrzad Zarghouni

Abbreviations

AVF: Arteriovenous fistula
AVG: Arteriovenous graft
PTA: Percutaneous transluminal angioplasty
VA: Vascular access

INTRODUCTION

The prevalence of chronic kidney disease and the need for hemodialysis are increasing in the United States [1, 2]. A careful program of vascular access (VA) surveillance and monitoring is essential for maintaining a functional arteriovenous fistula (AVF) or graft (AVG) [1, 3, 4] and maximizing its usable life. AVF and AVG dysfunction most commonly occurs due to thrombosis, stenosis along the venous outflow path, and/or stenosis at the arterial anastomosis. Thrombosis related to an underlying stenotic lesion is the most common cause of VA failure [1]. Stenosis is defined as greater than 50 % reduction in luminal diameter, and most frequently results from neointimal hyperplasia. Stenosis is more common in grafts than in fistulas, and more frequently affects the venous outflow than the arterial anastomosis. Hemodynamic and clinical findings of VA compromise, detailed below, include loss of palpable thrill or pulse, increased venous pressures at dialysis, arm swelling, and prolonged bleeding after needle removal. Non-maturation of a fistula, graft pseudoaneurysm formation, and development of steal syndrome are additional indications for VA interventions [1, 5, 6].

Endovascular approaches are typically the preferred first-line intervention for VA

D. Sridhar (✉) · M. Zarghouni
Department of Radiology, Division of Vascular and Interventional Radiology, New York University Langone Medical Center, 660 1st Ave, 7th Floor, Suite. 742, 10016 New York, NY, USA
e-mail: divya.sridhar@nyumc.org

M. Zarghouni
e-mail: mzarghouni@gmail.com

D.H. Hoffman · N.A. Lamparello
Department of Radiology, New York University Langone Medical Center, 660 1st Ave, 10016 New York, NY, USA
e-mail: david.hoffman@nyumc.org

N.A. Lamparello
e-mail: Nicole.Lamparello@nyumc.org

B. Taslakian et al. (eds.), *Procedural Dictations in Image-Guided Intervention*,
DOI 10.1007/978-3-319-40845-3_134

dysfunction. Compared to surgical intervention, endovascular procedures demonstrate decreased morbidity, increased patient comfort, and comparable results in many situations [5]. Initial sonographic evaluation and angiography are performed to define the graft or fistula anatomy and identify the cause of dysfunction. If a thrombus is present, pharmacomechanical thrombolysis is commonly performed, using thrombolytic agents. If a stenosis is identified in the outflow vein, central vein, or arterial anastomosis, percutaneous transluminal angioplasty (PTA) is typically performed, with the goal of restoring luminal diameter to less than 30 % residual stenosis [7, 8]. With the increasing availability of high-pressure and cutting balloons, PTA alone is often an effective treatment. In selected cases, stent placement may be indicated; although somewhat controversial, commonly accepted indications for stent insertion include central vein lesions, recurrent stenosis/failed angioplasty, venous rupture, and pseudoaneurysm, as well as contraindication to surgical revision [1, 5, 9–11].

COMMON INDICATIONS [1, 5]

- Thrombosis *(no palpable pulse or thrill)*
- Increased venous pressure or prolonged bleed after access needle removal
- Decreased palpable thrill
- AVF failure to mature by 3 months *(draining vein <6 mm)*
- Flow during dialysis <600 mL/min OR <1000 mL/min with >25 % drop in 12 months
- Stenosis on angiography with mean pressure gradient >10 mmHg
- Decreased clearance
- Graft pseudoaneurysm or primary fistula aneurysm
- Swelling
- Recirculation
- Arterial steal phenomenon with distal ischemia

COMMON CONTRAINDICATIONS [1, 5, 6]

- Infection of access site *(ABSOLUTE contraindication; typically with grafts)*
- Systemic infection
- Cardiopulmonary shunt: right to left, i.e., patent foramen ovale *(ABSOLUTE contraindication)*
- Uncorrectable coagulopathy
- Immature graft <30 days
- Contrast allergy
- Distal ischemia *(contraindication to increasing flow through AVF/AVG; may be an indication to occlude or limit flow)*
- Hemodynamically unstable patient *(especially with low baseline cardiac output; rapid arteriovenous shunting following angioplasty can result in heart failure)*

POSSIBLE COMPLICATIONS [1, 5, 12]

- Hematoma *(most common)*
- Infection
- Vein rupture or pseudoaneurysm formation
- Arterial dissection or rupture
- Embolic phenomena *(distal arterial, pulmonary embolism, rarely paradoxical emboli)*

PREPROCEDURAL ASSESSMENT AND PLANNING

- History, indications, and physical examination *(Appendix 1* in Chap. 149*)*
- Evaluation of diagnostic imaging studies (ultrasound or CT angiography): ultrasound of the upper extremity may be used before and during the procedure to assess anatomy, patency, and flow through AVF/AVG. CT angiography from the aortic arch and upper extremity may be helpful in cases of suspected compromised arterial inflow (due to atherosclerosis, dissection, or other etiology).

- Periprocedural management of coagulation status *(Appendices 2* in Chap. 150 *and 3* in Chap. 151*)*
- Antibiotic prophylaxis: Recommended if any implanted devices are placed (i.e., stents or coils), not recommended for PTA *(Appendices 4* in Chap. 152 *and 5* in Chap. 153*)*
- Imaging modality for guidance: Fluoroscopy, supplemented by ultrasound
- Positioning: Supine with upper extremity extended and abducted on armboard

PROCEDURE NOTE

Procedure: Right/Left upper extremity dialysis access fistulogram/graft angiogram with angioplasty [and/or thrombectomy and/or stent placement]
Staff: [_]
Fellow: [_]
Resident: [_]
Clinical Information: Describe history and list indications; e.g. end-stage renal disease requiring hemodialysis; [then list specific indication, i.e., high venous pressures, thrombosed graft, etc.]
Allergies: None known/Allergic to [specify/type of allergy]
Medications: List any relevant medications used
Contrast Used: (_) mL of [type] contrast media was used for intravascular injection
Field: Sterile
Procedure classification: Clean
Position: Supine
Monitoring: Intravenous access line was secured and vital signs were continuously monitored by nursing staff/anesthesia team throughout the procedure
Total fluoroscopy time: (_) minutes
Cumulative radiation dose: (_) mGy

Description of Procedure:
The risks, benefits, alternatives, and procedure itself were explained to the patient/patient's Power of Attorney/patient's legal guardian, and informed written consent was obtained. Time out was performed to confirm the correct patient, procedure and site. The site of the procedure was identified and marked.
Initial antegrade approach (unless findings suggest inflow lesion): The skin was prepped and draped in the usual sterile fashion. The outflow vein of the right/left arteriovenous fistula/graft was located by palpation/ultrasound and marked a few centimeters away from the arterial anastomosis in the direction of the venous outflow. The site of venous puncture was determined using combined information from palpation and ultrasound. Local anesthesia was administered. AV fistula/graft access was obtained using a (21)-gauge [type] needle and the Seldinger technique, with single-wall entry under direct ultrasound visualization/by palpation. Once needle access was achieved, a (0.018)-in. [type] guidewire was advanced through the needle, into the venous outflow under direct fluoroscopic visualization and a (6/7)-French (5)-cm vascular sheath was placed.
For thrombosed AVF/AVG only: (2–6) mg of tPA mixed with (2000–4000) units heparin were instilled throughout the thrombus via the sheath (and a 5-Fr diagnostic catheter). A (0.035) glidewire and (5)-French diagnostic catheter were gently advanced through the thrombus to the central veins, and venography was performed in the outflow veins and central veins above the thrombus. After initial central venography, mechanical thrombectomy was performed throughout the graft/fistula using a thrombectomy device/balloon sweeps/manual aspiration. Contrast study of the graft/fistula was performed after initial thrombectomy to identify stenoses and residual thrombus.
For patent AVF/AVG only: Venography was performed via the access sheath, initially with hand injection of (5) mL intravenous contrast. Digital subtraction venography was performed with (10–20) mL intravenous contrast to evaluate the graft/fistula, entire outflow tract, and central veins. A 0.035 glidewire and 5-Fr diagnostic catheter were advanced to the subclavian vein for central venography.

For hemodynamically significant stenosis: A guidewire was gently navigated across the stenosis. An (8) mm × (4) cm balloon (ideal balloon diameter >20–30 % of diameter of normal vessel adjacent to stenosis; ideal balloon length extends >5 mm into normal vessel on both sides of stenosis) was advanced over the guidewire and used to perform angioplasty across the stenosis in the (venous outflow tract/venous anastomosis/subclavian vein/etc.) with prolonged balloon inflation. Post-angioplasty venogram demonstrated improvement in stenosis/minimal improvement in stenosis/no change in stenosis. Due to minimal improvement in stenosis with initial angioplasty, repeat angioplasty was performed with a high-pressure/cutting/larger diameter balloon.

The venous outflow was then occluded using a tourniquet/internal balloon occlusion/manual pressure. Reflux/retrograde angiography was performed with brisk hand injection of (10) mL intravenous contrast and demonstrated patency/stenosis/occlusion of the arterial anastomosis. Digital subtraction angiography was performed with (10) mL intravenous contrast to confirm initial findings at the arterial anastomosis.

If intervention at arterial anastomosis is indicated due to stenosis or for any thrombosed AVF/AVG: Retrograde access into the AVF/AVG was achieved, a few centimeters upstream from the existing antegrade access and directed toward the arterial anastomosis. AV fistula/graft access was obtained using a (21)-gauge [type] needle and the Seldinger technique, with single-wall entry under direct ultrasound visualization/by palpation. Once needle access was achieved, a (0.018)-in. [type] guidewire was advanced through the needle, into the venous outflow under direct fluoroscopic visualization and a (5/6)-French (5)-cm vascular sheath was placed. The arterial anastomosis and inflow artery were cannulated gently using a (0.018/0.035) wire. A (2/3) mm angioplasty [OR 1-cm Fogarty] balloon was advanced over the wire across the arterial anastomosis. Angioplasty/balloon sweeps were gently performed across the arterial anastomosis. A catheter was gently advanced over the wire into the inflow artery, and repeat contrast study was performed post-treatment. Completion diagnostic angiography was performed from the arterial anastomosis to the central veins.

For angioplasty-induced vessel injury with extravasation: The angioplasty balloon was centered over the site of vessel injury and inflated for (3–5) min to tamponade the site. After 5 min, repeat angiography demonstrated no extravasation/persistent extravasation. A (size) [type] covered stent was advanced and deployed across the site of vessel injury due to persistent extravasation despite balloon tamponade.

All devices were then removed, and hemostasis was obtained at each access site using manual compression and placement of a suture. There was a/was no palpable thrill in the fistula after completion of the procedure.

The patient was transferred to the floor/recovery room following the procedure in a stable condition. Staff was present for the entire procedure.

Intra-Procedure Findings: List all relevant findings.

Immediate Complications: None encountered during or directly after the procedure. List complications if any.

Post-Procedure Plan

- Inform interventional radiology team if any bleeding is noted at vascular access site, distal extremity (hand or finger) changes in sensation or color, or extremity swelling or pain.
- Confirm patient is aware of next scheduled dialysis session.
- Remove any permanent sutures at next dialysis session (1–2 days).

Impression:

- Right/left upper extremity dialysis graft/fistula diagnostic angiography demonstrating stenosis/occlusion/thrombosis, successfully treated with thrombectomy/angioplasty/stent placement.

- The patient tolerated the procedure well and left the interventional unit in stable condition.
- The patient was unable to tolerate the procedure well which was canceled/terminated prematurely.
- List any other relevant or important information/finding.

References

1. Kidney Disease: Improving Global Outcomes (KDIGO) CKD Work Group. KDIGO 2012 Clinical Practice Guideline for the Evaluation and Management of Chronic Kidney Disease. Kidney inter., Suppl. 2013;3:1–150.
2. Whittier WL. Surveillance of hemodialysis vascular access. Semin Intervent Radiol. 2009;26(2):130–8.
3. Allon M, Robbin ML. Hemodialysis vascular access monitoring: current concepts. Hemodial Int. 2009;13 (2):153–62.
4. Gelbfish GA. Clinical surveillance and monitoring of arteriovenous access for hemodialysis. Tech Vasc Interv Radiol. 2008;11(3):156–66.
5. ACR-SIR practice guideline for endovascular management of the thrombosed or dysfunctional dialysis access. Reston, VA: Digest of Council Actions; 2006; amended 2014.
6. Mauro MA, Murphy KPJ, Thomson KR, Venbrux AC, Zollikofer CL, editors. Image-guided interventions. Philadelphia: Saunders Elsevier; 2008.
7. Gray RJ, Sacks D, Martin LG, Trerotola SO. Reporting standards for percutaneous interventions in dialysis access. J Vasc Interv Radiol. 2003;14(9 Pt 2): S433–42.
8. Saleh HM, Gabr AK, Tawfik MM, Abouellail H. Prospective, randomized study of cutting balloon angioplasty versus conventional balloon angioplasty for the treatment of hemodialysis access stenosis. J Vasc Surg. 2014;60(3):735–40.
9. Lorenz JM. Use of stents for maintenance of hemodialysis access. Semin Intervent Radiol. 2004;21(2):135–40.
10. Tordoir JH, Bode AS, Peppelenbosch N, van der Sande FM, de Haan MW. Surgical or endovascular repair of thromboses dialysis access: is there any evidence? J Vasc Surg. 2009;50(4):953–6.
11. Bent CL, Sahni VA, Matson MB. The radiological management if the thromboses arteriovenous dialysis fistula. Clin Radiol. 2011;66(1):1–12.
12. Sofocleous CT, Schur I, Koh E, Hinrichs C, Cooper SG, Welber A, et al. Percutaneous treatment of complications occurring during hemodialysis graft recanalization. Eur J Radiol. 2003;47(3):237–46.

Dialysis Fistulogram

135

Divya Sridhar, Nicole A. Lamparello, David H. Hoffman and Mehrzad Zarghouni

Abbreviations

AVG	Arteriovenous graft
AVF	Arteriovenous fistula
VA	Vascular access
CKD	Chronic kidney disease
GFR	Glomerular filtration rate

INTRODUCTION

Chronic kidney disease (CKD) is a serious condition associated with high risk for cardiovascular complications, infection, malignancy, and mortality. Its incidence and prevalence are increasing in the United States. KDIGO guidelines recommend initiation of dialysis in patients based upon the estimated glomerular filtration rate (GFR) (with <15 mL/min defined as stage 5 CKD), the rate of GFR decline, and the presence of signs and symptoms of end-stage renal disease [1, 2].

Approximately 300,000 patients in the United States rely on hemodialysis via vascular access (VA) to manage stage 5 CKD [3]. There are three major types of VA for hemodialysis: primary arteriovenous fistulas (AVFs), synthetic arteriovenous grafts (AVGs), and double-lumen cuffed tunneled catheters. VA function and patency are essential for patients on dialysis, and many studies have correlated inadequate completion of regular hemodialysis with increased patient morbidity and mortality [3, 4]. AVF is considered the first-line VA option due to its longevity, decreased risk of thrombosis and infection, and the lower morbidity and mortality associated with its use [5–7]; however, AVFs typically require 1–3 months to mature prior to use. By contrast, a major benefit of AVG creation is its

D. Sridhar (✉) · M. Zarghouni
Department of Radiology, Division of Vascular and Interventional Radiology, New York University Langone Medical Center, 660 1st Ave, 7th Floor, Suite. 742, 10016 New York, NY, USA
e-mail: divya.sridhar@nyumc.org

M. Zarghouni
e-mail: mzarghouni@gmail.com

N.A. Lamparello · D.H. Hoffman
Department of Radiology, New York University Langone Medical Center, 660 1st Ave, 10016 New York, NY, USA
e-mail: nicole.lamparello@nyumc.org

D.H. Hoffman
e-mail: david.hoffman@nyumc.org

B. Taslakian et al. (eds.), *Procedural Dictations in Image-Guided Intervention*,
DOI 10.1007/978-3-319-40845-3_135

near-immediate availability for access and use, in general days to weeks [2, 5].

Dialysis access angiography (fistulogram/ "graftogram") are performed to evaluate the patency and function of both AVFs and AVGs. Angiograms may be performed either as prospective surveillance or as diagnostic testing prompted by an abnormality (abnormal ultrasound, clinical exam, or clinical/physiologic symptoms) [2, 3, 7]. Abnormalities seen on dialysis access angiography may be amenable to endovascular treatment (see Chap. 134).

COMMON INDICATIONS [1–9]

- Increased venous pressure or prolonged bleed after access needle removal
- Decreased palpable thrill
- AVF failure to mature by 3 months *(draining vein < 6 mm)*
- Flow during dialysis <600 mL/min OR <1000 mL/min with >25 % drop in 12 months
- Stenosis on angiography with mean pressure gradient >10 mm Hg
- Decreased clearance
- Thrombosis *(no palpable pulse or thrill)*
- Graft pseudoaneurysm or primary fistula aneurysm
- Swelling
- Recirculation
- Arterial steal phenomenon with distal ischemia

COMMON CONTRAINDICATIONS [9, 10]

- Infection of access site *(absolute contraindication; typically with grafts)*
- Systemic infection
- Cardiopulmonary shunt: right to left, i.e., patent foramen ovale *(absolute contraindication)*
- Uncorrectable coagulopathy
- Immature graft <30 days
- Contrast allergy

POSSIBLE COMPLICATIONS [10–13]

- Hematoma
- Infection
- Venous or arterial injury *(rare)*
- Embolic phenomena *(rare)*

PREPROCEDURAL ASSESSMENT AND PLANNING

- History, indications, and physical examination *(Appendix 1* in Chap. 149*)*
- Evaluation of diagnostic imaging studies (ultrasound or CT angiography): ultrasound of the upper extremity may be used before and during procedure to assess anatomy, patency, and flow through AVF/AVG. CT angiography from the aortic arch and upper extremity may be helpful in cases of suspected compromised arterial inflow (due to atherosclerosis, dissection, or other etiology).
- Periprocedural management of coagulation status *(Appendices 2* in Chap. 150 *and 3* in Chap. 151*)*
- Antibiotic prophylaxis: Not routinely recommended *(Appendices 4* in Chap. 152 *and 5* in Chap. 153*)*
- Imaging modality for guidance: Fluoroscopy, supplemented by ultrasound
- Positioning: Supine with upper extremity extended and abducted on armboard

PROCEDURE NOTE

Procedure: Right/Left upper extremity dialysis access fistulogram/graft angiogram
Staff: [_]
Fellow: [_]
Resident: [_]
Clinical Information: Describe history and list indications; e.g. end-stage renal disease requiring hemodialysis; [then list specific indication, i.e. high venous pressures, thrombosed graft, etc.]
Allergies: None known/Allergic to [specify/type of allergy]

Anesthesia: Local anesthesia/rarely conscious sedation
Medications: List any relevant medications used (anesthesia, sedation)
Contrast Used: (_) mL of [type] contrast media was used for intravascular injection
Field: Sterile
Procedure classification: Clean
Position: Supine
Monitoring: Intravenous access line was secured and vital signs were continuously monitored by nursing staff/anesthesia team throughout the procedure
Total fluoroscopy time: (_) minutes
Cumulative radiation dose: (_) mGy

Description of Procedure:
The risks, benefits, alternatives and procedure itself were explained to the patient/patient's Power of Attorney/patient's legal guardian, and informed written consent was obtained. Time out was performed to confirm the correct patient, procedure and site. The site of the procedure was identified and marked.
Initial antegrade approach (unless pre-procedure findings strongly suggest isolated inflow lesion):
The skin was prepped and draped in the usual sterile fashion. The outflow vein of the right/left arteriovenous fistula/graft was located by palpation/ultrasound and marked a few centimeters away from the arterial anastomosis in the direction of the venous outflow. The site of venous puncture was determined using combined information from palpation and ultrasound. Local anesthesia was administered. AV fistula/graft access was obtained using a (21)-gauge [type] needle and the Seldinger technique, with single-wall entry under direct ultrasound visualization/by palpation. Once needle access was achieved, a (0.018)-inch [type] guidewire was advanced through the needle, into the venous outflow under direct fluoroscopic visualization and a (4/5)-French [micropuncture introducer or vascular access sheath] was placed. Venography was performed via the access sheath, initially with hand injection of (5) mL intravenous contrast. Digital subtraction venography was performed with (10–20) mL intravenous contrast to evaluate the graft/fistula, entire outflow tract, and central veins. A (0.035) glidewire and (5)-French diagnostic catheter were advanced to the subclavian vein for central venography.

The venous outflow was then occluded using a tourniquet/internal balloon occlusion/manual pressure. Reflux/retrograde angiography was performed with brisk hand injection of (10) mL intravenous contrast and demonstrated patency/stenosis/occlusion of the arterial anastomosis. Digital subtraction angiography was performed with (10) mL intravenous contrast to confirm initial findings at the arterial anastomosis.
For thrombosed AVF/AVG only: Do NOT perform contrast study via sheath before thrombectomy; doing so may result in inadvertent displacement of thrombus into the inflow artery with compromise of blood flow to the hand and/or pulmonary embolism. A 0.035 glidewire and 5-Fr diagnostic catheter may be gently advanced through the thrombus to the central veins to perform venography of the outflow veins and central veins above the thrombus prior to thrombectomy. Contrast study of the (graft/fistula) should be performed only after initial thrombectomy.
Retrograde cannulation: Most stenoses occur in the outflow veins, and reflux angiography combined with sonographic evaluation often provides adequate assessment of the arterial anastomosis; however, in specific cases of elevated concern for arterial inflow stenosis and/or arterial steal phenomenon, direct imaging of the inflow via retrograde cannulation of the AVF/AVG may be warranted [8].
If retrograde cannulation for imaging of the arterial anastomosis is indicated: Retrograde access into the AVF/AVG was achieved, a few centimeters upstream from the existing antegrade access and directed toward the arterial anastomosis. AV fistula/graft access was obtained using a (21)-gauge [type] needle and the Seldinger technique, with single-wall entry under direct ultrasound visualization/by palpation. Once needle access was achieved, a (0.018)-inch [type] guidewire was advanced through the needle, into the venous

outflow under direct fluoroscopic visualization and a (4/5)-French micropuncture introducer or vascular access sheath was placed. The arterial anastomosis and inflow artery were cannulated gently using a (0.018/0.035)-inch wire. A catheter was gently advanced over the wire into the inflow artery, and contrast study was performed.

An ALTERNATIVE approach to evaluate arterial inflow is direct cannulation of the artery proximal to the AVF/AVG: Antegrade access into the brachial/radial artery was achieved a few centimeters upstream from the arterial anastomosis using a (21)-gauge needle and the Seldinger technique with single-wall entry under direct ultrasound visualization/by palpation. Once needle access was achieved, a (0.018)-inch [type] guidewire was advanced through the needle, into the venous outflow under direct fluoroscopic visualization and a (3)-French inner dilator from a micropuncture introducer was placed. Contrast study was performed.

All devices were then removed, and hemostasis was obtained at each access site using manual compression. There was a/was no palpable thrill in the fistula after completion of the procedure.

The patient was transferred to the floor/recovery room/discharged home following the procedure in a stable condition. Staff was present for the entire procedure.

Intra-Procedure Findings: List all relevant findings.

Immediate Complications: None encountered during or directly after the procedure. List complications if any.

Post-Procedure Plan

- Inform interventional radiology team if significant oozing or bleeding at vascular access site, distal extremity numbness, extremity swelling, or pain.
- Confirm patient is aware of next scheduled dialysis session.

Impression:

- Right/left upper extremity dialysis graft/fistula diagnostic angiography demonstrating patency/stenosis/occlusion/thrombosis of the AVF/AVG.
- The patient tolerated the procedure well and left the interventional unit in stable condition.
- The patient was unable to tolerate the procedure which was canceled/terminated prematurely.
- List any other relevant or important information/finding.

References

1. Kidney Disease: Improving Global Outcomes (KDIGO) CKD Work Group. KDIGO 2012 Clinical Practice Guideline for the Evaluation and Management of Chronic Kidney Disease. Kidney Inter Suppl. 2013;3:1–150.
2. Whittier WL. Surveillance of Hemodialysis Vascular Access. Semin Intervent Radiol. 2009;26(2):130–8.
3. National Kidney Foundation. KDOQI Clinical Practice Guidelines and Clinical Practice Recommendations for 2006 Updates: Hemodialysis Adequacy, Peritoneal Dialysis Adequacy and Vascular Access. Am J Kidney Dis. 2006;48(suppl 1):S1–S322.
4. Hakim RM, Breyer J, Ismail N, Schulman G. Effects of dose of dialysis on morbidity and mortality. Am J Kidney Dis. 1994;23(5):661–9.
5. Santoro D, Benedetto F, Mondello P, Pipitò N, Barillà D, Spinelli F, et al. Vascular access for hemodialysis: Current perspectives. Int J Nephrol Renovasc Dis. 2014;8(7):281–94.
6. Dhingra RK, Young EW, Hulbert-Shearon TE, Leavey SF, Port FK. Type of vascular access and mortality in U.S. hemodialysis patients. Kidney Int. 2001;60(4):1443–51.
7. Bent CL, Sahni VA, Matson MB. The radiological management if the thromboses arteriovenous dialysis fistula. Clin Radiol. 2011;66(1):1–12.
8. Duijm LE, Overbosch EH, Liem YS, Planken RN, Tordoir JH, Cuypers PW, et al. Retrograde catheterization of haemodialysis fistulae and grafts: angiographic depiction of the entire vascular access tree and stenosis treatment. Nephrol Dial Transplant. 2009;24(2):539–47.

9. Zaleski G. Declotting, maintenance, and avoiding procedural complications of native arteriovenous fistulae. Semin Intervent Radiol. 2004;21(2):83–93.
10. Mauro MA, Murphy KPJ, Thomson KR, Venbrux AC, Zollikofer CL, editors. Image-guided interventions. Philadelphia: Saunders Elsevier; 2008.
11. Wu S, Ahmad I, Qayyum S, Wicky S, Kalva SP. Paradoxical embolism after declotting of hemodialysis fistulae/grafts in patients with patent foramen ovale. Clin J Am Soc Nephrol. 2011;6(6):1333–6.
12. Nikolic B. Hemodialysis fistula interventions: diagnostic and treatment challenges and technical considerations. Tech Vasc Interv Radiol. 2008;11(3):167–74.
13. Nassar GM. Endovascular management of the "failing to mature" arteriovenous fistula. Tech Vasc Interv Radiol. 2008;11(3):175–80.

Endovenous Thermal Ablation for Lower Extremity Venous Insufficiency

136

Abbas Chamsuddin

Abbreviations

CVD	Chronic venous disorder
GSV	Great saphenous vein
EVTA	Endovenous thermal ablation
RF	Radiofrequency

INTRODUCTION

Lower-extremity chronic venous disorder (CVD) is a common heterogeneous medical condition that decreases a patient's quality of life. The spectrum of CVD ranges from visually apparent abnormalities including varicose veins and spider telangiectasias with or without associated symptoms to severe edema, skin ulceration, and subsequent major disability. Venous hypertension caused by incompetent valves in the superficial veins is by far the most common cause of this condition. Traditionally treated with high ligation and stripping, minimally invasive procedures using endovenous thermal ablation techniques, such as endovenous laser ablation, have evolved. Endovenous thermal ablation (EVTA) of the saphenous veins has been used by physicians since the late 1990s as an alternative to surgical removal. While it was initially introduced as a treatment for great saphenous vein (GSV) insufficiency, EVTA is now being applied to many other venous segments in the lower extremities. The GSV, an important component of the superficial venous system, begins on the dorsum of the foot and ascends along the medial aspect of the leg to ultimately drain into the femoral vein near the groin crease. This vein resides in a space deep to the superficial and superficial to the deep fascia. It is the longest vein in the human body and the most commonly ablated. The use of detailed imaging and advances in the understanding of the anatomy are important for performing the endovenous ablation procedure successfully. EVTA utilizes primarily two techniques, laser and radiofrequency (RF) ablation, to achieve irreversible closure and ultimately fibrosis. Both procedures are associated with high success and low complication rates. The procedures are generally performed on an ambulatory basis with local anesthetic and typically require no sedation. The patients are fully ambulatory following treatment, and the

A. Chamsuddin (✉)
Interventional Radiology, Balamand University
Saint George University Medical Center, Beirut, Lebanon
e-mail: achamsuddin@yahoo.com

B. Taslakian et al. (eds.), *Procedural Dictations in Image-Guided Intervention*,
DOI 10.1007/978-3-319-40845-3_136

recovery time is short. Ablation is usually performed through a puncture of the vein below the knee joint with placement of the ablation fiber or probe in the venous lumen, injection of tumescent anesthesia, followed by delivery of thermal power to the lumen of the vein as the RF probe or LASER fiber are being retrieved.

COMMON INDICATIONS [1–3]

- Persistent symptoms due to incompetence of the great or small saphenous veins interfering with activities of daily living; such as aching, cramping, burning, itching, fatigue, and/or swelling during activity or after prolonged standing
- Skin changes associated with venous insufficiency:
  - Significant recurrent attacks of superficial thrombophlebitis
  - Ulceration from venous stasis
  - Atrophie blanche
  - Corona phlebectasia
  - Lipodermatosclerosis
  - Edema
  - Hemorrhage from a ruptured varix
- In addition to the indications, the following criteria should be met:
  - Failed conservative, nonoperative treatment; including mild exercise, avoidance of prolonged immobility, periodic elevation of legs, and compressive stockings
  - Anatomic criteria documented by duplex ultrasound: presence of significant venous reflux (>0.5 s) and anatomy amenable to endovenous ablation such as straight vein segment

COMMON CONTRAINDICATIONS [1–3]

No absolute contraindication is known for endovenous ablation however few conditions could exclude a patient from this therapy:

- Nonpalpable pedal pulses
- Severe uncorrectable coagulopathy
- Severe hypercoagulability disorders
- Sciatic vein reflux
- Inability to adequately ambulate after the procedure
- Deep vein thrombosis
- General poor health
- Pregnancy, planned pregnancy within 30 days of the procedure and nursing patients
- Extremely tortuous GSVs that would not allow endovenous catheterization and passage of the laser fiber as identified on pretreatment venous duplex ultrasound mapping
- Contraindications to use of local anesthetic such as liver dysfunction or allergy *(cold saline may be useful as an alternative)*

POSSIBLE COMPLICATIONS [1–4]

Although complications after endovenous ablation are rare, the following complications have been reported:

- Self-limiting ecchymosis with or without induration and pain; *100 %*
- Transient paresthesia and dysesthesia; *9 % (thigh), 51 % (leg)*
- Skin burn; *1–3 %*
- Deep venous thrombosis; *0–6 %*
- Superficial thrombophlebitis
- Nerve injury; *<1 %*
- Hematoma
- Feeling of "tightness" similar to that after a muscle sprain
- Arteriovenous fistula *(a few case reports)*
- Phlegmonous phlebitis
- Seroma
- Toxicity related to tumescent anesthesia *(i.e., from the use of large doses of lidocaine)*
- Device-related complication

PREPROCEDURAL ASSESSMENT AND PLANNING

- History, indications, and physical examination *(Appendix 1* in Chap. 149*)*
- Evaluation of diagnostic imaging studies such as venous duplex ultrasound to determine the

relevant venous anatomy and assess the access vessels

- Periprocedural management of coagulation status *(Appendices 2* in Chap. 150 *and 3* in Chap. 151*)*
- Antibiotic prophylaxis: Not routinely recommended [5] *(Appendices 4* in Chap. 152 *and 5* in Chap. 153*)*
- Imaging modality for guidance: Ultrasonography
- Positioning: Supine
- Vascular access: Saphenous vein

PROCEDURE NOTE [3]

Procedure: Endovenous laser/radiofrequency ablation of the right/left great saphenous vein
Staff: [_]
Fellow: [_]
Resident: [_]
Clinical History and Indications: Describe history and list indications
Allergies: None known/Allergic to [specify/type of allergy]
Anesthesia: Local anesthesia/Monitored conscious sedation *(rarely needed)*
Medications: List any relevant medications used (anesthesia, sedation)
Contrast Material: None
Field: Sterile
Procedure classification: Clean
Position: Supine
Imaging: Ultrasound
Monitoring: Intravenous access line was secured and vital signs were continuously monitored by nursing staff/anesthesia team throughout the procedure

Description of Procedure *(Endovenous laser ablation)*:
The risks, benefits, alternatives, and procedure itself were explained to the patient/patient's Power of Attorney/patient's legal guardian, and informed written consent was obtained. Time out was performed to confirm the correct patient, procedure and site. The site of the procedure was identified and marked.

With the patient in the supine position, the medial aspect of the left/right lower extremity was scrubbed from the level of the foot to the level of groin and draped in the usual aseptic manner. The skin and subcutaneous tissue overlying the greater saphenous vein below the level of the knee joint were infiltrated with lidocaine. The great saphenous vein was punctured under ultrasound guidance using a micropuncture needle. A (0.018) wire was advanced through the needle and the needle was exchanged for coaxial microcatheter. A (0.035) wire was advanced through the coaxial catheter and the catheter was exchanged for a (5)-French long vascular sheath. The vascular sheath was advanced over the wire under ultrasound guidance and its tip was positioned approximately 2 cm below the level of the saphenofemoral junction. A (980 nm/1470 nm) laser ablation fiber was advanced through the vascular sheath and the sheath was retrieved to accommodate the tip of the laser fiber approximately 2 cm below the saphenofemoral junction.

Tumescent anesthetic solution (consisting of 50 mL 1 % lidocaine with 440 mL normal saline and 10 mL sodium bicarbonate/or 50 mL lidocaine 1 % mixed with 450 mL Lactated Ringers) was then infiltrated around the entire shaft of the vein from the entry point to the most central location to be ablated (to collapse the vein therefore improve heat transfer to the vein wall and to separate the vein from the skin and other surrounding structures).

Endovenous ablation was then performed using (12) watt of continuous laser power as the fiber was being slowly pulled at the rate of (100) J per centimeter. Laser delivery was stopped as the tip of the laser fiber reached 2 cm from the entry point. The laser fiber and sheath were then removed and hemostasis was achieved by compression.

Sterile dressing was applied at the puncture site. The patient was then fitted with class II thigh-high compression hose.

The patient tolerated this procedure well and was transferred to the floor/recovery room/discharged home following the procedure in a stable condition. Staff was present for the entire procedure.

Power settings:

- GSV beginning at the saphenofemoral junction to treat the central most 10 cm: use 140 J/cm at 810 nm at a power setting of 14 W (10 mm/10 s pullback).
- GSV in the upper calf: use energy of approximately 100 J/cm (10 mm/7 s).
- GVF in mid and lower calf: use 70–84 J/cm when ablating GSV in mid and lower calf.
- Small Saphenous Vein: use 100 J/cm for the first 4 cm and 70–84 J/cm for the next 4 cm and then 56–70 J/cm thereafter.

Description of Procedure *(Endovenous radiofrequency ablation):*

The risks, benefits, alternatives, and procedure itself were explained to the patient/patient's Power of Attorney/patient's legal guardian, and informed written consent was obtained. Time out was performed to confirm the correct patient, procedure, and site. The site of the procedure was identified and marked.

With the patient in the supine position, the medial aspect of the left/right lower extremity was scrubbed from the level of the foot to the level of groin and draped in the usual aseptic manner. The skin and subcutaneous tissue overlying the greater saphenous vein below the level of the knee joint were infiltrated with lidocaine. The great saphenous vein was punctured under ultrasound guidance using a micropuncture needle. A (0.018) wire was advanced through the needle and the needle was exchanged for coaxial microcatheter. A (0.035) wire was advanced through the coaxial catheter and the catheter was exchanged for a (7)-French long vascular sheath. A (7)-French [type] endovascular radiofrequency ablation catheter was advanced through the vascular sheath and its tip was positioned approximately 2 cm below the saphenofemoral junction.

Tumescent anesthetic solution (consisting of 50 mL 1 % lidocaine with 440 mL normal saline and 10 mL sodium bicarbonate/or 50 mL lidocaine 1 % mixed with 450 mL Lactated Ringers) was then infiltrated around the entire shaft of the vein from the entry point to the most central location to be ablated (to collapse the vein therefore improve heat transfer to the vein wall and to separate the vein from the skin and other surrounding structures).

Radiofrequency ablation was carried out at (6.5)-cm intervals with (20) seconds per station, reaching a maximum catheter vein temperature of (121)°C. The procedure was concluded when the probe reached within 2 cm of puncture site. Catheters were then removed, and hemostasis was achieved by manual compression followed by application of a compression bandage. The patient was then fitted with class II thigh-high compression hose.

The patient tolerated this procedure well and was transferred to the floor/recovery room/discharged home following the procedure in a stable condition. Staff was present for the entire procedure.

Intra-Procedure Findings: List all relevant findings.

Immediate Complications: None encountered during or directly after the procedure. List complications if any.

Post-Procedure Plan [3]**:**

- A class II (30–40 mm Hg) full-thigh graduated support stocking or panty hose to be worn for at least 1 week at all times except when sleeping or during shower.
- Encourage patient to ambulate immediately after procedure (recommend 2 h of walking a day for 2 weeks) and resume normal activity.
- Avoid vigorous exercise for the first 2 weeks; hot tub, sauna or Jacuzzi for 6 months and long periods of immobility.
- Over-the-counter pain medications (Acetaminophen/NSAID) as needed for pain control. Pain should completely subside within a week.
- Perform clinical examination and duplex ultrasound follow-up at 1 week and 1, 3, 6, 9, and 12 months, and then yearly.

Impression:

- Endovascular LASER/radiofrequency ablation of the left/right [vein name] vein, as described above.
- The patient tolerated the procedure well and left the interventional unit in stable condition.
- The patient was unable to tolerate the procedure which was canceled/terminated prematurely.
- List any other relevant or important information/finding.

References

1. Khilnani NM, Grassi CJ, Kundu S, D'Agostino HR, Khan AA, McGraw JK, et al. Multi-society consensus quality improvement guidelines for the treatment of lower-extremity superficial venous insufficiency with endovenous thermal ablation from the Society of Interventional Radiology, Cardiovascular Interventional Radiological Society of Europe, American College of Phlebology and Canadian Interventional Radiology Association. J Vasc Interv Radiol. 2010;21(1):14–31.
2. Min RJ, Khilnani N, Zimmet SE. Endovenous laser treatment of saphenous vein reflux: long-term results. Vasc Interv Radiol. 2003;14(8):991–6.
3. Khilnani NM, Min RJ. Endovenous laser ablation. In: Kandarpa K, Machan L, editors. Handbook of interventional radiologic procedures. 4th ed. Philadelphia: Lippincott Williams & Wilkins; 2011. p. 439–49.
4. Van Den Bos RR, Neumann M, De Roos KP, Nijsten T. Endovenous laser ablation-induced complications: review of the literature and new cases. Dermatol Surg. 2009;35(8):1206–14.
5. Venkatesan AM, Kundu S, Sacks D, Wallace MJ, Wojak JC, Rose SC, et al. Practice guidelines for adult antibiotic prophylaxis during vascular and interventional radiology procedures. J Vasc Interv Radiol. 2010;21(11):1611–30.

Management of Visceral and Extremity Arteriovenous Malformations

137

Hearns W. Charles

Abbreviations

AVM	Arteriovenous malformation
ISSVA	International Society for the Study of Vascular Anomalies
IMA	Inferior mesenteric artery
PFA	Profunda femoris artery

INTRODUCTION

An exceedingly rare disease, arteriovenous malformations (AVMs) reflect part of the spectrum of vascular anomalies, classified by the International Society for the Study of Vascular Anomalies (ISSVA) [1]. Diagnosed at any age, there is growth tendency at the same rate as the individual, with possible growth acceleration at puberty, during pregnancy, and, in some cases, following trauma or intervention [2]. The clinical presentation can range from a cosmetic, asymptomatic birthmark to life-threatening congestive heart failure. Attributing any of associated varied symptoms to a vascular malformation can be challenging to the most experienced clinician, partly compounded by the relative rarity of these lesions. Patients seeking help from a number of physicians, often to disappointing outcomes, complications, and recurrence or deterioration of their presenting symptoms [3]. Physical examination is limited with visceral AVMs that often lack external signs of disease and may not be readily accessible. Presentation may be that of a soft tissue mass, with or without palpable pulsation or thrill. High-flow AVMs are typically non-tender to palpation and do not show much positional change, whereas low-flow lesions tend to enlarge when in a dependent position [2]. The advent of widespread cross-sectional imaging in medicine has sped the confirmation of the diagnosis following initial search of medical attention. CT and MRI, with angiography, provide much valuable diagnostic information, only helpful if the examination is dedicated to the lesion. More quantitative information of lesion flow dynamics has been described with ultrasound [4].

Angiographically, there is enlargement and tortuosity of the feeding arterial branches potentially leading to distal ischemia; enlargement of the draining veins; soft-tissue changes;

H.W. Charles (✉)
Department of Radiology, Division of Interventional Radiology, New York University Langone Medical Center, 660 First Avenue, 7th Floor, New York, NY 10016, USA
e-mail: hearns.charles@nyumc.org

B. Taslakian et al. (eds.), *Procedural Dictations in Image-Guided Intervention*,
DOI 10.1007/978-3-319-40845-3_137

generalized cardiovascular effects such as increased blood volume and a high-output cardiac state. Although high-output cardiac failure is often a concern of patients and referring physicians, it is actually quite uncommon, tending to occur with high-flow lesions in infancy or extremely extensive lesions in adults [2].

AVMs can occur anywhere in the mesenteric circulation resulting in gastrointestinal bleeding, mesenteric ischemia, and portal hypertension. Familial colonic angiodysplasia, the most common of visceral AVMs, can present with chronic anemia due to its intermittent nature of and slow bleeding. Embolization of lower gastrointestinal AVMs carries an increased risk of bowel ischemia. Higher flow mesenteric AVMs, complex and difficult to cure, can also cause shunting in the portal venous system, resulting in significant portal hypertension. Treatment needs to be staged, with the care of not inciting acute shunt closure lest it leads to acute portal vein thrombosis. Visceral involvement can also occur as part of a high-flow pelvic AVM with recruitment of blood supply from the mesenteric vessels, usually the inferior mesenteric artery (IMA). Drainage in this type of lesion is usually into the systemic venous circulation rather than the portal system [2].

The first point to be made for the management of visceral and other AVMs is the need for a multidisciplinary approach, involving a team of physicians (internists, surgeons, dermatologists, hematologists) and other healthcare workers (nurses, nurse practitioners, patient coordinators) in the overall care of the patient [3]. In general, embolization has become the primary treatment modality for AVMs. Although surgery plays a role, it should be reserved if complete resection of the lesion is feasible without resultant disability or significant deformity, and sizably large lesions worthy of debulking. Surgical ligation of feeding arteries, skeletonization procedures, is nearly always ineffective and tends to lead to development of new collateral pathways, rendering subsequent treatment more difficult. Combining preoperative embolization with surgical resection in accessible lesions has been used in many cases with excellent results. Treatment of the AVM nidus should be the primary focus of a successful procedure. Proximal occlusion of feeding arteries is equivalent to proximal surgical ligation, leading to inadequate treatment and renders further treatment more difficult. Distal embolic materials are available, with operator preference based generally on training and experience. These include liquid sclerosing agents, such as absolute ethanol; particles such as microspheres; liquid casting agents, such as n-butyl cyanoacrylate (n-BCA, Tru-fill, Cordis Inc.) acrylic adhesive, and ethylene vinyl alcohol copolymer (Onyx, EV3). Other ancillary embolization agents include standard and detachable coils, vascular plugs (such as the Amplatzer plug), and septal occluders [2]. These may be used to treat sizable associated arterial and venous aneurysms. Ancillary closure, temporary and permanent, of dilated, often aneurysmal outflow veins, may be necessary in some cases, especially in high-flow AVMs with persistent myriad inaccessible fine branches following successful embolization of major arterial feeders.

The treatment of visceral and other AVMs should be methodical and staged, with much operator and ancillary staff patience during each treatment session. General anesthesia is preferred for the patient, for comfort, optimal imaging, and close physiologic monitoring. This affords the operator to concentrate mostly on the treatment procedure. A Foley catheter is placed if the procedure is projected to take more than 2 h and for constant clearing of contrast from the urinary bladder in case of pelvic AVM embolization. Staging of treatment into multiple sessions has many advantages including some that were mentioned earlier. The primary goal is the elimination of symptoms or reduction of abnormal physiology related to the shunting (ischemia, high output). Complete eradication of the malformation radiologically is not expected, nor is it necessary in most cases [2].

COMMON INDICATIONS

- Associated symptoms (pain)
- Intestinal bleeding
- Symptomatic anemia

- Intestinal ischemia
- Portal hypertension
- High-output cardiac disease

COMMON CONTRAINDICATIONS

Absolute contraindications:
- Active infection

Relative contraindications:
- Coagulopathy (INR > 1.5)
- Thrombocytopenia (platelet count < 50–100)
- Anemia (hemoglobin < 8)
- History of allergic reaction to iodinated contrast
- Significant renal insufficiency

POSSIBLE COMPLICATIONS

- Access site complications *(e.g., bleeding, hematoma, pseudoaneurysm formation)*
- Nontarget embolization
- Contrast-induced nephropathy
- Contrast-induced allergic reaction

PREPROCEDURAL ASSESSMENT AND PLANNING

- History and physical examination
- Evaluation of diagnostic imaging studies (CT or MRI), for anatomic delineation
- Order blood analysis, dated <30 days from the procedure: complete blood count (CBC), complete metabolic profile (CMP), international normalized ratio (INR)
- Imaging modality for guidance: Fluoroscopy
- Positioning: Supine
- Arterial access: Common femoral artery

PROCEDURE NOTE

Procedure:

- Abdominal/pelvic angiogram
- Left and right upper leg angiogram
- Embolization [specify location] arteriovenous malformation (AVM).

Staff: [_]
Fellow: [_]
Resident: [_]
Clinical Information: Describe history and list indications
Allergies: None known/Allergic to [specify/type of allergy]
Anesthesia: Conscious sedation was administered and physiologic monitoring was carried out throughout the procedure by the radiology nursing staff
Medications: List any relevant medications used
Contrast Material: (_) mL of [type] nonionic contrast material
Field: Sterile
Procedure classification: Clean
Position: Supine
Total fluoroscopy time: (_) minutes
Cumulative radiation dose: (_) mGy

Description of Procedure:

Informed consent was obtained where the risks, benefits and alternatives to the procedure were explained to the patient.

Sterile technique and fluoroscopic guidance were used to catheterize the right common femoral artery using a (_)-French introducer sheath. Through this, a (_)-French catheter was advanced and used to catheterize the inferior abdominal aorta. Branch catheterization was carried out using an inner (_)-French microcatheter. Contrast examination was performed utilizing multiple views.

Vessels investigated [specify vessels; see examples below]:
- Posterior division, left/right hypogastric artery.
- Left/right external iliac artery.
- Left/right profunda femoris artery (PFA).
- Inferior/superior mesenteric artery.

Findings [specify findings; see examples below]:
- Over the left iliac wing, a few small arterial branches supply small foci of abnormal vascularity. Late appearance of small amorphous

areas of contrast pooling shows no arteriovenous communication. These findings correspond to a sizable area of signal abnormality and most likely reflect either a hemangioma versus a venous malformation.
- Small burden AVM is supplied by two small terminal branches of the left PFA. These branches were super-selectively catheterized using a 0.014-in Echelon catheter, through which embolization was performed using small aliquots of Onyx. There was resultant treatment of the AVM, with its lack of opacification at completion angiography
- Two other foci of AVM disease; moderately sized, at left mid-thigh, from a prominent and unexpected branch of the mid superficial femoral artery. This lesion is associated with a bi-lobed venous aneurysm. Small AVM, at left knee level, from a short truncal branch of the popliteal artery. These lesions lead to early venous opacification; these were not treated at this time.

Sterile technique and fluoroscopic guidance were used to catheterize the left common femoral artery using a (_)-French introducer sheath. Through this, a (_)-French catheter was advanced and used to catheterize the right common and deep femoral (PFA) arteries.

Findings [specify findings; see examples below]:
- Marked enlargement of the right deep external pudendal and medial circumflex arteries. These supply a large regional burden of AVM, proximal medial right thigh. Various individual branches of the deep external pudendal artery were super-selectively catheterized with a number of microcatheters, through which embolization was performed using small aliquots of 1:2 n-BCA: lipiodol adhesive.

Completion angiography shows [specify findings; see examples below]:
- Adequate treatment of the intended arterial territory (of the right deep external pudendal artery).
- Persistent large burden AVM disease from the right medial circumflex artery. This is associated with outflow venous aneurysmal disease. This arterial distribution will be treated in a few weeks.

Contrast examination of the right and left external iliac and common femoral arteries was performed, showing no disease.

The catheter and introducer sheath were then removed, with simultaneous deployment of a [type] arterial closure device, with supplemental manual compression applied to effect hemostasis. Patient tolerated the procedure well and was transferred to the floor/recovery room in a stable condition. Staff was present for the entire procedure.

Intra-Procedure Findings: Summarize all relevant findings.

Immediate Complications: None encountered during or directly after the procedure. List complications if any.

Post-Procedure Plan

- Keep patient in complete bed rest with the right/left leg extended for (_) hours.
- Check the (right groin) access site for any bleeding or hematoma formation every 15 min ×4, then every 30 min ×2, then every 1 h ×2.
- Check neurovascular exam: (right groin) access and popliteal, and ankle arterial pulses; every 15 min ×4, then every 30 min ×2, then every 1 h ×2.
- Inform interventional radiology team for any access site bleeding or hematoma formation.
- Monitor vital signs every 15 min ×4, then every 30 min ×2, then every 1 h ×2
- Notify Interventional Radiology team if systolic blood pressure $\geq$ 130 mm Hg or $\leq$90 mm Hg; or diastolic BP > 100 mm Hg.
- Notify interventional radiology team if heart rate $\geq$ 100 BPM or $\leq$ 60 BPM, at extension (_). If not during regular work hours, page beeper number (_).
- Remove Foley catheter when patient ambulatory.
- Resume diet and previous orders as needed and if not otherwise contraindicated.

- Encourage fluid intake and continue routine monitoring (intake/output) status.

Impression:

- Small burden AVM, [left lateral upper thigh/specify location], treated with (Onyx) embolization.
- Left lateral buttock [specify if otherwise needed] hemangioma versus venous malformation.
- Large burden AVM disease, [specify location], partially treated with glue embolization.

References

1. Based on Scientific Committee of the 11th Meeting of the International Society for the Study of Vascular Anomalies. Rome, Italy; 1996.
2. Rosen RJ, Nassiri N, Drury JE. Interventional management of high-flow vascular malformations. Tech Vasc Interventional Rad. 2013;16:22–38.
3. Legiehn GM, Heran MKS. A step-by-step practical approach to imaging diagnosis and interventional radiologic therapy in vascular malformations. Semin Intervent Radiol. 2010;27:209–31.
4. Rutherford RB. Noninvasive evaluation for congenital arteriovenous fistulas and malformations. Semin Vasc Surg. 2012;25:49–57.

Percutaneous Obliteration of Common Femoral Artery Pseudoaneurysm

138

Bedros Taslakian and Divya Sridhar

Abbreviations

PA Pseudoaneurysm

INTRODUCTION

Pseudoaneurysms (PAs) are one of the most common complications of femoral artery catheterization. In addition, arterial hemorrhage due to non-iatrogenic traumatic vascular injury or anastomotic leakage may also result in PA formation. A PA represents active hemorrhage contained within a hematoma, and is at constant risk of rupture if not diagnosed and treated expeditiously. Surgical repair is indicated in patients presenting with PAs due to previous vascular surgical interventions, infection, or non-iatrogenic trauma. Nonsurgical treatments for iatrogenic arterial PAs include compression, direct percutaneous thrombin injection, and endovascular stent graft placement. PA compression may be guided by palpation ("blind"), precompression ultrasound examination for localization with subsequent manual compression, or real-time ultrasound-guided compression using the transducer itself. Percutaneous thrombin injection under ultrasound guidance is the treatment of choice for noncomplicated femoral PAs, particularly those which have a narrow, long, and superficial neck amenable to compression. Simultaneous balloon occlusion of the artery across the site of arterial communication may be helpful in increasing safety of thrombin injection for a PA without a neck or with a short and wide neck. In the rare instance of thrombin failure due to a large arterial defect or in cases of accompanying arteriovenous fistula, a covered stent (stent graft) may be placed to repair the defect; however, consideration should be given to the position of the stent relative to the apex of hip flexion, as the excess motion may impact stent integrity and patency. The use of human thrombin is favored over bovine thrombin, as the latter has greater potential to induce allergic reactions. Autologous thrombin, which is cheaper than commercial bovine or human thrombin, can also be used; its application is simple, safe, and reliable.

B. Taslakian
Department of Radiology, New York University Langone Medical Center, 660 First Ave, New York, NY 10016, USA
e-mail: btaslakian@gmail.com

D. Sridhar (✉)
Department of Radiology, Division of Vascular and Interventional Radiology, New York University Langone Medical Center, 660 1st Ave, 7th Floor, Suite. 742, 10016 New York, NY, USA
e-mail: divya.sridhar@nyumc.org

B. Taslakian et al. (eds.), *Procedural Dictations in Image-Guided Intervention*,
DOI 10.1007/978-3-319-40845-3_138

COMMON INDICATIONS [1, 2]

- *Pseudoaneurysm compression:* Iatrogenic femoral PA with ALL of the following characteristics: small, <2 weeks old, long neck, intact overlying skin, no anticoagulation. Selected non-iatrogenic femoral PAs may also be appropriate for this treatment if mechanism resulted in similar vascular injury (e.g., small-caliber stab wound).
- *Direct percutaneous thrombin injection:* All iatrogenic femoral pseudoaneurysms can be potentially treated using this method. Selected non-iatrogenic femoral PAs may also be appropriate for this treatment.

COMMON CONTRAINDICATIONS [1, 3, 4]

Contraindications to pseudoaneurysm compression:
- Pain intolerant patients
- Painful pseudoaneurysms
- Morbid obesity
- Large pseudoaneurysm, obliterating adjacent vessels
- No compressible pseudoaneurysm neck
- Pseudoaneurysms with ipsilateral deep venous thrombosis

Contraindications to direct percutaneous thrombin injection:
- Previous exposure to bovine thrombin
- Aneurysmal sac <1 cm *(has higher rate of thrombin leakage and subsequent thrombosis of the femoral artery)*
- No compressible pseudoaneurysm neck *(unless adjunctive balloon occlusion used)*

Contraindications to both methods:
- Pseudoaneurysm associated with arteriovenous fistula
- Suspected pseudoaneurysm infection
- Breakdown of overlying skin
- Unstable patients
- Rupture or impending rupture

POSSIBLE COMPLICATIONS [1–8]

Complications encountered with pseudoaneurysm compression:
- Pain and pain-associated complications *(vasovagal reaction, atrial fibrillation, hypertension)*; *0–4.1 %*
- Pseudoaneurysm rupture; *0–0.9 %*
- Distal arterial embolization; *0–0.8 %*
- Ipsilateral deep venous thrombosis; *0–0.3 %*
- Pulmonary embolism; *rare*

Complications encountered with direct thrombin injection:
- Thromboembolic complications due to thrombin leakage into the femoral artery; *0–2.6 %*
- Allergy to the injected material; *0–0.4 %*
- Superimposed infection; *0.05–0.9 %*
- Pseudoaneurysm rupture; *0–0.8 %*
- Pain; *0–0.4 %*
- Deep venous thrombosis
- Reperfusion of previously completely thrombosed pseudoaneurysms *(i.e., treatment failure)*

PREPROCEDURAL ASSESSMENT AND PLANNING

- History, indications and physical examination *(Appendix 1* in Chap. 149*)*
- Evaluation of diagnostic imaging studies (ultrasound/CT angiography) to determine the relevant vascular anatomy and the location, shape, and size of the pseudoaneurysm

- Periprocedural management of coagulation status *(Appendices 2* in Chap. 150 *and 3 in* Chap. 151*)*
- Antibiotic prophylaxis: Not routinely recommended
- Imaging modality for guidance: Ultrasound
- Positioning: Supine

PROCEDURE NOTE

Procedure: Percutaneous obliteration of left/right common femoral artery pseudoaneurysm by direct ultrasound-guided compression/thrombin injection
Staff: [_]
Fellow: [_]
Resident: [_]
Clinical Information: Describe history and list indications
Allergies: None known/Allergic to [specify/type of allergy]
Anesthesia: Local anesthesia/conscious sedation
Medications: List any relevant medications used (anesthesia, sedation, thrombin/tissue adhesive agent)
Contrast Used: (_) mL of [type] contrast media was used for angiography/None
Field: Sterile
Procedure classification: Clean
Position: Supine
Monitoring: Intravenous access line was secured and vital signs were continuously monitored by nursing staff/anesthesia team throughout the procedure
Total fluoroscopy time: (_) minutes/not applicable
Cumulative radiation dose: (_) mGy/not applicable

Description of Procedure *(direct percutaneous intrapseudoaneurysm injection of thrombin):*
The risks, benefits, alternatives, and procedure itself were explained to the patient/patient's Power of Attorney/patient's legal guardian, and informed written consent was obtained. Time out was performed to confirm the correct patient, procedure, and site. The site of the procedure was identified and marked.

The patient was positioned supine. Baseline distal arterial pulses were determined bilaterally. Color-flow Doppler and grayscale ultrasound examination was performed to evaluate the pseudoaneurysm for size, complexity (number of lobes), neck location and dimensions, and hemodynamics. The relationship of the pseudoaneurysm with the supplying femoral artery was determined. Additional arterial injuries and arteriovenous fistula formation were excluded. The overlying skin was inspected to ensure it was intact, and to exclude necrosis and infection.

Thrombin Injection:
The ideal needle access site and trajectory were determined. The skin of the right/left groin was prepped and draped in the usual sterile fashion. [Balloon inflation for balloon-assisted thrombin injection should be performed at this time*]. Using real-time ultrasound guidance, a (25/22/21)-gauge needle was advanced into the pseudoaneurysm sac/junction of neck and sac (less preferred)/neck (not preferred). Then, thrombin was injected slowly and steadily (0.1–0.3 mL/s) under real-time color-flow Doppler ultrasound visualization. The formation of isoechoic to hyperechoic thrombus gradually filling the pseudoaneurysm was observed. Residual pockets showing vascular flow were identified, and the needle was redirected into these pockets for additional thrombin injection/ gentle pressure was applied to achieve complete thrombosis. A total of (_) units of thrombin were injected. Color-flow Doppler ultrasound examination showed complete/nearly complete thrombosis of the entire pseudoaneurysm and absence of high flow through the sac and the procedure was concluded.

Sterile dressing was applied and the patient was transferred to the floor/recovery room following the procedure in a stable condition. Staff was present for the entire procedure.

Balloon Placement and Inflation for Balloon-Assisted Thrombin Injection:
The contralateral common femoral artery, femoral head, and inguinal ligament were located by palpation/fluoroscopy/ultrasound and marked. The site of arterial puncture was determined using combined information from palpation, ultrasound, and fluoroscopy. Local anesthesia was administered. Common femoral artery access contralateral to the pseudoaneurysm was obtained using a (_)-gauge [type] needle and the Seldinger technique under direct ultrasound visualization/by palpation. Once good pulsatile arterial flow was detected, a (_)-inch [type] guidewire was advanced through the needle, into the aorta under direct fluoroscopic visualization, and a (_)-French vascular sheath was placed. A (_)-French [type] catheter and a (_)-inch [type] guidewire were navigated into the contralateral common iliac artery. Arteriography was performed by the manual injection of (_)-mL of contrast to localize the pseudoaneurysm. The wire was then advanced until its tip was distal to the femoral pseudoaneurysm. The diagnostic catheter was exchanged over the wire for a (_) × (_) mm balloon catheter. The balloon was positioned and inflated across the pseudoaneurysm neck.

Following the procedure the right/left femoral artery sheath was removed, and adequate hemostasis was achieved by compression for (_) minutes/using [type] vascular closure device. The lower extremity pulses were checked following the procedure and were [comparable to the pre-procedure pulses/specify if otherwise needed]. The patient was transferred to the floor/recovery room following the procedure in a stable condition. Staff was present for the entire procedure.

Notes:

- *Balloon occlusion of the pseudoaneurysm neck* is not routinely recommended due to its invasive nature and added complications. The application of this protocol is proposed in cases when the neck is <3 mm in length, wider than a point source [8], or otherwise unsuitable for effective percutaneous compression.
- *Pseudoaneurysm containing a single lobe:* a thrombin dose of 500–1000 IU is generally adequate [8]; inject thrombin slowly until flow in the PA ceases.
- *In patients with complex bi- or multilobed pseudoaneurysms:* Some authors recommend first injecting into the lobe farthest from the native femoral artery, with subsequent injection(s) into the lobe(s) communicating with the neck if they remain patent; in the believe that this minimizes the risk of propagation of thrombus into the femoral artery. By contrast, other authors recommend instead starting injection in the lobe closest to the artery, which should occlude flow to the distal lobe as it thromboses [8].

Description of Procedure *(real-time ultrasound-guided compression):*
The risks, benefits, alternatives, and procedure itself were explained to the patient/patient's Power of Attorney/patient's legal guardian, and informed written consent was obtained. Time out was performed to confirm the correct patient, procedure, and site. The site of the procedure was identified and marked.

Baseline distal arterial pulses were determined, bilaterally. The skin of the right/left groin was prepped and draped in the usual sterile fashion. Color-flow Doppler ultrasound examination was performed to evaluate the pseudoaneurysm for overall size, neck location, dimensions, and hemodynamics. The relationship of the pseudoaneurysm with the supplying femoral artery was determined. Additional arterial injuries and arteriovenous fistula formation were excluded. The overlying skin was evaluated to exclude necrosis and infection. The ideal trajectory for applying pressure was determined, with care taken to avoid gross compression of the pseudoaneurysm sac, femoral vein, and femoral artery. The ultrasound probe was then positioned directly over the pseudoaneurysm neck, and downward pressure was applied until flow into the pseudoaneurysm was observed to cease on color-flow Doppler imaging. Compression was performed intermittently, with assessment of residual flow within the pseudoaneurysm, using (6–20) min intervals.

The pseudoaneurysm neck was not clearly identified by color-flow Doppler examination, and ultrasound-guided direct compression of the pseudoaneurysm sac itself was performed until cessation of flow in the pseudoaneurysm was achieved.

After confirming absence of flow within the pseudoaneurysm, the procedure was concluded and sterile dressing was applied. The patient was transferred to the floor/recovery room following the procedure in a stable condition. Staff was present for the entire procedure.

Note: Pressure is held in cycles of 10–20 min, and the pseudoaneurysm is then reassessed. If flow persists, compression is held for another cycle, typically stopping after 1 or 2 attempts. Patients are then put on bed rest for 6 h, and duplex ultrasonography is performed 24–48 h later to confirm persistent thrombosis.

Intra-Procedure Findings: List all relevant findings.

Immediate Complications: None encountered during or directly after the procedure. List complications if any.

Post-Procedure Plan [1]:

- Keep patient in complete bed rest with the right/left leg extended for (_) hours *[recommended 2–12 h after thrombin injection, >6 h after ultrasound-guided compression].*
- Check the procedure site and lower extremity pulses every 15 min for 1 h, then every 30 min for 4 h; inform interventional radiology team if any complications are observed.
- Follow up Doppler ultrasound examination within 24 h of the procedure, at 3–10 days and then at 3 weeks–6 months.
- If contralateral side is catheterized for balloon-assisted occlusion; please follow post-procedural instructions in Chap. 75

Impression:

- Percutaneous obliteration of left/right common femoral artery pseudoaneurysm by direct ultrasound-guided compression/thrombin injection.
- The patient tolerated the procedure well and left the interventional unit in a stable condition.
- The patient was unable to tolerate the procedure which was canceled/terminated prematurely.
- List any other relevant or important information/finding.

References

1. Saad WEA, Waldman DL. Management of post-catheterization pseudoaneurysms. In: Mauro MA, Murphy KPJ, Thomson KR, Venbrux AC, Morgan RA, editors. Image-guided interventions. 2nd ed. Philadelphia: Saunders Elsevier; 2014. p. 247–55.
2. Kang SS, Labropoulos N, Mansour MA, Michelini M, Filliung D, Baubly MP, et al. Expanded indications for ultrasound-guided thrombin injection of pseudoaneurysms. J Vasc Surg. 2000;31(2):289–98.
3. Padidar AM, Kee ST, Razavi MK. Treatment of femoral artery pseudoaneurysms using ultrasound-guided thrombin injection. Tech Vasc Interv Radiol. 2003;6(2):96–102.
4. Stone PA, Campbell JE, AbuRahma AF. Femoral pseudoaneurysms after percutaneous access. J Vasc Surg. 2014;60(5):1359–66.
5. Krüger K, Zähringer M, Söhngen FD, Gossmann A, Schulte O, Feldmann C, et al. Femoral pseudoaneurysms: management with percutaneous thrombin injections—success rates and effects on systemic coagulation. Radiology. 2003;226(2):452–8.
6. Krueger K, Zaehringer M, Strohe D, Stuetzer H, Boecker J, Lackner K. Postcatheterization pseudoaneurysm: results of US-guided percutaneous thrombin injection in 240 patients. Radiology. 2005;236(3):1104–10.
7. Paschalidis M, Theiss W, Kölling K, Busch R, Schömig A. Randomised comparison of manual compression repair versus ultrasound guided compression repair of postcatheterisation femoral pseudoaneurysms. Heart. 2006;92(2):251–2.
8. Tsetis D. Endovascular treatment of complications of femoral arterial access. Cardiovasc Interv Radiol. 2010;33(3):457–68.

139 Retrieval of Intravascular Foreign Body

Karim Rebeiz and Peter Sawan

INTRODUCTION

Retained intravascular foreign bodies with the potential for embolization to the cardiopulmonary system carry a significant risk of morbidity and mortality. Therefore, when an intravascular foreign body is identified, endovascular extraction should be attempted. Several retrieval devices are available. Loop snares are the most commonly used retrieval devices, have the capability of maintaining their shape within the vessel, are easy to manipulate and require a free edge to grasp the foreign body. Basket snares and flexible grasping forceps, which have a powerful grasping capability, can be useful when an object is severely adherent or does not have an obvious free edge.

COMMON INDICATIONS [1–4]

- Misplaced or fractured endovascular device fragments *(e.g., arterial closure device, cardiac valve, sheaths, catheters, intravascular ultrasound catheters)*
- Misplaced or fractured pacemaker wire tips
- Misplaced or fractured guidewires
- Misplaced or migrated embolization coils
- Misplaced, fractured or migrated caval filters
- Malpositioned vascular stents
- Ingested foreign bodies migrated to the vascular system by transmural penetration

COMMON CONTRAINDICATIONS [1, 3]

- Firmly adherent foreign body
- Transmural perforation of the retained intravascular object
- Asymptomatic patient with a harmless location of the retained intravascular object
- Asymptomatic patient with a migrated foreign body into the extravascular space
- Significantly sized thrombus attached to the retained object with risk of embolization
- Severe coagulopathy that cannot be corrected
- Pregnancy

POSSIBLE COMPLICATIONS [1–5]

General (angiography-related) complications:
- Hemorrhage *(puncture-site hematoma, retroperitoneal hematoma if "high" puncture above inguinal ligament)*
- Pseudoaneurysm *(superficial femoral artery "low" puncture)*
- Arteriovenous fistula *(puncture-site artery)*
- Thrombosis of the access artery or vein

K. Rebeiz (✉) · P. Sawan
Department of Radiology, Memorial Sloan Kettering Cancer Center, 1275 York Ave, New York, NY 10065, USA
e-mail: krebeiz00@gmail.com

P. Sawan
e-mail: sawanpeter@gmail.com

B. Taslakian et al. (eds.), *Procedural Dictations in Image-Guided Intervention*,
DOI 10.1007/978-3-319-40845-3_139

- Distal embolization
- Contrast-induced allergic reaction
- Contrast-induced nephropathy
- Limb amputation *(rare)*
- Risks related to any minimally invasive procedure performed under conscious sedation *(e.g., allergy to medications)*

Procedure-specific complications:

- Failed endovascular retrieval and conversion to open surgical removal
- Failed endovascular retrieval leaving the foreign body in place
- Failed endovascular retrieval with pulmonary embolism from thrombotic debris around a retained foreign body
- Embolization of a thrombus attached to the retained object during manipulation
- Cardiac complications *(arrhythmias, ventricular and septal perforation, valvular damage, tamponade)*
- Arterial spasm or dissection
- Vessel perforation
- Vessel thrombosis
- Distal embolization into an irretrievable location
- Thrombus formation and thromboembolism in prolonged procedures

PREPROCEDURAL ASSESSMENT AND PLANNING

- History, indications, and physical examination *(Appendix 1* in Chap. 149*)*
- Evaluation of diagnostic imaging studies to determine the relevant vascular anatomy and the location, shape, and type of the retained intravascular foreign body
- Periprocedural management of coagulation status *(Appendices 2* in Chap. 150 *and 3 in* Chap. 151*)*
- Antibiotic prophylaxis: Not routinely recommended, unless infection is suspected
- Imaging modality for guidance: Fluoroscopy; combined with ultrasound for vascular access
- Positioning: Supine
- Venous access: Jugular vein, femoral vein, femoral artery [3]. If the object is peripheral or in arterial or venous branches, the best approach needs to be selected based on the location and accessibility of the object.

PROCEDURE NOTE

Procedure: Removal of intravascular foreign body [specify location and type if relevant]
Staff: [_]
Fellow: [_]
Resident: [_]
Clinical Information: Describe history and list indications
Allergies: None known/Allergic to [specify/type of allergy]
Anesthesia: Local anesthesia/conscious sedation
Medications: List any relevant medications used
Contrast Material: (_) mL of [type] contrast material was used for venography/arteriography.
Field: Sterile
Procedure classification: Clean
Position: Supine
Monitoring: Intravenous access line was secured and vital signs were continuously monitored by nursing staff/anesthesia team throughout the procedure
Total fluoroscopy time: (_) minutes
Cumulative radiation dose: (_) mGy

Description of Procedure *(intravenous foreign body retrieval through jugular or femoral approach, using a snare):*
The risks, benefits, alternatives, and procedure itself were explained to the patient/patient's Power of Attorney/patient's legal guardian, and informed written/verbal consent was obtained. Time out was performed to confirm the correct patient, procedure, and site. The site of the procedure was identified and marked.

[Choose one depending on the access site]

- The patient was positioned supine, with the neck turned to the contralateral side. The patient's left/right cervical and upper thoracic regions were prepped and draped in usual sterile fashion. Ultrasound examination was performed to determine the site of venous puncture. Local anesthesia was administered.

The left/right internal jugular vein was punctured under ultrasound guidance using a (_)-gauge [type] needle. Once good venous flow was detected, a (_)-inch [type] guidewire was advanced through the needle under direct fluoroscopic visualization. A small skin incision was made and a (_)-French, (_)-cm-long vascular sheath was advanced over the guidewire and positioned into [specify location].

- The skin of both groins were shaved, prepped, and draped in the usual sterile fashion. The right/left common femoral vein was located by palpation/ultrasound and marked. Local anesthesia was administered and a small skin incision was made. Femoral venous access was obtained using an (_)-gauge [type] needle under direct ultrasound visualization/by palpation. Once good venous flow was detected, a (_)-inch [type] guidewire was advanced through the needle, up through the femoral vein into the inferior vena cava under direct fluoroscopic visualization and a (_)-French, (_)-cm-long vascular sheath was placed into [specify location].

Then, a (_)-French [type] catheter was advanced into the [specify location/vein] over a (0.035)-in. [hydrophilic/type] guidewire. Venography was performed by injecting (_) mL of [type] contrast and digital subtraction angiography imaging was performed at (4–6) frames per second during suspended respiration in an anterior–posterior projection/[specify other projections if obtained] to evaluate the vein and exclude complications. Through the sheath, a vascular retrieval snare [specify type] was advanced with the guiding retrieval catheter, the snare was deployed and the free end of the retained foreign body was encircled. After grasping the foreign body, the guiding catheter was advanced to firmly entrap the retained object. Once the object was entirely within the retrieval device, it was pulled out along with the retrieval catheter through the vascular sheath while maintaining tension on the closed snare loop. The extracted object was inspected for integrity. Completion venography was performed to exclude complications.

The vascular sheath was removed and adequate hemostasis was achieved at the venotomy site by compression for (_) minutes. Sterile dressing was applied and the patient was transferred to the floor/recovery room following the procedure in a stable condition. Staff was present for the entire procedure.

Description of Procedure *(intra-arterial foreign body retrieval through a femoral approach, using a snare):*
The risks, benefits, alternatives, and procedure itself were explained to the patient/patient's Power of Attorney/patient's legal guardian, and informed written/verbal consent was obtained. Time out was performed to confirm the correct patient, procedure, and site. The site of the procedure was identified and marked.

The skin of both groins were shaved, prepped, and draped in the usual sterile fashion. The right/left common femoral artery was located by palpation/ultrasound and marked. Local anesthesia was administered and a small skin incision was made. Femoral arterial access was obtained using an (_)-gauge [type] needle under direct ultrasound visualization/by palpation. Once good arterial flow was detected, a (_)-inch [type] guidewire was advanced through the needle into the aorta and a (_)-French, (_)-cm-long vascular sheath was placed.

Then, a (_)-French [type] catheter was advanced into the [specify location/artery] over a (0.035)-in. [hydrophilic/type] guidewire. Angiography was performed by injecting (_) mL of [type] contrast and digital subtraction angiography imaging was performed during suspended respiration in an anterior–posterior projection/[specify other projections if obtained] to evaluate the artery and exclude complications. Through the sheath, a vascular retrieval snare [specify type] was advanced with the guiding retrieval catheter, the snare was deployed and the free end of the retained foreign body was encircled. After grasping the object, the guiding catheter was advanced to firmly entrap the retained object. Once the object was entirely within the retrieval device, it was pulled out along with the retrieval catheter through the vascular sheath while maintaining tension on the closed snare loop. The extracted object was inspected for integrity. Completion angiography was performed to exclude complications.

The vascular sheath was removed and adequate hemostasis was achieved at the puncture site by compression for (_) minutes/using a [type] vascular closure device. Sterile dressing was applied and the patient was transferred to the floor/recovery room following the procedure in a stable condition. Staff was present for the entire procedure.

Intra-Procedure Findings: List all relevant findings.

Immediate Complications: None encountered during or directly after the procedure. List complications if any.

Post-Procedure Plan [3]:

Standard post-angiogram management plan

- Keep patient in complete bed rest with the right/left leg extended for (_) hours *[adjust depending on the puncture site]*.
- Check the right/left groin/[specify the puncture site if different] for any bleeding or hematoma formation every 15 min for 1 h, then every 30 min for 1 h, then every hour for 4 h; inform interventional radiology team if any signs of bleeding are observed *[adjust depending on the puncture site]*.
- Check and document lower extremity pulses every 30 min for 2 h then every 1 h for 4 h *[adjust depending on the puncture site]*.
- Monitor vital signs every 15 min for 1 h, then every 30 min for 4 h; notify interventional radiology team if systolic blood pressure <95 mm Hg, or heart rate >110 beats/min.
- Resume diet and previous orders as needed and if otherwise not contraindicated.
- Continue adequate intravenous hydration and monitor fluid (intake–output) status.
- Check complete blood count and creatinine on the day following the procedure or as clinically indicated.
- Perform regular neurological examination when the procedure includes manipulation in the ascending thoracic aorta, aortic arch or brachiocephalic arteries.

Procedure-specific management plan:

- Place the patient on continuous cardiac monitoring for 4–6 h to detect arrhythmia or pericardial tamponade if any occurs.
- Consider heparin for 24–48 h post-procedure, if the patient is at high risk for thrombosis.

Impression:

- Removal of retained intra-arterial/intravenous foreign body as described above.
- The patient tolerated the procedure well and left the interventional unit in a stable condition.
- The patient was unstable and the procedure was canceled/terminated prematurely.
- List any other relevant or important information/finding.

References

1. Carroll MI, Ahanchi SS, Kim JH, Panneton JM. Endovascular foreign body retrieval. J Vasc Surg. 2013;57(2):459–63.
2. Suhocki PV. Foreign body retrieval. In: Mauro MA, Murphy KPJ, Thomson KR, Venbrux AC, Morgan RA, editors. Image-guided interventions. 2nd ed. Philadelphia: Saunders Elsevier; 2014. p. 801–5.
3. Speirs A, Sabharwal T. Retrieval of intravascular foreign bodies. In: Kandarpa K, Machan L, editors. Handbook of interventional radiologic procedures. 4th ed. Philadelphia: Lippincott Williams & Wilkins; 2011. p. 371–6.
4. Floridi C, Nocchi-Cardim L, De Chiara M, Ierardi AM, Carrafiello G. Intravascular foreign bodies: what the radiologist needs to know. Semin Ultrasound CT MR. 2015;36(1):73–9.
5. Tateishi M, Tomizawa Y. Intravascular foreign bodies: danger of unretrieved fragmented medical devices. J Artif Organs. 2009;12(2):80–9.

Part XXIII

Neurovascular Interventional Procedures: Head and Neck Interventions

Introduction by Michel Elias Mawad, Section Reviewer

Interventional and therapeutic procedures for the treatment of cerebrovascular disease have been rapidly evolving over the last 25 years at a very rapid pace. This rapid evolution is due primarily to maturing techniques and methods, improvements in the devices, increasing safety and predictability of the procedures and last but not least revolutionary advances in imaging technology, particularly the addition of in-room parenchymal imaging to vascular opacification.

This section addresses in concise and clearly written chapters many disease processes that the interventional therapist comes across every day.

For each chapter, the authors have appropriately discussed the background and rationale of the endovascular treatment, cited the relevant and recent references and described in a simple and clear style the various relevant techniques.

Additionally, the authors have very conveniently provided reporting templates that cover the various aspects and steps of the procedure. These templates are very useful for any operator, novice or highly experienced in the field, attempting to document the procedure particularly in today's environment of mandatory electronic medical record (EMR). In fact, these dictation templates can easily be adopted as favorite "Smart Text" used by many of us to appropriately describe our work. This will conveniently save precious time in our daily practice and, most importantly, it will standardize our reporting. This standardization in reporting is highly desirable and is becoming absolutely necessary.

The authors have attempted to cover the most important topics in interventional neurological procedures, i.e., acute stroke, arteriovenous malformations, carotid revascularization, aneurysm treatment, etc. However, the reader needs to keep in mind that this section represents a snapshot of the current techniques and trends; these trends will more than likely continue to evolve and change in the future as better devices are developed and as new data emerge on the efficacy or appropriateness of certain therapies. This section serves as a practical guide and an organizational tool in the daily practice of interventional neuroradiology.

Section Chapters

Brain Arteriovenous Malformation Embolization

140

Houssein Darwish, Mohammed Al-Garnawee and Tarek P. Sunna

Abbreviations

BAVM Brain arteriovenous malformation

INTRODUCTION

Brain arteriovenous malformations (BAVMs) are a major cause of intracranial bleed, morbidity, and mortality. They can be supra-tentorial and/or infra-tentorial. BAVMs can be ruptured or unruptured, that is, with symptoms resulting from mass effect, inflammation, altered hemodynamics from direct shunting, or recruitment of dilated perinidal capillary networks. BAVMs are described by nidus as the smallest unit and then it could be either compact or diffuse depending on the presence or absence of intertwining brain tissue. In accordance to the number of feeding vessels to a nidus, BAVMs can be further subdivided into: mono-compartmental or multi-compartmental. BAVMs could have multiple presentations ranging from asymptomatic to severe intracranial hemorrhage. Onadra et al. in 1990 studied patients with different presentations and found that the annual hemorrhage risk is 2–4 %, major morbidity 1.7 %, mortality 1 % and combined morbidity, and mortality 2.7 % per year [1].

The most commonly used grading system for BAVMs is the Spetzler-Martin grading system [2]. Embolization of BAVMs is the essence of our chapter. Multiple embolic agents were used during the 1990s. Ethylene vinyl alcohol copolymer in dimethyl sulfoxide solution (Onyx, Micro Therapeutics, Inc., Irvine, CA) was introduced in 1990 and received FDA approval for pre-surgical embolization of AVMs in 2005. Onyx is now the agent of choice for embolization of BAVMs [3].

COMMON INDICATIONS [4]

- Any BAVM that has been symptomatic whether presenting as seizures, ischemia, and/or bleeding

H. Darwish (✉)
Department of Neurosurgery, University of Virginia Health System, 258 Colonnade Drive, Charlottesville, VA 22903, USA
e-mail: had06_1982@hotmail.com

M. Al-Garnawee
Department of Surgery, Division of Neurosurgery, American University of Beirut Medical Center, Riad El-Solh, Beirut 10017 2020, Lebanon
e-mail: m.garnawee@gmail.com

T.P. Sunna
Department of Neurosurgery, University of Montreal, Montreal, QC, Canada
e-mail: tareksunna@hotmail.com

B. Taslakian et al. (eds.), *Procedural Dictations in Image-Guided Intervention*,
DOI 10.1007/978-3-319-40845-3_140

- Small or large BAVMs with the aim of total cure or under-staging before surgery/ radiosurgery
- BAVMs in eloquent areas that cannot be surgically resected
- Please note that although the design and conclusions of "A Randomized Trial of Unruptured Brain Arteriovenous Malformations (ARUBA)" trial are controversial, and its structure limits analysis of patients who could potentially benefit from treatment; it recommends against interventional therapy for patients with unruptured BAVMs [5].

COMMON CONTRAINDICATIONS [4]

Absolute contraindications:
- Hemodynamic instability with multisystem dysfunction
- BAVM with major intracranial bleed causing brain herniation and a resultant life threatening condition requiring emergency surgical decompression

Relative contraindications:
- Recent myocardial infarction
- Significant arrhythmias
- Prior history of allergy to intravenous contrast media
- Impaired renal function
- Tortuous blood vessels with difficulty in maneuvering and navigating the microcatheters

POSSIBLE COMPLICATIONS [4]

Angiography-related complications (see Chap. 75*)*
Procedure-specific complications:
- Rupture of a BAVM with an accidental closure of the draining veins before the feeding arteries
- Transient neurological disability
- Permanent neurological disability
- Non-disabling non-neurological complications
- Venous infarcts caused by venous embolus from the embolization material
- Air embolus
- Intracranial pseudoaneurysms
- Death

PREPROCEDURAL ASSESSMENT AND PLANNING

- History, indications, and physical examination *(Appendix 1* in Chap. 149*)*. Document indications of the procedure, lower extremity pulses, and vital signs
- Evaluation of diagnostic imaging studies (noninvasive vascular imaging), to determine the relevant anatomy, physiologic, and pathologic conditions
- Periprocedural management of coagulation status *(Appendices 2* in Chap. 150 *and 3* in Chap. 151*)*
- Antibiotic prophylaxis: Not routinely recommended *(Appendices 4* in Chap. 152 *and 5* in Chap. 153*)* [6]
- Imaging modality for guidance: Fluoroscopy; combined with ultrasound for arterial puncture
- Positioning: Supine
- Patient preparation:
  - Start intravenous fluids the night before angiography in order to ensure adequate hydration, combined with effective monitoring of fluid status
  - Insert a urinary catheter or ask the patient to void before the procedure depending on the estimated time of the procedure
  - Considerations for patients with specific diseases or conditions, patients on specific medications or patients with history of multiple comorbidities: obtain subspecialty consultation as needed

PROCEDURE NOTE

Procedure: Endovascular embolization of BAVM
Staff: [_]
Fellow: [_]
Resident: [_]
Clinical Information: Describe history and list indications

Allergies: None known/Allergic to [specify/type of allergy]
Anesthesia: General anesthesia
Medications: List any relevant medications used
Contrast Used: (_) mL of [type] contrast media
Embolic agent: List type, quantity
Field: Sterile
Procedure classification: Clean
Position: Supine
Monitoring: Intravenous access line was secured and vital signs were continuously monitored by nursing staff/anesthesia team throughout the procedure
Total fluoroscopy time: (_) minutes
Cumulative radiation dose: (_) mGy

Description of Procedure:
The risks, benefits, alternatives, and the procedure itself were explained to the patient/patient's Power of Attorney/patient's legal guardian, and informed written consent was obtained. The site of the puncture was identified and marked. Time out was performed to confirm the correct patient, procedure, and site.

The skin of both groins were shaved prepped and draped in the usual sterile fashion. The right/left femoral artery was located by palpation/ultrasound and marked. The site of arterial puncture was determined using combined information from palpation, ultrasound, and fluoroscopy. Local anesthesia was administered. Femoral artery access was obtained using a (_)-gauge [type] needle and the Seldinger technique, double-/single- wall entry under direct ultrasound visualization/by palpation. Once good pulsatile arterial flow was detected, a (_)-inch [type] guidewire was advanced through the needle, up the femoral artery, into the aorta under direct fluoroscopic visualization and a (_)-French, (_) cm long, vascular sheath was placed.

Then, six-vessel diagnostic angiography was performed (bilateral internal carotid, vertebral, and external carotid runs). The diagnostic angiography showed a large left/right (_) mm BAVM in [specify location] with feeders from [specify feeding arteries/branches] and multiple draining veins to the [specify draining vein/venous sinus]. Then after exchange with stiffer longer sheath, and (_)-French guiding catheter to give more support to the microcatheter, a (_) inch [type] microwire and a (_)-French [type] microcatheter were advanced. Intranidal/perinidal super-selective angiography run was done to confirm location of the microcatheter tip within the central part of the nidus*. [Embolic agent] was used under negative road map angiography to occlude the artery but not the draining vein. Angiography runs in between the boluses with tight blood pressure control throughout the procedure and post procedure were performed as well.

Following the procedure the right/left femoral artery sheath was removed and adequate hemostasis was achieved by (_) minute-compression/using [type] vascular closure device. The femoral pulses were checked following the procedure and were [comparable to the preprocedure pulses/specify if otherwise needed]. The patient was transferred to the floor/recovery room/neuro-ICU for close monitoring following the procedure in a stable/critical condition. Staff was present and scrubbed for the entire procedure.

***Note:** The operator should strive diligently to inject the embolic material in the nidus proper. Obliterating the feeding pedicle without obliteration of the nidus is not effective and should be avoided. Also, the operator should make sure the draining veins are not occluded during the embolization process.

Intra-Procedure Findings: List all relevant findings.
Immediate Complications: None encountered during or directly after the procedure. List complications if any.

Post-Procedure Plan [4]:

- *Standard postangiogram management plan:*
  - Keep patient in complete bed rest with the right/left leg extended for (_) hours.
  - Check the right/left groin access site for any bleeding or hematoma formation every 15 min for 1 h, then every 30 min for 1 h, then every 2 h for 4 h; inform interventional radiology team if any observed.

  - Check lower extremity pulses every 30 min for 2 h then every 2 h for 4 h and document findings.
  - Monitor vital signs every 15 min for 1 h, then every 30 min for 4 h; notify interventional radiology team if systolic blood pressure <95 mmHg, or heart rate >110 beat/minute.
  - Resume diet and previous orders as needed and if otherwise not contraindicated.
  - Heparin can be restarted within 2 h after removal of the catheter and puncture site compression, after documenting the absence of puncture site-related problems.
  - Continue adequate intravenous hydration and monitor fluid (intake-output) status.
  - Check puncture site after ambulation.
  - Check complete blood count, creatinine, and blood urea nitrogen on the day following the procedure or as clinically indicated.
- *Procedure-specific management plan:*
  - Transfer patient to the recovery room then to the Neuro-ICU.
  - Neuro-check every 1 h for 24 h.

Impression:

- Embolization of BAVM, as described above.
- The patient tolerated the procedure well and left the interventional unit in stable condition.
- The patient was unstable and the procedure was canceled/terminated prematurely.
- List any other relevant or important information/finding.

References

1. Ondra SL, Troupp H, George ED, Schwab K. The natural history of symptomatic arteriovenous malformations of the brain: a 24-year follow-up assessment. J Neurosurg. 1990;73(3):387–91.
2. Spetzler RF, Martin NA. A proposed grading system for arteriovenous malformations. J Neurosurg. 1986;65(4):476–83.
3. Jahan R, Murayama Y, Gobin YP, Duckwiler GR, Vinters HV, Vinuela F. Embolization of arteriovenous malformations with Onyx: clinicopathological experience in 23 patients. Neurosurgery. 2001;48(5):984–95.
4. Diagnostic cerebral angiography. In: Harrigan MR, Deveikis JP, editors. Handbook of cerebrovascular disease and neurointerventional technique. New York: Springer; 2013. p. 99–131.
5. Mohr JP, Parides MK, Stapf C, Moquete E, Moy CS, Overbey JR, et al. Medical management with or without interventional therapy for unruptured brain arteriovenous malformations (ARUBA): a multicentre, non-blinded, randomised trial. Lancet. 2014;383(9917):614–21.
6. Venkatesan AM, Kundu S, Sacks D, Wallace MJ, Wojak JC, Rose SC, et al. Practice guidelines for adult antibiotic prophylaxis during vascular and interventional radiology procedures. J Vasc Interv Radiol. 2010;21(11):1611–30.

Diagnostic Cerebral Angiography 141

Houssein Darwish, Michele Fouad Chemali and Mohammed Al-Garnawee

INTRODUCTION

Percutaneous techniques for blood vessel imaging are based on the Seldinger technique that started since 1953. Moniz and his colleague Almeida Lima, a neurosurgeon, performed the first angiogram on a living human patient in 1927 [1].

The transition from direct puncture of the cervical vessels to transfemoral artery arteriography began in the late 1960s and became widespread in the 1970s. Nowadays, it is used more for diagnosis of intracranial vascular abnormalities (aneurysms, arteriovenous malformations, vasculitis, and dural fistulas) as well as strokes. More than that, it is used as a bridge to plan for the proper intervention such as coiling, embolization, stenting, and mechanical embolectomy. Complications whether neurological or non-neurological have been reported ranging from 0.03 to 1.8 % [2].

COMMON INDICATIONS [3]

- Diagnosis of primary neurovascular disease *(e.g., intracranial aneurysms, arteriovenous malformations, dural arteriovenous fistulas, atherosclerotic stenosis, vasculopathy, cerebral vasospasm, acute ischemic stroke)*
- Planning for neurovascular interventional procedures
- Intra-operative assistance with aneurysm surgery
- Follow-up imaging after treatment *(e.g., after aneurysm coiling or clipping, treatment of arteriovenous fistulas)*

COMMON CONTRAINDICATIONS

Relative contraindications:
- Recent myocardial infarction
- Significant arrhythmias
- Significant serum electrolyte imbalance
- Prior history of allergy to intravenous contrast media
- Impaired renal function
- Uncooperative patient

Absolute contraindications:
- Hemodynamic instability with multisystem dysfunction

H. Darwish (✉)
Department of Neurosurgery, University of Virginia Health System, 258 Colonnade Drive, Charlottesville, VA 22903, USA
e-mail: had06_1982@hotmail.com

M.F. Chemali
Department of Surgery, American University of Beirut Medical Center, Riad El-Solh, 10017 2020, Beirut, Lebanon
e-mail: michele.chemali@gmail.com

M. Al-Garnawee
Department of Surgery, Division of Neurosurgery, American University of Beirut, Riad El-Solh, 10017 2020 Beirut, Lebanon
e-mail: m.garnawee@gmail.com

B. Taslakian et al. (eds.), *Procedural Dictations in Image-Guided Intervention*,
DOI 10.1007/978-3-319-40845-3_141

POSSIBLE COMPLICATIONS [2]

- Cerebral hemorrhagic *(subarachnoid and intracranial)* and ischemic events
- Air embolus
- Intracranial pseudoaneurysms
- Hemorrhage *(puncture site hematoma, retroperitoneal hematoma if "high" puncture above inguinal ligament)*
- Pseudoaneurysm *(superficial femoral artery "low" puncture)*
- Arteriovenous fistula
- Thrombosis of the femoral artery
- Distal embolization
- Contrast-induced allergic reaction
- Contrast-induced nephropathy
- Fever and chills
- Arterial perforation or dissection
- Catheter or guide wire breakage
- Limb amputation *(rare)*
- Mortality *(rare)*

PREPROCEDURAL ASSESSMENT AND PLANNING

- History, indications, and physical examination *(Appendix 1* in Chap. 149*)*; document indications of the procedure, lower or upper extremity pulses and vital signs
- Evaluation of diagnostic imaging studies to determine the relevant vascular anatomy and assess the access site
- Periprocedural management of coagulation status *(Appendices 2* in Chap. 150 *and 3* in Chap. 151*)*
- Antibiotic prophylaxis: Not routinely recommended *(Appendices 4* in Chap. 152 *and 5* in Chap. 153*)* [4]
- Imaging modality for guidance: Fluoroscopy; combined with ultrasound for arterial puncture
- Positioning: Supine
- Arterial access: Common femoral artery, left brachial artery, left axillary artery
- Patient preparation:
  - Start intravenous fluids the night before angiography in order to ensure adequate hydration, combined with effective monitoring of fluid status
  - Insert a urinary catheter or ask the patient to void before the procedure depending on the estimated time of the procedure
  - Considerations for patients with specific diseases or conditions, patients on specific medications or patients with history of multiple comorbidities: consult with the referring clinician, and obtain subspecialty consultation as needed

PROCEDURE NOTE

Procedure: Catheter-directed diagnostic cerebral angiography
Staff: [_]
Fellow: [_]
Resident: [_]
Clinical Information: Describe history and list the indications
Allergies: None known/Allergic to [specify/type of allergy]
Anesthesia: General anesthesia/Local anesthesia/Conscious sedation
Medications: List any relevant medications used
Contrast Used: (_) mL of [type] contrast media
Field: Sterile
Procedure classification: Clean
Position: Supine
Monitoring: Intravenous access line was secured and vital signs were continuously monitored by nursing staff/anesthesia team throughout the procedure
Total fluoroscopy time: (_) min
Cumulative radiation dose: (_) mGy

Description of Procedure:

The risks, benefits, alternatives, and the procedure itself were explained to the patient/patient's Power of Attorney/patient's legal guardian, and informed written consent was obtained. The site of the procedure was identified and marked. Time out was performed to confirm the correct patient, procedure, and site.

The skin of both groins were shaved, prepped, and draped in the usual sterile fashion. The right/left common femoral artery as well as the inguinal ligament were located by palpation/ultrasound and marked. The site of arterial puncture was determined using combined information from palpation, ultrasound, and fluoroscopy over the middle of the medial third of the femoral head. Local anesthesia was administered. Common femoral artery access was obtained using a (_)-gauge [type] needle and the Seldinger technique under direct ultrasound visualization/by palpation. Once good pulsatile arterial flow was detected, a (_)-inch [type] guide wire was advanced through the needle, into the aorta under direct fluoroscopic visualization and a (_)-French vascular sheath was placed.

A (_)-French [type] vascular catheter was introduced over a (_)-inch hydrophilic [type] and manipulated into the thoracic arch, then into the brachiocephalic trunk into the right common carotid artery. At this stage right common carotid run was performed to check for the position of the internal carotid artery. The catheter tip was then navigated trough the proximal part of the right internal carotid artery. Anteroposterior, lateral, and oblique views of the head run were obtained, showing [document findings].

Then the catheter was retrieved to the brachiocephalic trunk and the tip was manipulated into the subclavian artery and from there to the right vertebral artery. Head runs with anteroposterior and lateral views were obtained. Then the catheter tip was retrieved back to the aortic arch after confirming the absence of vertebral artery spasm. Left carotid and vertebral angiography was performed in the same fashion.

During angiography, double flushing was performed consisting of aspiration of the contents of the catheter with one 10-mL syringe of heparinized saline, followed by partial aspiration and irrigation with a second syringe of saline, to ensure clearing clots and air bubbles from the catheter. This was repeated every time a wire was removed from the catheter, prior to the injection of contrast.

Following the procedure the right/left femoral artery sheath was removed and adequate hemostasis was achieved by compression for (_) minutes/using [type] vascular closure device. The lower extremity pulses were checked following the procedure and were [comparable to the preprocedural pulses/specify if otherwise needed]. The patient was transferred to the floor/recovery room for close monitoring following the procedure in a stable condition. Staff was present for the entire procedure.

Intra-Procedure Findings: List all the relevant findings.

Immediate Complications: None were encountered during or directly after the procedure. List complications if any.

Post-Procedure Plan [3]:

- Keep patient in complete bed rest with the right/left leg extended for (_) h.
- Check the right/left groin for any bleeding and/or hematoma formation every 15 min for 1 h, then every 30 min for 1 h, then every hour for 4 h; inform interventional radiology team if any observed.
- Check lower extremity pulses and color every 30 min for 2 h then every 1 h for 4 h and document the findings.
- Monitor vital signs every 15 min for 1 h, then every 30 min for 4 h; notify interventional radiology team if systolic blood pressure <95 mmHg, or heart rate >110 beats/min.
- Transfer patient to the recovery room.
- Check puncture site after ambulation.
- Continue adequate intravenous hydration and monitor fluid (intake–output) status.
- Check complete blood count, creatinine, and blood urea nitrogen on the day following the procedure or as clinically indicated.

Impression:

- Cerebral angiography, as described above.
- The patient tolerated the procedure well and left the interventional unit in stable condition.
- The patient was unstable and the procedure was canceled/terminated prematurely.
- List any other relevant or important information/findings.

References

1. Krayenbühl H. History of cerebral angiography and its development since Egaz Moniz. In: Egas Moniz Centenary: Scientific Reports. Lisbon: Comissao Executiva das Comemoracoes do Centenario do Nascimento do Prof. Egas Moniz; 1977. P. 63–74.
2. Willinsky RA, Taylor SM, TerBrugge K, Farb RI, Tomlinson G, Montanera W. Neurologic complications of cerebral angiography: prospective analysis of 2,899 procedures and review of the literature. Radiology. 2003;227:522–8.
3. Diagnostic cerebral angiograpy. In: Harrigan MR, Deveikis JP, editors. Handbook of cerebrovascualr disease and neurointerventional technique. New York: Springer; 2013. P. 99–131.
4. Venkatesan AM, Kundu S, Sacks D, Wallace MJ, Wojak JC, Rose SC, et al. Practice guidelines for adult antibiotic prophylaxis during vascular and interventional radiology procedures. J Vasc Interv Radiol. 2010;21(11):1611–30.

Endovascular Management of Epistaxis

142

Bedros Taslakian and Hiba H. Sharafeldeen

Abbreviations

ECA	External carotid artery
SPA	Sphenopalatine artery
DPA	Descending palatine artery
IMA	Internal maxillary artery
ICA	Internal carotid artery

INTRODUCTION

Sixty percent of the population suffers from epistaxis during their lifetime. Epistaxis may affect any age group and is generally self-limiting. In most patients, epistaxis arises from the anteroinferior septal area (Little's area), which is supplied by branches of the external carotid artery (ECA)—the sphenopalatine artery, greater palatine artery, and superior labial artery [1]. The anterior and posterior ethmoidal branches of the ophthalmic artery usually arise from the internal carotid artery (ICA) anastomose with the nasal branches of the sphenopalatine artery, providing additional supply to this region [1]. Because this vasculature is readily accessible, hemorrhage from this region can usually be managed by local measures. In approximately 5 % of patients, epistaxis originates more posteriorly in the nasal cavity, causing these initial measures to fail [2]. If bleeding continues despite packing, or recurs after pack removal, subsequent treatment can consist of surgical ligation, endoscopic surgical procedures, or endovascular embolization of the arteries supplying the nasal fossa. The primary success rate of endovascular treatment is between 71 and 100 % [3].

Endovascular treatment of epistaxis was first presented as an alternative to surgery by Sokoloff et al. [4] and consisted of particle embolization of the ipsilateral internal maxillary artery (IMA). The technique was later refined by Lasjaunias et al., stressing the need for a standardized angiographic and therapeutic approach. It has gained increased acceptance, and several large series have been reported.

B. Taslakian (✉)
Department of Radiology, New York University Langone Medical Center, 660 First Ave, New York, NY 10016, USA
e-mail: btaslakian@gmail.com

H.H. Sharafeldeen
Department of Neurosurgery, American University of Beirut Medical Center, Riad El-Solh, 10017 2020, Beirut, Lebanon
e-mail: hs78@aub.edu.lb

B. Taslakian et al. (eds.), *Procedural Dictations in Image-Guided Intervention*,
DOI 10.1007/978-3-319-40845-3_142

COMMON INDICATIONS [5–7]

- Intractable epistaxis despite packing
- Recurrent epistaxis after packing removal, especially if posterior
- Traumatic epistaxis not controlled by less invasive measures
- Delayed epistaxis after trauma due to pseudoaneurysm formation
- Epistaxis due to arteriovenous malformation when either the lesion itself or its venous drainage pattern involves the oronasal cavity
- Refractory recurrent epistaxis in hereditary hemorrhagic telangiectasia
- Sinonasal neoplasm, especially juvenile nasopharyngeal angiofibroma *(embolization before surgery can reduce intraoperative bleeding, improve visualization of the surgical field, and allow for a more complete and uncomplicated resection)*

COMMON CONTRAINDICATIONS

- Filling of ECA-ICA anastomoses in the designated artery for embolization with the risk of cerebral infarction
- Bleeding from ethmoidal arteries, arising from the ophthalmic artery—even distal to the origin of the central retinal artery—with the risk of post-interventional blindness

Relative contraindications:

- Past history of allergy to intravenous contrast media
- Pregnancy
- Impaired renal function

POSSIBLE COMPLICATIONS [1, 5–9]

Angiography-related complications: Please refer to Chap. 75.

Procedure-specific complications:

- Necrosis of soft tissue of cheek or the tongue
- Trismus
- Numbness or swelling of cheek
- Temporofacial pain and headache
- Failure of embolization due to continued bleeding from the ethmoidal branches of the ophthalmic artery
- Blindness
- Generalized grand mal seizure
- Homolateral facial palsy
- Cerebrovascular accidents
- Facial atrophy

PREPROCEDURAL ASSESSMENT AND PLANNING

- History, indications, and physical examination *(Appendix 1* in Chap. 149*)*. Document indications of the procedure, lower or upper extremity pulses, and vital signs.
- Evaluation of diagnostic imaging studies to determine the relevant vascular anatomy and assess the access site. A diagnostic preembolization angiogram of the ICA and ECA may reveal specific abnormalities indicating the cause and location of the hemorrhage. These include contrast extravasation, a tumor blush, a vascular malformation, a traumatic pseudoaneurysm, or another unusual ICA source of epistaxis. Furthermore, angiography enables identification of vascular anomalies, variants, or anastomoses between the ECA and ICA or ophthalmic artery that could increase the risk of complications, such as stroke or blindness during embolization. These findings may influence the embolization protocol or even lead to aborting the procedure and referral to surgery
- Periprocedural management of coagulation status *(Appendices 2* in Chap. 150 *and 3* in Chap. 151*)*
- Antibiotic prophylaxis: Not routinely recommended
- Imaging modality for guidance: Fluoroscopy; combined with ultrasound for arterial puncture
- Positioning: Supine
- Arterial access: Common femoral artery
- The nose should be packed before the procedure and unpacked after the procedure by a specialist

PROCEDURE NOTE

Procedure: Endovascular treatment of epistaxis
Staff: [_]
Fellow: [_]
Resident: [_]
Clinical Information: Describe history and list indications
Allergies: None known /Allergic to [specify/type of allergy]
Anesthesia: Local anesthesia/Monitored conscious sedation/General anesthesia (preferred to protect airways in patients with uncontrolled bleeding)
Medications: List any relevant medications used
Contrast Material: (_) mL of [type] contrast material
Field: Sterile
Procedure classification: Clean
Position: Supine
Monitoring: Intravenous access line was secured and vital signs were continuously monitored by nursing staff/anesthesia team throughout the procedure
Total fluoroscopy time: (_) min
Cumulative radiation dose: (_) mGy

Description of Procedure:

The risks, benefits, alternatives, and the procedure itself were explained to the patient/patient's Power of Attorney/patient's legal guardian, and informed written consent was obtained. The site of the procedure was identified and marked. Time out was performed to confirm the correct patient, procedure, and site.

The skin of both groins were shaved, prepped, and draped in the usual sterile fashion. The right/left common femoral artery as well as the inguinal ligament were located by palpation/ultrasound and marked. The site of arterial puncture was determined using combined information from palpation, ultrasound, and fluoroscopy over the middle of the medial third of the femoral head. Local anesthesia was administered. Common femoral artery access was obtained using a (_)-gauge [type] needle and the Seldinger technique under direct ultrasound visualization/by palpation. Once good pulsatile arterial flow was detected, a (_)-inch [type] guidewire was advanced through the needle, into the aorta under direct fluoroscopic visualization and a (_)-French vascular sheath was placed.

Intravenous heparin was administered (5000-unit bolus, 1000 units/h thereafter). All catheters were flushed with pressurized heparinized normal saline solution (1 unit of heparin/mL).

A (_)-French [type] vascular catheter was introduced over a (_)-inch hydrophilic [type] and manipulated into the thoracic arch, then into the right common carotid artery. At this stage, right common carotid run was performed to check for the position of the internal and external carotid arteries. The catheter tip was then navigated through the proximal part of the right internal carotid artery. Anteroposterior, lateral, and oblique views of the head run were obtained, showing [document findings]. [**Note:** Internal carotid artery evaluation is performed to confirm supply to the ophthalmic artery and choroidal blush from the internal carotid artery, rule out an internal carotid artery source of bleeding, and check for extensive supply to nasal mucosa from the ethmoidal arteries].

Then the catheter was inserted into the external carotid artery, and angiography was performed showing [document findings] [**Note:** evaluation should rule out vascular anomalies and nonidiopathic causes of epistaxis and check for dangerous anastomoses between the ECA and ICA; also evaluate for significant supply from the facial artery to the nasal mucosa].

The same was performed on the left side and angiography of the left internal and external carotid artery showed [document findings].

Then, the guiding catheter was placed at the right/left external carotid artery origin, ipsilateral to the previously identified bleeding nostril. Coaxially, a (_)-French microcatheter was navigated selectively through the internal maxillary artery into [name the artery which was selected for embolization]. After confirming the bleeding site with selective angiography, embolization was performed with a suspension of polyvinyl alcohol (PVA) particles (250–350 μm) in contrast medium/injection of gelfoam pledgets proximally into the [name the artery].

During angiography, double flushing was performed consisting of aspiration of the contents of the catheter with one 10-mL syringe of heparinized saline, followed by partial aspiration and irrigation with a second syringe of saline, to ensure clearing clots and air bubbles from the catheter. This was repeated every time a wire was removed from the catheter, prior to the injection of contrast.

Following the procedure the heparin activity was reversed with protamine [specify dose] and then the right/left femoral artery sheath was removed and adequate hemostasis was achieved by compression for (_) min/using [type] vascular closure device. The lower extremity pulses were checked following the procedure and were [-comparable to the pre-procedure pulses/specify if otherwise needed]. The patient was transferred to the floor/recovery room for close monitoring following the procedure in a stable condition. Staff was present for the entire procedure.

Notes:

- Usually selective embolization of the sphenopalatine artery is recommended; coils should be avoided to occlude the sphenopalatine artery proximally.
- In patients with complex anatomy, catheterization of the pterygopalatine portion of the internal maxillary artery may also provide a safe and acceptable embolization point; if a significant supply is identified from the facial artery to the nasal mucosa, embolization beyond the submandibular artery can be performed; if no bleeding point is identified, embolization of the contralateral sphenopalatine artery—internal maxillary artery and the contralateral facial artery can be performed.
- Avoid using stiff guidewires or stiff microcatheters when catheterizing the arteries supplying the nasal mucosa. The operator should use soft micowires and soft-tip microcatheters to avoid inducing vasospasm in the arteries being embolized.
- It should be noted that insisting on very distal and superselective catheterization of the arteries can open dangerous anastomoses to the ophthalmic artery or intracranial circulation that can result in disastrous complications.
- A thorough knowledge of the complex vascular anatomy and the potential dangerous anastomoses is essential in planning and performing the procedure as well as avoiding complications.

Intra-Procedure Findings: List all relevant findings.

Immediate Complications: None encountered during or directly after the procedure. List complications if any.

Post-Procedure Plan:

- Transfer patient to the recovery room.
- Keep patient complete bed rest with the right/left leg extended for (_) h.
- Check the right/left groin for any bleeding and/or hematoma formation every 15 min for 1 h, then every 30 min for 1 h, then every hour for 4 h; inform interventional radiology team if any observed.
- Check lower extremity pulses and color every 30 min for 2 h then every 1 h for 4 h and document the findings.
- Monitor vital signs every 15 min for 1 h, then every 30 min for 4 h; notify interventional radiology team if systolic blood pressure <95 mmHg, or heart rate >110 beats/min.
- Nasal packs are usually left in place for 12–24 h and then removed by a specialist.
- Check puncture site after ambulation.
- Continue adequate intravenous hydration and monitor fluid (intake–output) status.
- Check complete blood count, creatinine, and blood urea nitrogen on the day following the procedure or as clinically indicated.

- Discontinue Intravenous access before discharge.

Impression:

- Embolization of [specify artery] for management of epistaxis, as described above.
- The patient tolerated the procedure well and left the interventional unit in stable condition.
- The patient was unstable and the procedure was canceled/terminated prematurely.
- The patient refused to undergo/complete the procedure.
- List any other relevant or important information/finding.

References

1. Koh E, Frazzini VI, Kagetsu NJ. Epistaxis: vascular anatomy, origins, and endovascular treatment. AJR Am J Roentgenol. 2000;174(3):845–51.
2. Viducich RA, Blanda MP, Gerson LW. Posterior epistaxis: clinical features and acute complications. Ann Emerg Med. 1995;25(5):592–6.
3. Tseng EY, Narducci CA, Willing SJ, Sillers MJ. Angiographic embolization for epistaxis: a review of 114 cases. Laryngoscope. 1998;108(4 Pt 1):615–9.
4. Sokoloff J, Wickbom I, McDonald D, Brahme F, Goergen TC, Goldberger LE. Therapeutic percutaneous embolization in intractable epistaxis. Radiology. 1974;111(2):285–7.
5. Cohen JE, Moscovici S, Gomori JM, Eliashar R, Weinberger J, Itshayek E. Selective endovascular embolization for refractory idiopathic epistaxis is a safe and effective therapeutic option: technique, complications, and outcomes. J Clin Neurosci. 2012;19(5):687–90.
6. Johnson MH. Vascular emergencies of the head and neck. In: Kandarpa K, Machan L, editors. Handbook of interventional radiologic procedures. 4th ed. Philadelphia: Lippincott Williams & Wilkins; 2011. p. 156–71.
7. Chewning RH, Wyse GM, Philippe G, Kieran PJM. Endovascular management of epistaxis. In: Mauro MA, Murphy KPJ, Thomson KR, Venbrux AC, Morgan RA, editors. Image-guided interventions. 2nd ed. Philadelphia: Saunders Elsevier; 2014. P. 720–4.
8. Wehrli M, Lieberherr U, Valavanis A. Superselective embolization for intractable epistaxis: experiences with 19 patients. Clin Otolaryngol Allied Sci. 1988;13(6):415–20.
9. Elahi MM, Parnes LS, Fox AJ, Pelz DM, Lee DH. Therapeutic embolization in the treatment of intractable epistaxis. Arch Otolaryngol Head Neck Surg. 1995;121(1):65–9.

Extracranial Carotid Artery Angioplasty and Stenting

143

Tarek P. Sunna, Fahed Zairi and Houssein Darwish

Abbreviations

CCA	Common carotid artery
ICA	Internal carotid artery
ECA	External carotid artery
CEA	Carotid endarterectomy
CAS	Carotid artery stenting
EPD	Embolic protection devices

INTRODUCTION

Balloon angioplasty of extracranial carotid artery stenoses to prevent stroke was first reported >30 years ago [1]. Thereafter, reports of carotid artery stenting (CAS), with or without embolic protection devices (EPDs), began to appear [2, 3]. CAS was developed to address the need for carotid revascularization in patients in whom open surgery is either difficult to perform or who are at high risk of complications.

Carotid artery stenting may be one of the most studied clinical procedures in medicine, but one of the primary confounders in assessing CAS outcomes has been the dynamic, evolving nature of the CAS procedure compared with the mature, stable carotid endarterectomy (CEA) procedure. CAS procedures today produce more favorable outcomes than those performed 15 years ago, and the dramatic improvement can be attributed to improved equipment as well as the increased experience of operators and endovascular teams.

More than three fourths of a million strokes occur each year, making it the third leading cause of death in the United States. Ischemic strokes, which are the most common, are often caused by atherosclerotic emboli from the carotid artery or aortic arch or are related to thromboembolism from the heart chamber. The incidence of asymptomatic extracranial carotid stenosis (50 %) in persons older than 65 years of age is estimated to be between 5 and 10 %, but less

T.P. Sunna (✉)
Department of Neurosurgery,
University of Montreal, Montreal, QC, Canada
e-mail: tareksunna@hotmail.com

H. Darwish
Department of Neurosurgery, University of Virginia
Health System, 258 Colonnade Drive,
Charlottesville, VA 22903, USA
e-mail: had06_1982@hotmail.com

F. Zairi
Department of Neurosurgery, Lille University
Hospital, Rue Emile Laine, 59000 Lille, France
e-mail: fahed.zairi@gmail.com

B. Taslakian et al. (eds.), *Procedural Dictations in Image-Guided Intervention*,
DOI 10.1007/978-3-319-40845-3_143

than 1 % have a critical stenosis (>80 %) [4]. Moreover, whereas 10–20 % of all strokes arise from atherosclerotic carotid artery stenosis, most symptoms are due to carotid artery plaque rupture and only a minority to carotid artery occlusion. Risk assessment can be affected by variables such as symptom status, stenosis severity, existence of plaque ulceration, and the nature of the plaque (lipid rich, sclerotic, homogeneous, or heterogeneous in composition) [5]. In the NASCET (North American Symptomatic Carotid Endarterectomy Trial), the 2-year stroke rate was 22 % among those with moderate (50–69 %) stenosis and 26 % with significant (70–99 %) carotid stenosis [6]. Therefore, as difficult as it might be, identifying which asymptomatic patients with CAS are at high risk of stroke is important.

COMMON INDICATIONS [7]

- Symptomatic, severe stenosis that is surgically difficult to access *(e.g., high bifurcation requiring mandibular dislocation)*
- Symptomatic, severe stenosis in a patient with a significant medical disease that would make the patient high risk for surgery
- Severe stenosis associated with contralateral carotid artery occlusion requiring treatment before undergoing cardiac surgery
- Severe underlying carotid artery stenosis revealed after recanalization of carotid occlusion after thrombolysis for acute stroke *(presumed to be the etiology of the treated occlusion)* or to enable thrombolysis for acute stroke
- Pseudoaneurysm
- Asymptomatic pre-occlusive lesion in a patient otherwise meeting criteria for treatment
- Symptomatic severe stenosis *and* one of the following conditions:
  - Significant tandem lesion that may require endovascular therapy
  - Radiation-induced stenosis
  - Restenosis after carotid endarterectomy
  - Refusal to undergo carotid endarterectomy after proper informed consent
  - Stenosis secondary to arterial dissection
  - Stenosis secondary to fibromuscular dysplasia
  - Stenosis secondary to Takayasu arteritis

COMMON CONTRAINDICATIONS [7]

- Asymptomatic stenosis of any degree, except in particular circumstances, as described above
- Symptomatic stenosis associated with an intracranial vascular malformation
- Symptomatic stenosis in a patient with a subacute cerebral infarction
- Symptomatic stenosis in a patient with a significant contraindication to angiography
- Absolute Contraindications:
  - Carotid stenosis with angiographically visible intraluminal thrombus
  - A stenosis that cannot be safely reached or crossed by an endovascular approach

POSSIBLE COMPLICATIONS [7]

Angiography-related complications: refer to Chap. 75.

Procedure-specific complications

- Cerebral hemorrhagic (subarachnoid and intracranial) and ischemic events
- Air embolus
- Intracranial pseudoaneurysms
- Distal embolization
- Mortality

PREPROCEDURAL ASSESSMENT AND PLANNING

- History, indications and physical examination *(Appendix 1* in Chap. 149*)*. Document indications of the procedure, lower or upper extremity pulses and vital signs.
- Evaluation of diagnostic imaging studies to determine the relevant vascular anatomy.

Baseline carotid duplex exam and confirmatory study (e.g., CTA, MRA, or catheter angiogram).

- Periprocedural management of coagulation status *(Appendices 2* in Chap. 150 *and 3* in Chap. 151*)*
- Antibiotic prophylaxis: Not routinely recommended *(Appendices 4* in Chap. 152 *and 5* in Chap. 153*)*
- Imaging modality for guidance: Fluoroscopy; combined with ultrasound for arterial puncture
- Positioning: Supine
- Arterial access: Common femoral artery, left brachial artery, left axillary artery
- Patient preparation:
  – Antiplatelet therapy [8–10]:
    ▪ Aspirin 325-mg PO QD for ≥3 days prior to the procedure and clopidogrel (Plavix®, Bristol-Myers-Squibb, NY, NY, USA) 75-mg PO QD for ≥3 days prior to the procedure.
    ▪ Or aspirin 325-mg PO QD for ≥3 days prior to the procedure and ticlopidine (Ticlid®, Hoffmann-La Roche, Basel, Switzerland) for ≥3 days prior to the procedure.
    ▪ Alternatively, a loading dose of Aspirin 325-mg PO and clopidogrel 300-mg PO can be given the day before or at least 5 h before the procedure.
    ▪ Stroke associated with carotid stenting is a major cause of morbidity and antiplatelet (aspirin and clopidogrel) resistance is becoming a recognizable entity as a potential cause for failure in stroke prevention. Up to 40 % and 15–48 % of patients may be resistant to aspirin and clopidogrel, respectively. Antiplatelet resistance can be routinely tested prior to stenting procedures using bedside tests (i.e., point of care analysis) that rapidly measures platelet function such as "verify now" (Accumetrics, CA, USA) system or the PFA-100™ System (Dade Behring, Germany). VerifyNow® results are reported in $P2Y_{12}$ reaction units (PRUs), with a lower PRU value corresponding to a higher degree of $P2Y_{12}$ receptor inhibition, and, hence, a decreased likelihood of platelet activation (i.e., hyper-response to clopidogrel) and aggregation; and a higher PRU value corresponding to a lower degree of $P2Y_{12}$ receptor inhibition and, hence, an increased likelihood of platelet activation and aggregation (i.e., hyporesponse to clopidogrel). Adjustments to the dose or type of $P2Y_{12}$ receptor antagonist might be required to keep PRU values within the 60–200 target $P2Y_{12}$ reaction units range.
    ▪ Ticagrelor and Cangrelor are newer antiplatelet agents that do not require metabolic activation to inhibit the $P2Y_{12}$ receptor, therefore are not subject to resistance and can be used as alternative antiplatelet agents.

✓ Place two peripheral intravenous lines
✓ Place Foley catheter
✓ NPO after midnight or 6 h prior to the procedure except for medications
✓ Hold routine antihypertensive medications on the morning of the procedure
✓ Make sure that all devices that may be needed are available in the interventional suite prior to the procedure

PROCEDURE NOTE

Procedure: Endovascular left/right extracranial carotid artery angioplasty and stenting
Staff: [_]
Fellow: [_]
Resident: [_]
Clinical Information: Describe history and list indications
Allergies: None known/Allergic to [specify/type of allergy]
Anesthesia: General anesthesia/Local anesthesia/ Conscious sedation
Medications: List any relevant medications used (sedation, heparin)
Contrast Used: (_) mL of [type] contrast media
Field: Sterile

Procedure classification: Clean
Position: Supine
Monitoring: Intravenous access line was secured and vital signs were continuously monitored by nursing staff/anesthesia team throughout the procedure
Total fluoroscopy time: (_) minutes
Cumulative radiation dose: (_) mGy

Description of Procedure: The risks, benefits, alternatives, and the procedure itself were explained to the patient/patient's Power of Attorney/patient's legal guardian, and informed written consent was obtained. The site of the procedure was identified and marked. Time out was performed to confirm the correct patient, procedure and site.

The skin of both groins were shaved, prepped and draped in the usual sterile fashion. The right/left common femoral artery as well as the inguinal ligament were located by palpation/ultrasound and marked. The site of arterial puncture was determined using combined information from palpation, ultrasound, and fluoroscopy over the middle of the medial third of the femoral head. Local anesthesia was administered. Common femoral artery access was obtained using a (_)-gauge [type] needle and the Seldinger technique under direct ultrasound visualization/by palpation. Once good pulsatile arterial flow was detected, a (_)-inch [type] guidewire was advanced through the needle, into the aorta under direct fluoroscopic visualization and a (_)-French vascular sheath was placed.

After 5 min, loading dose of intravenous heparin (70 U/kg) was given. Measured ACT was (_) seconds. Then, a (_)-French [type] vascular catheter was introduced over a (_)-inch hydrophilic [type] guidewire and manipulated into the thoracic arch, then into the right/left common carotid artery. At this stage common carotid run was performed to check for the position of the internal carotid artery. The catheter tip was then navigated trough the proximal part of the internal carotid artery. Anterior-posterior, lateral, and oblique contrast run views of right/left common carotid artery and internal carotid artery were obtained. Diameters of the common carotid artery, internal carotid artery, region of greatest stenosis, and the length of the plaque to be covered were (_), (_), (_), (_) mm, respectively. Then the diagnostic catheter was placed in the right/left common carotid artery/internal carotid artery. An exchange length (_)-inch stiff [type] catheter was placed in the carotid system to exchange the femoral sheath for a longer (_)-French, (_) cm [type] sheath. The exchange was performed under fluoroscopic guidance to make sure that the distal tip of the stiff wire was not pushing against the plaque. The distal end of the new sheath was positioned (_) cm proximal/distal to the carotid bifurcation. Then the exchange wire was withdrawn. Aspiration of (_) mL of blood was done through the sheath to confirm adequate flow and the absence of any clots. The sheath was then connected to continuous pressurized flushing system throughout the procedure. The high flow head run was performed before starting the stenting phase. In the stenting phase, a [type] embolic protection device was guided under fluoroscopy and was deployed (_) cm distal to the plaque under fluoroscopy slowly and carefully. After that, a gross neurological exam was performed. Again an angiogram was performed to check for any dislodgement of the plaque.

Following this, angioplasty was performed using a (_) × (_) mm [type] balloon. Pressure was continuously monitored during the slow inflation of the balloon. Atropine (_) mg was administered intravenously. Then the balloon was removed and neurological exam showed neurological deficit [specify]/no neurological deficit.

Under road map guidance a (_) × (_) mm [type] stent was deployed. This was followed by angiogram of the carotid tree and intracranial vessels. Post-stent-deployment angioplasty was performed using a (6-6.5) × (20) mm [type] balloon. The embolic protection device was then retrieved.

During angiography, double flushing was performed consisting of aspiration of the contents of the catheter with one 10-mL syringe of heparinized saline, followed by partial aspiration and irrigation with a second syringe of saline, to ensure clearing clots and air bubbles from the catheter. This was repeated every time a wire was removed from the catheter, prior to the injection of contrast.

Following the procedure, the right/left femoral artery sheath was removed and adequate hemostasis was achieved by compression for (_) minutes/using [type] vascular closure device. The lower extremity pulses were checked following the procedure and were [comparable to the preprocedural pulses/specify if otherwise needed]. The patient was transferred to the floor/recovery room for close monitoring following the procedure in a stable condition. Staff was present for the entire procedure.

Intra-Procedure Findings: List all relevant findings.
Immediate Complications: None encountered during or directly after the procedure. List complications if any.

Post-Procedure Plan [7–9]:

- Keep patient complete bed rest with the right/left leg extended for (_) hours.
- Check the right/left groin for any bleeding and/or hematoma formation every 15 min for 1 h, then every 30 min for 1 h, then every hour for 4 h; inform interventional radiology team if any observed.
- Check lower extremity pulses and color every 30 min for 2 h then every 1 h for 4 h and document the findings.
- Transfer patient to the recovery room.
- Monitor vital signs closely in the first 24–48 h; notify interventional radiology team if systolic blood pressure <95 mmHg or ≥140 mmHg, or heart rate >110 beats/minute. Hypertension after carotid stenting can predispose to intracranial bleeding.
- Check puncture site after ambulation.
- Continue adequate intravenous hydration and monitor fluid (intake–output) status.
- Check complete blood count, creatinine and blood urea nitrogen on the day following the procedure or as clinically indicated.
- Perform complete neurological exam in the recovery room every 15 min.
- Admit to neuro-ICU or step-down unit with neuro exams every 1 h.
- Antiplatelet therapy: Aspirin 325-mg PO QD indefinitely *and* Clopidogrel (Plavix®) 75-mg PO QD for 30 days after the procedure.
- For patients with hypotension: Hypotension after carotid artery stenting and angioplasty is usually self-limited and resolves within 1–2 days. A cardiac work-up should be done to exclude a myocardial infarction.

Impression:

- Angioplasty and stenting of right/left common/internal carotid artery, as described above.
- The patient tolerated the procedure well and left the interventional unit in stable condition.
- The patient was unstable and the procedure was canceled/terminated prematurely.
- The patient refused to undergo/complete the procedure.
- List any other relevant or important information/finding.

References

1. Kerber CW, Cromwell LD, Loehden OL. Catheter dilatation of proximal carotid stenosis during distal bifurcation endarterectomy. AJNR Am J Neuroradiol. 1980 Jul-Aug;1(4):348–9.
2. Roubin GS, Yadav S, Iyer SS, Vitek J. Carotid stent-supported angioplasty: a neurovascular intervention to prevent stroke. Am J Cardiol. 1996;78 (3A):8–12.
3. Theron JG, Payelle GG, Coskun O, Huet HF, Guimaraens L. Carotid artery stenosis: treatment with protected balloon angioplasty and stent placement. Radiology. 1996;201(3):627–36.
4. Goldstein LB, Adams R, Alberts MJ, Appel LJ, Brass LM, Bushnell CD, et al. Primary prevention of ischemic stroke: a guideline from the American Heart Association/American Stroke Association Stroke Council: cosponsored by the Atherosclerotic Peripheral Vascular Disease Interdisciplinary Working Group; Cardiovascular Nursing Council; Clinical Cardiology Council; Nutrition, Physical Activity, and Metabolism Council; and the Quality of Care and Outcomes Research Interdisciplinary Working Group. Circulation. 2006;113(24):e873–923.
5. Aichner FT, Topakian R, Alberts MJ, Bhatt DL, Haring HP, Hill MD, et al. High cardiovascular event rates in patients with asymptomatic carotid stenosis:

the REACH Registry. Eur J Neurol. 2009;16 (8):902–8.
6. Ferguson GG, Eliasziw M, Barr HW, Clagett GP, Barnes RW, Wallace MC, et al. The North American Symptomatic Carotid Endarterectomy Trial: surgical results in 1415 patients. Stroke. 1999;30 (9):1751–8.
7. Diagnostic cerebral angiograpy. In: Harrigan MR, Deveikis JP. Handbook of Cerebrovascualr Disease and Neurointerventional Technique. NewYork: Springer; 2013:99–131.
8. Enomoto Yukiko, Yoshimura Shinichi. Antiplatelet Therapy for Carotid Artery Stenting. Interv Neurol. 2013;1(3–4):151–63.
9. Ooi YC, Gonzalez NR. Management of extracranial carotid artery disease. Cardiol Clin. 2015;33 (1):1–35.
10. Fifi JT, Brockington C, Narang J, Leesch W, Ewing SL, Bennet H, et al. Clopidogrel resistance is associated with thromboembolic complications in patients undergoing neurovascular stenting. American Journal of Neuroradiology. 2013;34 (4):716–20.

Intracranial Aneurysm Coil Embolization

144

Mohammed Al-Garnawee, Faten El Ammar and Houssein Darwish

INTRODUCTION

The prevalence of intracranial aneurysms can reach up to 6 % [1] responsible for about 85 % of non-traumatic subarachnoid hemorrhages [2]. The pathophysiology of their formation is related to complex interaction between hemodynamic stress, vascular remodeling, and inflammatory response [3].

In addition to family history of aneurysms, many conditions are associated with development of intracranial aneurysms such as Autosomal Dominant Polycystic Kidney Disease, Ehlers–Danlos Syndrome type IV, alpha 1-Antitrypsin Deficiency, Marfan Syndrome, arteriovenous malformation, fibromuscular dysplasia, and sickle cell anemia [1, 4]. The majority of intracranial aneurysms are located in the anterior part of circle of Willis [5].

Despite the initial use of detachable balloons in 1974 by Serbinenko for the treatment of intracranial aneurysms, the essential contribution to endovascular management of such lesions was made by the introduction of Guglielmi detachable coils (GDCs) in 1991 [6–8]. Since the use of detachable coils in the treatment of the intracranial aneurysms was FDA approved, the endovascular techniques gradually started to replace surgical clipping [9]. The low rate of mortality and morbidity in addition to a small recurrence rate made such procedures the method of choice for treatment of both ruptured and unruptured aneurysms [10, 11].

COMMON INDICATIONS [12]

- Ruptured intracranial aneurysm
- Unruptured intracranial aneurysms:
  - In patients with high risk for surgery
  - In patients on systemic anticoagulation
  - Size is equal or greater than 2 mm
- Aneurysms in the posterior part of circle of Willis
- Cavernous segment of internal carotid artery aneurysm

RELATIVE CONTRAINDICATIONS [12, 13]

- Difficult vascular anatomy (wide-necked aneurysm, tortuous blood vessel)

M. Al-Garnawee
Division of Neurosurgery, Department of Surgery, American University of Beirut, Riad Elsolh, 10017 2020 Beirut, Lebanon
e-mail: m.garnawee@gmail.com

F.E. Ammar
Department of Neurology, American University of Beirut, Riad Elsolh, 10017 2020 Beirut, Lebanon
e-mail: faa41@aub.edu.lb

H. Darwish (✉)
Department of Neurosurgery, University of Virginia Health System, 258 Colonnade Drive, Charlottesville, VA 22903, USA
e-mail: had06_1982@hotmail.com

B. Taslakian et al. (eds.), *Procedural Dictations in Image-Guided Intervention*,
DOI 10.1007/978-3-319-40845-3_144

- Severe atherosclerosis which prevents access to the internal cerebral artery
- Coagulation disorders or heparin hypersensitivity
- Bacteremia at the time of embolization

POSSIBLE COMPLICATIONS [6]

Angiography-related complications: refer to Chap. 75.

Procedure-specific complications:

- Rupture of the aneurysm during coiling
- Coil herniation or migration
- Thromboembolic complications
- Recurrence and rebleed of the aneurysm

PREPROCEDURAL ASSESSMENT AND PLANNING

- History, indications, and physical examination *(Appendix 1* in Chap. 149*)*
- Evaluation of diagnostic imaging studies (CT angiography, MR angiography) to assess the size, site, and the neck-to-dome ratio of the aneurysm as well as the anatomy of the access vessels
- Periprocedural management of coagulation status *(Appendices 2* in Chap. 150 *and 3* in Chap. 151*)*
- Antibiotic prophylaxis: Not routinely recommended *(Appendices 4* in Chap. 152 *and 5* in Chap. 153*)* [14]
- Imaging modality for guidance: Fluoroscopy; combined with ultrasound for arterial access
- Positioning: supine
- Consults: Anesthesia and Cardiology

PROCEDURE NOTE

Procedure: Fluoroscopy-guided coil embolization of left/right [name artery] aneurysm
Staff: [_]
Fellow: [_]
Resident: [_]
Clinical Information: Describe history and list indications
Allergies: None known/Allergic to [specify/type of allergy]
Anesthesia: General anesthesia
Medications: List any relevant medications used
Contrast Used: (_) ml of [type] contrast media was used
Field: Sterile
Procedure classification: Clean
Position: Supine
Monitoring: Intravenous access line was secured and vital signs were continuously monitored by nursing staff/anesthesia team throughout the procedure
Total fluoroscopy time: (_) minutes
Cumulative radiation dose: (_) mGy

Description of Procedure:

The risks, benefits, alternatives, and the procedure itself were explained to the patient/patient's Power of Attorney/patient's legal guardian, and informed written consent was obtained. The site of the procedure was identified and marked. Time out was performed to confirm the correct patient, procedure, and site.

The skin of both groins were shaved, prepped, and draped in the usual sterile fashion. The right/left femoral artery as well as the inguinal ligament were located by palpation/ultrasound and marked. The site of arterial puncture was determined using combined information from palpation, ultrasound, and fluoroscopy over the middle of the medial third of the femoral head. Femoral artery access was obtained using a (_)-gauge [type] needle and the Seldinger technique, double-/single-wall entry under direct ultrasound visualization/by palpation. Once good pulsatile arterial flow was detected, a (_)-inch [type] guidewire was advanced through the needle, into the aorta under direct fluoroscopic visualization and a (_)-French vascular sheath was placed and attached to pressurized saline flush for continuous irrigation.

Then a (_)-French guide catheter was placed in the cervical internal carotid artery/extracranial vertebral artery and attached to pressurized saline flush for continuous irrigation. Angiography with three-dimensional reconstruction was done to obtain good working projections that display the details of the aneurysm including the dome to neck ratio and the relation to the parent vessels. After that three-dimensional road map was obtained, a (_)-French [type] microcatheter was advanced along the superimposed roadmap produced from the angiography into the aneurysm over a (_)-inch [type] microwire. The microcatheter was also connected to a pressurized irrigation system.

After accessing the aneurysm with the tip of the microcatheter, embolization was started by deploying the framing coils (type, size of coils) followed by filling coils (type, size of coils).

After each coil deployment, a checking angiography was done to see the coil loop, degree of aneurysm filling and rule out extravasation.

Finally, standard angiographic projections were done to check any distal thromboembolic occlusion and the guide catheter was removed.

Following the procedure, the right/left femoral artery sheath was removed and adequate hemostasis was achieved by compression for (_) minutes/using [type] vascular closure device. The lower extremity pulses were checked following the procedure and were [comparable to the preprocedural pulses/specify if otherwise needed]. The patient was transferred to the Neuro-ICU/recovery room for close monitoring following the procedure in a stable condition. Staff was present for the entire procedure.

Intra-Procedure Findings: List all relevant findings.

Immediate Complications: None encountered during or directly after the procedure. List complications if any.

Post-Procedure Plan: [12]

- Keep patient complete bed rest with the right/left leg extended for (_) hours.
- Admit patient to Neuro-ICU for close monitoring.
- Continue intravenous hydration and monitor accurate input–output.
- Perform full neurological exam every 1 h.
- Monitor vital signs every 15 min for the first hour, then every 30 min for the following 4 hours; notify interventional radiology team if systolic blood pressure <95 mmHg or >150 mmHg, or heart rate >110 beats/minute.
- Check the right/left groin for any bleeding and/or hematoma formation every 15 min for the first hour, then every 30 min for the second hour, then every 1 hour for the following 4 h. In the presence of any complication, inform the interventional radiology team.
- Observe the limb on the side of puncture, and check access site after ambulation.
- Check and document lower extremity pulses and color every 30 min for the first 2 hours then every 1 hour for the following 4 h.
- In case of ruptured aneurysm, specific management of subarachnoid hemorrhage should be initiated and transcranial Doppler should be requested.
- Follow up complete blood count, BUN, and creatinine on the day following the procedure or as clinically indicated
- The majority of patients with unruptured aneurysm can be discharged home on next day.
- Routine radiographic follow-up: magnetic resonance angiography at 6 months and 18 months and annually thereafter.

References

1. Gross B, Hage Z, Daou M, Getch C, Batjer H, Bendok B. Surgical and endovascular treatments for intracranial aneurysms. Curr Treat Options Cardiovasc Med. 2008;10(3):241–52.
2. Ajiboye N, Chalouhi N, Starke R, Zanaty M, Bell R. Unruptured cerebral aneurysms: evaluation and management. Sci World J. 2015;2015:954954.
3. Hashimoto T, Meng H, Young W. Intracranial aneurysms: links among inflammation, hemodynamics and vascular remodeling. Neurol Res. 2006;28(4):372–80.
4. Harrigan M, Deveikis JP. Intracranial aneurysms and subarachnoid haemorrhage. In: Harrigan M, Deveikis JP, editors. Handbook of cerebrovascular disease and neurointerventional technique. 2nd ed. Heidelberg: Springer; 2013. p. 483–569.

5. The International Study of Unruptured Intracranial Aneurysms Investigators. Unruptured intracranial aneurysms-risk of rupture and risks of surgical intervention. N Engl J Med. 1999;340(9):744.
6. Gkogkas C, Baker J, Norbash AM, Frerichs KU. Endovascular treatment of intracranial aneurysms. In: Proctor MR, editor. Minimally invasive neurosurgery, 1st ed. New York: Humana Press; 2005. P. 151–73.
7. Guglielmi G, Viñuela F, Dion J, Duckwiler G. Electrothrombosis of saccular aneurysms via endovascular approach. Part 2: preliminary clinical experience. J Neurosurg. 1991;75(1):8–14.
8. Ries T, Groden C. Endovascular treatment of intracranial aneurysms: long-term stability, risk factors for recurrences, retreatment and follow-up. Klin Neuroradiol. 2009;19(1):62–72.
9. Froehler M. Endovascular treatment of ruptured intracranial aneurysms. Curr Neurol Neurosci Rep. 2013;13(2):326.
10. Gallas S, Pasco A, Cottier J, Gabrillargues J, Drouineau J, Cognard C, et al. A multicenter study of 705 ruptured intracranial aneurysms treated with guglielmi detachable coils. AJNR Am J Neuroradiol. 2005;26(7):1723–31.
11. Rooij W, Sluzewski M. Procedural morbidity and mortality of elective coil treatment of unruptured intracranial aneurysms. AJNR Am J Neuroradiol. 2006;27(8):1678–80.
12. Harrigan M, Deveikis J. Intracranial aneurysm treatment. In: Harrigan M, Deveikis JP, editors. Handbook of cerebrovascular disease and neurointerventional technique. 2nd ed. Heidelberg: Springer; 2013. p. 189–241.
13. Ferrell AS, Agrawal A, Golshani K, Smith T, Britz GW. Intracranial aneurysms. In: Lanzer Peter, editor. Catheter-based cardiovascular interventions. Berlin: Springer; 2013. p. 771–86.
14. Venkatesan AM, Kundu S, Sacks D, Wallace MJ, Wojak JC, Rose SC, et al. Practice guidelines for adult antibiotic prophylaxis during vascular and interventional radiology procedures. J Vasc Intervent Radiol. 2010;21(11):1611–30.

Intracranial Stenting

145

Tarek P. Sunna, Houssein Darwish and Fahed Zairi

Abbreviations

CCA	Common carotid artery
ICA	Internal carotid artery
ECA	External carotid artery
VA	Vertebral artery
PTAS	Percutaneous transluminal angioplasty and stenting

INTRODUCTION

Stroke is one of the leading causes of morbidity and mortality in the United States [1] and along with transient ischemic attacks, afflicts approximately 900,000 people annually [2]. Intracranial atherosclerosis comprises 70,000–90,000 of these cases [3]. While medical therapy with aspirin has been shown to be safe and effective in treating symptomatic intracranial arterial stenosis in more than 50 % of cases [4], the rate of recurrent ischemic stroke ipsilateral to the stenotic artery is still approximately 12 % at 1-year follow-up. Unfortunately, surgery has, to date, not shown much promise in treating this disease [5]. Similarly, angioplasty provides only a temporary solution to a permanent problem and is associated with its own pitfalls, such as acute and chronic restenosis of the treated vessel and arterial dissection [6, 7]. The advent of flexible stents that could be deployed in intracranial vessels has greatly expanded the endovascular repertoire. Properly placed stents not only favorably alter intravascular dynamics, but also have the potential to reverse blood vessel stenosis, thereby increasing tissue perfusion, remodel deformed vasculature, and prevent recurrence of cerebrovascular pathology.

COMMON INDICATIONS [8]

- Symptomatic patients, who have failed medical therapy, with >50 % intracranial stenosis

T.P. Sunna (✉)
Department of Neurosurgery,
University of Montreal, Montreal, QC, Canada
e-mail: tareksunna@hotmail.com

H. Darwish
Department of Neurosurgery, University of Virginia
Health System, 258 Colonnade Drive,
Charlottesville, VA 22903, USA
e-mail: had06_1982@hotmail.com

F. Zairi
Department of Neurosurgery, Lille University
Hospital, Rue Emile Laine, 59000 Lille, France
e-mail: fahed.zairi@gmail.com

B. Taslakian et al. (eds.), *Procedural Dictations in Image-Guided Intervention*,
DOI 10.1007/978-3-319-40845-3_145

- There is insufficient evidence to make definite recommendations regarding endovascular therapy in asymptomatic patients with severe intracranial atherosclerosis. Stenting would be considered if maximal medical treatment did not prevent stroke or other symptoms
- It should be noted that the "Stenting versus Aggressive Medical Management for Preventing Recurrent Stroke in Intracranial Stenosis (SAMMPRIS) trial"[1] demonstrated superiority of medical therapy to percutaneous transluminal angioplasty and stenting (PTAS). As a result, the validity of stenting for intracranial atherosclerotic disease has become a subject of significant debate.

COMMON CONTRAINDICATIONS [9]

- Contraindications to antiplatelet therapy and/or anticoagulation
- Highly calcified lesions or anatomy which prevents endovascular access

POSSIBLE COMPLICATIONS [9]

Angiography-related complications: Please see Chap. 75.

Procedure-specific complications

- Cerebral hemorrhagic *(subarachnoid/ intracranial)* and ischemic events
- Air embolus
- Arterial perforation or dissection
- Catheter or guidewire breakage

PREPROCEDURAL ASSESSMENT AND PLANNING

- History, indications and physical examination *(Appendix 1* in Chap. 149*)*; document indications of the procedure, lower or upper extremity pulses and vital signs
- Evaluation of diagnostic imaging studies to determine the relevant vascular anatomy; baseline carotid duplex exam and a confirmatory study (e.g., CTA, MRA, or catheter angiogram)
- Periprocedural management of coagulation status *(Appendices 2* in Chap. 150 *and 3* in Chap. 151*)*
- Antibiotic prophylaxis: Not routinely recommended *(Appendices 4* in Chap. 152 *and 5* in Chap. 153*)* [10]
- Imaging modality for guidance: Fluoroscopy; combined with ultrasound for arterial puncture
- Positioning: Supine
- Arterial access: Common femoral artery, left brachial artery
- Patient preparation:
  - Antiplatelet therapy [11–13]
    - Aspirin 325-mg PO QD for ≥ 3 days prior to the procedure and Clopidogrel (Plavix®, Bristol-Myers-Squibb, New York, NY, USA) 75-mg PO QD for ≥ 3 days prior to the procedure
    - Or aspirin 325-mg PO QD for ≥ 3 days prior to the procedure and Ticlopidine (Ticlid®, Hoffmann-La Roche, Basel, Switzerland) for ≥ 3 days prior to the procedure
    - Alternatively, a loading dose of Aspirin 325-mg PO and clopidogrel 300-mg PO can be given the day before or at least 5 h before the procedure
    - Antiplatelet (aspirin and clopidogrel) resistance is becoming a recognizable entity as a potential cause for failure in stroke prevention. Up to 40 % and 15–48 % of patients may be resistant to aspirin and clopidogrel, respectively. Antiplatelet resistance can be routinely tested prior to stenting procedures using bedside tests (i.e., point of care analysis) that rapidly measures platelet function such as "verify now" (Accumetrics, CA, USA) system or the PFA-100™ System (Dade Behring, Germany). VerifyNow® results are reported in P2Y12 reaction units (PRUs), with a lower PRU value

[1] *N Engl J Med. 2011 Sep 15; 365(11):993-1003.*

corresponding to a higher degree of P2Y12 receptor inhibition, and, hence, a decreased likelihood of platelet activation (i.e., hyper response to clopidogrel) and aggregation; and a higher PRU value corresponding to a lower degree of P2Y12 receptor inhibition and, hence, an increased likelihood of platelet activation and aggregation (i.e., hyporesponse to clopidogrel). Adjustments to the dose or type of P2Y12 receptor antagonist might be required to keep PRU values within the 60–200 target P2Y12 reaction units range.

- Ticagrelor and Cangrelor are newer antiplatelet agents that do not require metabolic activation to inhibit the P2Y12 receptor, therefore are not subject to resistance and can be used as alternative antiplatelet agents.

- Place two peripheral intravenous lines
- Insert a Foley catheter
- NPO after midnight or 6 h prior to the procedure except for medications
- Hold routine antihypertensive medications on the morning of the procedure
- Make sure that all devices that may be needed are available in the interventional suite prior to the procedure

PROCEDURE NOTE

Procedure: Endovascular left/right [name artery] artery angioplasty and stenting
Staff: [_]
Fellow: [_]
Resident: [_]
Clinical Information: Describe history and list indications
Allergies: None known/Allergic to [specify/type of allergy]
Anesthesia: General anesthesia/Local anesthesia/Monitored conscious sedation
Medications: List any relevant medications used (sedation, heparin)
Contrast Used: (_) mL of [type] contrast
Field: Sterile
Procedure classification: Clean
Position: Supine
Monitoring: Intravenous access line was secured and vital signs were continuously monitored by nursing staff/anesthesia team throughout the procedure
Total fluoroscopy time: (_) minutes
Cumulative radiation dose: (_) mGy

Description of Procedure:

The risks, benefits, alternatives, and the procedure itself were explained to the patient/patient's Power of Attorney/patient's legal guardian, and informed written consent was obtained. The site of the procedure was identified and marked. Time out was performed to confirm the correct patient, procedure and site.

The skin of both groins were shaved, prepped, and draped in the usual sterile fashion. The right/left common femoral artery as well as the inguinal ligament were located by palpation/ultrasound and marked. The site of arterial puncture was determined using combined information from palpation, ultrasound and fluoroscopy over the middle of the medial third of the femoral head. Local anesthesia was administered. Common femoral artery access was obtained using (_)-gauge [type] needle and the Seldinger technique under direct ultrasound visualization/by palpation. Once good pulsatile arterial flow was detected, a (_)-inch [type] guidewire was advanced through the needle, up through the common femoral artery, into the aorta under direct fluoroscopic visualization and a (_)-French vascular sheath was placed.

After 5 min, a loading dose of intravenous heparin (70 U/kg) was given. Measured ACT was (_) seconds. Then, a (_)-French [type] vascular catheter was introduced over a (_)-inch hydrophilic [type] and manipulated into the thoracic arch, then into the right/left common carotid artery. At this stage, a common carotid run was performed to check for the position of the internal carotid artery. The catheter tip was then navigated trough the proximal part of the internal carotid artery. Anterior-posterior, lateral and oblique contrast run views of the right/left internal carotid artery were obtained. The catheter was then retracted into the subclavian artery and advanced into the vertebral artery and angiography was performed.

Angiography on the contralateral side was performed in the same way. The [name the artery] was selected for angioplasty and stenting.

The diagnostic catheter was placed in the right/left common carotid artery/internal carotid artery/vertebral artery. An exchange length (_)-inch stiff [type] catheter was placed in the carotid/vertebral system to exchange the femoral sheath for a longer (_)-French, (_) cm [type] sheath. The exchange was performed under fluoroscopic guidance to make sure that the distal tip of the stiff wire was not pushing against the plaque. The distal end of the new sheath was positioned [specify location]. Aspiration of (_) mL of blood was done through the sheath to confirm adequate flow and the absence of any clots. The sheath was then connected to continuous pressurized flushing system throughout the procedure. High flow head run was performed before starting the stenting phase.

Following this, angioplasty was performed using a (_) × (_) mm [type] balloon. Pressure was continuously monitored during the slow inflation of the balloon. (_) mg Atropine was administered intravenously. Then the balloon was removed and neurological exam showed neurological deficit [specify]/no neurological deficit.

Under road map guidance a (_) × (_) mm [type] stent was deployed across the lesion. This was followed by angiogram of the carotid tree and intracranial vessels including the posterior circulation.

During angiography, double flushing was performed consisting of aspiration of the contents of the catheter with one 10-mL syringe of heparinized saline, followed by partial aspiration and irrigation with a second syringe of saline, to ensure clearing clots and air bubbles from the catheter. This was repeated every time a wire was removed from the catheter, prior to the injection of contrast.

Following the procedure the right/left femoral artery sheath was removed and adequate hemostasis was achieved by compression for (_) minutes/using [type] vascular closure device. The lower extremity pulses were checked following the procedure and were [comparable to the preprocedure pulses/specify if otherwise needed]. The patient was transferred to the floor/recovery room for close monitoring following the procedure in a stable condition. Staff was present for the entire procedure.

Intra-Procedure Findings: List all relevant findings.

Immediate Complications: None encountered during or directly after the procedure. List complications if any.

Post-Procedure Plan [9]:

- Transfer patient to the recovery room.
- Perform complete neurological exam in the recovery room every 15 min.
- Keep patient complete bed rest with the right/left leg extended for (_) hours.
- Check the right/left groin for any bleeding and/or hematoma formation every 15 min for 1 h, then every 30 min for 1 h, then every hour for 4 h; inform interventional radiology team if any observed.
- Check lower extremity pulses and color every 30 min for 2 h, then every 1 h for 4 h and document the findings.
- Monitor vital signs every 15 min for 1 h, then every 30 min for 4 h; notify interventional radiology team if systolic blood pressure <95 mmHg, or heart rate >110 beats/minute.
- Check puncture site after ambulation.
- Continue adequate intravenous hydration and monitor fluid (intake–output) status.
- Check complete blood count, creatinine and blood urea nitrogen on the day following the procedure or as clinically indicated.
- Admit to the neuro-ICU or step-down unit with neuro exams every 1 h.
- Antiplatelet therapy [11, 12]
  - Aspirin 325-mg PO QD indefinitely *and* Clopidogrel (Plavix®) 75-mg PO QD for 30 days after the procedure.

  - Or Aspirin 325 mg PO QD indefinitely *and* Ticlopidine (Ticlid®) for 30 days after the procedure
- Most patients can be discharged from the hospital post-procedure day 1 or 2.

Impression:

- Angioplasty and stenting of [name of the artery] artery, as described above.
- The patient tolerated the procedure well and left the interventional unit in stable condition.
- The patient was unstable and the procedure was canceled/terminated prematurely.
- The patient refused to undergo/complete the procedure.
- List any other relevant or important information/finding.

References

1. Broderick J, Brott T, Kothari R, Miller R, Khoury J, Pancioli A, et al. The Greater Cincinnati/Northern Kentucky Stroke Study: preliminary first-ever and total incidence rates of stroke among blacks. Stroke. 1998;29(2):415–21.
2. Johnston SC. Clinical practice. Transient ischemic attack. N Engl J Med. 2002;347(21):1687–92.
3. Sacco RL, Kargman DE, Gu Q, Zamanillo MC. Race-ethnicity and determinants of intracranial atherosclerotic cerebral infarction. Northern Manhattan Stroke Study. Stroke. 1995;26(1):14–20.
4. Chimowitz MI, Lynn MJ, Howlett-Smith H, Stern BJ, Hertzberg VS, Frankel MR, et al. Comparison of warfarin and aspirin for symptomatic intracranial arterial stenosis. N Engl J Med. 2005;352(13):1305–16.
5. The EC/IC Bypass Study Group. Failure of extracranial-intracranial arterial bypass to reduce the risk of ischemic stroke. Results of an international randomized trial. N Engl J Med. 1985;313(19):1191–200.
6. Cruz-Flores S, Diamond AL. Angioplasty for intracranial artery stenosis. Cochrane Database Syst Rev. 200619;(3):CD004133.
7. Marks MP, Wojak JC, Al-Ali F, Jayaraman M, Marcellus ML, Connors JJ, et al. Angioplasty for symptomatic intracranial stenosis: clinical outcome. Stroke. 2006;37(4):1016–20.
8. Higashida RT, Meyers PM, Connors JJ 3rd, Sacks D, Strother CM, Barr JD, et al. Intracranial angioplasty & stenting for cerebral atherosclerosis: a position statement of the american society of interventional and therapeutic neuroradiology, society of interventional radiology, and the american society of neuroradiology. AJNR Am J Neuroradiol. 2005;26(9):2323–7.
9. Harrigan MR, Deveikis JP. Handbook of cerebrovascualr disease and neurointerventional technique. NewYork: Springer; 2013. p. 99–131.
10. Venkatesan AM, Kundu S, Sacks D, Wallace MJ, Wojak JC, Rose SC, et al. Practice guidelines for adult antibiotic prophylaxis during vascular and interventional radiology procedures. J Vasc Interv Radiol. 2010;21(11):1611–30.
11. Schleinitz MD, Olkin I, Heidenreich PA. Cilostazol, clopidogrel or ticlopidine to prevent sub-acute stent thrombosis: a meta-analysis of randomized trials. Am Heart J. 2004;148(6):990–7.
12. Bennett CL, Kiss JE, Weinberg PD, Pinevich AJ, Green D, Kwaan HC, et al. Thrombotic thrombocytopenic purpura after stenting and ticlopidine. Lancet. 1998;352(9133):1036–7.
13. Fifi JT, Brockington C, Narang J, Leesch W, Ewing SL, Bennet H, et al. Clopidogrel resistance is associated with thromboembolic complications in patients undergoing neurovascular stenting. Am J Neuroradiol. 2013;34(4):716–20.

146 Transcatheter Treatment of Acute Ischemic Stroke

Keith G. DeSousa and Eytan Raz

Abbreviation	
AIS	Acute ischemic stroke
TICI	Thrombolysis in cerebral infarction
LVO	Large vessel occlusion
DWI	Diffusion weighted imaging
AHA/ASA	American Heart Association/American Stroke Association
ICA	Internal carotid artery
MCA	Middle cerebral artery
NIHSS	National Institutes of Health Stroke Scale
ACA	Anterior cerebral artery

INTRODUCTION

Four significant multicenter trials were published in the New England Journal of Medicine that permanently and significantly changed the treatment paradigm for acute ischemic stroke (AIS) [1]. These trials, Multicenter Randomized Clinical Trial of Endovascular Treatment of Acute Ischemic Stroke in the Netherlands (MR CLEAN) [2], Endovascular Treatment of Small Core and Proximal Occlusion Ischemic Stroke (ESCAPE) [3], Extending the Time for Thrombolysis in Emergency Neurological Deficits-Intra-Arterial (EXTEND-IA) [4], and Solitaire With the Intention For Thrombectomy as PRIMary Endovascular Treatment (SWIFT PRIME) Trial [5] all provided data that showed efficacy of endovascular treatment for large vessel occlusions. This chapter serves as a guide for procedural dictation for routine stroke thrombectomy procedures. Keep in mind that there are multiple reperfusion strategies ranging from stent-retrievers to aspiration with large diameter distal access catheters. The current guidelines from the American Heart Association/ American Stroke Association (AHA/ASA)

K.G. DeSousa
Department of Radiology, New York University Langone Medical Center, 660 First Avenue, 7th Floor, New York, NY 10016, USA
e-mail: drkeith5@gmail.com

E. Raz (✉)
Department of Radiology, Divisions of Neuroimaging and Neurointervention, New York University Langone Medical Center, 660 First Avenue, 7th Floor, New York, NY 10016, USA
e-mail: eytan.raz@gmail.com

B. Taslakian et al. (eds.), *Procedural Dictations in Image-Guided Intervention*,
DOI 10.1007/978-3-319-40845-3_146

recommend the use of a stent-retriever [6]. Both options of aspiration and stent-retriever will be discussed here.

COMMON INDICATIONS [6, 7]

- Acute ischemic stroke with large vessel occlusion including internal carotid artery (ICA) or proximal middle cerebral artery (MCA) or anterior cerebral artery (ACA) as demonstrated with imaging
- National Institutes of Health Stroke Scale (NIHSS) >6
- ASPECTS of >6
- Treatment can be initiated within 6 h of symptom onset

COMMON CONTRAINDICATIONS [6]

- No evidence of large vessel occlusion (LVO) on imaging
- CT Perfusion or MRI Diffusion weighted (DWI) image showing large completed infarction
- Hemorrhage on imaging
- Patient too unstable to be brought to angiography suite

POSSIBLE COMPLICATIONS [2–5]

Angiography-related complications:

- Access site complications *(e.g., hematoma, retroperitoneal hemorrhage, arterial injury, thrombosis)*
- Contrast-induced allergic reaction
- Contrast-induced nephropathy
- Catheter or guidewire breakage
- Risks related to any minimally invasive procedure performed under conscious sedation *(e.g., allergy to medications)*

Procedure-specific complications:

- Intracranial hemorrhage (due to reperfusion injury or technical intra-procedural complications)
- Arterial dissection
- Propagation of thrombus or distal emboli
- Worsening stroke
- Death

PREPROCEDURAL ASSESSMENT AND PLANNING

- History, indications, and physical examination *(Appendix 1* in Chap. 149*)*
- Evaluation of diagnostic imaging studies (CT, CTA/CTP, MRI): to determine the extent of the infarct, presence of hemorrhage, location of vessel occlusion
- Periprocedural management of coagulation status *(Appendices 2* in Chap. 150 *and 3 in* Chap. 151*)*
- Antibiotic prophylaxis: Not routinely recommended *(Appendices 4* in Chap. 152 *and 5* in Chap. 153*)*
- Imaging modality for guidance: Fluoroscopy
- Positioning: Supine
- Arterial access: Common femoral artery
- Anesthesia: Multiple retrospective studies demonstrated better outcome if the patient is treated under conscious sedation rather than general anesthesia. Patients receiving general anesthesia had significantly increased in-hospital mortality and pneumonia compared to patients receiving conscious sedation. While ongoing prospective trials will most likely solve the dilemma, general anesthesia is certainly recommended in uncooperative patients where their poor cooperation may render the thrombectomy unsafe (i.e., perforation or dissection), patients with decreased level of consciousness (Glasgow Coma Scale <8), loss of ability to protect airways, and respiratory compromise. In those cases treated under general anesthesia, the anesthesiologists

should maintain adequate levels of blood pressure to avoid aggravation of brain hypoperfusion [8–10].

PROCEDURE NOTE

Procedure: Cerebral angiogram and thrombectomy
Staff: [_]
Fellow: [_]
Resident: [_]
Clinical Information: Describe history and list indications
Allergies: None known/Allergic to [specify/type of allergy]
Anesthesia: Local anesthesia with conscious sedation/General anesthesia
Medications: List any relevant medications used
Contrast Used: (_) mL of [type] contrast media was used for injection
Field: Sterile
Position: Supine
Monitoring: Intravenous access line was secured and vital signs were continuously monitored by nursing staff/anesthesia team throughout the procedure
Total fluoroscopy time: (_) minutes
Cumulative radiation dose: (_) mGy

Description of Procedure:

The risks, benefits, alternatives and the procedure itself were explained to the patient/patient's Power of Attorney/patient's legal guardian, and informed written/verbal consent was obtained. The site of the procedure was identified and marked. Time out was performed to confirm the correct patient, procedure, and site.

The CT of the brain was evaluated for evidence of hemorrhage or large territory completed infarction. CTA/MRA demonstrated [type of vessel occlusion/findings].

The skin of both groins were prepped and draped in the usual sterile fashion (shaving is avoided in the interest of time). The right/left femoral artery as well as the inguinal ligament were located by palpation/ultrasound and marked. The site of arterial puncture was determined using combined information from palpation/ultrasound/and fluoroscopy over the middle of the medial third of the femoral head. Local anesthesia was administered. Femoral artery access was obtained using a (_)-French micropuncture technique under direct ultrasound visualization/by palpation. Once good pulsatile arterial flow was detected, a (_)-inch [type] guidewire was advanced through the needle into the aorta under direct fluoroscopic visualization and a (_)-French vascular sheath was placed. A (_)-French [type] catheter over a (_)-Glidewire was navigated into [name the vessel] artery. Digital subtraction angiogram was obtained in frontal and lateral projections which revealed [relevant findings]. The catheter was then exchanged for a (_)-balloon guide catheter/long sheath over a (_) exchange wire. The balloon guide catheter/long sheath was hooked to continuous heparinized saline flush.

Option 1 (Stent-retriever):

Using roadmap guidance a (_) microcatheter was navigated over a (_) wire distal to the occlusion. A (_)-sized Stent-retriever was then deployed across the clot. After (_) minutes, the balloon was inflated and the Stent-retriever was removed. [Describe characteristics of thrombus removed, if any]. The balloon was then deflated. Digital subtraction angiogram was then obtained in frontal and lateral projections showing [discuss findings]. Thrombolysis in cerebral infarction (TICI) (_) recanalization was seen. The balloon guide catheter/long sheath was removed and groin hemostasis was obtained using [type] closure device.

Option 2 (Aspiration Catheter):

Using roadmap guidance, a (_) microcatheter was placed into a (_) aspiration catheter and navigated over a (_) guidewire to the level of the occlusion. Using care not to pass through the clot, the (_) aspiration catheter was carefully moved to the clot face. The (_) microcatheter and (_) wire were then removed. The (_) aspiration catheter was then hooked to the aspirator canister and was left on for (_) minutes. The balloon was inflated and the catheter was then withdrawn. The balloon was then deflated and digital subtraction angiogram was obtained in frontal and lateral projections revealing [discuss findings]. TICI (_) recanalization was obtained. The balloon guide catheter/long sheath was removed and groin hemostasis was obtained using [type] closure device.

The patient was transferred to the floor/recovery room/neuro-ICU following the procedure in a stable/critical condition. Staff was present for the entire procedure.

Intra-Procedure Findings: List all relevant findings.

Immediate Complications: None encountered during or directly after the procedure. List complications if any.

Post-Procedure Plan:

- Transfer patient to PACU/Stroke Unit/Intensive Care Unit as per institution protocol.
- Blood pressure parameters as per institution protocol.
- Post tPA protocol should be followed if patient received tPA.
- Bedrest for 6 h post-procedure with right/left leg straight.
- Check vital signs every 15 min for 1 h, every 30 min for 1 h then every 60 min for 4 h.
- Antiplatelet/anticoagulation as per neurology team.
- Follow up CT brain or MRI brain as per institution protocol.
- If bleeding/hematoma noted at groin access site, apply pressure and notify interventional team/primary team.

Impression:

- Thrombectomy of right/left [name the vessel] artery, as described above.
- The patient tolerated the procedure well and left the interventional unit in stable condition.
- The patient was unstable and the procedure was canceled/terminated prematurely.
- List any other relevant or important information/finding.

References

1. DeSousa KG, Potts MB, Raz E, Nossek E, Riina HA. Turning point of acute stroke therapy: mechanical thrombectomy as a standard of care. World Neurosurg. 2015;83(6):953–6.
2. Berkhemer OA, Fransen PS, Beumer D, van den Berg LA, Lingsma HF, Yoo AJ, et al. A randomized trial of intraarterial treatment for acute ischemic stroke. N Engl J Med. 2015;372(1):11–20.
3. Goyal M, Demchuk AM, Menon BK, Eesa M, Rempel JL, Thornton J, et al. Randomized assessment of rapid endovascular treatment of ischemic stroke. N Engl J Med. 2015;372(11):1019–30.
4. Campbell BC, Mitchell PJ, Kleinig TJ, Dewey HM, Churilov L, Yassi N, et al. Endovascular therapy for ischemic stroke with perfusion-imaging selection. N Engl J Med. 2015;372(11):1009–18.
5. Saver JL, Goyal M, Bonafe A, Diener HC, Levy EI, Pereira VM, et al. Stent-retriever thrombectomy after intravenous t-PA vs. t-PA alone in stroke. N Engl J Med. 2015;372(24):2285–95.
6. Powers WJ, Derdeyn CP, Biller J, Coffey CS, Hoh BL, Jauch EC, et al. American Heart Association/American Stroke Association focused update of the 2013 guidelines for the early management of patients with acute ischemic stroke regarding endovascular treatment: a guideline for healthcare professionals from the American Heart Association/American Stroke Association. Stroke. 2015;46(10):3020–35.
7. DeSousa KG, Haussen DC, Yavagal DR. Strategies for streamlining emergency stroke care. Curr Neurol Neurosci Rep. 2014;14(11):497.
8. McDonald JS, Brinjikji W, Rabinstein AA, Cloft HJ, Lanzino G, Kallmes DF. Conscious sedation versus general anaesthesia during mechanical thrombectomy for stroke: a propensity score analysis. Neurointerv Surg. 2015;7(11):789–94.
9. Wahlgren N, Moreira T, Michel P, Steiner T, Jansen O, Cognard C, et al. Mechanical thrombectomy in acute ischemic stroke: consensus statement by ESO-Karolinska stroke update 2014/2015, supported by ESO, ESMINT, ESNR and EAN. Int J Stroke. 2016;11(1):134–47.
10. Talke PO, Sharma D, Heyer EJ, Bergese SD, Blackham KA, Stevens RD. Republished: Society for Neuroscience in Anesthesiology and Critical Care expert consensus statement: anesthetic management of endovascular treatment for acute ischemic stroke. Stroke. 2014;45(8):e138–50.

Vertebral Artery Stenting 147

Tarek P. Sunna and Houssein Darwish

INTRODUCTION

Vertebral artery stenosis is associated with high morbidity and mortality, preceding brainstem infarction in up to 50 % of patients [1, 2]. Medical management includes both antiplatelet and anticoagulation therapies. However, in spite of maximum medical therapy, many patients exhibit refractory symptoms that necessitate revascularization procedures [3–5]. The combined rates of perioperative morbidity, mortality, and graft/anastomosis occlusion for surgical bypass procedures range from 11 to 25 % [6, 7]. Previously, primary angioplasty had been attempted in a limited number of symptomatic patients, resulting in various degrees of success associated with combined morbidity and mortality rates as high as 50 % [8]. Advances in catheter technology and clinical management of patients with vertebrobasilar disease have resulted in significantly improved access to and treatment of vertebrobasilar lesions.

T.P. Sunna (✉)
Department of Neurosurgery,
University of Montreal, Montreal, QC, Canada
e-mail: tareksunna@hotmail.com

H. Darwish
Department of Neurosurgery, University of Virginia
Health System, 258 Colonnade Drive,
Charlottesville, VA 22903, USA
e-mail: had06_1982@hotmail.com

COMMON INDICATIONS [9]

- Symptoms of vertebrobasilar insufficiency; must include at least two of the following symptoms: motor or sensory symptoms, dysarthria, imbalance, dizziness or vertigo, tinnitus, alternating paresthesia, homonymous hemianopia, diplopia, other cranial nerve palsies, and dysphagia
- MRI evidence of ischemic injury to the posterior circulation
- ≥ 50 % stenosis of the vertebral artery by CT, MRI or conventional angiography
- <50 % symptomatic stenosis with hypoplasia or stenosis affecting the contralateral vertebral artery

COMMON CONTRAINDICATIONS [9]

- Intraluminal thrombus

POSSIBLE COMPLICATIONS [9]

Angiography-related complications:

- Access site complications *(e.g., hematoma, retroperitoneal hemorrhage, arterial injury, thrombosis)*
- Contrast-induced allergic reaction
- Contrast-induced nephropathy
- Catheter or guidewire breakage

B. Taslakian et al. (eds.), *Procedural Dictations in Image-Guided Intervention*,
DOI 10.1007/978-3-319-40845-3_147

- Risks related to any minimally invasive procedure performed under conscious sedation *(e.g., allergy to medications)*

Procedure-specific complications:

- Cerebral hemorrhagic *(subarachnoid and intracranial)* and ischemic events
- Air embolus
- Arterial perforation or dissection
- Mortality

PREPROCEDURAL ASSESSMENT AND PLANNING

- History, indications, and physical examination *(Appendix 1* in Chap. 149*)*; document indications of the procedure, lower or upper extremity pulses and vital signs
- Evaluation of diagnostic imaging studies to determine the relevant vascular anatomy and assess the access site
- Periprocedural management of coagulation status *(Appendices 2* in Chap. 150 *and 3 in* Chap. 151*)*
- Antibiotic prophylaxis: Not routinely recommended *(Appendices 4* in Chap. 152 *and 5* in Chap. 153*)* [10]
- Imaging modality for guidance: Fluoroscopy; combined with ultrasound for arterial puncture
- Positioning: Supine
- Arterial access: Common femoral artery, brachial artery [1, 4]
- Patient preparation
  - Antiplatelet therapy:
    Aspirin 325-mg PO QD for $\geq$3 days prior to the procedure and Clopidogrel (Plavix®, Bristol-Myers-Squibb, New York, NY, USA) 75-mg PO QD for $\geq$3 days prior to the procedure.
    Or aspirin 325-mg PO QD for $\geq$3 days prior to the procedure and Ticlopidine (Ticlid®, Hoffman-La Roche, Basel, Switzerland) for $\geq$3 days prior to the procedure.
    Alternatively, a loading dose of Aspirin 325-mg PO and clopidogrel 300-mg PO can be given the day before or at least 5 h before the procedure.
    Antiplatelet (aspirin and clopidogrel) resistance is becoming a recognizable entity as a potential cause for failure in stroke prevention. Up to 40 % and 15–48 % of patients may be resistant to aspirin and clopidogrel respectively. Antiplatelet resistance can be routinely tested prior to stenting procedures using bedside tests (i.e., point of care analysis) that rapidly measures platelet function such as “verify now” (Accumetrics, CA, USA) system or the PFA-100™ System (Dade Behring, Germany). VerifyNow® results are reported in P2Y12 reaction units (PRUs), with a lower PRU value corresponding to a higher degree of P2Y12 receptor inhibition, and, hence, a decreased likelihood of platelet activation (i.e., hyper-response to clopidogrel) and aggregation; and a higher PRU value corresponding to a lower degree of P2Y12 receptor inhibition and, hence, an increased likelihood of platelet activation and aggregation (i.e., hyporesponse to clopidogrel). Adjustments to the dose or type of P2Y12 receptor antagonist might be required to keep PRU values within the 60–200 target P2Y12 reaction units range. Ticagrelor and Cangrelor are newer antiplatelet agents that does not require metabolic activation to inhibit the P2Y12 receptor, therefore are not subject to resistance and can be used as alternative antiplatelet agents.
  - Place two peripheral intravenous catheters
  - Place Foley catheter
  - Keep fasting (NPO) after midnight or 6 h prior to the procedure except for medications
  - Make sure that all devices that may be needed are available in the angiography suite prior to the procedure

PROCEDURE NOTE

Procedure: Fluoroscopy-guided endovascular left/right vertebral artery stenting
Staff: [_]
Fellow: [_]
Resident: [_]
Clinical Information: Describe history and list indications
Allergies: None known/Allergic to [specify/type of allergy]
Anesthesia: Local anesthesia/conscious sedation
Medications: List any relevant medications used
Contrast Used: (_) mL of [type] contrast media
Field: Sterile
Procedure classification: Clean
Position: Supine
Monitoring: Intravenous access line was secured and vital signs were continuously monitored by nursing staff/anesthesia team throughout the procedure
Total fluoroscopy time: (_) minutes
Cumulative radiation dose: (_) mGy

Description of Procedure:

The risks, benefits, alternatives, and the procedure itself were explained to the patient/patient's Power of Attorney/patient's legal guardian, and informed written consent was obtained. The site of the procedure was identified and marked. Time out was performed to confirm the correct patient, procedure and site.

The skin of left/right/both groins were shaved, prepped and draped in the usual sterile fashion. The right/left common femoral artery as well as the inguinal ligament were located by palpation/ultrasound and marked. The site of arterial puncture was determined using combined information from palpation, ultrasound and fluoroscopy over the middle of the medial third of the femoral head. Local anesthesia was administered. Femoral artery access was obtained using (_)-gauge [type] needle and the Seldinger technique, double-/single-wall entry under direct ultrasound visualization/by palpation. Once good pulsatile arterial flow was detected, a (_)-inch [type] guidewire was advanced through the needle into the aorta under direct fluoroscopic visualization and a (_)-French vascular sheath was placed. A loading dose of intravenous heparin (70 U/kg) was administered to reach an ACT of (_) seconds. Then (_) inch [type] guidewire with the diagnostic (_) French [type] catheter was inserted through the femoral sheath to the aortic arch and subsequently the right/left vertebral arteries were selectively catheterized. Anterior–posterior, lateral and oblique contrast run views of right/left vertebral artery were obtained. Diameters of the right/left vertebral artery, region of greatest stenosis, and the length of the plaque were (_), (_), (_) mm, respectively. Then, a (_) inch exchange length stiff [type] guidewire was placed to exchange the femoral sheath for a (_)-French, (_) cm [type] sheath. This was placed at the proximal part of the vertebral artery at V1. The exchange was done under fluoroscopic guidance to make sure that the distal tip of the wire was not pushing against the plaque. Then, the exchange guidewire was withdrawn. Aspiration of (_) mL of blood was done through the sheath to confirm adequate flow and absence of any clots. The sheath was then connected to continuous pressurized flushing system throughout the procedure. High flow head run was performed before starting the stenting phase. Then, an embolic protection device was guided under fluoroscopy and positioned (_) cm distal to the plaque and was deployed under fluoroscopy*. After that, a gross neurological exam and an angiogram were performed to check for any dislodgement of the plaque. Angioplasty was performed using a (_) × (_) mm [type] balloon. The blood pressure was continuously monitored during the slow inflation of the balloon. Then the balloon was removed and neurological exam showed deficit/no deficit. Under road map guidance, a (_) × (_) mm [type] stent was deployed across the lesion. This was followed by angiogram of the vertebral artery and intracranial posterior vascular tree.

Following the procedure, the right/left femoral artery sheath was removed and adequate hemostasis was achieved by compression for

(_) minutes/using [type] vascular closure device. The lower extremity pulses were checked following the procedure and were [comparable to the preprocedural pulses/specify if otherwise needed]. The patient was transferred to the floor/recovery room for close monitoring following the procedure in a stable condition. Staff was present for the entire procedure.

* **Note:** The use of distal protection devices in vertebral artery stenting is controversial. It is not easy nor safe to put both a balloon-mounted stent and a distal protection device in a small-caliber vertebral artery that requires stenting.

Intra-Procedure Findings: List all relevant findings.

Immediate Complications: None encountered during or directly after the procedure. List complications if any.

Post-Procedure Plan [9]:

- Transfer patient to the recovery room and perform neurological exams every 15 min for 1–2 h.
- Keep patient in complete bed rest with the right/left leg extended for (_) hours *[adjust depending on the puncture site]*.
- Check the right/left groin/[specify the puncture site if different] for any bleeding or hematoma formation every 15 min for 1 h, then every 30 min for 1 h, then every hour for 4 h; inform interventional radiology team if any observed *[adjust depending on the puncture site]*.
- Check lower extremity pulses and color every 30 min for 2 h then every 1 h for 4 h and document the findings.
- Monitor vital signs every 15 min for 1 h, then every 30 min for 4 h; notify interventional radiology team if systolic blood pressure <95 mm Hg or >140 mm Hg, or heart rate >110 beats/min.
- Check puncture site after ambulation.
- Continue adequate intravenous hydration and monitor fluid (intake–output) status.
- After adequate monitoring, admit to the Neuro-ICU or step-down unit with neuro exams every 1 h.
- Check complete blood count, creatinine and blood urea nitrogen on the day following the procedure or as clinically indicated.
- Antiplatelet therapy: Aspirin 325-mg PO QD indefinitely *and* Clopidogrel (Plavix®) 75-mg PO QD for 30 days after the procedure.
- For patients with hypotension, requiring dopamine infusion: Hypotension after vertebral artery stenting is usually self-limited and resolves within 1–2 days. However, cardiac work-up should be done to exclude a myocardial infarction.

Impression:

- Stenting of right/left vertebral artery, as described above.
- The patient tolerated the procedure well and left the interventional unit in stable condition.
- The patient was unstable and the procedure was canceled/terminated prematurely.
- List any other relevant or important information/finding.

References

1. Ausman JI, Shrontz CE, Pearch JE. Vertebrobasilar insufficiency. Arch Neurol. 1985;42:803–8.
2. Thompson JR, Simmons CR, Hasso AN. Occlusion of the intradural vertebrobasilar artery. Neuroradiology. 1978;14:219–29.
3. Berguer R, Morasch MD, Kline RA. A review of 100 consecutive reconstructions of the distal vertebral artery for embolic and hemodynamic disease. J Vasc Surg. 1998;27:852–9.
4. Berguer R, Bauer RB. Approach to the second segment of the vertebral artery. In: Vertebrobasilar arterial occlusive disease. Medical and surgical management. New York: Raven Press; 1984. p. 257–64.
5. Diaz FG, Ausman JI, Shrontz C. Surgical correction of lesions affecting the second portion of the vertebral artery. Neurosurgery. 1986;19:93–100.
6. Hopkins LN, Martin NA, Hadley MN. Vertebrobasilar insufficiency. Part 2: microsurgical treatment of intracranial vertebrobasilar disease. J Neurosurg. 1987;66:662–74.
7. Wilkins RH, Rengachary SS. Extracranial to intracranial bypass grafting: posterior circulation. In:

Neurosurgery, Vol. 2. New York: McGraw-Hill; 1985. p. 1281–92.
8. Dorros G, Cohn JM, Palmer LE. Stent deployment resolves a petrous carotid artery angioplasty dissection. AJNR. 1998;19:392–4.
9. Harrigan MR, Deveikis JP. Diagnostic cerebral angiograpy. In: Handbook of cerebrovascular disease and neurointerventional technique. NewYork: Springer; 2013. p. 99–131.
10. Venkatesan AM, Kundu S, Sacks D, Wallace MJ, Wojak JC, Rose SC, et al. Practice guidelines for adult antibiotic prophylaxis during vascular and interventional radiology procedures. J Vasc Interv Radiol. 2010;21(11):1611–30.

Wada Test

148

Eytan Raz and Keith G. DeSousa

INTRODUCTION

The provocative cerebral testing, also known as Wada test, is a procedure performed to evaluate the functional anatomy, which varies in different patients. The procedure was refined in the early 1960s in Montreal [1–3]. The basic principle of provocative cerebral testing is to determine the functional eloquence of cortical tissue using reversible pharmacological methods [4]. Before surgical resection, the Wada testing can be performed to isolate the function of a particular arterial territory, most often the speech and the memory functions. This, for example, can aid in the treatment of epilepsy, as it can give neuropsychologists information for memory testing prior to epilepsy focus resection. In order to perform the Wada test, a barbiturate (most often amobarbital) or propofol [5, 6] is injected in each internal carotid artery to identify the lateralization of primarily speech and memory [7]. This is preceded by a cerebral angiogram in order to evaluate the patient's vascular anatomy.

The neuropsychological testing, done after the injection of the medication, has a standard protocol that should be rigorously followed. There are two main standardized protocols for memory testing, the Montreal and the Seattle tests [8]. In the Montreal test, after the injection, a series of word cards and objects are shown to the patient, who is then tested for recall when the effect of the drug has dissipated. The Seattle test involves repeatedly displaying cards showing line drawings and sentences, which the patient is instructed to name and remember.

COMMON INDICATIONS [9–12]

- Preoperative evaluation before epilepsy surgery
- Preoperative evaluation before arteriovenous malformations treatment
- Preoperative evaluation before tumor surgical resection

COMMON CONTRAINDICATIONS [13, 14]

- Any contraindication to cerebral angiogram: Hemodynamic instability with multisystem dysfunction, uncorrectable coagulopathy, recent myocardial infarction, significant arrhythmias, significant serum electrolyte

E. Raz (✉)
Department of Radiology, Divisions of Neuroimaging and Neurointervention, 660 First Avenue, 7th Floor, New York, NY 10016, USA
e-mail: eytan.raz@nyumc.org

K.G. DeSousa
Department of Radiology, New York University Langone Medical Center, 660 First Avenue, 7th Floor, New York, NY 10016, USA
e-mail: drkeith5@gmail.com

B. Taslakian et al. (eds.), *Procedural Dictations in Image-Guided Intervention*,
DOI 10.1007/978-3-319-40845-3_148

imbalance, past history of allergy to intravenous contrast media, pregnancy, impaired renal function, and uncooperative patient
- Allergy to amobarbital
- If the patient has received medications with a carbonic anhydrase inhibitory effect (such as topomirate, zonisamide), which, if taken in the previous eight weeks, can make the amobarbital ineffective

POSSIBLE COMPLICATIONS [15–19]

Peculiar for Wada testing:
- Allergic reaction to amobarbital
- Injection of amobarbital in the posterior circulation, which can produce unconsciousness and apnea; keep in mind that this can happen through a posterior communicating artery but also through one of the rare carotid-basilar anastomoses such as the persistent trigeminal artery
- Cerebral edema may occur if the drug is mixed incorrectly
- Unpredictable severe emotional outbursts or disinhibited behavior may happen after the injection of intracarotid amobarbital

Similar complications to cerebral angiogram

- Ischemic-embolic events, related to injection of air or formations of clot or traumatic catheterization
- Access site complications *(e.g., hematoma, retroperitoneal hemorrhage, femoral artery pseudoaneurysm, femoral arteriovenous fistula, femoral artery thrombosis)*
- Contrast-induced allergic reaction
- Contrast-induced nephropathy
- Arterial perforation or dissection

PREPROCEDURAL ASSESSMENT AND PLANNING

- History, indications, and physical examination *(Appendix 1* in Chap. 149*)*
- Evaluation of diagnostic imaging studies (EEG, MRI, PET-MRI) to determine the location of the epileptogenic lesion, since that side is tested first. Also evaluate any images available in order to predict the circle of Willis variations.
- Periprocedural management of coagulation status *(Appendices 2* in Chap. 150 *and 3 in* Chap. 151*)*
- Antibiotic prophylaxis: Not routinely recommended *(Appendices 4* in Chap. 152 *and 5* in Chap. 153*)*
- Imaging modality for guidance: Fluoroscopy
- Positioning: Supine
- Arterial access: Common femoral artery
- Before beginning the procedure, contact must be made with the neurophysiology team
- Patients should do the neuropsychological testing using their primary language: if it is not English, arrangement should be done to have a translator in the room. Multilingual patients may have variable localization of language centers for the different languages and Wada testing may not be accurate.

PROCEDURE NOTE

Procedure: Cerebral angiogram and Wada test
Staff: [_]
Fellow: [_]
Resident: [_]
Clinical Information: Describe history and list indications
Allergies: None known/Allergic to [specify/type of allergy]
Anesthesia: Local anesthesia/conscious sedation
Medications: Amobarbital (Sodium Amytal), 20 mg/mL concentration, for a total of approximately 80–100 mg per hemisphere./Propofol … mg per hemisphere
Contrast Used: (_) mL of [type] contrast media
Field: Sterile
Procedure classification: Clean
Position: Supine
Monitoring: Intravenous access line was secured and vital signs were continuously monitored by nursing staff throughout the procedure
Total fluoroscopy time: (_) minutes
Cumulative radiation dose: (_) mGy

Description of Procedure:
The risks, benefits, alternatives, and the procedure itself were explained to the patient/patient's Power of Attorney/patient's legal guardian, and informed written consent was obtained. Time out was performed to confirm the correct patient and procedure.

The skin of both groins were shaved, prepped, and draped in the usual sterile fashion. The right/left femoral artery as well as the inguinal ligament were located by palpation/ultrasound and marked. The site of arterial puncture was determined using combined information from palpation, ultrasound, and fluoroscopy over the medial third of the femoral head. Local anesthesia was administered. Femoral artery access was obtained using (_)-gauge [type] needle and the Seldinger technique, double-/single-wall entry under direct ultrasound visualization/by palpation. Once good pulsatile arterial flow was detected, a (_)-inch [type] guidewire was advanced through the needle into the aorta under direct fluoroscopic visualization and a (_)-French vascular sheath was placed.

A (5)-French multipurpose catheter was introduced over a (_)-inch [type] Glidewire and used to selectively catheterize the right internal carotid artery. Digital subtraction angiography of the intracranial right internal carotid circulation was performed in frontal and lateral projections.

The left internal carotid artery was selectively catheterized. Digital subtraction angiography of the intracranial left internal carotid circulation was performed in frontal and lateral projections.

Arterial, capillary, and venous phase images were nonrevealing without angiographic evidence of cerebral aneurysm, arteriovenous malformation, intracranial vascular stenosis, mass effect, or veno-occlusive disorder related to the left or right internal carotid circulation. The veins of both hemispheres were well balanced.

Following angiographic evaluation, Wada testing was initiated with the administration of (100) mg of amobarbital/(_) mg Propofol into the left internal carotid artery followed by neuropsychological evaluation of right hemispheric functioning. After an appropriate recovery interval, the catheter was again placed within the right internal carotid artery, and neuropsychological testing of left hemispheric functioning performed after the administration of (75) mg of amobarbital/(_) mg Propofol into the right internal carotid artery.

The patient was discharged from the neuroangiographic suite in stable and unchanged neurologic condition following removal of the catheter and establishment of hemostasis in the right groin by manual compression. Staff was present for the entire procedure.

Intra-Procedure Findings: List all relevant findings.

- Unremarkable cerebral angiography. There was no angiographic evidence of cerebral aneurysm, arteriovenous formation, intracranial vascular stenosis, mass effect, or veno-occlusive disorder related to the right or left internal carotid circulations.
- Neuropsychological (Wada) testing consistent with left/right hemispheric dominance. Language functions were localized principally to the left/right hemisphere.
- The memory score of the left hemisphere was (_)/12.
- The memory score of the right hemisphere was (_)/12.

Immediate Complications: None encountered during or directly after the procedure. List complications if any.

Post-Procedure Plan:

Standard post-angiogram management plan:

- Keep patient in complete bed rest with the right/left leg extended for (_) hours *[adjust depending on the puncture site]*.
- Check the right/left groin/[specify the puncture site if different] for any bleeding or hematoma formation every 15 min for 1 h, then every 30 min for 1 h, then every hour for 4 h; inform interventional radiology team if any observed *[adjust depending on the puncture site]*.
- Check and document lower extremity pulses every 30 min for 2 h then every 1 h for 4 h *[adjust depending on the puncture site]*.

- Monitor vital signs every 15 min for 1 h, then every 30 min for 4 h; notify interventional radiology team if systolic blood pressure <95 mm Hg, or heart rate >110 beats/min.
- Resume diet and previous orders as needed and if otherwise not contraindicated.
- Continue adequate intravenous hydration and monitor fluid (intake-output) status.

Impression:

- Cerebral angiogram and Wada testing, as described above.
- The patient tolerated the procedure well and left the interventional unit in stable condition.
- The patient was unstable and the procedure was canceled/terminated prematurely.
- List any other relevant or important information/finding.

References

1. Wada J. Clinical experimental observations of carotid artery injections of sodium amytal. Igaku to Seibutsugaku. 1949;14:221–2.
2. Wada JA. Clinical experimental observations of carotid artery injections of sodium amytal. Brain Cogn. 1997;33(1):11–3.
3. Rovit RL, Gloor P, Rasmussen T. Intracarotid amobarbital in epileptic patients. A new diagnostic tool in clinical electroencephalography. Arch Neurol. 1961;5:606–26.
4. Branch C, Milner B, Rasmussen T. Intracarotid sodium amytal for the lateralization of cerebral speech dominance; observations in 123 patients. J Neurosurg. 1964;21:399–405.
5. Buchtel HA, Passaro EA, Selwa LM, Deveikis J, Gomez-Hassan D. Sodium methohexital (brevital) as an anesthetic in the Wada test. Epilepsia. 2002;43(9):1056–61.
6. Grote CL, Meador K. Has amobarbital expired? Considering the future of the Wada. Neurology. 2005;65(11):1692–3.
7. Bengner T, Haettig H, Merschhemke M, Dehnicke C, Meencke HJ. Memory assessment during the intracarotid amobarbital procedure: influence of injection order. Neurology. 2003;61(11):1582–7.
8. Dodrill CB, Ojemann GA. An exploratory comparison of three methods of memory assessment with the intracarotid amobarbital procedure. Brain Cogn. 1997;33(2):210–23.
9. Woermann FG, Jokeit H, Luerding R, Freitag H, Schulz R, Guertler S, et al. Language lateralization by Wada test and fMRI in 100 patients with epilepsy. Neurology. 2003;61(5):699–701.
10. Andelman F, Kipervasser S, Neufeld MY, Kramer U, Fried I. Predictive value of Wada memory scores on postoperative learning and memory abilities in patients with intractable epilepsy. J Neurosurg. 2006;104:20–6.
11. Cohen-Gadol AA, Westerveld M, Alvarez-Carilles J. Spencer DD intracarotid amytal memory test and hippocampal magnetic resonance imaging volumetry: validity of the Wada test as an indicator of hippocampal integrity among candidates for epilepsy surgery. J Neurosurg. 2004;101:926–31.
12. Lee GP, Westerveld M, Blackburn LB, Park YD, Loring DW. Prediction of verbal memory decline after epilepsy surgery in children: effectiveness of Wada memory asymmetries. Epilepsia. 2005;46:97–103.
13. Kipervasser S, Andelman F, Kramer U, Nagar S, Fried I, Neufeld MY. Effects of topiramate on memory performance on the intracarotid amobarbital (Wada) test. Epilepsy Behav. 2004;5(2):197–203.
14. Bookheimer S, Schrader LM, Rausch R, Sankar R, Engel J Jr. Reduced anesthetization during the intracarotid amobarbital (Wada) test in patients taking carbonic anhydrase inhibiting medications. Epilepsia. 2005;46(2):236–43.
15. Mikuni N, Takayama M, Satow T, Yamada S, Hayashi N, Nishida N, et al. Evaluation of adverse effects in intracarotid propofol injection for Wada test. Neurology. 2005;65(11):1813–6.
16. Beimer NJ, Buchtel HA, Glynn SM. One center's experience with complications during the Wada test. Epilepsia. 2015;56(8):e110–3.
17. Terzian H. Behavioural and EEG effects of intracarotid sodium amytal injection. Acta Neurochir. 1964;12:230–9.
18. Masia SL, Perrine K, Westbrook L, Alper K, Devinsky O. Emotional outbursts and post-traumatic stress disorder during intracarotid amobarbital procedure. Neurology. 2000;54(8):1691–3.
19. de Paola L, MÃ¤der MJ, Germiniani FM, Coral P, Zavala JA, Watzo DJ, et al. Bizarre behavior during intracarotid sodium amytal testing (Wada test): are they predictable? Arq Neuropsiquiatr. 2004;62(2B):444–8.

Part XXIV
Appendices

Author: Bedros Taslakian
Reviewer: Aghiad Al-Kutoubi

Appendix 1—Review of History and Physical Examination

149

Bedros Taslakian

General Interventional Procedures [1, 2]

Review and document the following:

- Chief complaint
- Pertinent medical and surgical history
- History of allergies including type and severity of allergic reaction
- Review of organ systems
- Pertinent laboratory results and imaging studies
- Current medications (prescribed and illicit)
- Directed physical examination
- Determine cardiopulmonary stability and request subspecialty consultation as necessary
- Review sedation or anesthesia requirements and request anesthesia consultation as necessary

Additional for Angiographic Procedures [1, 2]

Evaluate and document the following:

- Proposed puncture site and contraindications *(e.g., groin infection, common femoral artery aneurysm/pseudoaneurysm, inguinal hernia, fresh incision, and recent injury)*
- Extremity pulses, using a Doppler ultrasound probe when necessary
- Status of extremities *(e.g., color, perfusion, presence of swelling, ulceration)*
- Risk factors for contrast allergy *(e.g., previous allergic reaction to iodinated contrast, reaction to other allergens),* and type/severity of allergy
- Risk Factor for contrast-induced nephropathy *(e.g., preexisting renal dysfunction, diabetes, dehydration, hypotension, congestive heart failure, large contrast dose, advanced age, anemia, cardiovascular diseases, multiple myeloma)*

References

1. Taslakian B, Sebaaly MG, Al-Kutoubi A. Patient evaluation and preparation in vascular and interventional radiology: what every interventional radiologist should know (part 1: patient assessment and laboratory tests). Cardiovasc Intervent Radiol. 2016;39(3):325–33.
2. Taslakian B, Sebaaly MG, Al-Kutoubi A. Patient evaluation and preparation in vascular and interventional radiology: what every interventional radiologist should know (part 2: patient preparation and medications). Cardiovasc Intervent Radiol. 2016;39(4):489–99. doi: 10.1007/s00270-015-1239-4. [Epub 2015 Nov 25].

B. Taslakian (✉)
Department of Radiology, New York University Langone Medical Center, 660 First Ave, New York, NY 10016, USA
e-mail: btaslakian@gmail.com

B. Taslakian et al. (eds.), *Procedural Dictations in Image-Guided Intervention*,
DOI 10.1007/978-3-319-40845-3_149

150 Appendix 2—Society of Interventional Radiology Guidelines for Preprocedural Coagulation Parameter Surveillance Based on the Procedural Risk for Bleeding

Bedros Taslakian

Abbreviations

INR	International normalized ratio
aPTT	Activated partial thromboplastin time
TIPS	Transjugular portosystemic shunt
PICC	Peripherally inserted central catheter
IVC	Inferior vena cava

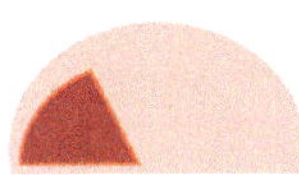

Procedures with Low Bleeding Risk [1–4]

Non-Vascular Procedures:

- Catheter exchange
- Thoracentesis
- Paracentesis
- Superficial drainage (excluding intrathoracic/ intraabdominal)
- Superficial aspiration (excluding intrathoracic/ intraabdominal)
- Superficial biopsy (excluding intrathoracic/ intraabdominal)
- Joint injection / aspiration
- Thyroid biopsy

Vascular Procedures:

- Dialysis access
- Venography
- Central line removal
- IVC filter placement
- PICC placement
- Non-tunneled venous catheter

Laboratory Testing & Correction Thresholds [1–4]

INR	Recommended Correct values to ≤ 2.0
aPTT	Recommended No consensus for values
Platelet	Not routinely recommended Transfusion if ≤ 50,000/ μL
Hematocrit	Not routinely recommended

B. Taslakian (✉)
Department of Radiology, New York University
Langone Medical Center, 660 First Ave, New York,
NY 10016, USA
e-mail: btaslakian@gmail.com

B. Taslakian et al. (eds.), *Procedural Dictations in Image-Guided Intervention*,
DOI 10.1007/978-3-319-40845-3_150

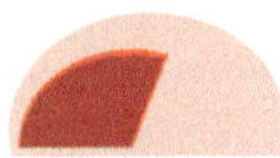

Procedures with Moderate Bleeding Risk [1–4]

Non-Vascular Procedures:

- Deep abscess drainage
- Deep biopsy (excluding renal)
- Cholecystostomy
- Percutaneous enteric tube (new tract)
- Spinal procedures

Vascular Procedures:

- Arterial interventions (access size ≤ 7 French)
- Complex venous interventions
- Chemoembolization
- Radioembolization
- Uterine fibroid embolization
- Tunneled venous catheter
- Transjugular liver biopsy
- Subcutaneous port device placement

Laboratory Testing & Correction Thresholds [1–4]

INR	Recommended Correct values to ≤ 1.5
aPTT	Recommended Correct values to ≤ 1.5 x control (73% consensus)
Platelet	Recommended Transfusion if ≤ 50,000/ μL
Hematocrit	Not routinely recommended

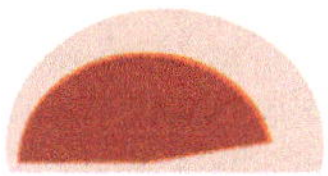

Procedures with Significant Bleeding Risk
Bleeding Difficult to Detect and Control [1–4]

Non-Vascular Procedures:

- Renal biopsy
- Biliary interventions (new tract)
- Nephrostomy tube placement
- Radiofrequency ablation

Vascular Procedures:

- TIPS

Laboratory Testing & Correction Thresholds [1–4]

INR	Recommended Correct values to ≤ 1.5
aPTT	Recommended Correct values to ≤ 1.5 x control
Platelet	Recommended Transfusion if ≤ 50,000/ μL
Hematocrit	Not routinely recommended

References

1. Taslakian B, Sebaaly MG, Al-Kutoubi A. Patient evaluation and preparation in vascular and interventional radiology: what every interventional radiologist should know (part 1: patient assessment and laboratory tests). Cardiovasc Intervent Radiol. 2016 Mar;39(3):325–33.
2. Taslakian B, Sebaaly MG, Al-Kutoubi A. Patient evaluation and preparation in vascular and interventional radiology: what every interventional radiologist should know (part 2: patient preparation and medications). Cardiovasc Intervent Radiol. 2016;39(4):489–99. doi: 10.1007/s00270-015-1239-4. [Epub 2015 Nov 25].
3. Patel IJ, Davidson JC, Nikolic B, Salazar GM, Schwartzberg MS, Walker TG, et al. Consensus guidelines for periprocedural management of coagulation status and hemostasis risk in percutaneous image-guided interventions. J Vasc Interv Radiol. 2012;23(6):727–36.
4. Patel IJ, Davidson JC, Nikolic B, Salazar GM, Schwartzberg MS, Walker TG, et al. Addendum of newer anticoagulants to the SIR consensus guideline. J Vasc Interv Radiol. 2013;24(5):641–5.

151 Appendix 3—Society of Interventional Radiology Preprocedural Management Guidelines for Current Antithrombotic Medications Based on the Procedural Risk for Bleeding

Bedros Taslakian

Abbreviations

INR	International normalized ratio
aPTT	Activated partial thromboplastin time
TIPS	Transjugular portosystemic shunt
PICC	Peripherally inserted central catheter
NSAIDs	Nonsteroidal anti-inflammatory drugs
CrCl	Creatinine clearance
LMWH	Low molecular weight heparin

B. Taslakian (✉)
Department of Radiology, New York University
Langone Medical Center, 660 First Ave, New York,
NY 10016, USA
e-mail: btaslakian@gmail.com

B. Taslakian et al. (eds.), *Procedural Dictations in Image-Guided Intervention*,
DOI 10.1007/978-3-319-40845-3_151

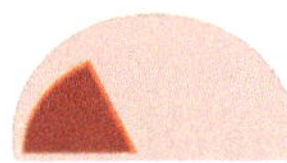

Procedures with Low Bleeding Risk [1–4]

Non-Vascular Procedures:

- Catheter exchange
- Thoracentesis
- Paracentesis
- Superficial drainage (excluding intrathoracic/ intraabdominal)
- Superficial aspiration (excluding intrathoracic/ intraabdominal)
- Superficial biopsy (excluding intrathoracic/ intraabdominal)
- Joint injection / aspiration
- Thyroid biopsy

Vascular Procedures:

- Dialysis access
- Venography
- Central line removal
- IVC filter placement
- PICC placement
- Non-tunneled venous catheter

Antithrombotic Drugs and Management Recommendations [1–4]

Clopidogrel	Withhold for 0-5 days
Aspirin	No need to withhold
Heparin[a]	No consensus (Check aPTT)
LMWH[b]	Withhold 1 dose or for 12 hours
Warfarin	Withhold for 3-5 days (correct INR to ≤ 2)
Fondaparinux	No need to withhold
Argatroban	No need to withhold
Bivalirudin	No need to withhold
Dabigatran	No need to withhold
NSAIDs[c]	No need to withhold
Abciximab	Withhold for 12–24 h
Eptifibatide	Withhold immediately pre-procedure

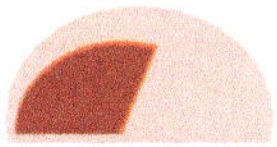

Procedures with moderate bleeding risk [1–4]

Non-vascular procedures:

- Deep abscess drainage
- Deep biopsy (excluding renal)
- Cholecystostomy
- Percutaneous enteric tube (new tract)
- Spine procedures

Vascular procedures:

- Arterial interventions (access ≤ 7 French)
- Complex venous interventions
- Chemoembolization
- Radioembolization
- Uterine fibroid embolization
- Tunneled venous catheter
- Transjugular liver biopsy
- Subcutaneous port device placement

Antithrombotic drugs and management recommendations [1–4]

Clopidogrel	Withhold for 5 days
Aspirin	No need to withhold
Heparin[a]	No consensus (correct aPTT to ≤ 1.5 control)
LMWH[b]	Withhold 1 dose or for 12 h
Warfarin	Withhold for 5 days (INR ≤ 1.5)
Fondaparinux	Withhold for: 2–3 days if CrCl ≥ 50 mL/min 3–5 days if CrCl ≤ 50 mL/min
Argatroban	Defer procedure until patient is off medication Urgent cases → withhold for 4 hours
Bivalirudin	Defer until off medication; urgent cases → withhold for: 2–3 hours if CrCl ≥ 50 mL/min 3–5 hours if CrCl ≤ 50 mL/min
Dabigatran	Defer until off medication; urgent cases → withhold for: 2–3 days if CrCl ≥ 50 mL/min 3–5 days if CrCl ≤ 50 mL/min
NSAIDs[c]	No need to withhold
Abciximab	Withhold for 24 h
Eptifibatide	Withhold for 4 h

Procedures with significant bleeding risk bleeding difficult to detect and control [1–4]

Non-vascular procedures:

- Renal biopsy
- Billiary interventions (new tract)
- Nephrostomy tube placement
- Radiofrequency ablation

Vascular procedures:

- TIPS

Antithrombotic drugs and management recommendations [1–4]

Clopidogrel	Withhold for 5 days
Aspirin	Withhold for 5 days
Heparin[a]	Withhold for 2–4 hours (correct aPTT to ≤ 1.5 control)
LMWH[b]	Withhold 2 doses or for 24 hours
Warfarin	Withhold for 5 days (correct INR to ≤ 1.5)
Fondaparinux	Withhold for: 2–3 days if CrCl ≥ 50 mL/min 3–5 days if CrCl ≤ 50 mL/min
Argatroban	Defer procedure until patient is off medication Urgent cases→withhold for 4 hours
Bivalirudin	Defer until off medication; urgent cases→ withhold for: 2–3 hours if CrCl ≥ 50 mL/min 3–5 hours if CrCl ≤ 50 mL/min
Dabigatran	Defer until off medication; urgent cases→withhold for: 2–3 days if CrCl ≥ 50 mL/min 3–5 days if CrCl ≤ 50 mL/min
NSAIDs[c]	*Short acting* → withhold for 24 hours *Intermediate-acting* → withhold for 2–3 days *Long-acting* → withhold for 10 days
Abciximab	Withhold for 24 hours
Eptifibatide	Withhold for 4 hours

Notes

[a]*Heparin (*unfractionated heparin)
[b]*LMWH:* recommendations are for therapeutic doses of LMWH
[c]*Short acting NSAIDs*: half-life 2–6 h (e.g., ibuprofen, diclofenac, ketoprofen, indomethacin); *intermediate-acting NSAIDs*: half-life 7–15 h (e.g., naproxen, sulindac, diflunisal, celecoxib); *long-acting NSAIDs*: half-life > 20 h (e.g., meloxicam, nabumetone, piroxicam)

References

1. Taslakian B, Sebaaly MG, Al-Kutoubi A. Patient Evaluation and preparation in vascular and interventional radiology: what every interventional radiologist should know (part 1: patient assessment and laboratory tests). Cardiovasc Intervent Radiol. 2016;39(3):325–33.
2. Taslakian B, Sebaaly MG, Al-Kutoubi A. Patient Evaluation and preparation in vascular and interventional radiology: what every interventional radiologist should know (part 2: patient preparation and medications). Cardiovasc Intervent Radiol. 2016;39(4):489–99. doi: 10.1007/s00270-015-1239-4. [Epub 2015 Nov 25].
3. Patel IJ, Davidson JC, Nikolic B, Salazar GM, Schwartzberg MS, Walker TG, et al. Consensus guidelines for periprocedural management of coagulation status and hemostasis risk in percutaneous image-guided interventions. J Vasc Interv Radiol. 2012;23(6):727–36.
4. Patel IJ, Davidson JC, Nikolic B, Salazar GM, Schwartzberg MS, Walker TG, et al. Addendum of newer anticoagulants to the SIR consensus guideline. J Vasc Interv Radiol. 2013;24(5):641–5.

152 Appendix 4—Surgical Procedures' Classification

Bedros Taslakian

Interventional procedures can be potentially classified as clean, clean-contaminated, contaminated, and dirty procedures by adapting the National Academy of Sciences/National Research Council (NAS/NRC) classification of surgical wounds. However, it should be taken into consideration that the infectious risks of open surgical procedures may differ considerably from those of interventional radiology procedures. Surgical prophylaxis is directed at preventing wound infection; whereas in vascular and interventional radiology, the access site, or instrumentation may potentially serve as a site of bacterial seeding and antibiotic prophylaxis is directed to diminish this risk [1–4].

Classification (risk of infection)	Criteria	Examples in vascular and interventional radiology
Clean (<5 %)	• No evidence of inflammation/infection **AND** • Uninterrupted aseptic technique **AND** • No entry into spaces potentially containing bacteria *(e.g., gastrointestinal, biliary, genitourinary, or respiratory tracts)*	Biopsy (excluding transrectal); angiography; venography; angioplasty/stenting; caval filter placement; varicocele embolization; central venous access; ablation; vertebroplasty/kyphoplasty; neurovascular interventions
Clean-contaminated (~10 %)	• No evidence of inflammation/infection **AND** • Uninterrupted aseptic technique **AND** • Gastrointestinal, genitourinary, biliary or respiratory tract entry	Nephrostomy or biliary drainage with sterile urine or bile in an unobstructed system and absence of prior intervention; gastrostomy/gastrojejunostomy; liver ablation/embolization/TIPS in patients with bilioenteric anastomosis; renal ablation in patients with ureteroenteric anastomosis
Contaminated (~20 %)	• Major break in aseptic technique **AND/OR** • Inflamed or colonized gastrointestinal, biliary, or genitourinary tract entry AND • Absence of frank pus	Nephrostomy in patients with obstructed urinary tract, bladder dysfunction, ureterointestinal anastomosis, bacteriuria, and/or nephrolithiasis; transrectal biopsy
Dirty (~39 %)	• Infected purulent site entry • Perforated viscus	Abscess drainage; nephrostomy or biliary drainage in patients with clinical infection (e.g., pyonephrosis, cholangitis)

B. Taslakian (✉)
Department of Radiology, Center for Biomedical Imaging, New York University Langone Medical Center, 660 First Ave, New York, NY 10016, USA
e-mail: btaslakian@gmail.com

B. Taslakian et al. (eds.), *Procedural Dictations in Image-Guided Intervention*,
DOI 10.1007/978-3-319-40845-3_152

References

1. Berard F, Gandon J. Postoperative wound infections: the influence of ultraviolet irradiation of the operating room and of various other factors. Ann Surg. 1964;160 (suppl 1):1–192.
2. McDermott VG, Schuster MG, Smith TP. Antibiotic prophylaxis in vascular and interventional radiology. AJR Am J Roentgenol. 1997;169(1):31–8.
3. Venkatesan AM, Kundu S, Sacks D, Wallace MJ, Wojak JC, Rose SC, et al. Practice guidelines for adult antibiotic prophylaxis during vascular and interventional radiology procedures. J Vasc Interv Radiol. 2010;21(11):1611–30.
4. Taslakian B, Sebaaly MG, Al-Kutoubi A. Patient evaluation and preparation in vascular and interventional radiology: what every interventional radiologist should know (Part 2: Patient Preparation and Medications). Cardiovasc Intervent Radiol. 2016;39(4):489–99. doi:10.1007/s00270-015-1239-4. [Epub 2015 Nov 25].

153 Appendix 5—Antibiotic Prophylaxis in Vascular and Interventional Radiology

Bedros Taslakian

Abbreviations

IV	Intravenous
IM	Intramuscular
mg	Milligram
g	Gram
IE	Infective endocarditis

Procedures and Classification	Routine prophylaxis recommended	Recommended antibiotic regimen
NON-VASCULAR PROCEDURES		
Percutaneous nephrostomy *(clean-contaminated, contaminated, dirty)*	Yes	*No consensus on first choice agent* • 1 g IV ceftriaxone or cefazolin • 1.5–3 g IV ampicillin/sulbactam • 1–2 g IV ampicillin + 1.5 mg/kg (or 120 mg) IV gentamicin *Penicillin-allergic patients:* vancomycin or clindamycin + aminoglycoside Continue until obstruction and clinical infection is resolved
Antegrade ureteral stenting *(clean-contaminated, contaminated)*	Yes	*No consensus on first choice agent* • 1 g IV ceftriaxone or cefazolin • 1.5–3 g IV ampicillin/sulbactam • 1–2 g IV ampicillin + 1.5 mg/kg (or 120 mg) IV gentamicin *Penicillin-allergic patients:* vancomycin or clindamycin + aminoglycoside

(continued)

B. Taslakian (✉)
Department of Radiology, New York University Langone Medical Center, 660 First Ave, New York, NY 10016, USA
e-mail: btaslakian@gmail.com

B. Taslakian et al. (eds.), *Procedural Dictations in Image-Guided Intervention*,
DOI 10.1007/978-3-319-40845-3_153

Procedures and Classification	Routine prophylaxis recommended	Recommended antibiotic regimen
		Continue until obstruction and clinical infection is resolved
Percutaneous biliary interventions *(clean-contaminated, contaminated, dirty)*	Yes	*No consensus on first choice agent* • 1 g IV ceftriaxone • 1 g IV cefotetan IV + 4 g IV mezlocillin *(such as in case of previous biliary interventions)* • 1.5–3 g IV ampicillin/sulbactam • 2 g IV ampicillin + 1.5 mg/kg IV gentamicin *Penicillin-allergic patients:* vancomycin or clindamycin + aminoglycoside
Percutaneous gastrostomy/gastrojejunostomy (pull technique) *(clean-contaminated)*	Yes	• 1 g IV cefazolin at the time of the procedure *Patients with head and neck cancer:* • 1 g IV cefazolin at the time of procedure + 500 mg cephalexin twice daily for 5 days orally or via enteric tube • 600 mg IV clindamycin at the time of the procedure + 600 mg clindamycin twice daily for 5 days orally or via enteric tube *Penicillin-allergic patients:* vancomycin or clindamycin
Percutaneous gastrostomy/gastrojejunostomy (push technique) *(clean-contaminated)*	No consensus	*Patients with head and neck cancer:* • 1 g IV cefazolin at the time of procedure + 500 mg cephalexin twice daily for 5 days orally or via enteric tube • 600 mg IV clindamycin at the time of the procedure + 600 mg clindamycin twice daily for 5 days orally or via enteric tube
Tube change	No	*Not applicable in cases of* routine tube change, in uninfected, unobstructed immunocompetent patients
Thermal ablation *(clean, clean-contaminated if bilioenteric or ureteroenteric anastomosis)*	No consensus[a]	*No consensus on first choice agent* • 1.5-3 g IV ampicillin/sulbactam (liver, renal, lung, adrenal) • 1 g IV cephazolin (liver, bone) • 1 g ceftriaxone IV (renal) *Penicillin-allergic patients:* vancomycin or clindamycin for gram-positive coverage and aminoglycoside for gram-negative coverage
Abscess drainage *(dirty)*	Yes[b]	*No consensus on first choice agent* • 1–2 g cefoxitin IV every 6 h • 1–2 g cefotetan IV every 12 h • 1 g ceftriaxone IV every 24 h • 3 g ampicillin/sulbactam IV every 6 h *Penicillin-allergic patients:* vancomycin or clindamycin for gram-positive coverage and aminoglycoside for gram-negative coverage
Fluid aspiration *(clean)*	No	*Not applicable in cases of* ascites, pleural effusion, lymphocele, or simple hepatic or renal cyst in the absence of clinical infection

(continued)

Procedures and Classification	Routine prophylaxis recommended	Recommended antibiotic regimen
Percutaneous biopsy *(Clean)*	No	Not applicable
Transrectal biopsy *(contaminated)*	Yes	*No consensus on first choice agent* • 80 mg gentamicin IM 30 min before procedure + 250 mg ciprofloxacin twice daily orally for 5 days • 500 mg ciprofloxacin twice daily orally for 4 days, starting the day before the procedure
Vertebroplasty/kyphoplasty *(clean)*	Yes	• 1 g IV cefazolin *Penicillin-allergic patients:* vancomycin or clindamycin
VASCULAR PROCEDURES		
Angiography, venography, arterial closure device *(clean)*	No	*Not applicable*
Thrombolysis *(clean)*	No	*Not applicable*
Inferior vena cava filter placement *(clean)*	No	*Not applicable*
Superficial venous insufficiency treatment *(clean)*	No	*Not applicable*
Varicocele embolization *(clean)*	No	*Not applicable*
Neurovascular interventions *(clean)*	No	*Not applicable*
Angioplasty with bare-metal stenting *(clean)*	Generally not recommended[c]	*Patient at risk for stent infection*[c] • 1 g IV cefazolin *Penicillin-allergic patients:* vancomycin or clindamycin
Central venous catheter placement *(clean)*	Generally not recommended[d]	*Patients at risk for catheter infection*[d] • 1 g IV cefazolin *Penicillin-allergic patients:* vancomycin or clindamycin
Aortic endografts *(clean)*	Yes	• 1 g IV cefazolin *Penicillin-allergic patients:* vancomycin or clindamycin
Peripheral artery endografts *(clean)*	Yes	• 1 g IV cefazolin *Penicillin-allergic patients:* vancomycin or clindamycin
Dialysis access endografts *(clean)*	Yes	• 1 g IV cefazolin *Penicillin-allergic patients:* vancomycin or clindamycin
Transcatheter arterial chemoembolization (TACE) *(Clean, clean-contaminated if bilioenteric anastomosis)*	Yes	*No consensus on first choice agent* • 1.5–3 g IV ampicillin/sulbactam • 1 g IV cefazolin + 500 mg IV metronidazole • 2 g IV ampicillin IV + 1.5 mg/kg gentamicin • 1 g IV ceftriaxone *Penicillin-allergic patients:* vancomycin or clindamycin + aminoglycoside *Absence of intact sphincter of Oddi*[e]: Tazobactam/piperacillin and consider bowel preparation

(continued)

Procedures and Classification	Routine prophylaxis recommended	Recommended antibiotic regimen
Solid organ embolization (renal/splenic) *(Clean, clean-contaminated)*	Yes[f]	• 1 g IV ceftriaxone *Penicillin-allergic patients:* vancomycin or clindamycin + aminoglycoside
Uterine artery embolization *(Clean, clean-contaminated)*	Yes	*No consensus on first choice agent* • 1 g IV cefazolin • 900 mg IV clindamycin + 1.5 mg/kg gentamicin • 2 g IV ampicillin • 1.5–3 IV g ampicillin/sulbactam *Penicillin-allergic patients:* vancomycin *History of hydrosalpinx:* 100 mg doxycycline twice daily for 7 days
TIPS *(Clean, clean-contaminated)*	Yes	*No consensus on first choice agent* • 1-2 g IV ceftriaxone once daily for 48 h • 1.5–3 g IV ampicillin/sulbactam *Penicillin-allergic patients:* vancomycin or clindamycin + aminoglycoside

[a]Many interventionalists continue to use prophylaxis, with special consideration in patients at risk (e.g., hepatic tumor ablation in cases where retrograde enteric bacterial communication with the biliary tract is present such as cases of bilioenteric anastomosis, biliary stent placement, and sphincterotomy; renal ablation in patients with ureteroenteric anastomosis or with ureteric stents; diabetes; immunosuppression). Prolonged administration for 5–10 days might be required in at risk patients.

[b]Patients referred for abscess drainage are typically being treated with empiric antimicrobial agent; the operator should ensure the appropriateness of empiric agent and may elect to administer a dose before the procedure if a long period of time has elapsed since the last dose. The regimens listed in the table are not recommendations for antibiotic prophylaxis, but empirical treatment prior to obtaining culture data, which requires knowledge of the most commonly encountered infectious organism based on the abscess location. In cases of pleural infection, aminoglycosides should be avoided (poor penetration of the pleural space and possibility of inactivation in the presence of pleural fluid acidosis)

[c]Prophylaxis is generally not recommend except in patients at risk: immune deficiencies (e.g., older age, chronic kidney disease, diabetes, immunosuppressive medications), using vascular sheath placed for >24 h, stenting a vessel that is often accessed (e.g., hemodialysis catheter), repeated endovascular procedures within 7 days, prolonged and complex procedures (e.g., multiple guidewire exchanges, access site hematoma, repeat puncture of the same vessel during a short time interval).

[d]Prophylaxis is generally not recommend except in patients at risk: immunocompromised populations such as patients receiving chemotherapy, neutropenic patients at the time of the procedure, patients undergoing a bone marrow transplant, prior history of catheter infection, and neonates.

[e]*Absence of intact sphincter of Oddi: (e.g., previous sphincterotomy, biliary drainage, history of bilioenteric anastomosis).*

[f]Routine prophylaxis remains controversial in the setting of embolization for control of trauma-induced organ bleeding. It is recommended if intent is to cause infarction or high likelihood of tissue infarction which may result significant volume of necrotic tissue.

Additional dosage information

- **Vancomycin dose:** 1 g IV over 45 min (due to long infusion time, start about 2 h before the procedure)
- **Clindamycin dose:** 600 mg IV over 15–30 min
- **Gentamicin (aminoglycoside) dose:** 1.2–1.5 mg/kg
- **Tobramycin (aminoglycoside) dose:** 1.5 mg/kg
- **Tazobactam/piperacillin dose:** 2.25 g

Timing of prophylaxis:

- Optimally for most procedures requiring prophylaxis → administration of a single dose within 1 h of the procedure.
- Allow 2 h for the administration of antimicrobial agents with prolonged infusion time such as vancomycin and fluoroquinolones.

(continued)

Procedures and Classification	Routine prophylaxis recommended	Recommended antibiotic regimen
• Patients being treated with empiric antimicrobial agent due to presence of a clinical infection → ensure the appropriateness of empiric agent and the need of a supplement dose before the procedure if a long period of time since the last dose has elapsed. • Complex or prolonged (>2 h) procedures → administering a supplemental dose during the procedure may be necessary based on the length of the procedure and the half-life of the antibiotic agent being administered. • Prophylactic antimicrobial agent can be discontinued within 24 h after intervention, unless clinical circumstances warrant continuation (e.g., procedures on obstructed viscus) or initiation of antibiotic therapy (e.g., abscess drainage, presence of clinical infection). In these cases, the antimicrobial agent should be adjusted according to the results of bacteriologic cultures. • The operator should request appropriate subspecialty consultation when necessary.		
Dose adjustment: • Many antibiotics are excreted by the kidneys and some by the liver and therefore can be nephrotoxic and hepatotoxic; dose adjustment might be required based on the agent and recent administration of a toxic agent. • Antimicrobial agents with predominant hepatic excretion are rarely used in interventional radiology (e.g., tetracycline, chloramphenicol, and sulfonamides). • Agents removed by dialysis: cephalosporins, most penicillins, aminoglycosides, and metronidazole. • Agents not removed by dialysis: vancomycin, mezlocillin, nafcillin, and clindamycin. • Renal and hepatic toxicity is often due to accumulation of the toxic drug → – If no antibiotic agents have been given previously → safe to administer a single normal dose. – If prolonged antibiotic therapy is anticipated → reduced dose may be administered at the usual interval or delayed intervals based on the level of renal or hepatic impairment.		
Antibiotic prophylaxis against infective endocarditis (IE) Prophylaxis is warranted only in the following high-risk patients • Prosthetic heart valves, including bioprosthetic and homograft valve • A prior history of IE • Unrepaired cyanotic congenital heart disease, including palliative shunts and conduits • Completely repaired congenital heart defects with prosthetic material or device during the first six months after the procedure • Repaired congenital heart disease with residual defects at the site or adjacent to the site of the prosthetic patch or device • Cardiac transplantation recipients who develop cardiac valvulopathy **Relevant procedures in vascular and interventional radiology:** • Antimicrobial prophylaxis is warranted for high-risk patients cited above in the setting of procedures likely to result in bacteremia with a microorganism that has the potential ability to cause endocarditis as follows • In patients undergoing an invasive respiratory tract procedure, such as drainage of an abscess or empyema – Antibiotic prophylaxis should contain an agent active against S. Viridans 2 g amoxicillin orally 2 g ampicillin IM or IV 1 g cefazolin IM or IV 1 g ceftriaxone IM or IV *Patients allergic to penicillin or ampicillin and able to take oral medications* → oral administration of one of the following agents: 2 g cephalexin, 600 mg clindamycin, 500 mg azithromycin, or 500 mg clarithromycin *Patients allergic to penicillin or ampicillin and unable to take oral medications* → 1 g cefazolin IM or IV or 1 g ceftriaxone IM or IV or 600 mg clindamycin IM or IV – If the infection is known or suspected to be caused by S. aureus → regimen should contain an agent active against S. aureus – If the infection is known or suspected to be caused by methicillin resistant strain of S. aureus → regimen should contain vancomycin • Routine prophylaxis is not warranted for gastrointestinal or genitourinary procedure • Patients with high-risk cardiac conditions and an established gastrointestinal or genitourinary tract infection warrant antimicrobial therapy with activity against enterococci (amoxicillin or ampicillin)		

(continued)

Procedures and Classification	Routine prophylaxis recommended	Recommended antibiotic regimen
• Patients with enterococcal urinary tract infection or colonization who are scheduled to undergo elective ureteral stent placement or urinary tract manipulation → eradicate the organism prior to the procedure (amoxicillin or ampicillin). • Patients who undergo an invasive procedure that involves infected skin or musculoskeletal tissue → therapeutic regimen should contain an agent active against Staphylococcus species and beta-hemolytic Streptococcus species, such as an anti-staphylococcal penicillin or a cephalosporin		
Notes • The specific antibiotic agent doses provided in this table are recommendations for normal adult patients. • When selecting the antimicrobial agent and dose, it is important to pay close attention to individual patient factors (e.g., advanced patient age, current medications, altered renal or hepatic function, medication allergy history, the intended procedure and its likely pathogens, and the dose and timing of the most recent antibiotic agent dose. • Interventional radiologist may consult with the infectious disease committee or consulting service, microbiology laboratory, and/or pharmacy for recommended medications and dosage.		

References

1. Beddy P, Ryan JM. Antibiotic prophylaxis in interventional radiology–anything new? Tech Vasc Interv Radiol. 2006;9(2):69–76.
2. Berard F, Gandon J. Postoperative wound infections: the influence of ultraviolet irradiation of the operating room and of various other factors. Ann Surg. 1964;160(suppl 1):1–192.
3. Bhatia SS, Spector S, Echenique A, Froud T, Suthar R, Lawson I, et al. Is antibiotic prophylaxis for percutaneous radiofrequency ablation (RFA) of primary liver tumors necessary? results from a single-center experience. Cardiovasc Intervent Radiol. 2015;38(4):922–8.
4. McDermott VG, Schuster MG, Smith TP. Antibiotic prophylaxis in vascular and interventional radiology. Am J Roentgenol. 1997;169(1):31–8.
5. Nishimura RA, Otto CM, Bonow RO, Carabello BA, Erwin JP 3rd, Guyton RA, et al. 2014 AHA/ACC guideline for the management of patients with valvular heart disease: a report of the american college of cardiology/american heart association task force on practice guidelines. J Thorac Cardiovasc Surg. 2014;148(1):e1–132.
6. Ryan JM, Ryan BM, Smith TP. Antibiotic prophylaxis in interventional radiology. J Vasc Interv Radiol. 2004;15(6):547–56.
7. Spies JB, Rosen R, Lebowitz AS. Antibiotic prophylaxis in vascular and interventional radiology: a rational approach. Radiology. 1988;166:301–87.
8. Sutcliffe JA, Briggs JH, Little MW, McCarthy E, Wigham A, Bratby M, et al. Antibiotics in interventional radiology. Clin Radiol. 2015;70(3):223–34.
9. Taslakian B, Sebaaly MG, Al-Kutoubi A. Patient evaluation and preparation in vascular and interventional radiology: what every interventional radiologist should know (part 2: patient preparation and medications). Cardiovasc Intervent Radiol. 2016;39 (4):489–99. doi: 10.1007/s00270-015-1239-4.
10. Venkatesan AM, Kundu S, Sacks D, Wallace MJ, Wojak JC, Rose SC, et al. Practice guidelines for adult antibiotic prophylaxis during vascular and interventional radiology procedures. J Vasc Interv Radiol. 2010;21(11):1611–30.
11. Wilson W, Taubert KA, Gewitz M, Lockhart PB, Baddour LM, Levison M, et al. Prevention of infective endocarditis: guidelines from the american heart association. a guideline from the american heart association rheumatic fever, endocarditis, and kawasaki disease committee, council on cardiovascular disease in the young, and the council on clinical cardiology, council on cardiovascular surgery and anesthesia, and the quality of care and outcomes research interdisciplinary working group. Circulation. 2007;116:1736–54.
12. Zarrinpar A, Kerlan RK. A guide to antibiotics for the interventional radiologist. Semin Interv Radiol. 2005;22(2):69–79.

Appendix 6—Interventional Radiology Preprocedural Documentation

154

Bedros Taslakian

The preprocedural documentation is an essential part of the interventional procedure and should be documented in the medical record of the patient before initiating the procedure or sedation. It provides a baseline record of the clinical status and documents the preprocedural diagnosis and indication for the procedure. It also provides a preprocedural check point to ensure that all laboratory results and imaging studies have been reviewed, contraindications for the procedure are excluded and consent is obtained [1]. A sample preprocedureal documental form is found below.

B. Taslakian (✉)
Department of Radiology, New York University
Langone Medical Center, 660 First Ave, New York,
NY 10016, USA
e-mail: btaslakian@gmail.com

B. Taslakian et al. (eds.), *Procedural Dictations in Image-Guided Intervention*,
DOI 10.1007/978-3-319-40845-3_154

Name:	Place patient label here
Hospital/medical record number:	
Date of birth:	

Summary of patient history and indication for procedure:
....
....

Physical examination findings (including vital signs):
....
....

Imaging findings:
....
....

Preprocedural diagnosis:
....

Planned procedure:
....

Laboratory findings:

Hematocrit:	**WBC:**	**Platelets:**	**Potassium*:** ....
Creatinine:**	**INR:**	**aPTT:**	....

*Procedures involving cardiac manipulation
**Procedures involving contrast media administration

Consent obtained:	⌑ Emergency	⌑ Written/verbal (risk/benefits/alternatives explained)
Anticoagulation/antiplatelet:	⌑ None	⌑ Specify ....
NPO status:	⌑ Not applicable	⌑ Specify ....
Allergies:	⌑ None known	⌑ Specify ....
Antibiotics prophylaxis:	⌑ Not applicable	⌑ Specify ....
Risk stratification (ASA class):	⌑ Not applicable	⌑ Specify ....
Vascular access site checked	⌑ Not applicable	⌑ Specify ....
Preprocedural pulses:	⌑ Not applicable	⌑ Specify ....

Interventional radiologist: .... **Signature:** .... **Date and time:**	**Additional relevant notes:** ....

Reference

1. Omary RA, Bettmann MA, Cardella JF, Bakal CW, Schwartzberg MS, Sacks D, et al. Quality improvement guidelines for the reporting and archiving of interventional radiology procedures. J Vasc Interv Radiol. 2003;14(9 Pt 2):S293–5.

155 Appendix 7—Immediate Procedure Note

Bedros Taslakian

Important to document in the medical chart immediately after the procedure. It provides a mean of communication with the medical staff before the final procedure report is completed [1].

Procedure(s) and brief description:

…………………………………………………………………………

…………………………………………………………………………

Samples obtained:

…………………………………………………………………………

…………………………………………………………………………

Implanted devices:

…………………………………………………………………………

…………………………………………………………………………

Results and findings:

…………………………………………………………………………

…………………………………………………………………………

Post-procedural diagnosis:

…………………………………………………………………………

…………………………………………………………………………

Post-procedure monitoring and treatment plan:

…………………………………………………………………………

…………………………………………………………………………

…………………………………………………………………………

…………………………………………………………………………

Complications:	☐ None encountered during or directly after the procedure	☐ Specify: ………………………… …………………………
Additional relevant notes	* Complete procedural report will follow * Please call/ page (_) for any questions or concerns regarding the procedure ………………………………………… …………………………………………	
Operator (1): **Operator (2):** **Assistant (1):** **Assistant (2):** **Date and time:**	…………………… …………………… …………………… …………………… ……………………	

B. Taslakian (✉)
Department of Radiology, New York University Langone Medical Center, 660 First Ave, New York, NY 10016, USA
e-mail: btaslakian@gmail.com

B. Taslakian et al. (eds.), *Procedural Dictations in Image-Guided Intervention*,
DOI 10.1007/978-3-319-40845-3_155

Reference

1. Omary RA, Bettmann MA, Cardella JF, Bakal CW, Schwartzberg MS, Sacks D, et al. Quality improvement guidelines for the reporting and archiving of interventional radiology procedures. J Vasc Interv Radiol. 2003;14(9 Pt 2):S293–5.

Appendix 8—Supplemental Reading Material 156

Bedros Taslakian

Books

1. Burke CT, Dixon RG, Mauro MA, Murphy KPJ, Thomson KR, Venbrux AC, Zollikofer CL, editors. High yield imaging: interventional. Philadelphia: Saunders Elsevier; 2010.
2. Gervais DA, Sabharwal T, editors. Interventional radiology procedures in biopsy and drainage. Heidelberg/New York: Springer; 2011.
3. Hong K, Georgiades K, editors. Percutaneous tumor ablation strategies and techniques. New York: Thieme Medical Publishers; 2010.
4. Kandarpa K, Machan L, editors. Handbook of interventional radiologic procedures. 4th ed. Philadelphia: Lippincott Williams & Wilkins; 2011.
5. Mauro MA, Murphy KPJ, Thomson KR, Venbrux AC, Morgan RA, editors. Image-guided interventions. 2nd ed. Philadelphia: Saunders Elsevier; 2014.
6. Mauro MA, Murphy KPJ, Thomson KR, Venbrux AC, Zollikofer CL, editors. Image-guided interventions. Philadelphia: Saunders Elsevier; 2008.
7. Valji K, editor. Vascular and interventional radiology. 2nd ed. Philadelphia: Saunders/Elsevier; 2006.
8. Valji K, editor. The practice of interventional radiology with online cases and videos. Philadelphia: Saunders Elsevier; 2010.

Practice Guidelines

1. American College of Radiology. Illustrated breast imaging reporting and data system (BI-RADSTM), 3rd edn. Reston, VA: American College of Radiology; 1998.
2. American College of Radiology. ACR practice guideline for performance for magnetic resonance image-guided breast interventional procedures. Reston, VA: American College of Radiology; 2011.
3. American College of Radiology. ACR practice parameter for the performance of stereotactic-guided breast interventional procedures. Reston, VA: American College of Radiology; 2014.
4. American College of Radiology. ACR standard practice guideline for performance of ultrasound-guided percutaneous breast interventional procedures. Reston, VA: American College of Radiology; 2009.
5. American College of Radiology. ACR–SIR–SPR practice parameter for performance of arteriography. Reston, VA: American College of Radiology; 2014.

B. Taslakian (✉)
Department of Radiology, New York University Langone Medical Center, 660 First Ave, New York, NY 10016, USA
e-mail: btaslakian@gmail.com

B. Taslakian et al. (eds.), *Procedural Dictations in Image-Guided Intervention*,
DOI 10.1007/978-3-319-40845-3_156

6. Angle JF, Nemcek AA Jr, Cohen AM, Miller DL, Grassi CJ, D'Agostino HR, et al. SIR Standards Division. Quality improvement guidelines for preventing wrong site, wrong procedure, and wrong person errors: application of the joint commission "universal protocol for preventing wrong site, wrong procedure, wrong person surgery" to the practice of interventional radiology. J Vasc Interv Radiol. 2009;20(7 Suppl): S256–62.
7. Angle JF, Siddiqi NH, Wallace MJ, Kundu S, Stokes L, Wojak JC, et al. Society of Interventional Radiology Standards of Practice Committee. Quality improvement guidelines for percutaneous transcatheter embolization: Society of Interventional Radiology Standards of Practice Committee. J Vasc Interv Radiol. 2010;21(10):1479–86.
8. Aruny JE, Lewis CA, Cardella JF, Cole PE, Davis A, Drooz AT, et al. Society of Interventional Radiology Standards of Practice Committee. Quality improvement guidelines for percutaneous management of the thrombosed or dysfunctional dialysis access. J Vasc Interv Radiol. 2003;14(9 Pt 2):S247–53.
9. Baerlocher MO, Saad WE, Dariushnia S, Barr JD, McGraw JK, Nikolic B; Society of Interventional Radiology Standards of Practice Committee. Quality improvement guidelines for percutaneous vertebroplasty. J Vasc Interv Radiol. 2014;25(2):165–70.
10. Bakal CW, Sacks D, Burke DR, Cardella JF, Chopra PS, Dawson SL, et al. Quality improvement guidelines for adult percutaneous abscess and fluid drainage. J Vasc Interv Radiol. 2003;14(9 Pt 2):S223–5.
11. Bakal CW. Quality improvement for diagnostic neuroangiography and other procedures. J Vasc Interv Radiol. 2003;14(9 Pt 2): S255–6.
12. Barr JD, Connors JJ 3rd, Sacks D, Wojak JC, Becker GJ, Cardella JF, et al. SIR Standards of Practice Committees. Quality improvement guidelines for the performance of cervical carotid angioplasty and stent placement. AJNR Am J Neuroradiol. 2003;24(10):2020–34.
13. Brown DB, Nikolic B, Covey AM, Nutting CW, Saad WE, Salem R, et al. Society of Interventional Radiology Standards of Practice Committee. Quality improvement guidelines for transhepatic arterial chemoembolization, embolization, and chemotherapeutic infusion for hepatic malignancy. J Vasc Interv Radiol. 2012;23(3):287-94.
14. Brown DB, Singh H, Cardella JF, Aruny JE, Cole PE, Oglevie SB, et al. Society of Interventional Radiology Standards of Practice Committee. Quality improvement guidelines for diagnostic infusion venography. J Vasc Interv Radiol. 2003;14(9 Pt 2):S289–92.
15. Caplin DM, Nikolic B, Kalva SP, Ganguli S, Saad WE, Zuckerman DA. Quality improvement guidelines for the performance of inferior vena cava filter placement for the prevention of pulmonary embolism. J Vasc Interv Radiol. 2011;22(11):1499–506.
16. Citron SJ, Wallace RC, Lewis CA, Dawson RC, Dion JE, Fox AJ, et al. Society of Interventional Radiology; American Society of Interventional and Therapeutic Neuroradiology; American Society of Neuroradiology. Quality improvement guidelines for adult diagnostic neuroangiography. Cooperative study between ASITN, ASNR, and SIR. J Vasc Interv Radiol. 2003;14(9 Pt 2): S257–62.
17. Connors JJ 3rd, Sacks D, Becker GJ, Barr JD. Carotid artery angioplasty and stent placement: quality improvement guidelines to ensure stroke risk reduction. J Vasc Interv Radiol. 2003;14(9 Pt 2):S317–9.
18. Dariushnia SR, Haskal ZJ, Midia M, Martin LG, Walker TG, Kalva SP, et al. Society of Interventional Radiology Standards of Practice Committee. Quality improvement guidelines for transjugular intrahepatic portosystemic shunts. J Vasc Interv Radiol. 2016;27(1):1–7.
19. Dariushnia SR, Wallace MJ, Siddiqi NH, Towbin RB, Wojak JC, Kundu S, et al. Quality improvement guidelines for central venous access. J Vasc Interv Radiol. 2010;21 (7):976–81.

20. Grassi CJ, Swan TL, Cardella JF, Meranze SG, Oglevie SB, Omary RA, et al. Society of Interventional Radiology Standards of Practice Committee. Quality improvement guidelines for percutaneous permanent inferior vena cava filter placement for the prevention of pulmonary embolism. J Vasc Interv Radiol. 2003;14(9 Pt 2):S271–5.
21. Gupta S, Wallace MJ, Cardella JF, Kundu S, Miller DL, Rose SC. Quality improvement guidelines for percutaneous needle biopsy. J Vasc Interv Radiol. 2010;21(7):969–75.
22. Heran MK, Marshalleck F, Temple M, Grassi CJ, Connolly B, Towbin RB, et al. Joint quality improvement guidelines for pediatric arterial access and arteriography: from the Societies of Interventional Radiology and Pediatric Radiology. J Vasc Interv Radiol; 2010. 21(1): 32–43.
23. Hoggard J, Saad T, Schon D, Vesely TM, Royer T. Guidelines for venous access in patients with chronic kidney disease. A Position Statement from the American Society of Diagnostic and Interventional Nephrology, Clinical Practice Committee and the Association for Vascular Access. Semin Dial. 2008;21(2):186–91.
24. Itkin M, DeLegge MH, Fang JC, McClave SA, Kundu S, Janne d'Othee B, et al. Multidisciplinary practical guidelines for gastrointestinal access for enteral nutrition and decompression from the Society of Interventional Radiology and American Gastroenterological Association (AGA) Institute, with endorsement by Canadian Interventional Radiological Association (CIRA) and Cardiovascular and Interventional Radiological Society of Europe (CIRSE). J Vasc Interv Radiol. 2011;22(8):1089–106.
25. Kaufman JA, Kinney TB, Streiff MB, Sing RF, Proctor MC, Becker D, et al. Guidelines for the use of retrievable and convertible vena cava filters: report from the Society of Interventional Radiology multidisciplinary consensus conference. J Vasc Interv Radiol. 2006;17(3):449–59.
26. Khilnani NM, Grassi CJ, Kundu S, D'Agostino HR, Khan AA, McGraw JK, et al. Cardiovascular Interventional Radiological Society of Europe, American College of Phlebology, and Society of Interventional Radiology Standards of Practice Committees. Multi-society consensus quality improvement guidelines for the treatment of lower extremity superficial venous insufficiency with endovenous thermal ablation from the Society of Interventional Radiology, Cardiovascular Interventional Radiological Society of Europe, American College of Phlebology and Canadian Interventional Radiology Association. J Vasc Interv Radiol. 2010;21(1):14–31.
27. Martin LG, Rundback JH, Wallace MJ, Cardella JF, Angle JF, Kundu S, et al. Society of Interventional Radiology (SIR). Quality improvement guidelines for angiography, angioplasty, and stent placement for the diagnosis and treatment of renal artery stenosis in adults. J Vasc Interv Radiol. 2010;21(4):421–30; quiz 230.
28. Omary RA, Bettmann MA, Cardella JF, Bakal CW, Schwartzberg MS, Sacks D, et al. Quality improvement guidelines for the reporting and archiving of interventional radiology procedures. J Vasc Interv Radiol. 2003;14(9 Pt 2):S293–5.
29. Patel IJ, Davidson JC, Nikolic B, Salazar GM, Schwartzberg MS, Walker TG, et al. Consensus guidelines for periprocedural management of coagulation status and hemostasis risk in percutaneous image-guided interventions. J Vasc Interv Radiol. 2012;23(6):727–36.
30. Patel IJ, Davidson JC, Nikolic B, Salazar GM, Schwartzberg MS, Walker TG, et al. Addendum of newer anticoagulants to the SIR consensus guideline. J Vasc Interv Radiol. 2013;24(5):641–5.
31. Rajan DK, Patel NH, Valji K, Cardella JF, Brown DB, Brountzos EN, et al. CIRSE and SIR Standards of Practice Committees. Quality improvement guidelines for percutaneous management of acute limb ischemia.

J Vasc Interv Radiol. 2009;20(7 Suppl): S208–18.
32. Ramchandani P, Cardella JF, Grassi CJ, Roberts AC, Sacks D, Schwartzberg MS, et al. Quality improvement guidelines for percutaneous nephrostomy. J Vasc Interv Radiol. 2003;14(9 Pt 2):S277–81.
33. Saad WE, Wallace MJ, Wojak JC, Kundu S, Cardella JF. Quality improvement guidelines for percutaneous transhepatic cholangiography, biliary drainage, and percutaneous cholecystostomy. J Vasc Interv Radiol. 2010;21(6):789–95.
34. Spies JB, Bakal CW, Burke DR, Cardella JF, Drooz A, Edwards ME; Society of Interventional Radiology Standards of Practice Committee. Angioplasty standard of practice. J Vasc Interv Radiol. 2003;14(9 Pt 2): S219–21.
35. Stokes LS1, Wallace MJ, Godwin RB, Kundu S, Cardella JF; Society of Interventional Radiology Standards of Practice Committee. Quality improvement guidelines for uterine artery embolization for symptomatic leiomyomas. J Vasc Interv Radiol. 2010;21(8):1153–63.
36. Vedantham S, Sista AK, Klein SJ, Nayak L, Razavi MK, Kalva SP, et al. Society of Interventional Radiology and Cardiovascular and Interventional Radiological Society of Europe Standards of Practice Committees. Quality improvement guidelines for the treatment of lower extremity deep vein thrombosis with use of endovascular thrombus removal. J Vasc Interv Radiol. 2014;25 (9):1317–25.
37. Venkatesan AM, Kundu S, Sacks D, Wallace MJ, Wojak JC, Rose SC, et al. Practice guidelines for adult antibiotic prophylaxis during vascular and interventional radiology procedures. J Vasc Interv Radiol. 2010;21 (11):1611–30.
38. Walker TG, Kalva SP, Yeddula K, Wicky S, Kundu S, Drescher P, et al. Clinical practice guidelines for endovascular abdominal aortic aneurysm repair: written by the Standards of Practice Committee for the Society of Interventional Radiology and endorsed by the Cardiovascular and Interventional Radiological Society of Europe and the Canadian Interventional Radiology Association. J Vasc Interv Radiol. 2010;21(11):1632–55.
39. Wallace MJ, Chin KW, Fletcher TB, Bakal CW, Cardella JF, Grassi CJ, et al. Quality improvement guidelines for percutaneous drainage/aspiration of abscess and fluid collections. J Vasc Interv Radiol. 2010;21(4):431–5.

Review Articles

1. Behrens G, Ferral H. Transjugular liver biopsy. Semin Intervent Radiol. 2012;29 (2):111–7.
2. Chadha M1, Ahuja C. Visceral artery aneurysms: diagnosis and percutaneous management. Semin Intervent Radiol. 2009;26 (3):196–206.
3. Covey AM, Brown KT. Percutaneous transhepatic biliary drainage. Tech Vasc Interv Radiol. 2008;11:14–20.
4. Dohan A, Guerrache Y, Boudiaf M, Gavini JP, Kaci R, Soyer P. Transjugular liver biopsy: indications, technique and results. Diagn Interv Imaging. 2014;95 (1):11–5.
5. Dyer RB, Regan JD, Kavanagh PV, Khatod EG, Chen MY, Zagoria RJ. Percutaneous nephrostomy with extensions of the technique: step by step. Radiographics. 2002;22 (3):503–25.
6. Funaki B. Tunneled central venous catheter insertion. Semin Intervent Radiol. 2008;25 (4):432–6.
7. Gupta S, Nguyen HL, Morello FA Jr, Ahrar K, Wallace MJ, Madoff DC, et al. Various approaches for CT-guided percutaneous biopsy of deep pelvic lesions: anatomic and technical considerations. Radiographics. 2004;24(1):175–89.
8. Gupta S, Seaberg K, Wallace MJ, Madoff DC, Morello FA Jr, Ahrar K, et al. Imaging-guided percutaneous biopsy of mediastinal lesions: different approaches and anatomic considerations. Radiographics. 2005;25(3):763–86.

9. Imbrogno BF, Ray CE. Splenic artery embolization in blunt trauma. Semin Intervent Radiol. 2012;29(2):147–9.
10. Kalambokis G, Manousou P, Vibhakorn S, Marelli L, Cholongitas E, Senzolo M, et al. Transjugular liver biopsy–indications, adequacy, quality of specimens, and complications—a systematic review. J Hepatol. 2007;47(2):284–94.
11. Krokidis M, Hatzidakis A. Percutaneous minimally invasive treatment of malignant biliary strictures: current status. Cardiovasc Intervent Radiol. 2014;37(2):316–23.
12. Lee J, Darcy M. Renal cysts and urinomas. Semin Intervent Radiol. 2011;28(4):380–91.
13. Madoff DC, Denys A, Wallace MJ, Murthy R, Gupta S, Pillsbury EP, et al. Splenic arterial interventions: anatomy, indications, technical considerations, and potential complications. Radiographics. 2005;25(Suppl 1):S191–211.
14. Maher MM, Kealey S, McNamara A, O'Laoide R, Gibney RG, Malone DE. Management of visceral interventional radiology catheters: a troubleshooting guide for interventional radiologists. Radiographics. 2002;22(2):305–22.
15. Nitschke AM, Ray CE Jr. Percutaneous neurolytic celiac plexus block. Semin Intervent Radiol. 2013;30(3):318–21.
16. Stassen NA, Bhullar I, Cheng JD, Crandall ML, Friese RS, Guillamondegui OD, et al. Selective nonoperative management of blunt splenic injury: an Eastern Association for the Surgery of Trauma practice management guideline. J Trauma Acute Care Surg. 2012;73(5 Suppl 4):S294–300.
17. Taslakian B, Sebaaly MG, Al-Kutoubi A. Patient evaluation and preparation in vascular and interventional radiology: what every interventional radiologist should know (Part 1: Patient assessment and laboratory tests). Cardiovasc Intervent Radiol. 2016;39 (3):325–33.
18. Taslakian B, Sebaaly MG, Al-Kutoubi A. Patient evaluation and preparation in vascular and interventional radiology: what every interventional radiologist should know (Part 2: Patient preparation and medications). Cardiovasc Intervent Radiol. 2016;39 (4):489–99. doi: 10.1007/s00270-015-1239-4.
19. Thabet A, Kalva SP, Liu B, Mueller PR, Lee SI. Interventional radiology in pregnancy complications: indications, technique, and methods for minimizing radiation exposure. Radiographics. 2012;32(1): 255–74.

Index

B. Taslakian et al. (eds.), *Procedural Dictations in Image-Guided Intervention*,
DOI 10.1007/978-3-319-40845-3

R

S

Printed by Printforce, the Netherlands